Smallpox

WITHDRAWN

Smallpox
A History

S. L. KOTAR *and* J. E. GESSLER

McFarland & Company, Inc., Publishers
Jefferson, North Carolina, and London

LIBRARY OF CONGRESS CATALOGUING-IN-PUBLICATION DATA

Kotar, S. L.
Smallpox : a history / S. L. Kotar and J. E. Gessler.
p.   cm.
Includes bibliographical references and index.

ISBN 978-0-7864-6823-2
softcover : acid free paper ∞

1. Smallpox — History.   I. Gessler, J.E.   II. Title.
RC183.1.K68 2013   614.5'21— dc23   2013006946

BRITISH LIBRARY CATALOGUING DATA ARE AVAILABLE

Front cover images: A posting from the local Medical Society
supported the Board of Education's stance on requiring vaccination
in the classroom, but did not go so far as to make vaccination
mandatory. Such half-way measures only complicated the situation
and left the debate open for future lawsuits (*Salt Lake Tribune,*
January 11, 1900); background © 2012 Shutterstock

Manufactured in the United States of America

*McFarland & Company, Inc., Publishers
Box 611, Jefferson, North Carolina 28640
www.mcfarlandpub.com*

This book is proudly dedicated to Jimmy and Rosalynn Carter,
who through their creation and work at the Carter Center
in Atlanta, Georgia, selflessly devote themselves to
"Waging Peace. Fighting Disease. Building Hope."

Table of Contents

Preface

A paragraph in a local 19th century newspaper presented an interesting scenario under the heading of "Burial of Small-Pox":

Funeral Notice: Died at Sierra City, California, February 22, 1888, Small-Pox. As the deceased has no friends in town, his enemies are invited to assemble at Spencer & Moore's hall at 8 o'clock, to dance on his coffin. The funeral exercises will be under the auspices of the Butte's Band, which will pipe its level best for the occasion. Tickets, $1. P.S.— The wake will continue ad libitum at the close of the dance.

The notice indicated that a scourge of smallpox had just succeeded in being stamped out. With the quarantine lifted, virtually the entire town turned out to celebrate, including 35 persons who had recovered from the disease. The dance program included, the "Small-pox Polka," the "Virus Jig," the "Vaccination Reel," and the "Quarantine Quadrille."[1]

While the article was meant to be amusing, smallpox was no laughing matter. Although its origins are obscure, the speckled disease seemingly plagued mankind from "time immemorial," leaving staggering death rates, horrifying scars and blindness in its wake.

Few, if any, persons living in the 21st century have ever seen a case of variola major or variola minor as the two strains of the disease are more specifically designated. Combating it began almost as soon as it appeared among our ancient ancestors. Most early treatments relied upon superstition and pseudoscience, but long before smallpox became an international scourge brilliant minds developed surprisingly effective methods for preventing, if not curing the disease. These methods of inoculation never became widespread, and over the course of centuries smallpox was spread from its relatively small containment throughout the globe. Religious travelers to and from Mecca, Crusaders, slave traders, merchants and explorers all played a part in importing it throughout Africa, the Middle East, India and finally to Europe and the New World. Statistical evidence of early smallpox is nearly impossible to obtain and accounts of the disease come from vague, firsthand accounts. It was not until Europeans began colonizing distant lands that identification, containment, treatment, "cures" and records assumed paramount importance.

Smallpox was known as a disease that spared neither commoner nor royalty, and the dread of it became so great that children were not considered part of the family until they had successfully contracted and passed through the contagion. Thereafter they were immune from further attacks and safe to be included.

Inoculation, or the passage of live smallpox virus from one person to another, either by inhaling dried crusts or through implantation into the skin, provided immunity but made the recipient a carrier, capable of infecting healthy persons. Often decried by religious practitioners as an offense against God under the belief that smallpox existed as a punishment to humans and ought to be accepted as such, scientists pursued inoculation as the only means at their disposal to prevent epidemics and high death totals.

Edward Jenner, who became known as the Father of Immunology, developed the method of "vaccination" in 1798 by extracting matter from cows suffering from the related disease, cowpox, and inserting it under the skin of healthy individuals to initiate a mild disease similar to but not exactly like smallpox. When the person recovered, immunity from variola was achieved. This technique eliminated the threat of carriers, thereby providing a preventive for the deadly disease.

While it would appear that Jenner's brilliant discovery, carried across the globe, would all but eliminate smallpox as a threat, condemnation of his idea was fast and furious. Nineteenth century authorities from scientists to clerics debunked the operation, crying out that people would become beasts from having animal matter inserted into their bodies or that, as God had created smallpox, humans ought to suffer from it without complaint. This group, who would later become known as anti-vaccinationists, were so successful that smallpox continued to be a scourge, nearly devastating entire populations, including the indigenous populations of North America. As hard as it is to believe, debate against vaccination carried over well into the 20th century and it was not until a massive global effort, years after man had walked on the moon, that the World Health Organization declared smallpox eradicated.

This book details the history of smallpox, its spread, mutations and deadly effects. More important, however, it was our intent to chronicle the medical, political and moral considerations of combating the Speckled Disease through the words of those directly involved in the struggle. Contemporary accounts of those who faced the daily threat of death: those who researched the virus, performed the operations, compiled the data (occasionally speculative in nature), penned the editorials and saw loved ones suffer the untold agonies of the disease are the real story. Conquering smallpox took inestimable courage, insight, inspiration and a dedication almost beyond belief. The achievements of these people, including plunges backward into the depths of prehistory as well as breakthroughs launching their world brethren into heights farther than the stars, are staggering. It is therefore up to us, and the generations that follow, to acknowledge our deep gratitude for what they achieved and what they sacrificed.

1

Smallpox "from time immemorial"

> From time immemorial this domestic animal [the cow] has been consecrated among ancient nations as an object of worship; to all it is now an object of grateful admiration. What then is due to that philosopher, who has drawn new and heretofore unexplored sources of happiness from this salutiferous animal.[1]

Throughout history, combating deadly diseases has inspired human ingenuity and sharpened the senses of the curious, placing science and the natural world on a par with religion and superstition. Smallpox was a killer: whether in ancient or modern times, it was the responsibility of mankind to seek a preventive. The journey would be arduous, fraught with twists and turns, breakthroughs and back steps. Scientists and theologians would occasionally be on the same side, at other times stand diametrically opposed; politicians who passed laws would be accused of depriving men of personal freedom; doctors would save millions of lives with new techniques yet lose battles on individual levels. Combating the invisible world slowly evolved into diagnosing that which would become visible under the use of a powerful lens.

Along the slow path toward eradication, soldiers would use smallpox as germ warfare, some with regret, others with a cold heart. Prisoners of war would carry disease with them into enemy territory; men in the ranks died more frequently from disease than from bullets. Some physicians would have statues dedicated to them; others would contract the disease and die. In the name of humanity, many health care professionals worked gratuitously, just as others who had taken the same oaths charged exorbitant prices for their services. First inoculation and then vaccination vied with home remedies and patent medicines; places of quarantine were homes and pesthouses. Flags of red or yellow designated areas of contagion; miasmas were thought to create disease; and infectious persons walked the streets without regard to spreading the "loathsome disease."

Smallpox came during the epoch designated "Before Christ" and wasn't globally eradicated until late in the 20th century. The story is one of human triumph and human tragedy, perhaps fittingly encapsulating the best and the worst of *Homo sapiens*.

The plague referred to as smallpox (commonly hyphenated as "small-pox" or spelled as two words well into the 20th century) became extinct in the world from the simple application of a vaccine originally taken from cows infected with a disease called "cowpox." A historical killer known throughout Asia, Africa and the Middle East from "time immemorial," smallpox became the only disease ever to be eradicated from planet Earth.

Also known by the Latin name "Variola" (from *varius,* changing color, because it disfigured the skin)[2] smallpox was a highly contagious disease unique to humans. Bishop Marius of Avenches first used the word "variola" around the 6th century to describe an epidemic then raging in Italy and France. Five centuries later, Constantinus Africanus expressly limited the word to mean smallpox. The actual English word "smallpox" was adapted from French usage. At the end of the 15th century, syphilis was the great killer the French called *la grosse vérole*; "variola" thus became *la petite vérole*. Consequently, "pox" became "small," while syphilis was referred to as the "great pox," "great" differentiating the size of the lesions. Additionally, "small" denoted that smallpox was generally regarded as a disease of children, while "great" referred to the adult nature of syphilis, a sexually transmitted disease.[3] A definition from 1865 described the medical name *variola* as being derived from the Latin *varus*, meaning a blotch or pimple, while the popular affix "pox" was Saxon for bag or pouch, creating a combination literally meaning a small bag filled with pus.[4]

Before the development of germ theory, the use of high-powered microscopes and analysis of DNA, the only available method of diagnosis for early scientists was from symptoms. Physicians examined the patient, listened to complaints and correlated observations to known diseases. In the case of smallpox, any disease that produced fever with pocks or skin eruptions in a characteristic pattern were believed to be of the same family. In the case of chicken pox and syphilis, long believed related to variola, this assumption was incorrect. Chicken pox was caused by a herpesvirus and syphilis by a spirochaete bacteria.

Variola (smallpox) and related viruses belong to the family of *Poxviridae*, the subfamily of *Chordopoxvirinae* and the genera *Orthopoxvirus*. Species were traditionally named on the basis of the host animal from which they were derived. All species of *Orthopoxvirus* share a large conserved central part of their genomes, but each bears significant differences. Of the nine known species, raccoonpox is the only indigenous *Orthopoxvirus* yet discovered in the Americas. The nine known are listed below:

Species of the genus Orthopoxvirus

Name	*Creatures Affected*
Variola	Humans (eradicated in 1977)
Vaccinia	Humans, cows, pigs, rabbits, buffalo
Cowpox	Humans, cows, rats, cats, large felines, gerbils, elephants, rhinoceroses
Monkeypox	Monkeys, great apes, humans, anteaters, squirrels
Ectromelia	Mice, voles
Camelpox	Camels
Taterapox	*Tatera kempi* (gerbils)
Raccoonpox	Raccoons
Uasin Gishu disease	Horses[5]

Smallpox was caused by two virus variants, variola major, the most deadly form with a mortality rate of 20–40 percent and variola minor, a mild type with a mortality rate of 1 percent.[6] Until late in the 19th century variola major predominated, and was justly termed a "loathsome disease." Survivors of variola major were left with deep pitting and disfiguring scars on the face, but, by far, the most debilitating aftereffect was blindness. In the 17th century, nearly two-thirds of the pauper blind had been rendered sightless by smallpox.[7] Not insignificantly, the disease was accompanied by a distinctive, offensive odor that mortified patients and was excessively disagreeable to those who attended them.

In 1842, the *Lexicon Medicum; or Medical Dictionary* definition of smallpox instructed physicians that contraction of the disease came from breathing air impregnated with the effluvia arising from the bodies of those afflicted. The four stages were described as febrile, eruptive, maturative, and declination or scabbing. Eruptions were commonly preceded by a redness in the eyes; soreness in the throat; pains in the head, back, and loins; weariness and faintness; alternate fits of chilling and heat; thirst; nausea; inclination to vomit; and a quick pulse. The disease attacked people of all ages, but the young of both sexes were more likely than those of advanced age to contract it and die. Smallpox appeared in any season but was more prevalent in the spring and summer.

About the third or fourth day from the first seizure, eruptions appeared in little red spots on the face, neck, and breast, frequently preceded or attended by a rosy efflorescence similar to that of measles but with a continuation of fever. The eruptions continued to increase in size and number for 3 to 4 days, at the end of which they were dispersed over several parts of the body.

When the pustules were thick and numerous on the face, the face swelled and the eyelids closed, previous to which there was a hoarseness and difficulty swallowing, accompanied by considerable saliva. (In infants, rather than salivating, they were prone to diarrhea.) About the eleventh day the swelling of the face subsided, followed by a reduction of swelling in hands and feet, after which the pustules broke and discharged their contents. They then became dry and fell off in crusts, leaving the skin a brown-red color, which appearance continued for many days. Where the pustules were large they tended to leave pits behind; those small and few in number might clear completely. In infants, convulsive fits were apt to occur, which either proved fatal before any eruption appeared or ushered in a malignant species of the disease.

Smallpox usually proved fatal from the eighth to the eleventh day, but in some cases death was protracted until the fourteenth to the sixteenth day. The disease left behind a predisposition to inflammatory complaints, particularly opthalmial and visceral but more especially of the thorax, and not infrequently excited scrofula into action that might otherwise have lain dormant in the system.

There is no irrefutable date or place of origin for the beginning of smallpox. As a disease, smallpox is not self-perpetuating. Having once survived, the human host is not susceptible to another attack. Therefore, variola virus could only persist in a community where enough humans were present to establish a continuous passage of infection. Without the introduction of new members, once the population had been exposed, the contagion ended. Because of this, with worldwide vaccination in the 20th century the disease was finally eradicated by the elimination of vulnerable hosts.

Presuming variola to have been present for perhaps 3,000 years, the question remains how it originated. The World Health Organization postulates two theories: either early humans contracted a form of smallpox from rodents and the virus subsequently mutated into variola, affecting only humans; or early humans suffered from a mutant "proto-variola" that evolved into the disease. In the first scenario, all existing strains of *Orthopoxvirus* have a genome pattern distinct from variola, suggesting that what we know today as variola has remained virtually unchanged for 3,000 years. In the second, no evidence of a "proto-virus" has ever been found, making this hypothesis unlikely.[8]

Uncertainty throughout the ages brought forth diverse opinions, from superstition (Native Americans suggested it arose from "invisible darts of angry fate, pointed against them for their young people's vicious conduct") to Dr. Joseph Lister, the scientist responsible for antiseptic technique, who suggested smallpox might have originally been caused by human ancestors being bitten by or eating some venomous creature.[9] Historically, ancient writings mentioned diseases that might have been an early form of smallpox, but exact indications of epidemics are lacking. Unmistakable descriptions of smallpox do not appear until the 4th century A.D. in China, the 7th century in India and the Mediterranean, and the 10th century in southwestern Asia.[10]

Present-day epidemiologists place its origin in northeastern Africa about 10,000 B.C. although, peculiarly, no written reports from ancient physicians, the Talmud or the Bible confirm this. Palaeopathologists who inspected the bodies of several mummies deducted that their skin appeared covered with lesions similar to those of smallpox; the oldest mummy presenting "dome-shaped vesicles" lived during the 20th Dynasty (1200–1100 B.C.). Eruptions believed to be smallpox were also discovered on the face of the Egyptian pharaoh Ramses V, who died in 1157 B.C. If, indeed, these individuals suffered from smallpox, this sets the date over 1,000 years earlier than any substantiated outbreaks.[11]

In India, a disease similar to smallpox, but not positively identified as such, was described in the ancient Ayurveda texts ("the complete knowledge for long life"), a system of metaphysics involving the "five great elements": earth, water, fire, air and ether.[12] An English physician of the British East India Company, J.Z. Holwell, suggested that smallpox had existed in India from "time immemorial" and stated that the disease was mentioned in the *Atharva Veda*, the most ancient of Sanskrit writings. Contemporary authorities[13] note the word *masurika*, meaning "smallpox," had been found in Indian medical texts since the beginning of the Christian era, but not in the *Atharva Veda*. The first appearance of *masurika*, referencing a severe and sometimes fatal disease, did not appear until the 7th century A.D. The only suggestion of an earlier appearance of smallpox in the Indian subcontinent was the epidemic that struck Alexander's army in 327 B.C. The appearance of "scabs" was mentioned, but a definitive diagnosis is impossible to make from that vague description.

It is speculated that smallpox was brought to India by Egyptian traders in the 1st millennium B.C., but there is no reliable evidence of its existence before the *Susruta Samhita*, begun before the Christian era and therein described only as a trivial skin disease.[14] Early 20th century research described the first book on smallpox to have been written by Ahrow, a priest and physician who lived in Alexandria, Egypt, in A.D. 683. He wrote 30 works on physic, concentrating on the treatment of disease. Ahrow advised swimming, drinking ice water in large quantities, taking small doses of saffron and warming medicines. In cases of high fever, he suggested the room be kept cool.[15]

Modern authorities believe Huns from the north introduced smallpox into China, possibly as early as 250 B.C., although it is considered more likely to have originated between A.D. 25 and 49. By the 2nd century A.D., smallpox had spread through the Chinese agricultural settlements of the Huang Ho valley, and by the 4th century it had become an endemic (ever-present) disease (as opposed to "epidemic," meaning a sudden outbreak having a known beginning and end) in both China and Korea. The ancient physician Ko Hung accurately described smallpox in his work, *Handbook of Medicines for Emergencies,* in A.D. 340.

By the beginning of the 13th century, fear of the disease may have affected how the Mongols planned their invasion of the country. The situation was little changed by the 17th century when the Manchus used only soldiers who had previously suffered from smallpox to scout weaknesses in the Great Wall. The Tibetan Dalai and the Panchen Lamas feared visits to Beijing because of this contagion. When the Panchen Lama finally accepted an invitation from Emperor Ch'ien-Lung, he quickly contracted the disease and died. Smallpox became epidemic in Tibet and tragically remained a serious threat until 1940, when vaccination was introduced.[16]

Chinese and Korean sailors were probably responsible for bringing smallpox to Japan between A.D. 552 and 582. After sailors suffered repeated exposure during the 7th and 8th centuries, an infected sailor spread the disease in 735, nearly destroying Nara, a city with half a million persons. Shinto and Buddhist priests argued over which religion best protected the inhabitants. In 748 the *Nara Daibutsu,* or the great bronze statue of Buddha, was completed, having been commissioned by the emperor to end the epidemics of smallpox.

No major outbreaks occurred in Japan until the 10th century, when the disease was established as endemic. The years 915, 925, 947, 993 and 998 witnessed great loss of life. Epidemics persisted although they were widely spaced: 1209, 1277, 1311, 1361, 1424, 1452, 1454, 1522 and 1550. The 17th century proved to be the worst, with numerous outbreaks reaching as far as the royal family.[17]

Smallpox was endemic in many parts of southwestern Asia beginning in the 6th century. Early in the 7th century, Arab armies, united by Mohammed's teachings, began their war of conquest, inadvertently carrying smallpox with them to Persia, across western Asia and northwestern Africa and into Spain, which was conquered in 710.[18]

The earliest records indicate a (re)introduction of the disease into Africa as possibly occurring in A.D. 568 when Ethiopian troops were exposed during the "Elephant War" at Mecca, eventually carrying it back to their homeland. During the 11th century as Islam became a significant factor, pilgrims making the round trip to Mecca likely contracted the disease and spread it on their return. Arab traders colonizing the eastern coast may also have brought smallpox. By 1589, when the Portuguese became a presence among the coastal towns, they reintroduced the disease, causing an epidemic along the coasts of Kilwa and Mombasa.

By the 17th century, the disease was widespread in Africa, having been brought into the interior by slave traders. The southern coast was free of the disease when the Dutch settled Cape Town in 1652, but in 1713 a ship returning from India sent ashore infected laundry, starting an outbreak. The indigenous Hottentots and Bushmen immediately fell victim. A second importation from Ceylon in 1775 devastated several entire tribes, and in 1767 a Danish ship instigated a third epidemic. European settlers, protected by variolation (see below), were spared the worst of the disease but the natives suffered high mortality rates.

Slave traders continued to spread smallpox, not only to African ports free from smallpox but also into the lands where they sold their human cargoes. Smallpox remained a severe endemic disease in northern Africa, while six epidemics were recorded in Ethiopia and the Sudan in 1811–1813, 1838–1839, 1865–1866, 1878–1879, 1885–1887 and 1889–1890.[19]

According to the World Health Organization's publication "Smallpox and Its Eradication" (1988), there were "no unequivocal records of smallpox in Europe before the 6th century A.D.," although empirical evidence suggested the disease was a major component of the "Plague of Athens" in 430 B.C. The affliction was said to have originated in Ethiopia and spread to Egypt and Libya before being transported across the Mediterranean to the port of Piraeus and on to Athens. Other ancient outbreaks, although unconfirmed, suggest that a smallpox epidemic prevented the Carthaginians from gaining control of Sicily at the siege of Syracuse in 395 B.C. and that the "Antonine Plague" afflicted the Roman army fighting in Mesopotamia in A.D. 164.

In the 5th century, Nicaise, the Bishop of Rheims, who was said to have suffered from smallpox, was beheaded by the Huns in A.D. 452 and later became the patron saint of Europeans suffering from smallpox.[20]

Endemic Smallpox

Within the first millennium of the Christian era, smallpox was established as an endemic disease on the southern and western outskirts of Europe, but it had not made ingress into central and northern Europe. During the 11th and 12th centuries, the Crusades of southwestern Asia spread smallpox, but it was not until the 15th century that the disease was endemic in many parts of Europe, although with little widespread devastation in either Spain or Italy. During this 100-year period, smallpox came to be regarded in France as a disease primarily affecting children. This is significant because it indicated an underlying, widespread endemic presence.

When smallpox was first introduced into "virgin soil," where none of the inhabitants had previously been exposed, the contagion struck young and old alike, wiping out a huge percentage of the population. Leaders were struck down and commerce destroyed, resulting in starvation. As the living were unable to bury the large numbers of the dead, other diseases set in, complicating the disaster. Survivors were not only left disfigured, traumatized and often homeless, the inexplicable trauma was also known to cast doubt on indigenous religious beliefs. In the years following major epidemics, communities suffered from low birthrates, requiring the passage of generations before the population rebounded. An example would be the tragic aftereffects of smallpox on Native Americans.

After smallpox became endemic, or ever-present, epidemics tended to occur in cycles. Since survivors of smallpox were conferred with life-long immunity, the population would not be susceptible to another major outbreak until several generations had been born and raised or the community was increased by immigration of unexposed individuals. When contagion was reintroduced, these vulnerable groups were the first to suffer. Considering smallpox a disease of children indicated that most adults had been exposed and were therefore exempt from a second attack.

Smallpox in the 15th century tended to be less violent than it would be in the 17th, 18th and mid–19th centuries, possibly because the strain then in circulation was of a milder form. This reprieve from the most deadly strain (variola major) would repeat itself in the early 20th century, when an even less drastic form (variola minor) would become epidemic across much of the world.

By the 16th century, smallpox had extended over much of the European continent except, perhaps, Russia. It also represented a time when important scientific works were published, among them Girolamo Fracastoro's *De Contagione et Contagiosis Morbis* (1546). He indicated that smallpox could be transmitted from person to person through fomites (contaminated articles such as clothing) or through the air. He also considered smallpox primarily a disease of children.[21]

It is interesting to compare the World Health Organization's research with a leading medical authority from 1781. Dr. Black, an English physician, conjectured that smallpox was introduced into Europe from Arabia. In his comprehensive thesis, he set a time of about the six hundredth year of the Christian era when smallpox and measles, then unknown "in any part of the globe frequented by Europeans," were "exported from the deserts of Arabia when Mahomet's followers sallied forth to propagate his religious doctrines." Black speculated that many centuries later, the Crusades "were instrumental in diffusing this exotic venom more widely over Europe." He concluded that, by the latter half of the 10th century, smallpox was relatively common in most of the Arab-controlled areas of North Africa and Europe.

Even then, it took many centuries before the scourge became widely distributed, causing

Black to question the extraordinary circumstance that smallpox and measles, two highly contagious diseases, "could have been circumscribed, and [their] ravages confined for several thousand years to a small corner of the globe." He ultimately left the question unanswered.[22] An earlier work, *An Historical Account of the Rise and Progress of Smallpox,* written by William Hillany, M.D., of Bath, England, dating from 1740, described the first known appearance of smallpox as the time of the destruction of Alexandria and the burning of its famous library by Amrow Ebnai Aks, general of the Saracen army in the reign of Omar Chatab the Second, successor of Mohammed.[23]

Dr. L.M. Hanna, in his study, *Vaccenia, a Prophylactic Against Variola* (1882), quoted the writings of Procopias, who lived in the middle of the 6th century. Procopias speculated that the earliest smallpox originated at Pelusium, Egypt, in A.D. 544 and eventually spread to Constantinople. Hanna noted that ancient medical writers typically dated the beginning of smallpox as 569, the year of the birth of Mahomet. In that year, the Abyssinian army appeared before Mecca and laid siege to the city but was unexpectedly disbanded on what authorities at the time believed to be an outbreak of smallpox.[24]

Smallpox Gods and Preventive Measures

Chinese in the 12th century made the observation that, once having contracted smallpox, children were immune from a second infection. They developed the technique (insufflation) of drying smallpox scabs and directing persons to inhale the powder as a way of securing immunity. This was traditionally done to children three years of age. After contracting a mild form of the disease, it was rare to find an individual more than 20 years old who did not have protection. The Chinese achieved the same purpose by dressing children in shirts worn by smallpox patients, thus exposing them to the disease. The Brahmins used a similar technique by applying to the skin ropes made of hair that were soaked in the poison of smallpox.[25]

Among Chinese religious tenets was the belief in a female divinity presiding over smallpox, inflicting the malignant disease on whomsoever she pleased. She was given the title of "Pearl Mother," for the purpose of securing her good will in hopes the disease might therefore be mitigated. For the same reason, pox pustules were spoken of as "pearly," and the illness went by the name of "the heavenly blossoms."[26]

Another Chinese name for the goddess of smallpox was *T'ou-Shen Niang-Niang.* Tradition traced her worship to an 11th century Buddhist nun who was credited with introducing variolation into China. From the 18th century, *Sitala* (*Shitala*) *mata* was an Indian goddess closely associated with smallpox; temples and shrines were erected to her throughout India. In Africa, the male smallpox deity was called *Sopona* (later referred to as *Obaluaye* ("King of the Earth") or *Omolu.* Introduced from northern Africa at the beginning of the 18th century, he was popular in southwest Nigeria, Benin and Togo.[27]

By the 17th century, the Turks and Greeks used a method called "variolation," which involved inserting live serum from smallpox pustules under the skin of a healthy person to induce a mild case of the disease. Upon recovery, individuals were rendered immune. Similar techniques were practiced in Asia and Africa.[28]

The translation of a centuries old Indian manuscript written by a native prince indicated that some Brahmins also practiced vaccine inoculation. The operation was performed by means of a thread impregnated with smallpox virus run across the forearm of a child. Apparently, only offspring whose parents worshipped the Bhowany, a female deity and protectress of those with smallpox, were treated. The goddess was generally represented riding an ass; as payment, the father of the child to be inoculated offered corn for the ass to eat. The ceremony was repeated as soon as pustules appeared.[29]

Preventive measures slowly evolved to include inoculation with year-old smallpox matter. Inoculators (those performing the operation) traveled across India pricking the skin of the patients' arms with a small metal instrument using "variolous matter" taken from pustules recovered from the previous year's inoculators. Dr. J.Z. Holwell confirmed the success of the procedure in a report to the College of Physicians, London, in 1767.[30] As important as these steps were, collectively they reached only a small percentage of the population and lacked significant impact on overall public health.

A Killer Without Regard to Person or Rank

Although smallpox was primarily a killer of children after it had become endemic, its virulence attacked susceptible adults without regard to social standing. Anne of Cleves, Henry VIII's fourth wife, survived smallpox but was scarred, as was Charles IX of France, whose nose was so badly deformed it appeared twice the normal size. Louis XIV contracted the disease, as did Louis XV, Tsar Peter II of Russia, Queen Ulrika Eleonora of Sweden, Emperor Joseph I of Austria, King Luis I of Spain: all died from it. Mary II of England perished from smallpox in 1694, at 32 years of age.[31] Early American history cites accounts of how Pocahontas died three years after her marriage, succumbing to smallpox.[32]

Upon the death of a monarch it was customary to examine the body to determine cause of death. An oft-repeated story held that after Louis XV's demise, the king's attendants fled in superstitious dread, prompting the first gentleman of the bedchamber to demand that the chief surgeon proceed by himself. The doctor replied, "My Lord Duke, your office renders it imperative upon you to hold the head of the deceased during the process; I declare to you that if the corpse is opened, neither you, nor I, nor any one of those assisting, will be alive eight days afterwards." The duke, "it need not be added, said no more about the matter."[33]

In Japan, a red picture of *Tametomo*, a 12th century hero reputed to have defeated a smallpox demon, was hung in sick rooms to ward away symptoms. This carried over into practice as subsequent Japanese physicians hung red cloth in the rooms of smallpox sufferers. As the idea developed, the chamber and bedding were furnished in red and patients wrapped in gowns of the same color. The concept of red possessing healing powers transferred to Europe in the 12th century. King Charles V of France, who reigned from 1364 to 1380, was clothed in a red shirt, stockings and veil. Queen Elizabeth I of England, who recovered from smallpox, was wrapped in a red blanket during her illness in 1562.[34] The idea of using the color red to alleviate symptoms or scarring persisted into the 1930s. In 1920, for instance, a Dr. Vincent of Ohio "discovered that a red ray in the room of the patient" would lessen the danger of the disease and leave fewer scars.[35] No scientific data has ever been presented to prove the theory.

Instances such as these prompted the origin of hanging a red flag outside the home of infected persons to warn others that smallpox raged within. When smallpox became endemic in the United States red flags served the same purpose. Other methods, such as that used in Bordeaux, required black paper with the words "petite verole" in large white characters to be affixed to the door of every house where the disease existed.[36]

2

Enter Inoculation

> Besides the security afforded by inoculation, we learn that the Circassians and Georgians were induced to this practice by an additional and powerful motive, avarice, in order to preserve the beauty of their female children, and to sell them at higher prices to the rich Turks and Persians as mistresses.[1]

The four deadliest diseases spreading pandemics throughout the Old World were plague, leprosy, syphilis and smallpox. By the 17th century, smallpox had surpassed the others to become the swiftest and most deadly of infectious diseases. Heavily populated cities suffered the most due to the inevitability of exposure to carriers in the form of immigrants, traders, seamen, soldiers and slaves. Due to isolation, those living in rural areas were often spared, and even when one family developed the disease, it often died out before victims could spread it. This saved many who lived off the beaten track, but as transportation improved and political factions eased, resulting in fewer armed conflicts, distant territories once thought immune were caught in the waxing and waning cycles of smallpox.

The year 1628 marked the first major epidemic in England. The disease became so prevalent that it was a commonly held belief that children should not be regarded as permanent members of the family, for the purposes of inheritance, until they had recovered from smallpox.[2] Understandably, people were desperate for a means of preventing or alleviating the disease. In 1663, thirty-five years after the initial outbreak, an enterprising concocter advertised a cure-all, the likes of which would resound across the quasi-medical system throughout the 18th and 19th centuries:

> The famous and approved Pectorall Lozenges, made by Mr. *Theophilus Buckworth,* for the Cure of Consumptions, Coughs, Catarhes, Asthmaes, Strongness of Breath, Hoarseness, Colds in generall, Ptisicks, and all other distempers of the Lungs, (being likewise a sovereign Antidote against the Plague, Small-pox, and other contagious Diseases,) are to he had at the said *Theophilus Buckworth's* house on *Mile-end Green...*

All of this, sealed with his "Coat of Armes," was available for the pricey sum of 2s 6d.[3] Adding familiar names to an advertisement was likely even more effective than a coat of arms. In 1681, Dr. Pordages began his pitch by stating, "Having some years been acquainted with the Ingenious Dr. Bacon, then of Bristol, but now of Winchester-street London, he has imparted to me a secret (with success experienced on thousands, if called for in time) for cure of the Small-Pox...." He promised to cure "those whose Pox is stuck in, and those who have been speechless; it removes all pains and sickness in four or six hours after the first Administration...." Stating his promises were presented without the least "hyperbole," the doctor left the form and manner of the remedy to the imagination.[4]

THe famous and approved Pectorall Lozenges, made by Mr *Theophilus Buckworth*, for the Cure of Consumptions, Coughs, Catarhes, Astmaes, Strongness of Breath, Hoarseness, Colds in generall, Ptisicks, and all other distempers of the Lungs, (being likewise a sovereign Antidote against the Plague, Small-pox, and other contagious Diseases,) are to be had at the said *Theophilus Buckworth*'s house on *Mile-end Green* ; and for convenience of such as live remote, Quantities of them are sealed up with his *coat* of Armes, and **2 s 6 d** upon every Paper, which are to be had at Mr. *Rooks* at the Lamb and Bottle in St. *Pauls* Church-yard, Mrs. *Seils* over against St. *Dunstans* Church in *Fleetstreet*, Mr. *Clark* at the Entrance of the Royall Exchange, Mr, *Millwards* at *Westminster-Hall Gate*, Mr. *Place* at *Grayes-Inne Gate Holborn*, Mr *Cranford* at the Gun in St. *Pauls Church-yard*, Mr. *Magnes* in *Covent-Garden*, Mr. *Sowersby* near the *New-Market*, Booksellers. Mr. *Hayes* at the Crosse-Daggers in *Moor-Fields*, Mr. *Mainstone* at the Goat near *Ivy- Bridge* in the *Strand*, and no where else.

Pectorall miracle lozenges promised a cure for almost everything that ailed the human body, including smallpox. Nostrums such as this were promoted by medical men as well as hucksters. Most potions were cathartics; taken in excessive doses they occasionally led to death. During smallpox epidemics in the 19th century, Coroner's Inquests were held over the bodies of those thought to have been poisoned by such over-the-counter "remedies" (from *The News, Published for the Satisfaction and Information of The People of Privilege* (London), February 4, 1663).

Not to be outdone, in 1712, one doctor offered his services for a new, albeit, unspecified treatment:

A Physician who has found out an easier and safer way of curing the Small-Pox than what is generally practiced, offers to Cure the Poor gratis of that Distemper. All therefore who are desirous of his Assistance send a note of their Habitation to Old Man's Coffee-house Charing-Cross, and they shall be attended on once a Day at least till they are past Danger. N.B. Such as send early and before the Small-Pox are come out upon them, will find the greater benefit by his Method.[5]

Young men, hoping to establish a practice by good will, typically placed such advertisements offering free care or new methods or both. The alternative to a private physician (and the even more common self-treatment) was the hospital. In 1746, a smallpox hospital was established at King's Cross, but beds were limited, and as the concept of hospitalization was frightening to the ordinary man, most opted to stay at home.

Spurious claims notwithstanding, in the early 1700s the technique of variolation (commonly referred to as engrafting, inoculation, insertion or transplantation) was the only known method of achieving personal protection. Sporadically practiced in the Orient, variolation was the process by which variola virus (the species of *Orthopoxvirus* that caused smallpox in humans) was transmitted from an infected person to a healthy one via a technique called arm-to-arm transfer. This involved placing a point or needle into an eruption and then inserting it under the skin of the person to be inoculated, with the expectation a mild case of smallpox would develop. Upon recovery, inoculated persons were presumed to have permanent immunity.

Variolation presented serious drawbacks, the most obvious of which was that the induced disease had the potential to become a full-blown attack. Most people who had variolation suffered only mild symptoms (as compared to natural smallpox), including severe

ADVERTISEMENTS.

AN Excellent Secret to take away Warts; Being a noble Mineral Tincture, which fafely and without Trouble takes away the largeft and moft ugly Warts from the Hands, or other Parts of the Body, fo as never to return again, rendring the Places on which they grew as fmooth and fair, as if no fuch Excrefcence had ever been. It's a ftupendious Medicine, and takes away Warts very fóon and with the greateft Safety, Certainty and Eafe imaginable. Is Sold only at Mr. *Ailcraft's*, a Toy-Shop, at the *Blue-Coat-Boy*, againft the *Royal-Exchange* in *Cornhill*, at 2 s. 6 d, a Bottle, containing enough to take away fifty Warts, with Directions.

THE Famous LOZENGES, being effectual in all Scorbutick Cafes; they eafe Pains in the Head and Stomach, caufe a good Appetite, purifie the Blood, and give fpeedy Relief in Rheumatifms, Dropfie, and Gout, and totally deftroy the very Seed of Worms.

They cure Agues and Fevers of all Sorts, give prefent Eafe in the Cholick, Stone and Gravel, cleanfe the Body after hard Drinking; as alfo after the Small-Pox, Meafles, and Child-bearing, and are a more general Cathartick Medicine than any yet known.

Prepar'd only by R. *Owner*, Apothecary, at the Peftle and Mortar, in *Eaft Smithfield*.

The top advertisement promotes "An Excellent Secret" to take away warts, being "a noble Mineral Tincture." The bottom advertisement, taken out by R. Owner, Apothecary, East Smithfield, London, promises his Famous lozenges will purify the blood, give speed relief from Rheumatism, Dropsie, Gout and destroy the "very Seed of Worms." Additionally, they cleansed the Body After Hard Drinking, "as also after the Small-Pox, Measles, and Child-bearing" (from *A Review of the State of the British Nation* (London), May 15, 1708).

local lesions with a generalized and at times extensive rash. A far more wide-ranging problem stemmed from the fact that persons inoculated with true (live) smallpox became carriers of the disease, capable of infecting individuals who had not previously contracted smallpox or who had not undergone variolation. As a public health preventive, the system worked only if entire towns or cities underwent inoculation. The idea of creating carriers was not well established in the 1700s and variolation served as the gold standard by which 18th century citizens protected themselves. Although the technique was known in Great Britain, the procedure did not make significant inroads until 1718, when it was promoted in an astonishing fashion: neither by a doctor nor by a man.

It is probable Mary Pierrepont, the eldest daughter of Evelyn, Duke of Kingston, never imagined she would have her name inscribed in the medical annals of her native country, but such was the case. Born at Thoresby, in Nottinghamshire around 1690, she received a classical education under the same preceptors as did Viscount Newark, her brother. Suffering smallpox as a child left Mary's face scarred, and it is likely this personal experience promoted a lifelong fascination with the disease.

In 1712, Mary married Edward Wortley Montagu, Esq., eldest son of Ann Wortley, wife of the Honourable Sidney Montagu, second son of Lord Sandwich, who died "in the arms of victory" during the battle of Solebay, during the reign of Charles II. A son, Edward Wortley, was born to the couple before Mr. Montagu received an ambassadorship to the Porte (Turkey). The family journeyed over the continent of Europe to Constantinople. In

Turkey, Lady Mary devoted considerable attention to studying the customs of the Turkish people.[6] Primary among them was the method of "engrafting." In a letter to Sarah Chiswell, dated April 1, 1717, she described her observations.

> Apropos of distempers, I am going to tell you a thing that I am sure will make you wish yourself here. The smallpox, so fatal and so general amongst us, is here entirely harmless by the invention of engrafting (which is the term they give it). There is a set of old women who make it their business to perform the operation. Every autumn, in the month of September, when the great heat is abated, people send to one another to know if any of their family has a mind to have the smallpox. They make parties for this purpose, and when they are met (commonly fifteen or sixteen together) the old woman comes with a nutshell full of the matter of the best sort of smallpox and asks what veins you please to have opened. She immediately rips open that you offer to her with a large needle (which gives you no more pain than a common scratch) and puts into the vein as much venum as can lie upon the head of her needle, and after binds up the little wound with a hollow bit of shell, and in this manner opens four or five veins. The Grecians have commonly the superstition of opening one in the middle of forehead, in each arm, and on the breast to mark the sign of the cross, but this has a very ill effect, all these wounds leaving little scars, and it is not done by those that are not superstitious, who choose to have them in the legs or that part of the arm that is concealed. The children of young people play together all the rest of the day and are in perfect health till the eighth. Then the fever begins to seize 'em and they keep their beds two days, seldom three. They have very rarely above twenty or thirty [pock marks] in their faces, which never mark, and in eight days' time they are as well as before their illness. Where they are wounded there remains running sores during the distemper, which I don't doubt is a great relief to it. Every year thousands undergo this operation, and the French ambassador says pleasantly that they take the smallpox here by way of diversion as they take the waters in other countries. There is no example of any one that has died in it, and you may believe I am very well satisfied on the safety of the experiment since I intend to try it on my dear little son. I am patriot enough to take pains to bring this useful invention in England, and I should not fail to write to some of our doctors very particularly about it if I knew any one of 'em that I thought had virtue enough to destroy such a considerable branch of their revenue for the good of mankind, but that distemper is too beneficial to them not to expose to all their resentment the hardy weight that should undertake to put an end to it. Perhaps if I live to return I may, however, have courage to war with 'em. Upon

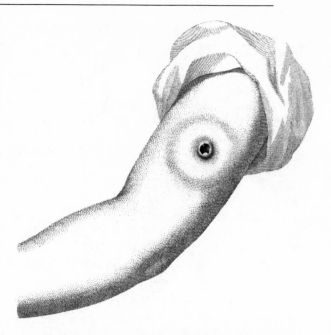

This illustration from Jenner's *An Inquiry into the Causes and Effects of Variolae Vaccinae*, p. 38A, represents the pustule taken from William Pead, a boy of 8 years who was inoculated March 28. On the sixth day he complained of pain in the axilla, and on the seventh was affected with the common symptoms of a patient sickening with the smallpox from inoculation. The efflorescent blush around the part punctured in the boy's arm was characteristic of that which appeared on variolous inoculation. The drawing was made "when the pustule was beginning to die away, and the areola retiring from the centre."

this occasion, admire the heroism in the heart of your friend, etc.[7]

Lady Mary was as good as her word. In the spring of 1717, she had her son inoculated at Constantinople by Dr. Maitland, an English surgeon and physician to the mission of the Porte.[8] The child became the first publicized English person to undergo the operation. She wrote, "The boy [Edward Wortley] was engrafted last Tuesday, and is at this time singing and playing, and very impatient for his supper.... I cannot engraft the girl [her daughter]; her nurse has not had the small pox."

Edward's inoculation would prove more beneficial than anticipated. When, at age six, the child ran away from Westminster school, the family offered a £20 reward plus expenses for his return. The notice describing him advised there were "two marks by which he is easily known, viz, on the back of each arm, about two or three inches above the wrist, a small roundish scar, less than a silver penny, like a large mark of the smallpox."

In 1717, Montagu received "orders of recal" and the family returned to England. Determined to see the preventive become widespread, Lady Mary persuaded Dr. Maitland to introduce the method of engrafting to the English public. Under her considerable patronage and buoyed by her indomitable spirit and faith in the procedure, he set up practice and began offering smallpox inoculation to his patients. Instead of finding their efforts lauded, the "heathen practice" was attacked by two of the most powerful groups in England — the clergy and the medical fraternity.

Physicians condemned the procedure as a "hazardous experiment," arguing that in the small portion of variolous poison, "inveterate hereditary diseases might be communicated." Many "divines and foolish bigots" preached against the practice as "impious, and an insult to the divine decrees," claiming it bore a stronger resemblance to magic than physic, "and to crown this fiery rhapsody, that the devil had inoculated Job."[9]

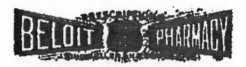

SMALLPOX IS DUE TO IGNORANCE AND PREJUDICE

Vaccination against smallpox has stood every test during 125 years. Few physicians have ever seen a case in anyone ever vaccinated. Ignorance and prejudice are the only excuses for smallpox epidemics. We keep our vaccine in cold storage, ready for use by your physician. A drop of prevention is worth an acre of smallpox. Consult your physician. When the physician writes a prescription, bring it to us to be filled. We are specialists at this work.

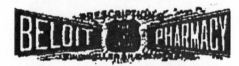

Madison and Beloit
Forest 350

Historically, doctors and apothecaries were often accused of promoting vaccination for their own pecuniary means, causing their sincerity to be called into question. While advertisements against vaccination appeared more often in the press, occasionally one in support of the procedure can be found. In the case of the Beloit Pharmacy, its defense of vaccination went hand in hand with the desire to sell vaccine, "kept in cold storage, ready for use by your physician" (from the *Forest Park Review* [IL], September 8, 1928).

Other "zealous churchmen" considered inoculation repugnant to religion and felt it their duty to interfere. Their most common idea held that inoculation was a daring attempt to interrupt the eternal decrees of Providence. In 1722 a Mr. Massy preached in St. Andrew's Church, Holborn, England, that "all who infused the variolous ferment were sorcerers, and that inoculation was the diabolical invention of Satan." Further, one of the rectors of Canterbury, the Reverend Theodore de la Faye, in a sermon preached in 1751, denounced the procedure as the offspring of atheism and drew a parallel between resignation to the divine will and inoculation.[10]

Undeterred by these attacks, Lady Mary persisted in her efforts, fortunately enlisting the support and cooperation of a prominent physician, Richard Mead. In 1720, when an epidemic threatened London, Mead wrote the treatise "A Short Discourse Concerning Pestilential Contagion and the Methods Used to Prevent It," supporting inoculation. Within the year, the text was reprinted seven times and an eighth edition appeared in 1722. In conjunction with Sir Hans Sloane, physician to the king and president of the Royal Society, who had conducted extensive research on engrafting, permission was obtained in 1721 to experiment on seven condemned criminals from Newgate Prison.[11] Dr. Mead and Mr. Maitland supervised the inoculations and all seven prisoners recovered from their mild cases of smallpox, receiving a pardon from the king for their service. In April 1722, two royal princesses, Amelia and Caroline, were inoculated under Dr. Sloane's supervision. Acceptance by the royal family quickly made the operation more palatable to British minds.

The following year, Lady Mary had her own young daughter inoculated by inserting matter in slight incisions on both arms. This prompted a letter to Lady Mary, in the spring of 1722, in which her friend Lady Mar triumphantly observed, "I suppose that the same faithful historians give you regular accounts of the growth and spread of the inoculation of the small-pox, which is becoming almost a general practice attended with great success." It certainly proved to be such in Bohemia, where Dr. Johann Adam Reiman carried out successful inoculations.

Acceptance was not universal, however, and in 1723, Lady Mary's sister's son, Gower, died of the disease. Ruing the unnecessary loss of life, she wrote to Lady Mar in July: "I think she has a great deal of regret it [*sic*], in consideration of the offer I made her, two years together, of taking the child home to my house, where I would have inoculated him with the same care and safety I did my own. I know nobody that has hitherto repented the operation; though it has been very troublesome to some fools who had rather be sick by the doctor's prescriptions, than in health in rebellion to the College [of Physicians]."

Mr. Maitland had his own problems, publishing a second edition of his "Account of Inoculating the small-pox," vindicating himself from Dr. Wagstaffe's "Misrepresentations of That Practice," to which Maitland added his account of inoculating the small-pox.[12]

Among Lady Mary's greatest supporters was Dr. Richard Steele. An article in the *Plain Dealer* (London), July 3, 1724, written by Steele, attracted great attention by his absolute praise of her:

> We are indebted to the Reason and Courage of a Lady, for the introduction of this Art, which gives such Strength in its Progress, that the Memory of its Illustrious Foundress will be render'd Sacred by it, to future ages.
> This Ornament of her Sex, and Country, who ennobles her own Nobility, by her learning, Wit, and Frequency, even among those obstinate Proedestinarians; and brought it over, for the Service and the Safety, of her Native England; where she consecrated its first effects on the Persons of her own fine Children! And has already receiv'd this Glory from it. That the Influence of her example has reach'd as high as the Blood Royal; And our noblest and most ancient Families, in Conformation of her happy Judgment, add the daily Experience of those who are most dear to them.[13]

Inoculation existed as the primary method of protection from smallpox for eighty years, although fears and prejudices prevailed against so novel a practice. In 1723, during a smallpox epidemic, opponents attributed the outbreak to inoculation. In defense, Dr. James Jurin, inoculation's "fostering patron," observed that mortality from the present outbreak had occurred in January and February, but that no person had been inoculated before the 27th of March.

As secretary of the Royal Society, Dr. Jurin collected a tremendous amount of firsthand data on the efficacy of inoculation, but as deaths from the palliative procedure increased, or were thought to increase (in fact, while the death rate from natural smallpox remained stable at a ratio of 1:6, the death rate for inoculated persons stood at 1:48–60)[14] the "public disgust" in England brought the operation into discredit. Not so on the island of St. Kitts in the West Indies, where 300 Negroes were inoculated and not one died.

Dr. Short's Table, derived from the London Bills of Mortality from January 1, 1728, to 1743, a period of 15 years, presented averages in the following proportions (while causes of death were not given, smallpox typically struck the very young):

London Deaths, 1728–1743

Years of Age	Died
Under 2 years	9,910
From 2–5 years	2,411
5–10	980
10–20	851
20–30	2,000
30–40	2,471
40–50	2,510
50–60	2,231
60–70	1,675
70–80	1,200
80–90	634
90–100	117[15]

Physicians slowly acknowledged the advantages of inoculation, and in 1746 a small charitable hospital was erected at Pancras in the environs of London for the double purpose of inoculation and to receive indigents afflicted with smallpox. Of the 1,800 inoculated there over the course of several years, only eight died from the operation. In 1759, a total of 593 were inoculated at Pancras, many of whom were adults, with only one death. The following table provides more specific data:

Diseases and Casualties of the Week
(London), June 3–6, 1748

Cause of Death	Number of Deaths
Consumption	104
Dropsy	15
Fever	67
Convulsion	118
Small Pox	31
Sudden death	2
Teeth	21
Thrush	1
Drowned	2

Cause of Death	*Number of Deaths*
Found dead	4
Killed by a blow	1
Overlaid (one disease added to another)	3

During the same time frame, 125 males and 120 females were christened (total 245), while 230 males and 222 females were buried (total 452).[16]

The Suttonian Art of Inoculation

Robert Sutton was a practicing surgeon in Suffolk who developed what became known as the "Suttonian System" of inoculation for smallpox. Born in 1707, he apprenticed to a surgeon named John Turner and after completing his study opened a practice at Kenton. In 1756, he asked surgeon John Rodbard to inoculate his oldest son, Robert Junior. The boy developed a serious case of smallpox and it is likely this incident inspired the patriarch to develop his own technique.

Although inoculation in England at the time was not the standard of practice, Sutton achieved immediate success. After renting a house where he could administer the treatment, in April 1757, he advertised terms that included board, nursing, tea, wine, fish and fowl, charging £7/7 per month, £5/5 for farmers, 10/6 for nonboarders,"[17] a hefty price by any standards. Business was good and by October he operated two houses, claiming "remarkable success with this method in the spring."[18]

His area of practice increased and by February 1759, Sutton claimed his technique had achieved the greatest success, "never having lost one patient or had one so bad as to be blind with it." By September, the boast increased to "never having had one bad symptom."[19] Success drew imitators and he dropped his fee to £5/5s, but "for the benefit of the lower class of people" he offered easier terms.[20]

Sutton's technique was reputed to have been performed without any incision and "that the most curious eye could not discern where the operation had been performed for the first 48 hours," and that he was always careful to be sure the patient received the infection required for true protection.

Sutton's technique was actually a minor revision of the inoculation technique practiced at the midpoint of the 18th century combined with a dietary regime and padded with puffing. In his book, *The Inoculator or Suttonian System of Inoculation, Fully Set Forth in a Plain and Familiar Manner,*[21] Robert's son Daniel described the operation, writing, "The charged lancet is held slantwise to $\frac{1}{16}$" deep in the skin." With careful administration, the smallpox matter was injected with minimal, if any, distress to the patient. The patient then put on his clothes without any dressing covering the wound.[22]

The regimen consisted of having the patient abstain from meat and alcohol for two weeks prior to inoculation in order to weaken constitutions considered too strong to properly accept the operation. After surgery, the patient was to exercise in the open air until developing a fever, at which time he was treated with cold water and fed warm tea and thin gruel. Once eruptions appeared, the patient was ordered to get up and walk around the garden. Regular purges were administered and a "secret remedy" given to try to control symptoms of the mild case of smallpox. No formula was ever offered for the "secret remedy," but contemporaries conjectured that it contained mercury and antimony.[23] (In the 18th and 19th centuries, mercury was a commonly administered heavy metal used for venereal and eruptive diseases, having two effects: a stimulus on the constitution and a "specific" on a diseased part of the body. Antimony, a metal of metallic luster "generally containing a small portion of arsenic," was widely used to combat fevers.[24] Both are now known to be deadly poisons and proof of the maxim "the cure is worse than the disease."

Sutton's son Robert, also a practicing physician, joined him in late 1762 or early 1763, before opening his own houses for inoculation. As testimony to the temper of the times and the speculative nature of inoculation, Robert Sutton was threatened with prosecution by the parish authorities of Debenham in June 1763.

Daniel moved to Ingatestone, Essex, setting up his practice on the London to Harwich road in 1763. His business of inoculation met with local opposition but the following year when a smallpox epidemic broke out in Maldon, a subscription was raised to pay for his services; in consequence he inoculated 70 gentlemen and tradesmen and 417 poor people. Within three weeks, no further cases of smallpox were reported.[25]

With his reputation established, Robert, Junior, hired the Reverend Robert Houlton, M.A., at a considerable salary of 200 guineas per year to promote him. Always wise to have the backing of religious individuals, Houlton earned his salary by preaching praises of the Suttonian System, going so far as to have his sermons printed and distributed.[26] In June 1766, a month after hiring Houlton, Mr. Ristch, first surgeon to the King of Poland, visited Robert, Junior, reportedly being surprised at the "slightness of the operation."[27] Over a five-year period, Robert, Junior, inoculated more than 20,000 people at Ingatestone.[28]

When inquiries from Vienna and Brussels concerning the Suttonian System were received, the Physicians and Surgeons to his Majesty the King investigated the technique, concluding that its success was due to the rules laid down regarding diet and exposure of patients to cool air. They also noted others used a similar method with success. Eventually, six of Robert Sutton's sons practiced inoculation, including Henry, who worked at Suffolk and Joseph Sutton, who went to Bordeaux in 1763, offering to treat Louis XV when he was dying of smallpox.[29]

The Suttonian System was wildly popular and equally lucrative, made more so by the "system" of offering residential care. Had Lady Mary Montagu known the extent to which practicing physicians earned considerable fortunes by performing inoculations, she would surely have changed her not unfounded belief they would resist the operation, as it would "destroy such a considerable branch of their revenue" from treating smallpox. Daniel Sutton alone earned 2,000 guineas in 1764 and 6,000 guineas in 1786.[30]

Aside from personal administrations, the Suttons and their agent, Reverend Houlton, licensed physicians to perform the system. By early 1769, the *Dublin Journal* reported that over 40,000 individuals throughout England had been inoculated, with not more than 100 lost. Along with Samuel Sparrow and Charles Blake, the team taught and authorized others, including John Blakely, surgeon of the King's County Hospital.[31] The same year, Houlton and Blake were invited to Counties Cavan, Monaghan, Leitrim and Longford and other areas of Ireland to inoculate for the smallpox; they warned potential patients to "beware of Imposters."[32] By December 1769, they claimed 32 "partners" practicing the "new Mode of Inoculation." Among that number were seven surgeons of county hospitals.[33] Houlton himself, "having executed his Commission from England," announced he would be in Dublin until the following summer and persons "inclined to be Inoculated by Mr. Houlton" were requested to apply at Mrs. Aderine's in York Street.[34] John Lee, M.D., was the first physician to introduce the Suttonian method of inoculation in Paris.[35]

Not surprisingly, imitators were soon on the scene. The same year the Suttonian System was advertised in Dublin, the "Arnoldian Art of Inoculation" made its appearance. As with the Suttons, Joseph Arnold warned the public that Mr. John Byrne of Kildare was his only authorized agent.[36] Letters between supporters of the Suttonian and Arnoldian systems became acrimonious, with Joseph Arnold taking out an advertisement to defend himself while casting aspersions against the Suttonian System:

INOCULATION

Whereas it has been currently reported, that in order to procure Patients to Inoculate for the Small Pox, I lately advertised my Intentions of Inoculating for the Measles; this is to assure the Public, that I had not the least Concern in said Advertisement, but am informed it was the famous Doctor Howard, in Conjunction with the Rev. Mr. Houlton who is generally known by the Name of the Bogg'd Inoculator. This Howard it is said also has lately taken out his Degree in Physic at Rheames in France. O Tempora! O Mores! JOSEPH ARNOLD.

With both sides vying for favor, published testimonies like the following were typical:

INOCULATION

Mrs. Morgan of William Street, has lately employed Mr. Arnold to Inoculate her Children, "Twins" being under the Age of five Months, which had the Small Pox in a mild and favourable Manner, and she with the greatest Gratitude, in Justice to Mr. Arnold's Care and Assiduity in attending them, takes the Liberty thus publicly to express her sincere Thanks. Dublin, Feb. 5th, 1770. ANN MORGAN.[37]

Nor were profiteers left out of the inoculation business. In May 1782, Mrs. Adrian advertised her "Italian Cream of Roses." Used not only to keep the skin from "tanning and freckling, occasioned by walking and riding in the sun," it was also prescribed by "Dr. Sutton the Inoculator, in particular, to be used in and after the Small Pox, in order to preserve the face from being pitted with that malignant disorder."[38]

Few would object to physicians augmenting their income by performing smallpox inoculation, but exorbitant fees raised ethical questions. During the course of their careers, the Suttons charged between £3 3s and £7 7s, with the money to be paid before the surgery and to include room and board. Inoculation in the home cost £1 3d,[39] but that still constituted a very large amount of money and remained out of the reach of many. During their lifetimes, the Suttons, particularly Robert, would be criticized for their high charges; ultimately, this would cost them a more revered place in the medical history of inoculation. Physician's fees would remain an issue well into the "Vaccination Era."

The Suttonian technique (as opposed to the entire "System") of making minute punctures in the skin and administering small amounts of lymph did succeed in making the procedure more acceptable and less dangerous and many practitioners adopted this method.

Worldwide reaction to inoculation continued to favor the operation. Dr. Fronchin introduced inoculation into Amsterdam in 1748, beginning experiments on his own son. Before 1754, the technique was adopted in several other towns in Holland. Haller and Tissot introduced the practice into Switzerland and later Dr. Gatti, professor of medicine in Italy, inoculated 1,000 "without a single miscarriage." In 1755, an inoculating hospital was established in Stockholm and of 1,000 inoculated in Sweden before 1764, not one died. Denmark adopted the practice about the same time.[40]

In France, where opposition was particularly strong, Charles de La Condamine, a mathematician and geographer, began an inoculation campaign in 1754, claiming that nearly one million deaths could have been averted had France followed England's lead. When

Louis XV died of smallpox on May 19, 1774, dread of the disease finally opened the eyes of the public and medical profession, ushering in the beginnings of this medical practice.

A letter from Parma in 1764 demonstrated its acceptance when the duke signed his consent that the prince, his son, be inoculated, it was supposed, "in consequence of the Loss of a Consort and a Daughter whom he tenderly loved, and who might possibly have been still living had Recourse been had to the same Operation."[41]

Dr. Black's Observations (1781, cited in chapter 1) argued that 2,000 lives a year might be saved in London if physicians went to private residences and inoculated children under the age of five. Citing Dr. Short's statistics above, he demonstrated that the greatest number of deaths occurred in that age group, the general consensus being that "those more stricken in years, and the aged, will trust, as usual, to Providence."

Black's point was made to dispute the writing of Baron Thomas Dimsdale (see below) in the latter's own book, in which he argued against the propriety of inoculating at home and suggested instead the creation of a large "Inoculating Hospital." A reviewer of both texts, signed "A Friend to General Inoculation in London," concurred with Black: "To think of crowding together all the young infants *under* that age [5 years], with their mothers and nurses, into an Inoculating Hospital, could only be the scheme of a man worthy to be confined in a dark room and a straw bed. So much for Baron Dimsdale's Inoculating Hospital for the great hive of society, *the Poor and middling Tradespeople.*"[42] Eventually, a combination of both techniques would evolve and be put into practice.

The Great Inoculators

William Watson (1715–1787) was appointed physician to the Foundling Hospital, London, in 1762. Already a practitioner of the Suttonian System (further simplifying it and omitting the residential treatment), he followed the dictate that all children admitted to the hospital be inoculated against smallpox. In 1766, Sir John Pringle (1707–1782) introduced Watson to Jan Ingen-Housz (1730–1799). Pringle had met the Breda-born Ingen-Housz while serving as physician-general to the British army then stationed near Breda during the War of Austrian Succession. He introduced him to medicine and encouraged him to go to England.

Watson espoused the cause of inoculation and Ingen-Housz became an ardent convert. After practicing at the Foundling Hospital, he expanded his practice, eventually joining another inoculator, Thomas Dimsdale (1712–1800), a Hertfordshire physician. Dimsdale criticized the Suttons for permitting their freshly inoculated patients to circulate among the uninoculated, for fear of unintentionally spreading contagion. He rightly believed that the only sure way to prevent cross-contamination was to inoculate everyone. Together with Ingen-Housz they put this idea into practice, successfully inoculating two entire Hertfordshire parishes, Little Berkhampstead and Bayford. This ended a devastating cycle of inoculation and contamination that had sustained an epidemic of smallpox for three years that reached a mortality rate of 20 percent.[43]

In 1768, Dimsdale traveled to St. Petersburg to perform the "Dimsdale method" of inoculation on Catherine the Great, Tsarina of Russia — but not without potential danger, this time to the physician. He had relays of horses ready in case the operation did not succeed and he was set upon by her subjects. The entire matter was kept secret until her favorable recovery, at which time he and the system were looked upon with higher regard.[44] For his services, Dimsdale received the rank of baron, £10,000 and a pension of £500 per year.[45]

The same year Dimsdale went to Russia, Sir John Pringle recommended that Ingen-Housz go to Vienna. Arriving in May, he successfully inoculated the children of Empress Maria Theresa. She rewarded him with the appointment of court physician and councilor, which carried with it a life-long pension of 5,000 gulden per year. Once established, the doctor went to Florence, where he inoculated Emperor Joseph's brother Leopold, Grand Duke of Tuscany, as well as his family. As part of his duties, Ingen-Housz also taught the practice of inoculation to the Hapsburg physicians.[46]

Despite its acceptance as a personal preventive, engrafting was never fully adopted by the English, in part because people were "inoculated by ignorant Operators; by Imposters and Pretenders to the real method, who know not the Smallpox from a common rash,"[47] and the disease continued to ravish both city and countryside.

The beginning of the anti-inoculation movement (that would later develop into the anti-vaccination movement) argued that, however useful the technique had been to individuals, it "has been productive of much injury to the community at large." Proponents offered data from the Bills of Mortality to substantiate their own claims, stating that after 1750, when Lady Mary Wortley Montagu argued in its favor, the number of deaths from smallpox actually increased:

Years	Died of Small Pox	Total Deaths
From 1702 to 1712	12,368	213,973
From 1712 to 1722	20,990	245,404
From 1722 to 1732	23,309	274,042
From 1732 to 1742	19,929	271,832
From 1742 to 1752	17,554	241,376
From 1752 to 1762	21,144	204,632
From 1762 to 1772	24,369	235,124
From 1772 to 1782	23,399	231,452[48]

More specifically, with death an everyday occurrence, a notice from June 3–6, 1748, presented an idea of how difficult life was for those living in an age characterized by filth, disease and disaster:

London "Diseases and Casualties" for the Last Week of 1759

Disease	Number of Deaths	Disease	Number of Deaths
Convulsions	113	Small Pox	25
Consumption	81	Teeth	17
Fever	46	Dropsy	10
Aged	35	Measles	7

The returns reflected an increase of 55 burials from the previous week.[49] Yearly totals three years later reveal a staggering loss of life:

Partial List of Disease and Casualties (London)
December 14, 1762 to December 13, 1763

Convulsions	6,338	Drowned	105
Small-Pox	5,582	Killed themselves	34
Consumption	4,892	Executed	18
Malignant Fevers	3,414	Excessive Drinking	8
Aged	1,836	Worms	7
Teeth	890		

Only one cause of death ranked higher than smallpox: convulsions. On the lower but no less tragic end were a wide variety of causes reflective of the era. A total of 15,133 persons were christened, and 26,143 were buried.[50]

If life was grim, there were occasional rewards for health care workers. In 1753, *Alexander's Feast* by George Frideric Handel, with a concerto on the organ by Mr. Stanley, was performed at the King's Theatre in the Haymarket before the presidents, vice-presidents, and governors of the Small-Pox Hospital.[51]

Finally, in 1793, John Haygarth offered a comprehensive plan of "systematic inoculation throughout the country, isolation of patients, decontamination of potentially contaminated fomites, supervised inspectors responsible for specific districts, rewards for observance of rules for isolation by poor persons, fines for transgression of those rules, inspection of vessels at ports, and prayers every Sunday."[52] His ideas, applied to a new technique, would later be incorporated — and argued about — well into the 20th century.

3

Smallpox in the New World

We are told by one of the black robe
The Devil inoculated Job.
Suppose 'tis true, what he does tell,
Pray, Neighbors, did not Job do well?[1]

The above rhyme from 1774 was a play on a sermon given by the Reverend Massey in 1722. Contending that the Devil was the first inoculator and Job his first patient, the minister preached, "So went Satan forth from the presence of the Lord, and smote Job with boils from the sole of his foot unto his crown."[2]

In the 52 years that passed between the religious aspersions cast on the process of inoculation and the stanza poking fun at it, it is clear that colonial attitudes radically changed. This does not mean that after half a century all Americans embraced the technique, for they did not. The struggle for acceptance, first of variolation and then of vaccination, was long and daunting. It involved not only how early settlers viewed God, but also how they, in turn, were judged by the indigenous peoples of North and South America. Thrown into the mix were devastating and recurring epidemics of smallpox, ever-volatile political situations, the idea of mandatory public health legislation and the hard practicalities of war.

Dr. Black's 1805 "History of Smallpox" offered the contention that the first infection in North America was carried into Mexico in 1520 by a "[N]egro" slave of Spain, and killed off half the population.[3] Contemporary authorities generally offer the island of Hispaniola in the year 1507 as receiving the first infusion of smallpox. Brought by Spanish seamen, the disease caused devastation; in 1517, an outbreak occurring in African slaves spread to the Amerindian population, killing about one-third of them. Of greater magnitude, those involved in the African slave trade (beginning around 1503) spread the disease through Cuba, Puerto Rico, the Caribbean Islands and Mexico.[4]

Cortez sailed from Cuba to the coast of Mexico, then moved inland, reaching Tenochtitlán in November 1519. Narváez followed in 1520. According to reports from the period, among the latter's crew was a Negro suffering from smallpox; introduction of the disease into the unprotected population resulted in horrific suffering and death throughout the indigenous population. So many Aztec warriors were lost that those left had little ability to prevent further inroads by the invaders, making conquest inevitable. Equally significant from a military standpoint, the Spaniards appeared immune to the disease (from previous exposure or inoculation), giving the impression they possessed almost magical powers.

By September 1520, smallpox claimed victims in the Valley of Mexico and, quickly swept into Tenochtitlán. Before these ravages had quieted death toll estimates suggest that half the population of Mexico perished within six months. With resistance impossible, the disease progressed into Guatemala and the Yucatan Peninsula. Continuing its southward progression, smallpox reached the Inca Empire between 1524 and 1527, killing approximately 200,000 out of 6 million inhabitants, including the Inca emperor. An interior conflict broke out over who was to become the successor. Political intrigue, disease and the overwhelmingly unsettled nature of their once-stable economies made the Inca susceptible to Pizarro's invading troops in 1533.

Similar devastation wrecked South America, where smallpox was introduced in 1555. Five years later, the introduction of infected African slaves caused fresh outbreaks. Close behind them were the Portuguese, who reinfected the remaining natives during the years 1562–1563. By 1588, the entire South American continent suffered from unchecked epidemics. Portuguese missionaries did not introduce variation until 1728, leaving a period of 173 years for the disease to decimate the population. Even then variation was not widely practiced, leaving people unprotected through the 18th century.[5]

Explorers conquering other areas of the globe introduced smallpox into Greenland. The first known epidemic there occurred in 1734, killing two-thirds of the population. Iceland also suffered great epidemics of the disease and by 1797, during the 18th such outbreak, 18,000 out of a population of 50,000 were destroyed.[6]

The image of death—in this case, death from smallpox, scarlet fever and other diseases—is represented here by a winged skeleton, the harbinger of death. One of the most deadly diseases ever to infect humans, smallpox persisted with little resistance from "time immemorial." In many countries, infants and children were not considered members of the family until they had passed through the scourge of the Speckled Disease (illustration from the *Salt Lake City Tribune,* October 3, 1900).

Smallpox Among Native Americans

Smallpox arrived in the New World with the earliest settlers, literally jumping ship from the Old World. Colonization along the eastern seaboard occurred almost a century after that of Central and South America, but it did not take long for the disease to gain a foothold. Repeating the pattern of exposure among indigenous people, the earliest victims of this contact were Native Americans. Lacking any type of immunity, entire settlements were quickly obliterated. As pioneers moved inland, they unintentionally carried the disease with them, but on occasion, smallpox was used as a weapon of conquest.

In his work "Magnalia," Cotton Mather described the fate of Native Americans after exposure to the colonists. "The Indians in these parts had newly, about every year or two before, been visited with such a prodigious pestilence; as carried away not a tenth, but nine parts of ten (yea, 'tis said nineteen of twenty) among them."[7]

Elizabeth A. Fenn, in her book, *Pox Americana: The Great Smallpox Epidemic of 1775–82*,[8] makes the point that, although early numbers of Indian casualties were staggering, accurate numbers are impossible to obtain and may have, by the horror of witnessing the sight of devastated villages, been exaggerated by early witnesses. What is incontestable is that the Amerindians were totally susceptible to the smallpox infection and died, not only from disease but also from its terrible aftermath. In an all-too-familiar pattern destined to be played out throughout the world over three centuries, once a large segment of the population became ill, everything from commerce to basic housekeeping ground to a standstill. No one earned a living, few gathered or prepared food, and fewer still were available to tend the sick. Those who might have survived the initial attack perished from lack of nutrition and sanitation. The grim reality was that, until individuals developed a natural immunity from exposure or were inoculated, a safety net simply did not exist.

The earliest immigrants brought just such immunity with them, but successive generations were by and large left unprotected. As long as communities remained small and somewhat isolated from outside influences, widespread epidemics were rare. Even when they did occur, transmission outside the settlement did not progress with the rapidity of epidemics in densely populated European cities where travel was facilitated by paved roads and public conveyances.

It is important to note that the lack of immunity in colonial children posed an unanticipated risk that did not become evident until the sons of wealthy landowners traveled to Europe. Whether they crossed the Atlantic for pleasure, to establish connections with relatives or for higher education, they were immediately exposed to smallpox in the major cultural cities. Contracting the disease often proved fatal, ironically fostering the establishment of institutions of higher learning in America.

The first epidemic to strike the eastern seaboard came in the years 1617–1619, killing many Indians along the Massachusetts coast. Thus weakened in numbers, they posed less of a threat to the settlers who arrived at Plymouth in 1620.[9] Fourteen years later, in 1634, smallpox struck again. William Bradford wrote of the appalling condition of the Connecticut Indians suffering from smallpox during the 1634 epidemic:

> They fell sick of ye small poxe, and died most miserably; for a sorer disease cannot befall them; they fear it more than ye plague; for usually they that have this disease have them in abundance, and for wante of bedding and lining and other helps, they fall into a lamentable condition, as they lye on their hard mats, ye poxe breaking and mattering, and running one into another, their skin cleaving to the matts they lye on; when they turn them, a whole side will flea of at once, and they will be all of a gore blood, most fearful to behold; and then being very sore, what with could and other distempers, they dye like rotten sheep.[10]

Although the English were afraid of the infection, "seeing this woefull and sadd condition" they assisted in procuring wood and water, brought food and buried the dead. "By the marvelous providence of God," none of the English caught the disease, though they tended the Indians for weeks on end.[11] On February 1, 1634, John Winthrop added his own observation in his diary: "Such of the Indians' children as were left were taken by the English. Most whereof did die of the pox soon after."[12]

Aiding in the dissemination of smallpox was the Indians' fear of this unimaginable killer. Once an epidemic struck, survivors, many of whom were sick, fled the poisoned area, carrying contamination on their bodies and within their possessions. Perhaps of greater significance than fear were the cultural differences between British and Spanish invaders. The former were likely to drive the Indians away while the latter used force to enslave them.

Thus, smallpox victims along the East Coast tended to spread the disease deeper into the country while disease in the West was kept more closely confined.

Smallpox Used in Germ Warfare

One of the earliest instances of what has come to be known as "germ warfare" (as opposed to traditional weaponry) occurred during the French and Indian Wars, 1754–1763. Lord Jeffrey Amherst served as Commander-in-Chief of the British forces from 1758 to 1763, warring against the French and Native Americans to secure Canada for His Majesty, George III. So revered was the officer that Amherst, Massachusetts, was named after him.

With the defeat of the French in 1763, Amherst encountered a rebellion of the Ottawa Indians led by Chief Pontiac in what has become known as "Pontiac's Rebellion." The Indians expected the British to continue providing supplies in exchange for cooperation. Amherst, however, rebelled against the idea of "bribery" and refused to continue the tradition. Rumors over the centuries have long implicated "Lord Jeff," as he was called, in distributing smallpox-tainted blankets among the Indians as a means of extermination.

In a landmark study called the "British Manuscript Project" (1941–1945), under the auspices of the Library of Congress, letters and documents from the era were preserved on microfilm. This enabled a close examination that categorically revealed Amherst's loathing of the Indians and his desire to "Extirpate this Execrable Race" (Amherst to Colonel Henry Bouquet, July 16, 1763). A letter not found in the collection but cited by Francis Parkman[13] quotes Amherst as writing, "Could it not be contrived to send the *Small Pox* among those disaffected tribes of Indians? We must on this occasion use every stratagem in our power to reduce them." The fact that smallpox had been reported at Fort Pitt provides a strong indication that obtaining disease matter was well within the realm of possibility (Bouquet to Amherst, June 23, 1763).

Historian J.C. Long states that Pontiac's attacks on forts at Detroit and Presqu'Isle "aroused Amherst to a frenzy, a frenzy almost hysterical in its impotence." In a letter from that officer to Sir William Johnson, Amherst said, "It would be happy for the Provinces that there was not an Indian settlement within a thousand Miles of them, and when they are properly punished, I care not how soon they move their Habitations, for the Inhabitants of the Woods are the fittest Companions for them, they being more nearly allied to the Brute than to the Human Creation."[14]

Later evidence taken from the *Journal of William Trent* includes an entry for May 24, 1763. Trent, commander of local militia at Pittsburgh during Pontiac's siege of the fort, stated, "[W]e gave them two Blankets and an Handkerchief out of the Small Pox Hospital. I hope it will have the desired effect." Contemporary reports indicate that smallpox did, indeed, break out among the Indians.[15]

The Spread of Smallpox Among Native American Populations

The situation regarding smallpox in Canada mirrored that of the territories that would become the United States. French settlers introduced smallpox around 1635. That year it spread to the Montagnais living near Quebec City, quickly decimating the native population and spreading into the Algonquins, Hurons, and other tribes inhabiting "New France."[16]

During the 1630s and 1640s, smallpox spread throughout the St. Lawrence-Great Lakes region, killing half of those belonging to the Huron and Iroquois confederations. A Canadian smallpox epidemic in 1702–1703 resulted in 3,000 deaths; thirty years later another destroyed 1,800. In pre–Revolution times, nearly half the Cherokees succumbed to smallpox epidemics from 1738 to 1739, followed by the epidemics of 1759–1760, 1780, 1783 and 1806. Among the Cherokee, it was believed disease resulted from "the violation of social sanctions or as simply a form of social opposition between humans or between humans and supernatural forces." They considered disease, particularly that introduced by the white man, and the dwindling of animal and plant life to be a direct result of the invaders who destroyed sacred places. This situation was exacerbated in 1777, when they ceded Tugalo, on the Georgia–South Carolina border (believed by them to be the first place created by the Provider). They, along with most Native Americans, believed that social and spiritual balance could not be achieved until the whites left their land.[17]

In 1759, similar numbers were lost to smallpox among the Catawbas. The third Canadian epidemic resulted in 2,600 deaths in 1757. During the American Revolution, smallpox appeared among the Piegan tribe with equal devastation.[18] In the summer of 1781, the Piegan Blackfeet raided a Shoshone village. As described by Saukamappee, one of the warriors, "Our war hoop instantly stopt, our eyes were appalled with terror; there was no one to fight with but the dead and the dying, each a mass of corruption." David Thompson, the explorer who recorded the oral history, added that the Piegan took no scalps but plundered the village and returned home. Two days later, smallpox broke out among the Piegan.

That same summer, the Piegan communicated the disease to the Western Cree and the Assiniboine, with whom they traded. On October 22, 1781, at a Hudson Bay Company trading post on the North Saskatchewan River, the first Indian with smallpox appeared; thereafter, numerous reports of casualties poured in. By 1782, three-fifths of the Indian population had died and trading houses became centers of contagion.

Smallpox continued to spread, covering the American Southwest and Southeast as well as the Northern Plains and Canada. The Comanche, "who engaged in a spirited horse and slave trade with their Shoshone kinfolk in western Wyoming and Montana," were the likely carriers. In turn, the Shoshone infected those in the Canadian interior as well as the tribes of the upper Missouri River. The disease was to linger. In 1805, Meriwether Lewis and William Clark observed numerous villages abandoned by the Mandans and Hidatsas that had been destroyed by the Sioux and smallpox. When they returned through the Cascades in 1806, they stopped at a Chinook village where smallpox scars were evident; one old woman told them the disease had struck 28–30 years before, placing the appearance during the time of the sweeping pandemic.

A "winter count" by a Sioux recorder indicated that among the Sioux "many died of smallpox"; in all, thirteen different winter counts reflected the presence of smallpox. Eyewitness accounts indicated that the pandemic began in 1775 ended in 1782 at Hudson Bay and the Northern Plains. The disease, however, was far from conquered.

Inhabitants of the Pacific Northwest felt the scourge of smallpox dating from the period 1787–1795. In 1787, the explorer Nathaniel Portlock discovered a Tlingit village on the southeast coast of what is now Alaska so completely destroyed by smallpox only nine individuals remained.

In her study, from which the above data is drawn, Elizabeth Fenn suggested that smallpox traveled westward from the Shoshones, following trade routes to the sea. She also offers the possibility that Spanish explorers introduced smallpox to the natives. During the period 1775–1779, four vessels were known to have sailed north from San Blas, Mexico, and infected seamen could have unknowingly passed on the contagion. Russian sailors also frequented the northwestern coast during this period, and as smallpox had been epidemic on the Asian Kamchatka peninsula in 1768, possibly lingering into 1774, they might have been responsible for introducing the disease.[19]

The period following the Revolution further opened the territory of south-central Canada to Indian traders but these rough men presented an entirely different picture than the colonial settlers of Massachusetts. The riches to be gained from beaver, otter pelts and hides induced men to obtain them at any cost and during the period 1789–1793 their "irregularity" in pursuing such wealth along the Assinboine River induced the Indians to form "a resolution to extirpate the traders."

In the book *Voyages from Montreal on the River St. Laurence, Through the Continent of North America, to the Frozen and Pacific Oceans, in the Years 1789 and 1793*[20] the author writes that nothing but calamity could have saved the traders from destruction and this came in the form of smallpox, "which spread its destructive and desolating power as the fire consumes the dry grass of the field." As the disease destroyed families and entire tribes, the horrid scene "presented to those who had the melancholy and afflicting opportunity of beholding it, a combination of the dead, the dying, as such as, to avoid the fate of their friends around them, prepared to disappoint the plague of its prey, by terminating their own existence." To aggravate the calamity, the putrid carcasses were first mangled by starving dogs, then dragged from the huts and devoured by wolves. Further:

> Nor was it uncommon for the father of a family whom the infection had not reached, to call them around him, to represent the cruel sufferings, and horrid fate of their relations, from the influence of some evil spirit who was preparing to extirpate their race; and to incite them to baffle death, with all its horrors, by their own poniards. At the same time, if their hearts failed them in this necessary act, he was himself ready to perform the deed of mercy with his own hand, as the last act of his affection, and instantly to follow them to the common place of rest and refuge from human evil.[21]

Among the northeast Native American population, death from disease was staggeringly high. A conservative estimate placed it at 55 percent. In specific regions, catastrophic mortality rates reached from 84 percent to 95 percent of the population. Compounding the problem was the sporadic nature of epidemics; groups had little opportunity to recover before smallpox struck again. "This situation, in conjunction with war, slavery, and other cultural disruptions resulting from contact [with the white settlers] sent Indian populations into a precipitous decline."[22]

After an 18-year period of relative freedom from smallpox, the disease struck Mexico City in 1779. First appearing in August, by December it had afflicted 44,286 people. An estimated 60,000 persons underwent inoculation, likely saving many lives. But just as Europeans discovered that inoculation often turned individuals into carriers, this bitter lesson was destined to be relearned, as those undergoing the operation quickly spread it throughout the countryside. The explorer Alexander von Humboldt noted, "A great part of the Mexican youth was cut down that year." By early 1780, the disease had burned itself out, leaving behind an estimated 18,000 dead.

As traders, indigenous peoples and missionaries crisscrossed the land, smallpox traveled with them, reaching the frontier provinces of Texas and New Mexico in the fall and winter of 1780–81. Among the New Mexico mission Indians, the epidemic killed 5,025; adding non-mission populations would make the number significantly higher.[23] The Yavapais people of the Great Plains were decimated by the disease, likely losing the majority of young people born after 1781; such serious losses eventually forced them to alter their form of government into one less formal and structured.[24]

For the Native Americans as a whole, contact with whites not only led to massive population decreases, but also disrupted cultural systems. Following periods of high mortality were steep drops in fertility, preventing any meaningful recovery. Equally important was the loss of influential elders; routine tasks associated with food gathering, settlements and hygiene were lost or corrupted in the ensuing recovery periods.

In light of such drastic alterations, beliefs in spirituality also underwent changes. As the people confronted the dilemma of abandonment, anxiety about religious matters greatly affected them. Complicating matters was the presence of missionaries in their "campaign to Christianize America." Early efforts by Jesuit priests were directed toward shamans, whose duties were not only religious but also medical, they being expected to diagnose, treat and interpret the cause of illness.

In some cases, interference proved beneficial — at least from a medical standpoint. Among some northern Iroquoians and Algonquians, one traditional means of ridding the body of impurities was the sweat lodge. This required gathering people in a confined space, inadvertently facilitating the transmission of smallpox. Additionally, extensive perspiration led to dangerous dehydration. The use of medical herbs also contributed to the problem, as many were cathartics, emetics or diuretics.

Not unlike their European counterparts, Native Americans sought redress in rituals. When the shaman failed to discover the right combination to cure the suffering, blame was placed on individuals supposed to be "witches." Charged with provoking epidemics and other crimes, these victims were occasionally tortured or killed to ward off bad spirits. Occasionally, Jesuit priests fell into this category and suffered a like fate.[25]

Colonial Laws Enacted for Public Health

It was not uncommon for the early settlers to set aside days of humiliation and prayer, and even colonial governments made covenants with God for their safekeeping. Colonists were aware that immigrants (and, not inconsequentially, African slaves) carried disease to the new land. In order to stem the tide of epidemics, the first quarantine measures were adopted in 1647, when the Puritans attempted to isolate infected seamen arriving from Barbados. This plan was adopted by other coastal towns and given sanction by the Crown.

It was almost twenty years later that land quarantine regulations were added to those of maritime rules. The first instance of such an act was recorded in the town records of East Hampton, Long Island, on March 2, 1662. Under this statute, no Indian infected with smallpox was allowed into town under penalty of 5 shillings or "that they be whipped until they be free of the small poxe." The same penalty applied to any English or Indian servant who went to wigwams housing infected persons.[26]

Outbreaks of smallpox occurred in Boston in 1640, 1660, and from 1677 to 1680. A year into the latter epidemic the Salem selectmen passed their first quasi-official ordinance:

It is ordered that William Stacy who is sick of the small pox doeth not presume to Come aboard till three weeks after this date be expired and that he be very careful [that] when [the] time be expired he shift his Clothes and doe not frequent any Company till he be wholly cure of that infection.[27]

A combined maritime-land act of 1701–1702 empowered the selectmen of individual towns to protect their citizens by removing infected persons into what amounted to isolation houses, with nurses and necessities provided by the sick person. In the case of a child being ill, the parents were expected to cover costs, while a master was expected to pay for the care of his servants. An important aspect of an early statute involving charity care stated that if the individual suffering from smallpox was unable to pay for his treatment, "the town or place whereto they belonged" was to cover the charge.

In what today would be called "out of network coverage," if a townsman became sick away from his residence and his care fell upon those of another municipality, the selectmen of his town were to lay the charge for his care before justices of the peace, who were empowered to adjust and pay the accounts. For homeless persons without means to provide for themselves, their health care was to be paid out of the colonial treasury. Furthermore, justices were empowered to impress "convenient housing, lodging, nursing, [at]tendance, and other necessities" for the sick.[28]

Ten years after the epidemic of 1721 (see below), "An Act to Prevent Persons from Concealing the Small Pox" was enacted in the Massachusetts colony. In what would set the standard for other colonies, the head of the house was required to inform the selectmen of any person on his premises with smallpox. Additionally, a red flag was to be flown from a pole outside the residence, warning others of contagion within. This flag was to remain outside until the selectmen judged the premises cleansed and free from disease. In an indication of how seriously the matter was regarded, the penalty for ignoring the law was the staggering sum of £50, a fine that would have crippled most household incomes. Under this statute, selectmen issued a "prodigious" number of quarantine warrants, actively impressing houses and nurses to isolate and care for the sick.[29] Quarantine worked only if ingress and egress were controlled. In 1764–1765, the law was strengthened to authorize local authorities to appoint or impress guards to keep people from entering or leaving infected premises without a specific license issued by the selectmen.[30]

South Carolina enacted legislation similar to that of Massachusetts in 1738. Called "An Act for the Better Preventing of the Spreading of the Small Pox in Charleston," it required that when a person "in any house or plantation" discovered himself infected with smallpox, he was to report that fact to the master, who was then responsible for posting a warning at the nearest public road as well as on the nearest parish house or church. As in Boston, failure to do so would result in a fine of £50. Authorities could also impress men to stand guard around dwellings wherein smallpox was present.[31]

Without official sanction, New York adapted vague maritime laws into land quarantine or copied those established in East Hampton, Long Island. Official legislation did not occur until 1755, when authority was granted for land quarantine based on maritime laws.[32] In 1771, the Huntington, New York, authorities voted that "the Trustees should have full power to make any Prudential rules and orders in the Town Concerning the small pox and any other thing that shall seem to be needful."[33] As a landlocked state, Pennsylvania did not have any maritime laws upon which to base land quarantine and consequently that state did not have any statutes for quarantine until after the Revolutionary War.[34]

As a preventive, quarantine was seldom effective, as demonstrated by the well-chronicled spread of disease in England and Europe during the 1700s. Even when guards were placed outside dwellings and hefty fines levied against violators, it was impossible to isolate every sick person. Physicians, exposed by contact, went from house to house by common roads, providing the means by which airborne and physical transmission were possible. Ministers, apothecaries, tradesmen and well-wishers also aided the spread of smallpox. Clearly, a more substantial method of prevention was required. In the American colonies, just such a technique would be introduced by a very unlikely source.

4

Cotton Mather and Smallpox Inoculation in the American Colonies

> The town is become almost an Hell upon Earth, a City full of Lies, and Murders, and Blasphemies, as far as Witnesses and Speeches can render it so; Satan seems to take a strange Possession of it, in the epidemic Rage, against that notable and powerful and successful way of saving the Lives of People from the Dangers of the Small-Pox. What can I do on this Occasion, to get the miserable Town dispossessed of the evil Spirit which has taken such an horrible Possession of it? What besides Prayer and Fasting, for it?[1]

The scourge of smallpox was particularly well known to the colonists in Boston, Massachusetts. Before the disease struck with particular virulence in 1721, the citizens there had endured outbreaks in 1640, 1660, 1677–1680 and 1702. In the earliest days, people born across the Atlantic were immune, usually having suffered the disease as a child. Those born in the colonies, however, had no such protection and were easily susceptible. When smallpox became endemic and larger numbers acquired immunity, smallpox reverted to its more familiar threat as a killer of infants, children and individuals migrating into the city from outlying areas.

On April 22, 1721, the British ship HMS *Seahorse* arrived from Barbados. Within a day of passing through inspection, a crewman demonstrated the telltale symptoms of smallpox and was quarantined in a house near the harbor. A red flag was placed outside, warning, "God have mercy on this house." By early May, nine other crewmen exhibited symptoms. They, too, were quarantined, but by that time, smallpox had spread outside the protected zone, reaching into the city.[2] One of those destined to affect, and be affected by, the outbreak was a man named Cotton Mather.

Cotton Mather, a one-time medical student and Congregational clergyman, is known to Americans today as the religious fanatic primarily responsible for the Salem witch trials in the late 1600s. Nearly lost in history is the fact that his name should also be associated with the introduction of smallpox inoculation to America.

Born in Boston, Massachusetts, February 12, 1663, he was the eldest child of Increase Mather and Maria Cotton. A bright student, he entered Harvard at the age of 12, graduating in 1678. Assuming teaching duties that he carried out between 1678 and 1685, Mather began the study of theology, but due to a speech impediment, he abandoned the effort and studied medicine. Later conquering his disability, Mather finished his religious studies and was elected assistant pastor in his father's church, the North Church of Boston, in 1681. He was ordained in 1685, and three years later, when his father went to England as an agent for the colony, he was left in charge of the largest congregation in New England, a post he held the rest of his life.

When the Boston clergy were asked for advice in regard to the Salem witchcraft cases, Mather had already written *Memorable Providences Relating to Witchcraft and Possessions* (1689). He drafted their reply, upon which the prosecutions were based. Mather used his influence to bring the suspected individuals to trial, attended courtroom hearings, investigated the cases and wrote sermons on witchcraft.

Mather received a master of arts degree from Harvard University in 1681, a doctor of divinity degree from the University of Glasgow in 1710, and was made a Fellow of the Royal Society in 1713.[3] Extremely well educated, he had reached his 58th year when the massive epidemic of smallpox struck Boston in April 1721. At this period in England, Lady Mary Montagu was promoting inoculation for smallpox by having the operation tested on criminals, but it was far from an accepted preventive. Mather himself had gained some familiarity of the technique from one of his slaves in 1706: "I had from a servant of my own an account of its being practiced in Africa. Inquiring of my Negro-man, Onesimus, who is a pretty intelligent fellow, whether he had ever had the smallpox, he answered both yes and no. He told me that he had undergone the operation which had given something of the smallpox and would forever preserve him from it, adding that was often used in West Africa."[4]

Mather later deepened his knowledge by reading the observations of Dr. Emanuele Timoni (spelled "Emanuel Timonius" by Boylston), a graduate of Padua and Oxford and a Fellow of the Royal Society, London. Living in Constantinople, Timoni learned of the Turkish practice of inoculation; in 1713 and 1715, he wrote letters to Dr. Woodward of the Royal Society of London. Jacob Pylarini, a Venetian physician (described as the Venetian consul at Smyrna by Boylston, who spelled the name "Jacobus Pylarinus"; various other spellings of both Timoni and Pylarini appear throughout the 19th century), also communicated with the Royal Society and published a text in 1715, *A New and Safe Method of Exciting the Small-Pox by Transplantation,* that described inoculation similar to that of Timoni. The material was published in the *Philosophical Transactions.*[5] Timoni described the operation:

> They make choice of as Healthy a Young Person as they can find, that has the *Small Pox* of the best sort upon him, an the Twelfth or Thirteenth Day of his Discomfiture. With a needle they prick some of the larger *Pustules,* and press out the Matter coming from them into some convenient Vessel of Glass (or the like) to receive it, which ought first of all to be washed very clean with warm Water. A convenient quantity of this Matter being thus collected, it is to be stop'd close, and kept warm in the bosom of the Person that carries it (who ought rather to be some *other Person,* than what visited the Sick Chamber for it, lest the Infection of the *Small Pox* be convey'd in the *Garments,* as well as in the *Bottle,* and the intended Operation be hurt by the *Infection* being first conveyed another way, and so it should be conveyed as soon as may be to the Person that is waiting to be the Patient. The Patient being in a warm Chamber, is to have several small Wounds made with a Surgeon's Three edged Needle, or with a *Lancet,* in two or more Places of the Skin (the best Places are in the Muscles of the *Arm*) till some drops of Blood follow: And immediately let there be dropt out a drop of the Matter in the Glass, on each of the Places; and mix'd well with the Blood that is issuing out. The Wound should be covered with half a Walnut shell, or any such concave Vessel, and bound over that the matter may not be rub'd off by the Garments for a few Hours; And now let the Patient (having Fillets on the Wounds,) keep House, and keep warm, and be careful of his Diet; The Custom at *Constantinople* is to abstain from Flesh and

Broth for Twenty Days or more. They chuse to perform the Operation either in the beginning of *Winter* or *Spring*.[6]

The concept stimulated Mather's scientific interest and he familiarized himself with all matters concerning smallpox. Thomas Sydenham's treatise, "Methodus Curandi Febres" (1666), asserted that "noxious miasmas" arising from the earth into the air were responsible for epidemics. While this was hardly a new concept, being espoused by the ancient authority Rhazes (A.D. 865–925), the idea of poisoned air causing disease existed as medical canon well into the 19th century. Where Sydenham differed from Rhazes and the later Italian authority Girolamo Frascastoro (see chapter 27) came in the treatment of the disease. While the two former scientists advocated heat therapy to drive away infectious humors, the 17th century expert argued against it, believing that heat therapy with steam and blankets exacerbated the condition and led to further contagion.[7]

Mather, influenced by Sydenham, became a believer in the concept of poison air and added to the literature by penning "The Venomous Miasmas of the Small-Pox," asserting that the disease entered the body by way of inspiration. His primary concern, however, lay in the belief that inoculation was the way to save lives, and he began a quest to introduce a practice "never used ... in our Nation." The effort nearly proved to be his undoing.

In what would seem to be the antithesis of his own religious foundations, Cotton Mather composed a letter and mailed copies to individual Boston physicians, hoping to gain support for the new preventive of inoculation. In what may be considered one of the earliest and most significant writings on medical matters in North America, it read as follows:

No. 1 June 24, 1721
SIR,

YOU are many ways endeared unto me, but in nothing more than the very much good which a gracious god employs you and honours you to do to a miserable world.

I design it as a testimony of my respect and esteem, that I now lay before you the most that I know (and all that was ever published in the world) concerning a matter, which I have been an occasion of its being pretty much talked about. If, upon mature deliberation, you should think it advisable to be proceeded in, it may save many lives that we set a great value on. But if it be not approved of, still you have the pleasure of knowing exactly what is done in other places.

The Gentlemen, my two authors, are not yet informed, that among the [illegible] 'tis no rare thing for a whole company, of a dozen together, to go to a person sick of the small-pox, and prick his pustules, and inoculate the humour, even no more than the back of one hand, and go home, and be a little ill, and have a few [pocks], and be safe all the rest of their days. Of this I have in my neighbourhood a competent number of living witnesses.

But see, think, judge; do as the Lord our healer shall direct you; and pardon this freedom of,

> Sir,
> Your hearty friend and servant,
> Co. Mather

Dr. Boylstone[8]

Mather's reference to a matter "pretty much talked about" likely referred to the stiff resistance his ideas had received from the religious community (including his own parishioners), who believed smallpox was a punishment from God. Many felt that to experiment on the human body, particularly by such a new and unknown technique (and perhaps even to prevent disease), ran contrary to the wishes of their deity and was sure to bring further calamity.

Only one physician, Zabdiel Boylston (frequently spelled with an "e" at the end), responded. Boylston was the eldest son of Thomas Boylston, an Englishman who had obtained the degree of doctor of medicine at the University of Oxford. Thomas settled in Brookline, Massachusetts, in 1635; Zabdiel was born in 1680. After studying under his father's tutorage, Zabdiel began his own practice, in time earning a small fortune and the distinction of being a naturalist as well as a healer.

After conferring with Mather and reading the works of Timoni and Pylarini, Boylston became convinced the procedure had merit. On June 26, 1721, he wrote, "I inoculated my son, Thomas, of about six, my Negro-man, thirty-six, and Jackey, two and a half Years old." These treatments are considered the first inoculations in United States history. He performed the operation on others in July, and on August 12 of the same year he inoculated Mather's son, Samuel. During the epidemic, Boylston inoculated 248 persons, while 39 were credited to Drs. Raby and Thompson, in Roxbury and Cambridge. Out of that number, 6 died.[9]

"Fullfreighted with Nonsense..."

Among his peers, Dr. Boylston stood alone. Other Boston medical men, led by William Douglass (a Scottish physician and the only man in Boston with a doctor of medicine degree), Dr. Dalhonde, a French physician, and John Checkley, an apothecary who had a personal feud with Mather, formed the Society of Physicians Anti-Inoculators. This group considered inoculation as introducing of the plague and accused those who practiced it as being no better than murderers. Douglass, whom Mather had left off his list when soliciting assistance from the medical community, resented the slight, no less than a clergyman meddling in matters outside his realm of expertise.

The open antagonism between Mather and Douglass exacerbated reaction to Boylston's experiments, compelling him to publish a defense in the *Boston Gazette*. He argued the "new Practice" was recommended by "Gentlemen of Figure and Learning," and that after the operation, the patient need not fear disfiguring facial scars or a recurrence of smallpox, those facts being "fully cleared up" by the gentlemen referenced.

In what would seem to be a contradiction of principals, Mather, the extreme conservative, defended inoculation while Douglass and his group, the younger and far more liberal Boston constituents, questioned, perhaps with insincere conviction, whether their enemies trusted science more than the hand of God.

On July 21, His Majesty's justices of the peace and town physicians confronted Boylston and charged him with "the most dangerous Consequence" of spreading the smallpox infection. He was ordered to stop the practice, but with a show of contempt and the backing of the Puritan oligarchy, the doctor refused to follow their order and continued his work.

What followed next replayed events in Great Britain but on a much larger scale. When England, Wales and Scotland faced smallpox epidemics, editorials and political cartoons by anti-inoculators played out with humor and wit as well as uncertainty. In the small confines of Boston, however, fear-mongering assumed epic proportions, nearly paralyzing the inhabitants. A war of words ensued, with Douglass, writing under the pseudonym "W. Philanthropos," in the July 17–24 edition of the *Boston News-Letter,* calling Boylston ignorant and illiterate. Cotton Mather, his father, Increase Mather, and four clergymen known as the "Inoculation Ministers," defended Boylston, entreating Bostonians to "treat one another with decency and charity, meekness and humility."

For himself, Boylston published "A Faithful Abridgment of Two *Accounts* from the

Philosophical Translations" (the work of "Timonius" and "Pylarinus") in a booklet entitled "Some Account of What Is Said of Inoculation or Transplanting the Small Pox." In "Remarks" that followed, he substantiated his inoculation by beginning:

> Let it be considered, That these Communications come from Great Men, and Persons of Great Erudition and Reputation, and are addressed unto very Eminent Persons. Let it be also considered, that with the Approbation of the ROYAL SOCIETY (as Illustrious a Body as are in the World) their Secretary the celebrated Dr. *Halley,* has publish'd these things, as worthy to come into the notice of Mankind."

He described the story told by "Negroes" of how they learned the "Way," by which they "take the Juice of the *small pox,* and *Cut the Skin,* and put in a drop; then by'nd by a little *Sick,* then few *Small Pox;* and no body dye of it: no body have *Small Pox* any more."

In defending himself against those who considered the epidemic as punishment from God, or who questioned whether God would even wish his scourge cured, Boylston added, "Here is a Discovery, that is a great *Blessing to Mankind,* and should be thankfully receiv'd.... The Case in short we take to be this. 'Almighty GOD in His great Mercy to Mankind, has taught us a *Remedy,* to be used when the dangers of the *Small Pox* distresses us.'" He concluded by writing, "I Enquire, whether any sort of Practice the whole Art of Physick ever came to us with a stronger Recommendation than this of Inoculation or Transplantation."[10]

The infighting only got worse. On August 7, 1721, a new weekly publication called the *New England Courant* sided with Douglass, accusing the Inoculation Ministers of being "profoundly ignorant of the Matter," a play on words, as "matter" was also the medical term used to signify smallpox pus taken for inoculation. The editor followed with a sarcastic piece entitled "Project for Reducing the Eastern Indians by Inoculation," a "matter" that would lose its humor in 1763.

The *Courant* was written and published by James Franklin. Serving as his apprentice was his younger brother, Benjamin. It is not clear whether Benjamin Franklin wholeheartedly supported the attack against inoculation or merely followed his brother's dictates, but in later years he, like many other Revolutionaries, became an ardent supporter of the operation.

The Reverend Thomas Walter (Cotton Mather's nephew) used more inflammatory rhetoric to counter the print attacks. Writing under the non de plum "Your Friends and Well-Wishers to Our Country and All Good-Men," he called the *Courant* that "notorious, Scandalous Paper ... fullfreighted with Nonsense, Unmannerliness, Railery, Prophaneness, Immorality, Arrogancy, Calumnies, Lyes, Contradictions" and conspired to have James jailed for four weeks. In his absence, Benjamin continued to publish the paper by himself.

While learned men quarreled, smallpox continued to escalate. In August, 26 persons died; by September, the number climbed to 101; and in October, over 400 persons had perished. With the "War of Pamphlets" ever escalating, on November 14 a small bomb was hurled through the window of Mather's house, containing this note: "Cotton Mather, you dog, dam you! I'l [*sic*] inoculate you with this; with a pox to you." Mather's nephew was in the room, recuperating from his own inoculation. Fortunately, the fuse failed to ignite the incendiary and no one was hurt.

On August 4, 1721, Charles Maitland and Dr. Mead inoculated convicts from Newgate Prison. When word of the success of the operation and its subsequent acceptance in England crossed the Atlantic, some of the apprehension in Boston subsided. The smallpox plague eventually died out and life returned to normal. Years later, when another outbreak occurred,

William Douglass had the operation performed on himself; he remained unrepentant, however, over Mather and Boylston, whom he considered to have acted irresponsibly.[11]

Dr. Boylston visited England in 1725 or 1726, where he was attended with "every honourary distinction which he wished." He was chosen a member of the Royal Society and developed lasting friendships with many notable men of medicine, including Dr. Watts, with whom he frequently corresponded. In 1726, he published "An Historical Account of the Small-pox Inoculated in New England, Upon All Sorts of Persons, Whites, Blacks, and of all Ages and Constitutions: With Some Account of the Nature of the Infection in the Natural and Inoculated Way, and their Different Effects on Human Bodies: With Some Short Directions to the Unexperienced in this Method of Practice." The work was "Humbly Dedicated to Her Royal Highness the Princess of Wales." The princess had long been interested in inoculation and it was through her intervention with the King that Lady Mary Montagu was able to have the prisoners turned over to Maitland and Mead for the test in London.

Boylston returned to Boston and continued his practice, eventually retiring to the patrimonial estate at Brookline and dying June 2, 1766.[12] For his own part, although his reputation remained sullied in his own lifetime and well beyond by his association with devils and demons, Cotton Mather has been described as being "the first significant figure in American medicine."[13]

5

"This Distemper Is the King of Terrors": Smallpox and the American Revolution

This I suppose will find you, at Boston, growing well on the Small Pox. This Distemper is the King of Terrors to America this year. We shall suffer as much by it as We did last Year by the Scarcity of Powder. And therefore I could wish that the whole People was inoculated.[1]

The Founding Fathers had one thing in common they would rather not have shared: firsthand experience with smallpox. Franklin's exposure to the dread disease came during the 1721 epidemic in Boston where the young printing apprentice assisted his brother in publishing searing anti-inoculation articles. The younger Franklin eventually changed his mind about the usefulness of the preventive and became a strong and powerful advocate.

While it is likely Franklin lost friends to the disease in Boston, a much more tragic loss awaited him. The second of his two sons, Francis Folger, was born in 1732. "Franky" was the apple of his parents' eye and apparently a very clever child, for at the age of two years his father advertised for a tutor. Two years later, however, Franky contracted smallpox and died of the disease. On his tombstone, the family inscribed the touching sentiment, "The delight of all who knew him."

With proponents and adversaries of inoculation still waging a virtual war, accusations soon spread that the boy had died from the disease contracted by inoculation. Franklin was finally forced to explain the circumstances, replying that the child had never been inoculated at the onset of the epidemic because he was suffering from flux (diarrhea). He argued that Franky "reciev'd the distemper in the common way of infection," adding "inoculation was a safe and beneficial practice."[2]

In 1759, Franklin solicited his friend, William Heberden, a London physician, to write a text supporting inoculation. Heberden complied and the text was published under the title "Some Account of the Success of Inoculation for the Small-Pox in England and America, Together with Plain Instructions by Which Any Person May Be Enabled to Perform the Operation and Conduct the Patient Through the Distemper." Distributed without cost, Franklin's introduction read as follows:

A small Pamphlet wrote in plain language by some skillful Physician, and publish'd, directing what preparations of the body should be used before the inoculation of children, what precautions to avoid giving the injection at the same time in the common way, and how the operation is to be performed, the incision dress'd, the patient treated, and on the appearance of what symptoms a Physician is to be called, &c. might be encouraging parents to inoculate their own children, be a means of removing that objection of the expence, render the practice much more general, and thereby save the lives of thousands.

For his own part, Heberden offered the opinion that "it would be better to have inoculation performed by any body, or in any manner, than to suffer this disease to come on in the common way, though assisted with all the helps which art can afford." Some of the statistics included in the pamphlet included those below:

Mortality from Smallpox and Variolation, 1759

Had the Small-pox in the common way		Of these died		Received the distemper by Inoculation		Of these died	
Whites	Blacks	Whites	Blacks	Whites	Blacks	Whites	Blacks
5059	485	452	62	1974	139	23	7[3]

More substantially, Franklin helped found the Pennsylvania Hospital, ensuring free inoculations were made available to the poor.[4]

George Washington and Smallpox

By the mid–18th century, smallpox was a devastating endemic disease found everywhere in the world but Australia (where it would finally make an unwelcome appearance in 1789) and several small islands set off from major shipping routes.[5] On a smaller and more specific scale, the disease touched the life of one particular individual, the loss of whom would certainly have affected, if not ultimately changed, the outcome of the Revolutionary War.

In 1751, 19-year-old George Washington accompanied his brother Lawrence to Barbados. It was hoped the trip and change of scenery would improve Lawrence's cough, a typical "remedy" prescribed for those suffering from tuberculosis. The newly arrived Washingtons were invited to the house of Gedney Clarke, an influential merchant, planter and slave trader with ties to the family. On November 3, George wrote in his diary, "We went,— myself with some reluctance, as the smallpox was in his family." His reticence was soon justified, as he wrote on November 17, "Was strongly attacked with the smallpox." He was confined for nearly one month, being too ill to write in his diary, as his next notation did not appear until December 12.[6]

The fact that George Washington survived made him immune from future epidemics but gave him a healthy respect for the disease and the devastation wrought by its insidious power. The lessons learned would affect his personal and professional life, carrying over to his days as commander of the Continental Army when he would be a major proponent of inoculation.

In that opinion he had good company. During yet another smallpox epidemic in Boston, John Adams underwent variolation in the winter of 1764 under the direction of Drs. Nathaniel Perkins and Joseph Warren. Two years later, in 1766, the 23-year-old Thomas Jefferson underwent inoculation in Philadelphia.

Smallpox was a common killer in coastal cities such as Boston, Philadelphia and Charleston, as they received an influx of seamen and passengers from the continent. As early as the 1660s, incoming vessels were quarantined until crews were inspected for smallpox.

Boston established quarantine stations in 1717, and New York City followed by 1755. A 1738 law in Charleston dictated that victims of smallpox be isolated at home. Interestingly, legislation for the public good was accepted without large-scale protest over the loss of personal freedom. Such acceptance did not carry over to inoculators, who, as private citizens, were looked upon with suspicion.[7]

Smallpox was less prevalent in more inland areas such as Virginia, which experienced no epidemics prior to 1747. The threat remained ever present, however. But when the technique of variolation was introduced in Norfolk County in 1768, it elicited riots in protest. Riots continued the following year when Dr. Archibald Campbell's house was burned as a result of the technique's being performed there. Thomas Jefferson, then a practicing lawyer, became involved in defending the victims.[8]

Despite suspicions about inoculation, George Washington's second cousin, John Smith, began a smallpox inoculation hospital in 1767 and continued practicing the operation until his death in 1771. (Further north, James Latham became the first Canadian to practice arm-to-arm transfer when he inoculated soldiers of his regiment in Quebec City.)[9] Washington's stepson, John Parke Custis, was inoculated at Baltimore in 1771, and Martha Washington received the inoculation in 1776. Washington's brothers, John Augustine and Samuel, had their families inoculated in 1777, and slaves at Mount Vernon were also protected by the procedure.

The Washingtons' support for smallpox protection ran contrary to the rest of the colony for in 1769 a Virginia statute prohibiting inoculation unless specifically approved by the county courts was made into law. Residents feared the procedure would introduce the disease into their cities and counties, while others fought the medical advancement by citing the religious tenet that if the Lord chose to inflict mankind with epidemics, it was the duty of the faithful to accept without question or fight.

The attempt to prohibit inoculation became a national issue immediately before and during the Revolutionary War. In the summer of 1775, shortly after assuming command of the army at Cambridge, Massachusetts, General Washington wrote to the president of the Continental Congress that he was "particularly attentive to the least Symptoms of the Small Pox," promising he would "continue the utmost Vigilance against this most dangerous disease." Aside from quarantine in a hospital created for that purpose, there was little he could do,[10] as the idea of mass inoculation at the time was unpopular and impossible to implement. That subject and the disease itself would become major issues during the war.

In the fall of 1775, Continental soldiers were moved northward toward Quebec with the object of taking the city out of British hands. By early December, smallpox had begun to infect the soldiers, a situation exacerbated by freezing temperatures and an inability to quarantine infected persons. The debilitated soldiers made an attack on December 31. The attack was complicated by a devastating blizzard, and the Americans were repulsed and forced to spend the winter in ill-supplied, disease-ridden camps.

When the British troops were reinforced on May 6, 1776, nearly 900 out of 1,900 Continental soldiers were sick, many suffering from smallpox, including Major General John Thomas. Facing disparate numbers of British soldiers after their five-month siege, the American army took 1,500 men and retreated up the St. Lawrence River, abandoning those unable to keep pace.

On May 11, the army reached Sorel, 50 miles northeast of Montreal. Reinforcements arrived, but with all semblance of quarantine lost, the fresh troops were quickly infected. General Thomas died of the disease on June 1. By June 11, General Philip Schuyler wrote to General Washington, warning that further reinforcements would "rather weaken than strengthen our Army, unless they had already had smallpox."

The Northern Army of the Continental forces further retreated along the Richelieu River, stopping at Isle aux Noir, near the north entrance of Lake Champlain, where smallpox was so virulent lice and maggots crawled over sufferers and mass graves were filled with 30–40 victims per day. Fearing disease more than the enemy, General John Sullivan ordered a further move, eventually stopping at Ticonderoga, New York.[11]

In a letter to his wife, John Adams wrote of these survivors:

> Our Army at Crown Point is an Object of Wretchedness, enough to fill a humane Mind, with Horror. Disgraced, defeated, discontented, dispirited, naked, undisciplined, eaten up with Vermin — no Cloaths, Beds, Blankets, no Medicines, no Victuals, but Salt Pork and flour.... I hope that Measures will be taken to cleanse the Army at Crown Point from the small-pox, and that other Measures will be taken in New England, by tolerating and encouraging Inoculation, to render that Distemper less terrible.[12]

The disease was not fully eradicated until September, after taking the lives of approximately 1,000 soldiers.

Disease continued to play an ominous role in the rebellion as outbreaks of smallpox appeared in and around Boston in 1774. After the Battles of Lexington and Concord on April 19, 1775, the Americans laid siege to the city, confining the British soldiers with the local population. Over the course of eleven months, the disease raged, primarily infecting the Americans, who had little resistance. Foreign soldiers were better adapted to survive as most came from overcrowded European cities where they contracted smallpox in childhood, thus giving them immunity.

Rumors were rampant that the British planned on sending persons exposed to smallpox through the lines in the hope of infecting and thus disabling the Americans. It had long been suspected (and perhaps known as fact) that such a tactic had succeeded after the French and Indian War by no less a renowned and respected general than Jeffrey Amherst. Many argued that to introduce disease among the Indians was one thing, but to purposely condemn members of their own European race to a horrible, agonizing death was quite another.

The question seemed to have been put to rest on December 3, 1775, as four British deserters escaped the city and reported to General Washington's headquarters, where they stated that General Howe, the British commander, had deliberately infected some people, leaving Boston "with a design to spread the Small-Pox among the Troops."[13]

The idea of inoculating the entire Continental Army presented a daunting problem, not the least of which was the fear evinced by Washington's own soldiers, many of whom would have deserted before submitting to the mandatory injection of pustule matter into their bodies. Instead of challenge prevailing resistance, Washington ordered strict quarantine of anyone showing signs of the disease and forbad those fleeing the city entrance into camp as the only means in his power of preventing widespread contamination. In the short term this tactic worked, for on March 17, 1776, the British withdrew from Boston. Washington then sent a force of 1,000 smallpox-immune troops to occupy the city.

With Boston freed, people returned in large numbers, turning the city into "a hospital with the small-pox." When the epidemic peaked in July, the town selectmen set aside the prohibition against inoculation and established a 12-day window in which people could receive protection. They also enacted strict quarantine, which ultimately proved effective, as the disease burned itself out by mid–September.[14]

Many Africans enslaved by the colonists felt British success in the war better served their chances for freedom and black men joined their ranks by the thousands, often with tragic results. In January 1776, smallpox appeared in Virginia, hitting the black recruits of Lord Dunmore's army at Tucker's Point with particular virulence. Lacking previous exposure and thus immunity afforded European-born soldiers, they died by the hundreds.

After a massive inoculation effort, Dunmore moved his base of operations to Gwynn Island in late May, leaving behind the graves of 300 people. Matters did not improve with a change of scenery, Dunmore reporting, "There was not a ship in the fleet that did not throw one, two or three or more dead overboard every night." Diseased bodies floated to shore, often amounting to a dozen per day.

Notwithstanding, Africans continued to apply for service with the British at the rate of six to eight a day; most soon became infected by smallpox and joined others, literally rotting alive. Shallow graves soon dotted the island. Compounding the atrocity, a report from Gloucester published June 15 stated, "His Lordship, before the departure of the fleet from Norfolk harbour, had two of those wretches inoculated and sent ashore, in order to spread the infection, but it was happily prevented."[15]

When the British were driven from the island in early July 1776, the fleet commander reported the "distress and confusion" of the hasty retreat beyond his powers to describe.[16] When the Virginia militia retook the island later in July, they encountered bodies in a state of putrefaction strewn about a two-mile wide area, "without a shovelful of earth upon them." Fear of contagion prompted the rebels to set fire to the hospital huts, burning to death those still inside. The death toll on the island was placed at "near 500 souls."[17]

Public opinion was not the only problem Washington faced when deciding on widespread inoculation of the army. Variolation actually caused the onset of the disease. Although it was hoped the resulting infection would be mild, it incapacitated the soldier for weeks, making him unavailable for active service. In May 1776, sensitive to the fact that spring campaigning was about to begin in earnest, Washington issued the command that no inoculations were to take place. Violators were to be severely punished.

Confirming the oft-expressed sentiment that the Continental Army had more to fear from smallpox than from the sword of the enemy, soldiers continued to die from the disease. Heavy losses in the Jersey campaign and low morale forced the commander to revisit his orders concerning inoculation. As the army went into winter quarters, Washington decided to begin a massive inoculation program for all units joining the ranks.

On April 23, 1777, the Continental Congress resolved "that Dr. James Tilton be authorized to repair to Dumfries in Virginia, there to take charge of all Continental soldiers that are or shall be inoculated, and that he be furnished with the necessary medicines." It was further ordered that inoculation centers be established at Colchester and Alexandria for the inoculation of troops from the Carolinas. Unfortunately, this ran counter to the law of Virginia, where inoculation had been illegal since 1769.

Washington, who was aware of the law, wrote to his brother: "Surely that impolitic Act, restraining Inoculation in Virginia, can never be continued. If I was a Member of that Assembly, I would rather move for a Law to compel the Masters of Families to inoculate every Child born within a certain limitted time under severe Penalties."[18]

To escape Virginia law, some colonial officers moved their inoculation centers to Frederick, Maryland, thus placing the military outside the state's jurisdiction. In Virginia, justices were of a mixed mind as to how and when to enforce the law. As originally written, authorities were given leeway to make exceptions upon specific requests by locals. In 1777, Benjamin Harrison desired to have his family inoculated at his home, Glanville, situated near Marshall.

He was forced to apply to the Fauquier Court for permission. This was granted, at the same time widening the scope of permission to other families "if they think proper."

Due to overwhelming protest by citizens in the county who not unreasonably feared inoculations would produce an epidemic, on April 29 the justices rescinded the order: "For reasons appearing to the Court, it is ordered that no person be Inoculated for the smallpox in this County for the Future." Protests in favor finally compelled the court in May to grant leave "to any of the Inhabitants ... to inoculate their Families with the smallpox, where any of them shall have the disorder in the natural way." In other words, if one member of the family contracted the disease by exposure, others in the familial circle could use matter obtained from that person to inoculate their immediate kin. (Considering the belief that human-to-human transfer was believed to pass on heredity diseases or other contaminations, this stipulation was not as unreasonable as it sounds.) The Virginia law was repealed in October 1777, with the stipulation that those wishing to be "immunized" first had to have the consent of a majority of the inhabitants within a two-mile radius."[19]

During 1779, as the war progressed through the South, civilians became victims of disease, occasionally spread by the influx of recruits. German "Waldeckers" coming to fight for the British, contracted smallpox in Jamaica and infected those on Pensacola Bay. By mid–October, the Indian village of Little Tallassee had been reduced by smallpox, while the cities of Charleston and Savannah were plagued with it for two years.

Promised freedom by the king's officers if they took up arms against those in rebellion, African men continued to join the British ranks. They soon fell victim to smallpox, however, becoming a burden to their erstwhile benefactors. By the summer of 1781, with the tides of war turning against him and 700 infected black men who had come downriver on his hands, one English general envisioned a way to rid himself of the problem while aiding the war effort. Hoping an epidemic would weaken those in resistance, he coldly wrote, "I shall distribute them about the Rebell Plantations." This, or a subsequent plan, was put in place as an American warned, "The British have sent from Yorktown a large number of negroes, sick with the small pox, probably for the purpose of communicating the infection to our army." If victory at the cost of betraying their sacred word to the blacks in an act of barbarism was the aim, it did not succeed, for the war soon concluded with the British surrender on October 19, 1781.[20]

The end could not have come too soon for Andrew Jackson, a youth of 14, who, with his brother Robert, joined the Continental Army. Andrew served as a courier and his brother participated in the Battle of Hanging Rock, South Carolina. Later betrayed by Tory neighbors, the boys were taken prisoner and placed in the Camden city jail beside nearly 200 other sick and starving patriots. Smallpox broke out and both Jacksons contracted the disease.

Their mother, Elizabeth Jackson, arranged for their release by having them exchanged for British soldiers, but Robert died two days later. Andrew survived, only to become an orphan a short time later when his mother died of cholera attempting to rescue her two nephews being held aboard a pestiferous prison ship in Charleston harbor.[21]

The Significance of Inoculation

By the turn of the 18th century and into the 19th century, smallpox had become endemic across the Old World and the New World, with epidemics occurring in most populated cities. As a general rule, epidemics were generational. The reason for this was twofold. First, between the intervening twenty or thirty years, fresh exposure to smallpox could not cause massive sickness because most of the population had already developed immunity, either by contracting the disease or by being inoculated. There were sure to be isolated cases but no large loss of life. Second, the passing decades provided enough time for young people surviving the last epidemic to mature, marry and bear children. If there were no mass inoculations during periods of relative health (people typically ignored preventives when not directly confronted with disease), new exposure to the virus from any event as seemingly innocuous as contaminated laundry to the appearance of an infected stranger had the potential to strike the exposed, beginning the cycle all over again.

It is fair to say that inoculation spared many thousands of lives and was far safer than contracting the disease in the normal way. The mortality rate after variolation was 0.5–2 percent, compared with 20–30 percent after natural smallpox, while the technique generally produced a less severe rash.[22] When inoculation of entire towns was begun during an epidemic, the cycle of contamination from victim to healthy person was prevented, thus abating and ultimately breaking the transmission of disease. During the 1700s, world populations grew to an extent impossible without inoculation.

That the technique of inoculation resulted in the death in a small percentage of cases was also true. This occurred on three levels. First, the operation *caused* smallpox, rarely, but significantly, killing or severely maiming the patient. Second, people inoculated with smallpox became carriers of the disease and were capable of infecting others. (Because of this, inoculators often chose out-of-the-way locations in which to establish their clinics.) Recently inoculated persons were believed to have caused epidemics in Weimer (1788), Hamburg (1794) and Berlin (1795). Third, inoculation provided false security. In an era when it was difficult to prove that immunity by inoculation had been successful ("taken"), individuals believing themselves immune from smallpox tended to discount the danger of exposure. By interacting with the afflicted, those improperly engrafted were likely to be stricken. Together, these serious problems led to vitriolic and occasionally violent uprisings against the introduction of any virus into the human system, critically delaying widespread prophylactic measures.

Inoculation had been the first stage in defeating smallpox, but its day had come and gone. This recognized, if controversial, preventive since the proverbial "dawn of time" was about to be replaced by a far safer and more effective method and by 1840 inoculation was outlawed in Great Britain.

By the very end of the 1700s, a small corner of the globe had already seen the beginning of what was to become one of the most significant discoveries known to humankind: vaccination. It would not only change how medical science looked at, prevented and cured disease, it would ultimately alter the landscape of death.

6

The Father of Immunology

Don't think, try; be patient, be accurate. — Dr. John Hunter to Edward Jenner, 1798[1]

In the June 29–July 2, 1798, issue of the *London Evening Mail* a seemingly innocuous advertisement appeared:

This day is published, with plates coloured from Nature, price 7s. 6d. in boards,

AN INQUIRY into the CAUSES and EFFECTS of the VARIOLAE VACCINAE, a Disease discovered in some of the Western Counties of England, particularly Gloucestershire, and known by the name of the Cow-Pox; with Observations on the origin of the Small-pox, and on the subject of Inoculation.

By EDWARD JENNER, M.D. F.R.S., &c.

Printed and sold by Sampson Low, No. 7, Berwick-street, Soho; Law, Ave-Maria Lane; and Murray and Highley, Fleet-street.

This discovery was destined to change the world.

Edward Anthony Jenner (May 17, 1749–January 26, 1823) was the eighth of nine children born to Sarah and Stephen Jenner in Berkeley, Gloucestershire, England. Edward's father was the vicar of Berkeley (Church of England). Orphaned at the age of five, Edward was raised by his older sister Mary, who married G.C. Black, the incoming vicar. Edward was educated at the school in Wotton-under-Edge and Cirencester. At the age of thirteen, he was apprenticed to Daniel Ludlow, a surgeon of Chipping Sodbury, South Gloucestershire. During this time, Jenner was inoculated against smallpox. After eight years of training, he went to London, studying under John Hunter (1728–1798), a prominent Scottish anatomist and surgeon at St. George's Hospital. The two became lifelong friends.

Jenner returned home to Berkeley in 1772 and set up a medical practice, becoming involved in two medical societies, one held at the Fleece Inn at Rodborough, originating in 1770, and the second meeting at the Ship Inn at Alveston, dating from 1780. His early research included the purification of tartar emetic, a moderately poisonous chemical used in the treatment of parasites and the study of heart disease. From autopsies of patients who had complained of chest pain, he correlated fatty deposits around the large arteries with angina (pain or pressure in the chest caused by inadequate blood flow and oxygenation to the heart muscle).[2] He also connected narrowing of the mitral valve opening (stenosis) to what is now known as rheumatic heart disease.[3]

Jenner married Catherine Kingscote in 1788, when he was 39 and she 27 years of age. They had three children: Edward (1789), who died of tuberculosis in 1810; Catherine (1794); and Robert Fitzhardinge (1797), who died unmarried.[4]

As a country physician, Jenner was well aware of a disease known as "cowpox" (typically hyphenated in the 18th and 19th centuries and also known as "kine pox"), described in the *Lexicon Medicum; or Medical Dictionary*[5] from 1842 as follows:

Variola Vaccina. *Vaccinia.* The cow-pox. Any pustulous disease affecting the cow may be called cow-pox, whether it arises from an over-distention of the udder, in consequence of a neglect in milking the cow, or from the sting of an insect, or any other case.

The genuine cow-pox appears on the teats of the cow, in the form of vesicles, of a blue colour approaching to livid. These vesicles are elevated at the margin and depressed at the centre. They are surrounded by inflammation. The fluid they contain is limpid. The animals are indisposed; and the secretion of milk is lessened. Solutions of the sulphates of zinc and copper are a speedy remedy for these pustules; otherwise they degenerate into ulcers, which are extremely troublesome. ... The obstinacy attending these cases is owing to the friction of the pustules, in consequence of milking.

The origin of cowpox was supposed to be a transfer of horse "grease," or the material found in horses' hooves, through dirt or the hands of farriers, to the hooves or bodies of cows. In *An Inquiry into the Causes and Effects of the Variolae Vaccinae,* Jenner wrote this:

There is a disease to which the Horse, from his state of domestication, is frequently subject. The Farriers have termed it *the Grease.* It is an inflammation and swelling in the heel, from which issues matter possessing properties of a very peculiar kind, which seems capable of generating a disease in the Human Body (after it has undergone the modification which I shall presently speak of), which bears so strong a resemblance to the Small Pox, that I think it highly probable it may be the source of that disease.

The *Lexicon* supported Jenner's theory, stating that disease "which originates from the grease in the horse's heel, is called the *genuine cow-pox;* all other kinds are *spurious.*"

"Grease" was actually an inflammation of the fetlocks caused by the bacterium *Dermatophilus congolensis* that produced lesions on the horse.

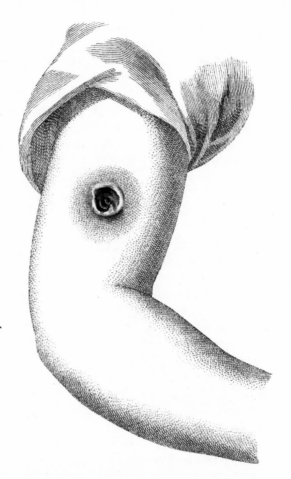

This illustration from Jenner's *An Inquiry into the Causes and Effects of Variolae Vaccinae,* p. 37A, represents the pustule taken from John Baker, a 5-year-old child. He was inoculated March 16, 1798, with matter taken from the hand of Thomas Virgoe, a servant who had been infected from a mare's heels. Jenner noted there was some variation in the appearance of this pustule: "Although it somewhat resembled a Small-pox pustule, yet its similitude was not so conspicuous as when excited by matter from the nipple of the cow, or when the matter has passed from thence through the medium of the human subject." The experiment was made to ascertain the progress and subsequent effects of the disease when thus propagated. He added, "We have seen that the virus from the horse, when it proves infectious to the human subject is not to be relied upon as rendering the system secure from variolous infection, but that the matter produced by it upon the nipple of the cow is perfectly so."

During the 19th century, a poxvirus ("horsepox") was an occasional cause of this syndrome. In 1801, it was demonstrated that lesions from "grease," taken from the hands of a man who had been treating horses, produced typical vaccine lesions in children and lesions like cowpox on the teats of inoculated cows. Children treated with grease material resisted variolation, meaning they had developed some immunity to smallpox.[6] By 1842, medical research indicated that protection obtained by farriers was imperfect. It was speculated that the virus underwent "modification" during passage through the cow, creating "a more abundant source of this inestimable fluid, than its original element the horse."[7]

Modern research indicates that both cowpox and some cases of horsepox were contracted by infected rodents, "or, as Jenner suggested, may have been transferred accidentally from horses to cows or vice versa, by man." In 1781, D. Baxby suggested that horsepox was a disease distinct from that contracted by cross infection. Horsepox became extinct about the end of the 19th century. Baxby believed vaccinia virus caused horsepox.[8]

In the late 1700s, it was an established fact that symptoms similar to those described above appeared on the hands of dairymaids or milkers, attended with febrile symptoms and sometimes tumors in the axilla. Other parts of the hand, where the cuticle was abraded, were also liable to the same affliction. This disease was termed "cowpox" (typically hyphenated as "cow-pox") felt to be a close relation to smallpox but presenting a much milder and seldom fatal form. Farmers commonly believed that those affected with cowpox were subsequently immune from contracting smallpox and many families purposely exposed themselves to the disease as a means of preventing the more virulent disease.

Prior to Dr. Jenner's work, there were a number of documented accounts relating to the successful transfer of immunity by cowpox, including the work of Mr. Fewster in 1765; Mr. Bose in 1769; Mr. Nash, a medical practitioner, in 1781; Mr. Jensen and Peter Platt of

[13]

CASE IV.

MARY BARGE, of Woodford, in this parish, was inoculated with variolous matter in the year 1791. An efflorescence of a palish red colour soon appeared about the parts where the matter was inserted, and spread itself rather extensively, but died away in a few days without producing any variolous symptoms *. She has since been repeatedly employed as a nurse to Small-pox patients, without experiencing any ill consequences. This woman had the Cow Pox when she lived in the service of a Farmer in this parish thirty-one years before.

* It is remarkable that variolous matter, when the system is disposed to reject it, should excite inflammation on the part to which it is applied more speedily than when it produces the Small Pox. Indeed it becomes almost a criterion by which we can determine whether the infection will be received or not. It seems as if a change, which endures through life, had been produced in the action, or disposition to action, in the vessels of the skin; and it is remarkable too, that whether this change has been effected by the Small Pox, or the Cow Pox, that the disposition to sudden cuticular inflammation is the same on the application of variolous matter.

CASE

This copy from Jenner's text, *An Inquiry into the Causes and Effects of Variolae Vaccinae*, p. 13, represents Case IV, a study of Mary Barge, of Woodford, who was inoculated with variolous matter in 1791.

Holstein, who vaccinated three children with cowpox in 1791. In 1784, when smallpox broke out in Schonwade, these children were the only ones spared from the disease.[9]

Benjamin Jesty was a farmer who lived at Yetminster and later moved to Downshay. In 1774, he made the observation that two milkmaids, Ann Notley and Mary Read, were immune from smallpox after having previously suffered from cowpox. Wishing to test the theory, he took his wife and two small sons to a neighboring farm, where he inoculated them using matter from infected cows. His method consisted of using his wife's knitting needle to hold the matter as he injected it in their arms. All survived, although Mrs. Jesty's arm became much inflamed. They family subsequently proved immune to smallpox. The Jennerian Society honored Mr. Jesty in 1805.[10] At the time, however, these cases remained anecdotal and achieved no widespread acknowledgment by the medical community.

Jenner studied the incidence of smallpox around the countryside, taking particular note of those individuals who had previously contracted cowpox. His observations convinced him local superstition held validity: cowpox did, in fact, prevent smallpox. If that was true, inoculation of cowpox matter would prove of far greater benefit than inoculation with smallpox, as the person receiving immunity would not be a carrier of smallpox and thus pose no risk to the uninoculated. His task, then, required that he substantiate theory with fact.

In May 1796, a dairymaid named Sarah Nelmes presented with a rash on her hand that Dr. Jenner diagnosed as cowpox. She confirmed this by stating that one of her animals, a Gloucester cow named Blossom, had recently contracted cowpox. On May 14, 1796, Jenner took a bold step by inoculating a boy of eight years named James Phipps, son of his gardener. After making several scratches on the lad's arm, he effected an arm-to-hand transfer of matter from one of Sarah's pocks. James became mildly ill with cowpox but recovered within the week. Later exposure to smallpox proved his immunity.[11]

Progression of Vaccination on the Skin

After the insertion of cowpox under the skin, a papule (a small bump or pimple) appeared on the third day. Within 2–3 days, it became vesicular (developed small blisters) later called the "Jennerian vesicle." The vesicle soon became pustular (caused by the introduced viral infection) and the surrounding area became erythematous (redness of the skin, a "rash") to a much greater degree than was found in the skin lesions of true smallpox. The rash reached a maximum between 8 and 12 days (typically between the 9th and 10th days), concurrent with draining, enlarged and sore lymph nodes and mild fever. If inspection of the "Jenner-

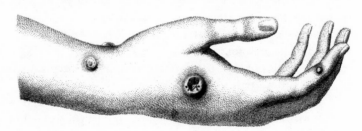

This illustration from Jenner's text, *An Inquiry into the Causes and Effects of Variolae Vaccinae*, p. 32A, represents the pustules on the hand of Sarah Nelmes, a dairymaid, who was infected from cows in May 1796. Jenner noted the pustule was expressive of the true character of the "Cow Pox" as it commonly appeared upon the hand. The two small pustules on the wrist also arose from application of the virus, while the pustule on the forefinger indicated the disease was in an early stage.

ian pustule" on the 7th day revealed a "major reaction" (became large and inflamed) the procedure was considered a success. The pustule dried from the center outward, becoming a brown or black scab that fell off in about three weeks.[12]

"The Vaccine Clerk to the World"

The 1798 publication of Edward Jenner's *An Inquiry into the Causes and Effects of the Variolae Vaccinae* struck an immediate nerve. The public responded to the vaccine (the word "vaccine" was taken from the Latin *vacca,* for cow) with enthusiasm, partly from the fact that Jenner refused to patent his discovery, fearing doing so would raise the cost beyond the reach of the poorer classes. Medical societies and colleges took a more guarded approach. The author provided additional evidence in his 1799 pamphlet, *Further Observations on the Variolae Vaccinae, or Cow-Pox,* but independent research was needed. It was not long in coming. On August 1, 1799, George Pearson, M.D.F.R.S., published *A Statement of the Progress in the Vaccine Inoculation; and Experiments to Determine Some Important Facts Belonging to the Vaccine Disease*, in the *Philosophical Magazine* (London). This particular article followed up on previous writings, stating that "through the recommendation of the *Surgeon-general, Thomas Keate, Esq.*, the new practice has been introduced into the army; of which a valuable report has been already communicated." He also noted that he had been granted permission to practice the *new inoculation* in certain situations where great numbers would have been inoculated by the old method. Cases from these sources and from private practice "form a valuable body of Evidence, by means of which the professional public will be enabled (I do not say precisely) the value of the *new practice.*"

Receiving matter from two principal milk farms near London where the *vaccine* disease had broken out six months previously, Pearson introduced the vaccine to London, where "at the fewest, 2000 persons" passed through the cowpox inoculation. From this wide sample, he concluded the following:

1. On the high end, one in 200 inoculated persons died from the disease, primarily because the practice is often trusted in the hands of persons not sufficiently acquainted with the treatment fit for different states of the human constitution.
2. The constitutional fever which occurs in the cow-pox is more considerable than Dr. Jenner's account, although was extremely slight.
3. The eruptions which did occur, in many instances, could not be distinguished from small-pox, but they were seen much less frequently this summer than in the spring and winter preceding.
4. The inoculated arms manifested a much more extensive spreading of the red areola around the inoculated part, but no danger seemed to attend such a state.
5. There were contradicting reports of people contracting small-pox after inoculation.

The facts were summed up with the statement, "I think we may safely conclude, that the cow-pox inoculation is attended with advantages sufficient to force its way speedily into general practice, and that of course it will supercede and ultimately extinguish the small-pox." Pearson ended his paper by stating that the following facts were established:

1. A constitution which has undergone the small-pox, is unsusceptible of again undergoing this disease.

2. A constitution which has not undergone the small-pox, but which has undergone the cow-pox, is unsusceptible of undergoing the small-pox.
3. A constitution which has not undergone the cow-pox, but which has undergone the small-pox, is unsusceptible of undergoing the cow-pox.[13]

The difference between variolation (the engrafting of variola virus) and vaccination was the substitution of cowpox, an entirely different strain of *Orthopoxvirus*. Cowpox vaccination produced a local lesion at the site of entry, but, except in extremely rare instances, it did not infect the unvaccinated. Nor was it capable of transforming into natural smallpox.[14]

Jenner's research also showed that the cowpox vaccine, "in passing from one human subject to another (arm-to-arm transfer) ... lost none of its protective properties." Success quickly led to the realization that vaccinating thousands of people might be impractical, as many physicians dwelling in major cities did not have access to fresh cowpox vaccine.[15] Jenner spent much of the rest of his life supplying cowpox matter to doctors around the world, at one time joking that he had become "the Vaccine Clerk to the World."[16]

As with variolation, a second and potentially far more dangerous situation arose when others, either less careful or less skilled, began harvesting and dispensing cowpox vaccine. Additionally, people working in smallpox hospitals or those administering variolation often tainted cowpox matter used in vaccination, leading to claims that the new vaccine was no safer or was possibly ineffective or both.

Complications from Cowpox Vaccination

1. Abnormal skin eruptions, not serious;
2. *Eczema vaccinatum* (itchy, red rash that weeped or oozed serum) that were occasionally severe;
3. Progressive vaccinia that occurred in persons with compromised immune systems that rarely had fatal results;
4. Accidental infection as noted above. This either came from improper procurement where the matter was contaminated with bacteria, contamination in storage or improper technique in the administration. This was the most common type of complication and while symptoms appeared frightening, they were usually not serious.[17]

These complications would later be used by legions of anti-vaccinationists well into the 20th century.

Four other, more insidious, influences also delayed the immediate widespread application of the vaccine. As Lady Mary Montagu had prophesied eighty years earlier, there were many doctors who did not wish to lose a substantial portion of their income by the eradication of smallpox. Then, too, the recognized medical authorities looked askance at the momentous discovery of a country doctor, finding it distasteful that a mere unknown without standing in their community should have provided the world with a preventive long sought but never substantiated by one of their own.

The very nature of the vaccine, derived from cows, also proved unnerving to many, and political cartoons filled the papers. James Gillray was one such artist who depicted engravings of people growing cow's heads from their bodies. Robert Hooper, M.D., F.L.S., author of the *Lexicon Medicum* (1842), perhaps best summed up the counter argument: "That the vaccine fluid, fraught with such unspeakable benefits to mankind, derives its origin from this humble source, however it may mortify human pride, or medical vanity, is confirmed by the observations and experiments of competent judges." Hooper further added, "This theory, that the preservative against variolous contagion is perfect when it issues from the fountainhead, and comes immediately from the hands of Nature, is consonant with reason, and consistent with analogy. Thus, one obstacle more to the universal adoption of the practice is removed."

In that, Dr. Hooper erred, as men of the day denounced the vaccine on religious grounds, stating they would not be treated "with substances originating from God's lowlier creatures."[18] Notwithstanding these loud and vigorous denunciations, Edward Jenner's discovery would not be denied the world.

"This inestimable discovery"

The wreath of conquest, and the voice of fame,
Have crown'd the warrior, and proclaim'd his name.
Say what fair leaf shall bind the brow of those,
Whose gen'rous labours lessen human woes:—
Who wield no sword,—who wake no orphan's tears,
—But snatch our infants from untimely biers![1]

Dr. Jenner continued his trials of inoculation at Berkley with good success, publishing *A Continuation of Facts and Observations Relative to the Variolae Vaccinae* in 1800, while George Pearson continued to publish updates on his own experiments. Others rapidly joined their ranks. On June 14, 1800, the surgeon Richard Dunning of Plymouth Dock published the pamphlet *Some Observations on Vaccination, or the Inoculated Cow-Pox*, in the hope that "some good might be produced by an 'attempt to remove prejudices.'"[2] Jenner and Dr. Woodville jointly produced "A Comparative Statement of Facts and Observations Relative to the Cow Pox," at a price of 5 shillings, released in October of the same year.[3] (Woodville's work in support of cow lymph as a protective was still being quoted in 1880, when the value of vaccination was being seriously questioned.)[4]

Good news traveled quickly and by October 1800, Professor Jean DeCarro (also spelled deCarro) reported on his success with the vaccine inoculation from Vienna. Stating that "there never was, perhaps, so disastrous an epidemic at Vienna as that we have now," he mentioned that the people "think so much now of the cow-pock, against which they had been exceedingly incredulous," adding the vaccination inoculation at Geneva "is exceedingly rapid." The purpose of his letter was to question the exact method of administration, either that of puncture (favored by Jenner and Pearson) or incision (favored by Woodville). In another published letter, John Branson of Doncaster noted that he had "inoculated upwards of 500 for the vaccine disease, without any unpleasant symptoms."

More testimonials followed. Dr. J.M. Nowell of Boulogne, correspondent of the Committee of Medicine, who had been commissioned to compile data on experiments respecting the vaccine inoculation in Paris, reported that since the London Vaccine Institution had introduced the vaccine into France, it had "triumphed over that coalition of prejudices, interests, and passions, which had armed against it even the supreme authority." His studies concluded that cowpox was actually a species of smallpox, which differed from the human variety only by its origin and the peculiar character of mildness.

So convinced was he of benefits derived from cowpox Nowell offered a premium for every poor person who could prove he contracted smallpox after being inoculated "with care" by the vaccine. He added, "I should not be afraid to risk my whole fortune at present on this head." The physician added a codicil that would prove highly important over the next two hundred years: "I cannot too strongly recommend to practitioners to bestow more care on this operation and to repeat it if the least doubt should remain; otherwise there will be some danger of seeing persons attacked with the small-pox after being supposed secured from that disease by the vaccine. It is to errors of this kind that the obstacles opposed to the introduction of the common inoculation in the north of England were to be ascribed."

The last paragraph of his letter bears repeating:

> This inestimable discovery has triumphed over all obstacles as well as every prejudice in England. Sophisms have been refuted by facts; and it is contrary to the rules of good logic to reply to facts by hypotheses. The celebrated Dr. David, of Rotterdam, wrote to me in the month of October last, that the experiments which he repeated with the matter sent from Boulogne have been attended with the most complete success; and Dr. Jenner, the author of this noble discovery, informed him at that period, that more than 50,000 persons have been already inoculated with the vaccine in England; that a third of that number had been exposed to every test possible without the small-pox ever taking effect: and, in the last place, for five years, during which time he has been constantly employed in repeating the experiments, no one has ever yet refuted this theory, or weakened the conclusions he has drawn from it.[5]

By 1800, over 100,000 people worldwide had received the cowpox vaccination. In the spring of 1801, Dr. Jenner was presented with a gold medal by the Medical Officers of the Navy for his work on vaccination. The award featured Apollo, the god of physic, introducing a young seaman recovering from the new inoculation to Britannia, who in return, extended a civic crown on which was written "Jenner."[6]

The House of Commons issued a lengthy study in 1802 on Dr. Jenner's petition respecting his important discovery of "Vaccine Inoculation." Three different heads of inquiry were investigated: the utility of the discovery; the right of the petitioner to claim the discovery; and the advantage, in point of medical practice and pecuniary emolument, which he derived from it. The conclusions were definitive. Medical authorities affirmed Jenner's authorship of the discovery; the cowpox inoculation was proven to be a preventive of smallpox; and that, had Jenner kept the secret for himself instead of offering it to the world free of charge, he might have become "the richest man in these kingdoms." As it was, Jenner was an acknowledged "loser" on the pecuniary side by abandoning his practice to publish and diffuse research on the subject.[7]

An early proponent of vaccination was John Clinch, a classmate of Jenner's at Reverend Dr. Washbourn's school in Cirencester, Gloucestershire. Both went to London to study under John Hunter; Clinch then practiced in Dorset before moving to Newfoundland. Although far removed from his friend, he obviously kept in touch, because in December 1796 he requested a supply of the new vaccine. Receiving dried lymph from either Edward or the Reverend George C. Jenner (Edward's nephew, also a doctor) in lines of impregnated threads, Clinch began the work of vaccination in 1797; by the end of 1801, he had vaccinated 700 people. Clinch and Benjamin Waterhouse of Boston, were credited as being the first vaccinators in North America.[8] By 1802, G.C. Jenner himself had used the vaccine inoculation over 3,000 times in persons from early infancy to 80 years of age, as well as women in every stage of pregnancy, with perfect success.[9]

In ever-conflicted France, the "war between partisans of the Vaccine system, and the Friends to the old plan of Inoculation" assumed a serious aspect. Enemies of vaccination asserted that it induced pain in the bowels, complaints in the throat, and scarlet and military fevers. "The patrons of the Cows," however, were not to be silenced "by such objections, and a furious reply is preparing."[10]

The following year, Dr. Herz, a Jewish physician in Berlin, gave "great offense to all the friends and promoters of vaccination" by his "Epistle to Dohmeyer." Terming vaccination a "Brutal inoculation," he was of the opinion that human nature would, by the prevalence of it, become brutalized.[11]

Meanwhile, supporting evidence poured in. At Lord Egremont's Petworth, 200 people from infancy to advanced old age were successfully inoculated under the care of Dr. Jenner, it being noted "from the great patronage which this most valuable discovery has received both from rank and science, there is little doubt of its speedy and general introduction into the highest circles; it is much to be wished that measures similar to the above were taken to introduce the benefits of it to the lower; which would more than any other means accelerate the extirpation of that most melancholy disease the Small Pox. Was the inoculation of parishes for the Cow Pock to become general, the principal means of circulation for the Small Pox, namely, the want of care as well as cleanliness in the poor, would become extinct."[12] Toward this end, noting that 45,000 individuals in the United Kingdom died annually from smallpox, the Contributors to the Public Dispensary, Edinburgh, announced that henceforth, all children in the city and neighborhood were to be inoculated free of charge.[13]

The fourth of Jenner's pamphlets, *The Origin of the Vaccine Inoculation,* published in 1801, clarified facts concerning improper inoculations using spurious infections from a cow's udder (as opposed to actual cowpox matter) that resulted in failures to provide protection. He also defended his hypothesis of permanent immunity against claims the procedure lost effectiveness after several years. In this, he was actually incorrect, for later 19th century studies concluded that vaccination had to be reinforced every 5–10 years.[14]

Adding more data to the growing regulations, Dr. Jenner also offered a golden rule for vaccination: "Never to take the virus from a vaccine pustule, for the purpose of inoculation, after the efflorescence is formed around it. I wish this efflorescence to be considered as a sacred boundary over which the lancet should never pass."[15]

The same year (1802) the first fever hospital opened in London in Gray's Inn Lane under the name, "House of Recovery," patterned after the example of several provincial towns. Unfortunately, London did not establish any hospitals for infectious diseases for nearly three-quarters of a century.

Vaccination Travels the Globe

In January 1802, the Commission at Copenhagen published a report of 297 cases made by its members and 408 submitted from practicing physicians. They concluded that vaccination protected against smallpox for at least twelve weeks; that it was attended with no considerable danger; patients did not suffer from the inoculation; and the cow-pox produced the infection by the mere contact of the matter on the place of inoculation.[16]

Further testimony came from the Dutch surgeon A. van der Velden from the journal *Algemeene Konsten Letter-Bode* (1802),[17] managers and physicians of the London Foundling Hospital and Dr. Macdonald at "Hamburgh" [*sic*]. Physicians at the court of Vienna patronized the discovery, as did the Italian republic under the direction of Dr. Sacco of Milan, who treated 12,000 persons and succeeded in stopping fatal ravages of smallpox.[18] In order to avoid the long wait of receiving vaccination from abroad, Sacco secured the cooperation of local herdsmen and procured the infection from cows in a nearby pasture by repeatedly soaking a thread in the mature pustules. He went on to test 300 individuals by exposing them to smallpox, none of whom contracted the disease.[19]

In Spain, during the same period, 7,000 persons were inoculated at Catalonia. Don Diego de Bances published an octavo volume dealing with the use of vaccination, drawn from results of 600 Spanish cases. He was so convinced of the practice he invited his professional brethren to extend the procedure by every means in their power, offering to supply them with matter "fit for use, gratis." In Madrid, Dr. Don Pedro Hernandez published a work attesting that of some one thousand infant patients, he did not know of one individual that "suffered in the operation."[20]

Distribution of smallpox vaccine throughout the Spanish empire was largely the work of Francisco Xavier de Balmis, court physician to King Carlos IV. After the daughters of King Carlos recovered from smallpox, he had the rest of his family vaccinated. At government expense, the king mounted the "philanthropic expedition of vaccination," commissioning Balmis to introduce smallpox vaccination to Spanish colonies in North and South America, and, if possible, to the Spanish Philippines. At the time, this was the largest vaccination program ever attempted. Balmis took aboard his ship 22 abandoned or orphaned children selected from Coruna and surrounding areas. The plan was to vaccinate the boys in pairs during the voyage so fresh pustules would always be available. On the first leg of his journey, Balmis reached the Canary Islands and Puerto Rico.

Unfortunately, by the time he arrived at Caracas, Venezuela, South America, only one child still had a visible pustule. Using matter from the boy, he began vaccinating the population. All 22 of the children aboard survived the ordeal and were eventually settled in Mexico, where they were adopted and educated at the expense of the Spanish government.[21]

Balmis' work over the years 1803–1807 reached staggering proportions — more than 100,000 people in Latin America were directly or indirectly vaccinated through his efforts. His techniques reached as far as Mexico and the territory that would become Texas. In 1806, dried scabs and vials of pus, taken from the open sores of a child in Mexico City, were delivered to Manuel Antonio Cordero y Bustamante, governor of the Spanish provinces surrounding the missions of San Antonio. The governor's physicians lanced the skin of several hundred European-Americans and Indians living in the area, then rubbed diluted matter into the wounds. They developed cowpox and thus immunity from smallpox.[22]

Attempts were made to introduce the vaccine to India, but as the matter had to be transported from Constantinople to Bassorah [sic] and thence to Bombay, it became unfit during the passage.[23]

Transmitting matter (vaccine) across great distances continued to be a problem. In 1802, when arm-to-arm transfer was not practical, attempts were made to save it on threads, lancets and pieces of glass. Matter stored in this way did not survive lengthy trips, but in 1802, Dr. DeCarro discovered that matter impregnated in lint remained moist and viable. This enabled him to send it to Persia (present-day Iran) where vaccination achieved great success. At the same time, the East India Company assisted in introducing vaccination to the British settlements there.[24]

As early as 1804, calls began for an act of the British Parliament to require those who practiced inoculation (arm-to-arm transfer with smallpox matter) to perform vaccination solely with cow pock matter. The reason centered around the fact that engrafted individuals became carriers: "Since Inoculation with Small-pox matter has been known, what a scourge has the Small-pox been to this nation! More die of it since, than they did before it was known. *Because it was not universally adopted,* the infection took place where otherwise it might not." One author lamented the fact that 30,000 British subjects died annually from the disease, whereas only 7,000 were saved by use of the cow pock matter. In France and other nations, more than half a million were preserved by inoculation with cow pock matter.[25]

The subject of the prevalence of vaccination was broached again in 1806, when the House of Commons, noting Jenner's beneficence in offering his discovery to the public gratis, observed, "In this country, in which the discovery originated, the progress of vaccination had been checked, partly by prejudice, and partly by the artifices of interested persons, in consequence of which, the annual deaths by Small-Pox, in London, which had been reduced from 1811 to 611, had again risen to 1685." It was hoped the College of Physicians would study the effectiveness of the vaccine and report on the causes that retarded its progress.[26]

Smallpox Used in Germ Warfare—Again

During the war between France and England, an article appearing in *La Citoyen* [*sic*] *Francois* in 1804 debated whether the British were plotting a similar sort of germ warfare that had proven so effective against Native Americans in the French and Indian Wars:

[A] nation which sends sacks with cotton and wool on our coast, to infect the brave Army of England with the plague; and which troops to employ men of all factions and of all sects, [so] by it the misery of France can be produced. We advise, therefore, our countrymen to be upon their guard, even in using the vaccine discovery, because we have had from good authority, that the English cows are subject to madness, and many shocking diseases as known upon the Continent, among animals of that species; and that their milk is one of the causes of the natural brutality of Englishmen, of their unsociable characters, of their spleen, of their suicides, &c.—Who can answer but that by introducing among us the vaccine inoculation, we do not introduce among the human species all the diseases of English cows, and augment the mass of human sufferings already so many and so great?[27]

Despite such rants, Napoleon was a major supporter of smallpox vaccination and after Dr. Jenner's intervention he released several Englishmen who had been jailed in France in 1804, reportedly remarking, "Ah, Jenner, I can refuse him nothing."[28]

8

"The state of medicine is worse than that of total ignorance"

One fact in such cases is worth a thousand arguments.— Dr. Benjamin Waterhouse's exclamation upon the success of his early vaccination experiment.[1]

The title statement, written by Thomas Jefferson in a letter to William Green Munford, June 18, 1799, typified what many 18th century Americans felt about doctors and the medical arts. Ironically, Jefferson would become one of the earliest Americans to support the new technique of vaccination developed by Edward Jenner.

Already a supporter of inoculation, having received variolation in 1766, and having his daughters inoculated just two months after the death of his wife, Martha, in 1782, Jefferson became fascinated with the new cowpox immunization. His involvement with the discovery started with a letter written by Dr. Benjamin Waterhouse dated December 1, 1800.

Benjamin Waterhouse (March 4, 1754–October 2, 1846) was born in Newport, Rhode Island, to Timothy and Hannah Waterhouse. His father was a chairmaker and a member of the governor's council. Benjamin was apprenticed to a local doctor at age 16, the most common way for a youth to learn the healing arts in the 18th century and well into the 19th century, and one reason why highly educated men like Jefferson scorned the profession. Dr. Robley Dunglison, Jefferson's own physician and the first professor of medicine at the University of Virginia School of Medicine, quoted Jefferson as remarking, "It is not to physic that I object so much as physicians."[2]

Clearly, young Waterhouse had the means and desire for more than the transfer of knowledge from teacher to student, as he went to Europe at age 21, studying for a time under Dr. John Fothergill in London. He was also educated in Leyden, where he received his medical degree. As an example of how lives touch one another, while in Holland he lodged with John Adams.

Waterhouse returned to the newly established United States in 1782 and briefly practiced medicine at Newport before joining the medical school at Harvard as professor of Theory and Practice of Physic along with John Warren and Aaron Dexter.[3] As a European-trained physician, he was intimately familiar with Edward Jenner's work on smallpox vaccination, exchanging letters with colleagues in England, including Jenner. On March 16, 1799, Waterhouse published a report on the method and effectiveness of the operation in the Boston *Sentinel*. His opinion on Jenner's technique stated this: "On perusing this work I was struck with the unspeakable advantages that might accrue to this country, and indeed to the human race at large, from the discovery of a mild distemper that would ever after secure the constitution from that terrible scourge, the smallpox."[4]

Determined to pursue the matter, Waterhouse wrote to Dr. John Haygarth, one of England's authorities on contagious diseases, and requested a sample of cowpox. He received a thread soaked with cowpox matter on July 4, 1800. Placing it in a sealed glass vial, four days later he vaccinated his 5-year-old son, Daniel, who is credited with being the first American so treated. Waterhouse then vaccinated several other family members and servants, including a 12-year-old boy. In order to test the efficacy of the preventive, he sent the boy to Dr. William Aspinwall's Smallpox Hospital in Brookline, where he was exposed to the contagion. After twelve days, the child returned home with, according to Waterhouse, little more than a sore arm.[5]

Eager to promote the success of his experiment, Waterhouse sent his friend John Adams his treatise, "A Prospect of Exterminating the Small Pox, Part 1." By this time, Adams was president of the United States. On September 10, 1800, Adams responded by writing he had read the paper with pleasure and would communicate it to the American Academy of Arts and Sciences. Waterhouse did not wait long for an answer from the academy. On December 1, 1800, he sent his work to Thomas Jefferson, then vice president of the United States:

Sir,

Having long regarded Mr. Jefferson as one of our most distinguished patriots & philosophers, I conceived that a work which had for its end the good of the community would not be unacceptable to him.—Under that impression, I have sent him "a prospect of exterminating the smallpox," and am with the utmost consideration and respect his very humble servant Benj Waterhouse.

Jefferson received the letter December 24 and responded the following day:

Washing, Dec. 25, 1800

Sir,

I received last night, and have read with great satisfaction, your pamphlet on the subject of the kine-pox, and pray you will accept my thanks for the communication of it.

I had before attended to your publications on the subject in the newspapers and took much interest in the result of the experiments you were making. Every friend of humanity must look with pleasure on this discovery, by which one evil more is withdrawn from the condition of man; and must contemplate the possibility, that future improvements and discoveries may still more and more lessen the catalogue of evils. In this line of proceeding you deserve well your country; and I pray you accept my portion of the tribute due to you, and assurance of high consideration and respect, with which I am, Sir

Your most obedient, humble servant,

Thomas Jefferson

Jefferson and Waterhouse began a correspondence related to smallpox. After Jefferson became president, Waterhouse sent him vaccine matter to test in Washington. Jefferson gave the samples to Dr. Gantt. Edward Gantt (chaplain of the Senate from December 9, 1800, through November 6, 1804) was well known to Jefferson. Princeton educated, Gantt graduated with a bachelor of arts in 1726. After studying under Dr. Benjamin Rush in Philadelphia and in Edinburgh, the Scottish city famous for innovations in the healing arts, he received his medical degree. Gantt practiced in Somerset County, Maryland, before being ordained a minister in England in 1770.

From Cambridge, Massachusetts, on June 25, 1801, Waterhouse wrote a "card," or informational letter, beginning, "Dr. Waterhouse takes this method, most respectfully, to suggest something to his brethren at a distance, in which the honor of the profession, and the cause of humanity are particularly concerned." Acknowledging that Americans were ill-disposed to believe "what happened a good while ago, or a great way off," he defended the technique of vaccination and in lieu of no one else coming forward, proposed to establish a "Medical Philosophical Society" to test and disseminate data on the successful prevention of smallpox. He requested physicians to forward their experiences with kine pox to him (patient names, ages, dates and places of abode being absolutely necessary) and asked individuals willing to take part in his studies to repair to the hospital at Brookline to see if "they can take the smallpox, after having gone fairly through the kine pox." Waterhouse concluded by asking "printers throughout these states" to insert his card, "and Patriotism will carry it to their credit."[6]

The first three tests using Waterhouse's lymph failed, presumably because the live matter had become ineffective during transport. On July 28, 1801, Jefferson suggested Waterhouse "put the matter into a phial of the smallest size, well corked and immersed in a larger one filled with water and well corked." This, he hoped, would prevent heat from corrupting the matter. He closed by adding, "I know of no one discovery in medicine equally valuable. Accept assurance of my great esteem and respect." With his letter he re-enclosed a treatise by Dr. Lettsom (see below).

Jefferson's hypothesis on transport and his suggestion on how to preserve live matter proved entirely successful and explained the three earlier failures. That summer, he requested that Dr. Wardlaw vaccinate those at Monticello, but the doctor replied that he was too busy. Acting as vaccinator, Jefferson performed the operation on 20 of his family members and a number of others at his estate.[7] In a letter dated August 21, Jefferson informed Waterhouse of his success, the latter replying the news had given him "pleasure inexpressible." Waterhouse added that no further vaccine need be sent from Boston, as the strain established in Virginia would suit the need.

Establishing his own legacy in the annals of American medicine, in August and September 1801, the Founding Father sent fresh matter to Washington, Petersburg, Richmond, and throughout Virginia, hoping that by successful vaccinations he could convince not only the medical community but also the citizens of the state to accept and undergo the operation. Through the intermediary John Vaughn, the president learned that Dr. John Redman Coxe had performed vaccine inoculation in Philadelphia. On November 5, Jefferson responded to Vaughn, writing that over the two-month period of July and August he had inoculated between 70 or 80 of his own family, including his two sons-in-law, as well as any of his neighbors who wished to avail themselves of the opportunity, the total reaching about 200 persons.[8]

In this letter, Jefferson meticulously described the results of the operations, concluding from observation that the eighth day after inoculation was the best for securing fresh matter. He regretted the fact he had no access to variolous matter by which to test those he vaccinated and thus prove resistance to smallpox, and he asked Dr. Coxe to send him some "so carefully taken and done up, that we may rely on it; you are sensible of the dangerous security which a trial with effete matter might induce."

Coxe complied, and Jefferson quickly put his patients to the test. On Christmas Day, 1801, a year to the day he first wrote Waterhouse (Jefferson did not celebrate that holiday[9]), the president informed him that his own vaccinations were proven successful, "and consequently those in Virginia who received the matter from me are now in security."[10]

Dr. Coxe later publicized conclusions to his vaccinations, stating, "The result was a uniform opposition to the variolous contagion." Among those successfully inoculated was his three-week-old infant, who was exposed to a man "full of the variolous eruption" for a quarter of an hour without becoming infected. Dr. Coxe subsequently communicated with

George Farquhar, M.D., of Jamaica, who informed him that after procuring matter from England, vaccination was immediately begun. Twelve hundred people were successfully vaccinated in the parish of Trelawny; significantly, Farquhar noted that during their convalescence, patients were able to follow their usual avocations. In order to ascertain its effectiveness, each person previously inoculated with cowpox underwent the same operation with variolous matter, and in no instance did disease follow.[11]

Thomas Jefferson and "Little Turtle"

Early in 1802, the second edition of *Observations on the Cow Pock,* by John Coakley Lettsom, M. and LL.D, member of several academies and literary societies, appeared in London. This pamphlet of 8vo., containing 80 pages, cost 3 shillings. The first edition had been distributed only among the author's friends and "not exposed to sale," but the pamphlet subsequently would become widely influential, not only in England but also in the United States.

Lettsom began by reflecting on the animal and the man responsible for the new discovery of the cowpox vaccination:

> An animal, whose lactarious fountains afford in our infancy a substitute for that of the parent, and from which we draw, through life, a considerable portion of our nutriment, is destined, by the sagacity of one enlightened philosopher, to protect the human species from the most loathsome and noxious disease to which it is subjected. In reflecting upon its ravages, the mind revolts with horror; not merely from its fatal devastation, but likewise from the deformity it inflicts upon its victims, by rendering the fairest sublunary being, that god-like countenance, impressed by the Creator, an object of compassion, if not of disgust.

Lettsom's vaccination work embraced the following axioms:

I. It prevents the accession of the most fatal malady under heaven — the variolous infection.
II. It is not infectious or contagious.
III. It is believed, that it never has been fatal, and never will be.
IV. It creates no blemish, or mark, on the human frame.
V. It conveys no constitutional disease.

Furthermore, the author contended that of 60,000 persons inoculated with the cowpox, only four died. Doubting even that small number as accurate, he added, "It must, however, be acknowledged, that many mistakes have been committed by practitioners; matter has been taken from the chicken-pox *(varicella),* and too frequently from the purulent fluid round the scab of the Cow-pox, or in the variolous pustule; and in either case it is needless to say, inoculation under such circumstances is no security against the small-pox."

Next cited was a report of the Medical Committee of Paris, which confirmed that of 72 persons under observation who had been vaccinated and exposed to the contagion, none took the infection. (Lettsom added that the number in England exceeded 50,000, "or perhaps even double.") The committee thus verified the observations of English physicians, concluding vaccine was "an effectual preservative against the small-pox." Lettsom also remarked on the practice of Dr. Woodville in France, the institution founded by Dr. Pearson for vaccine inoculation and Dr. Waterhouse's experiments and successful practices in America.

Lettsom's pamphlet continued with a "combat" directed against those who denied the practice "on account of its origin; many persons conferring upon it the epithet of a *beastly disease,* and branding its promoters as persons possessed with the *cow mania.*"[12]

Being made aware that his work was extensively and favorably reviewed in *European Magazine,* Lettsom wrote to the editor, noting he could not "but feel an high sense of the Writer's kindness." Significantly, he included part of a letter received from Professor Waterhouse, of Cambridge, Massachusetts. The details of this and a succeeding letter provide interesting details of Thomas Jefferson's continuing involvement with smallpox vaccination and the treatment of Native Americans, in this instance Little Turtle.

Little Turtle was a warrior of the Miami tribe living in the area that is now Indiana. After coming to prominence during the Revolution, when he defeated the Frenchman Augustin de La Balme in 1780, Little Turtle became a leader of the Western Confederacy, which included the Shawnees under Blue Jacket and the Delawares under Buckongahelas. After the Northwest Territory was created in 1787, the goal of the Western Confederacy was to keep the Ohio River as a boundary between the westward expanding pioneers and the Indians.

In the border war that followed, Little Turtle and Blue Jacket defeated General Josiah Harmar's troops in October 1790. By 1791, after the Ottawas and Wyandots joined them, the combined forces defeated General Arthur St. Claire in the worst defeat ever suffered by American soldiers at the hands of Native Americans. In June 1794, General Anthony Wayne's troops defeated the confederacy, the war ending with the Treaty of Greenville.[13]

Chief Little Turtle went on to counsel peace with the United States and in the winter of 1801–1802, he and a delegation met with President Thomas Jefferson in Washington. Waterhouse's letter to Lettsom described the president's contributions to the Indians, adding the following:

> [T]he President exclaimed to little turtle, how the *Great Spirit* had made a donation to the enlightened White Men; first to one [Dr. Jenner] in England, and from him to *one* [Waterhouse] in Boston, of the means to prevent them from ever having the small-pox (which had occasioned great fatality among the race); and, such confidence had the copper coloured King in the words of his *Father,* the President, that he submitted to be inoculated, together with the rest of the warriors, by the hands of the Rev. Dr. Garitt [Gantt], Chaplain to Congress. On their departure, the President caused them to be supplied with the vaccine matter, and gave their Interpreter an abstract of the letter of instructions which I had written to the President.
>
> Not long since fifteen more Chiefs came down to Washington to receive the same blessing from the Clergyman who had inoculated *Little Turtle* and the other warriors.[14]

In the September 1802, issue of *European Magazine,* Lettsom submitted a second letter, this one dated July 12, 1802. It came from Dr. Thornton, "resident in that new metropolis" (Washington), offering further particulars of the meeting between Jefferson and Little Turtle:

> The President of the United States has been very instrumental in propagating this useful knowledge in various parts of this country, and gave some of the matter to little turtle, the celebrated Indian Chief, who commanded at the defeat of our General St. Clair. By a letter from the Interpreter, the Indians among the Miamis has inoculated *three hundred,* and they were arriving from all quarters to be inoculated.

The letter added that Thornton thought as many more would receive the matter before his letter arrived in England, adding his hope "that this disease will no longer be among the enemies of these poor people."

On a side note, Thornton described Little Turtle as "most polished and refined, as well as astute." When a previous attempt to compile a vocabulary of the Indian language taken by Monsieur Volney was found inadequate due to his "making use of the Roman alphabet only," Thornton "took a very extensive vocabulary from him [Little Turtle] of the Miamis language for the President, referred to in England as, 'the present Supreme Magistrate of the United States.'"

In praising "he who now occupies the chair of the late illustrious Washington," Thornton described Jefferson as having "the urbanity of a good heart" in his dealings with Little Turtle, noting that by influencing a great mind, he had "not only been the preserver of the lives of the Indians, by the introduction of vaccine inoculation, but has taught the wandering tribes to cultivate the soil, rather than to roam the woods for subsistence, he has domesticated them by the introduction of the spinning-wheels, and various other implements of domestic and agricultural utility; and has thus prepared them to receive the beneficent principles of the Christian religion."

Hearing praise of the president not only from his correspondents in Boston, Washington, and New York, Thornton also received "heartfelt eulogies" from his friends in Philadelphia. His letter concluded: "When we consider the fatality of the small-pox among the Indians, no man of feeling, however remote from the seat of his government, can refrain from approbation of his provident attention to the lives, and to the instruction, of a despised, but not a degraded, race of human beings."

John Lettsom owned a medal of Jefferson, described as having the head of the president on the obverse, with the inscription, "*Th. Jefferson, President of the U.S. 4 March 1801,*" and on the reverse, Minerva, the right hand supporting the cap of Liberty, the left holding a book; on a leaf was inscribed, "*Declari Independence,*" with Trophies; under which was "*Constitution.*" Over the book was a dove with an olive branch, inscribed, "Exurge — To commemorate July 4, 1776." With it, Lettsom intended to ornament a new edition of his book, *Observations on the Cow-Pock,* thus promoting a patron of the great Jennerian discovery of vaccination. He concluded his discussion by remarking that the late empress of Russia, who had encouraged inoculation of the smallpox before vaccination was established, had a female inoculated with the cow-pock, "to whom she gave the surname of Vaccinavitz."[15]

The Battle for Vaccination in the Early Years of the Republic

Reflections on the Vaccine as given by Mr. Ring:
On the 3rd day it resembles a flea bite; on the 6th, a crystal; on the 10th a pearl; on the 12th a rose-a rose without thorns!— The vesicle which it displays, may be considered a gem of inestimable value; and the fluid it contains a precious balm.[1]

Benjamin Waterhouse comes down through history as a bit of an enigma. His early work with vaccination and persistence in seeing the preventive spread throughout the country was lauded in his own time and he is credited with being the first American physician to inoculate with the cowpox vaccine.

His work in promoting the vaccine in Boston often placed him in conflict with the Boston medical establishment, including the Massachusetts Medical Society and John Warrer, Harvard's professor of anatomy and surgery. This "clique" vilified and persecuted Waterhouse,[2] doing everything in their power to prevent his establishment of a vaccine institution in that city. They ultimately succeeded in defeating his efforts, but failed to prevent a public test of Jenner's vaccination.

On August 16, 1802, the Boston Board of Health determined to put Waterhouse's beliefs to the test. They appointed a committee of seven of the most respected doctors in the city and vaccinated 19 children at the health office. On November 9, they sent the subjects to Noddle's Island, where they were twice inoculated with variolous matter and exposed to the smallpox contagion for 20 days. The committee concluded, "The cow-pox prevented their taking the small-pox, and they do therefore consider the result of the experiment as satisfactory evidence that the cow-pox is a complete security against the small-pox."[3]

The result of the Boston experiment did little, if anything, to improve Dr. Waterhouse's reputation. Professional nitpicking and jealousies were not uncommon and might have been overlooked but for the charges of Waterhouse's pecuniary interests in vaccination. Unlike Edward Jenner, who freely offered his discovery to the world so that there would never be a question of the poor being able to afford protection, it was circulated that Waterhouse took a different path. In contrast to his cooperation with Thomas Jefferson, he refused to share vaccine matter with local physicians, and when he did, his demand to receive a share of the profits derived from the operation put him at odds with his peers.

Accusations flew "fast and furious," and the matter was often fought out in the newspapers. Defenders claimed Waterhouse only wished to be sure the technique was performed by qualified doctors, a questionable stance since Jefferson, to whom he sent vaccine, was not a physician. Jefferson was, however, a very influential politician, and soliciting him to his side was sure to garner laurels. On the other hand, it is difficult to see how Waterhouse could have created a monopoly on vaccine matter, considering its use in other parts of the country. The only claim he might have had was that his matter was pure and proven, not an insubstantial point considering that improper handling, cross-contamination or incorrect technique in harvesting matter frequently resulted in failed protection or, worse, caused full-blown cases of smallpox.

Notwithstanding, Waterhouse was lauded in England and in 1804 the second part of his work, "A Prospect of Exterminating the Small Pox," was reviewed as being "in every respect worthy of the excellent reputation which the author has so long and so deservedly sustained both at home and abroad." The same reviewer added that Waterhouse's "unwearied exertions to introduce, disseminate and defend this inestimable substitute for the Small Pox, give him a just and elevated distinction among those who have laboured in this field, and signalized their zeal in the cause of humanity."[4]

In 1810, Waterhouse petitioned the legislature of Massachusetts to reimburse him for his efforts in disseminating and promoting vaccination in his own and other states. He claimed the work had impoverished him, but his pleas fell on deaf ears and he was ultimately humiliated by being forced to withdraw his request.

It is unfortunate Waterhouse's name became sullied, as it finally led to his expulsion as a professor at Harvard in 1812. In a letter to a friend in England, he wrote:

> For the honor of my country I am ashamed to tell Dr. Jenner how I have been treated by our Legislature respecting remuneration. I have received nothing but abuse, nay, more, I have been intrigued out of my place as physician to the U.S. Marine Hospital, with 500 sterling a year, and given me by Jefferson as a reward for my labors in vaccination; and this merely in consequence of his going out and others coming in, so that, at 56 years of age, I have now to contrive and execute some new plan to supply this deficiency.[5]

He continued his medical career by the intervention of President James Madison, who named him medical superintendent of New England's nine military bases. Elizabeth Oliver, his first wife, whom he married in 1788, died in childbirth in 1815. Together they had six children. He remarried in 1819, to Louisa Lee, and died at his home in Cambridge in 1846.

Like Jenner, the claim that Waterhouse was the first to introduce cowpox vaccination in America did not go unchallenged. A letter written July 24 and published in the *Philosophical Magazine* (London), August 31, 1803 (vol. 16), written by Nath. H. Rhodes, stated:

> In the winter of the year 1799 Dr. John Chichester, a practitioner of the first distinction in Charleston, South Carolina, and to whom I have been pupil, received vaccine matter from his learned friend and former teacher, Dr. Pearson, accompanying the first publications written on the cow-pox by Dr. Jenner and himself. With this matter several persons were inoculated, but the disease was produced in one case only. This was a mulatto boy named Robert, about seven or eight years old, the property of Thomas Tunno, esq. merchant. The small-pox matter was subsequently inserted, in the most careful manner, without effect. It was some time after the occurrence of the above case, before those which have been published as the first instances in America really happened.
>
> It may be proper to notice that my late worthy master Dr. Chichester was not supported by the approbation of his brethren in his introduction of the vaccine inoculation in America, notwithstanding the high authorities above mentioned who first proposed it to the public.

Rhodes added in a P.S. that "the error concerning the inoculation of the cow-pox in America would not have happened if Dr. Chichester's account had not failed in getting to Europe."

Another individual vying for the honor of being the first to introduce vaccination to

America was Dr. William Yates. Born November 13, 1767, to the manor of Sapperton, Bur-ton-on-Trent, England, he was cousin to Prime Minister Sir Richard Peel and to the philan-thropist John Howard. Although the elder son and a baronet, Yates studied medicine under Sir James Earle at St. Bartholomew's Hospital, London. His early interest lay in the treatment of the insane, and at his manor he treated a considerable number of "pauper lunatics." After an unfortunate accident, when one of his patients took the life of another inmate "under shocking circumstances" and then committed suicide, Yates closed his asylum.

Having previously developed a fascination with the new concept of vaccination, he made the personal acquaintance of Edward Jenner and studied under him. Desirous for a change of scenery after the horrific accident and equally determined to bring the medical advancement to America, he obtained a generous supply of lymph matter from Dr. Jenner and sailed for the United States, arriving in Philadelphia in June 1799.

Immediately upon reaching the city, he engaged himself "with all the zeal and philan-thropic mind, to disseminate the knowledge of the then-new discovery." According to the *Evening Post* (as quoted in the *New York Daily Times*, March 20, 1857), "it is certain that he was the first to introduce into America this great boon to humanity, although the credit of its first introduction has been generally accorded to another. He knew this, but had a morbid dislike to publicity, and never publicly contradicted it."

Yates was credited with inoculating thousands with the vaccine virus and according to family history, he may have been the physician who personally vaccinated John Adams during one of his trips to Philadelphia.[6] Interestingly, the first method used by Dr. Yates to vaccinate patients was by having them apply the lymph to their hands and between the fingers, in imi-tation of the natural way "cow-pox" was acquired by the milkmaids of England.[7]

William Yates was a friend of Judge Cooper, founder of Cooperstown, New York, and father of James Fennimore Cooper, the American author. Yates married Hanna Palmer in 1801, and the pair returned to Europe for a yearlong honeymoon. After turning over the manor and title to his brother, the couple returned to New York, where they purchased a large estate in Butternuts. He died March 7, 1857, after traveling in subzero temperatures to attend a patient. On the return trip, his feet froze and gangrene set in. His obituary lauded him as being the first who introduced vaccination to the United States.[8]

Another early pioneer introducing the kine pox vaccine into the United States was Dr. Valentine Seaman. A friend of chief justice John Jay and Edward Jenner, it was claimed that his children were the first individuals vaccinated in the country. According to the *New York Times* of August 8, 1897, Seaman's faith in Jenner's discovery brought the threat of death on him by angry New York mobs. As the only Quaker physician in the city, his determination never flinched as he continued his vaccination work. Future famous New Yorkers Valentine Mott and John C. Cheesman began as office boys under his tutelage. For many years, Seaman was the chief surgeon at the New York Hospital.

A Subject of High Importance

In a new country bursting at the seams with democratic ideas and desirous of expanding into uncharted territories, it would be logical to assume that medical advancements would be embraced with enthusiasm. Yet, "out with the old, in with the new" was more represen-tative of the Old World than the New World. Americans seemed suspicious of scientific advancement, at least as it pertained to the smallpox vaccine, and acceptance did not come easily. Much convincing was required and the newspapers of Boston, Philadelphia and Baltimore were filled with learned articles espousing the technique of vaccination.

The January 21, 1802, edition of the *Carlisle Eagle* began, "Finding much, on this subject [vaccine], in the public prints both of this, and the other States of the Union, we thought it our duty to call the attention of our readers to it." Describing the subject as one of "high importance," rather than mere curiosity, the author described Dr. Alexander Herman Mac-Donald's work on vaccination. The work was published in October 1800, in both English and German, and the eminent physician (a native of Holland, then working in Hamburg), concluded with "a most animated address to fathers and mothers on the subject."

Dr. Waterhouse's studies were also chronicled, noting that when using fluid direct from the arm of an infected person he had but few failures, but while using matter stored on a thread it was sometimes injured by heat, particularly in the summer months. Three hospitals were being established, principally for the purpose of testing the Kine Pox, at Rochester, Franklin and Waterford.

The article also included details in the work done in Philadelphia by Dr. John Redman Coxe, confirming, "Those persons whom he *vaccinated,* (a convenient term adopted by physicians, to this new or *jenner* mode of inoculation) would not afterwards take the *variolus* infection." To the laboring classes, the advantages of the inoculation were invaluable, as it seldom required nursing or confinement, was equally safe at all seasons and "never prove[d] mortal." In conclusion, Coxe stated the operation required "but to be known in order to insure its speedy diffusion in every part of the world."

Of importance, some of the notes and statistics included in Coxe's "Practical Observations on Vaccination: or Inoculation for the Cow-Pox" were submitted by Thomas Jefferson, who later received a letter from the Royal Jennerian Society, London, recognizing his promotion of the vaccine in the United States.[9]

Like others before him, Dr. Coxe's prediction proved premature. In 1803, to confront the "weakness and perversion" of some men governed by "invincible ignorance, prejudice, pride, and envy" who "not only deny their assent, but reprobate *established facts,*" the physicians of Philadelphia, led by Dr. Samuel Agnew of Gettysburg, Pennsylvania, were compelled to run a statement in the newspaper to the effect that "Inoculation for the Kine or Cow pock IS A CERTAIN PREVENTIVE OF THE SMALL POX" and they "RECOMMENDED IT TO GENERAL USE."[10]

In what would become a battle, at times fought with invectives and acrimonious charges within and without the medical community, smallpox continued to rear its ugly head. Throughout the 19th century, small paragraphs like the following were tucked in between matters of political and commercial significance; in this case, a resolution to move the seat of government from Lancaster to Philadelphia and a shipping notice that the *Sally, Commerce* and *Lexington* had arrived at Baltimore: "The town of Marblehead, which has been so dreadfully afflicted with the small pox for upwards of three months, is happily relieved from the contagion; eighty-three grown persons died."[11]

What makes this particularly interesting is that this excerpt is from the *Courier and Evening Gazette*, a London newspaper, clearly revealing international interest in the havoc wrought by smallpox. Similar notices ran in out-of-town American newspapers. A typical notice in the *Sprig of Liberty* (PA), on December 13, 1804, ran: "A Hudson paper informs that the small pox continues its ravages in Newyork [*sic*], notwithstanding the advantages permitted by the vaccine institution. In one week lately, ten died, and in the next 11, being about one forth of the whole number of natural deaths in that city."

On April 11, 1805, in the same newspaper, a writer under the pseudonym "Aurora" bemoaned the lack of acceptance across the country: "The mortality in this city and neighborhood, by Small Pox, in the present year, we are informed, has been as great as before the discovery of the Vaccination preventive; and we find that in New England the same indifference, or the same unfortunate prevalence of prejudice against the influence of science and experiment, has been in many instances, fatal to adults." What "Aurora" failed to mention was the expense of the new procedure. Prices charged by local physicians ranged from £3 in Philadelphia to £5 15 shillings, a cost well out of the reach of most families. Benjamin Franklin observed the problem with some distress, writing, "The *expense* of having the operation perform'd by a Surgeon, has been pretty high in some parts of *America*."[12] Matters would hardly improve. A notice in the *Star and Banner* (PA) for June 4, 1852, noted, "The Doctors of Boston have raised their charges. Sickness will soon become one of the luxuries of life which a poor man cannot afford."

American supporters continued to pound home the acceptance of vaccination overseas, hoping to impress their fellow citizens into action on a personal and public level. Through the medium of the Philadelphia Medical Museum, in November 1807, people were informed that after nine years of experience, the Royal College of Physicians, London; the Royal College of Physicians, Edinburgh and Dublin; the Royal College of Surgeons in London, Dublin and Edinburgh, all declared the kine pox to be a certain preventive of smallpox.

In an interesting argument made December 26, 1804, supporting vaccination over inoculation, Horatio G. Jameson of Gettysburg put forth that, in English law, the crime for larceny was death, noting that law, in general, was replete with cruelty. "So long as people are ignorant of a better remedy, they are perfectly justifiable in punishing with death ..." but given an alternative such as the workhouse, the more humane remedy was its substitution for death. He likened inoculation to the punishment of death and vaccination to confinement, remarking that both operations offered some risk but the latter was far more successful and expedient.

In combating the vociferous religious opposition to vaccination that continued to stymie general acceptance among the population, he used equally strong language:

> It is the greatest ignorance imaginable to assert, as many do, that as God sends it, we are justifiable in taking our chances; but that same beneficent being, who has created all, has provided remedies for all our evils, means for the removal of our pains and sickness, with minds capable of directing us gradually to ascertain and discover them, and in proportion as the mind is evolved and expanded, so is more required of us — and it is not improbable that had not the vanity and wickedness of men engaged them so much in wars and other follies, they might have discovered many means of smoothing and rendering human life more agreeable.[13]

In agreement with the sentiments of Jameson, who, three years later, demanded his peers "*blush* for their *folly* or their *ignorance*" in failing to grasp the benefits of vaccination,[14] Thomas Jefferson crafted instructions for Meriwether Lewis prefatory to what would become known as the Lewis and Clark Expedition. Writing in June 1803, he ordered the explorer to "carry with you some matter of the kine-pox; inform those of them with whom you may be, of its efficacy as a preservative from the smallpox; & encourage them in the use of it."[15]

Jefferson continued his quest for knowledge on the subject, actually exchanging letters with Edward Jenner:

To Dr. Edward Jenner Monticello, May 14, 1806

Sir, — I have received a copy of the evidence at large respecting the discovery of the vaccine inoculation which you have been pleased to send me, and for which I return you my thanks.

Having been among the early converts, in this part of the globe, to its efficiency, I took an early part in recommending it to my countrymen. I avail myself of this occasion of rendering you a portion of the tribute of gratitude due to you from the whole human family. Medicine has never before produced any single improvement of such utility. Harvey's discovery of the circulation of the blood was a beautiful addition to our knowledge of the animal economy, but on a review of the practice of medicine before and since that epoch, I do not see any great amelioration which has been derived from that discovery. You have erased from the calendar of human afflictions one of its greatest. Yours is the comfortable reflection that mankind can never forget that you have lived. Future nations will know by history only that the loathsome small-pox has existed and by you has been extirpated.

Accept my fervent wishes for your health and happiness and assurances of the greatest respect and consideration.[16]

A major development in the eradication of smallpox was a mere seven years away. Where this movement would take the country perhaps only Jefferson, the skeptic, could have guessed. What he might not have foreseen was that other words he wrote to Jenner in 1806 would be quoted by Professor Viktor Zhdanov of the USSR at the 11th World Health Assembly in 1958, when he proposed the eradication of smallpox within ten years: "It is owing to your discovery ... that in the future the peoples of the world will learn about this disgusting smallpox disease only from ancient traditions."[17]

10

Testimonies to the
High Value of Esteem

Within this tomb hath found a resting place
  The great physician of the human race —
Immortal Jenner! whose gigantic mind
  Brought life and health to more than half mankind.

Let rescued infancy his worth proclaim,
  And lisp out blessings on his honoured name;
And radiant beauty drop one grateful tear,
  For beauty's truest friend lies buried here.
                    — The epitaph on Edward Jenner's tomb[1]

Almost overnight, Dr. Edward Jenner became a living legend. Attending a levee late in 1799, he had the honor of presenting to his majesty his treatise on smallpox.[2] Jenner would have the privilege of attending another of the king's levees in early March 1802, where he was again presented to the monarch.[3] On May 21, 1802, the *Edinburgh Advertiser* announced, "The liberality of the County of Gloucester was exemplified by the donation of a most elegant vase of Dr. Jenner, as a testimony to the high value they set upon his discovery on INOCULATION for the Cow pox — a discovery which equals that of the immortal HARVEY, in its effect on the philosophy of medicine, and surpasses it in the benefits it brings to mankind." Nor did it fail to note, with due pride that, "as a national concern, it elevates the scientific credit of GREAT BRITAIN to a height that EUROPE, notwithstanding all her vast discoveries of late, must look up to with generous envy."

That same year, in discussing whether to give Jenner a £10,000 tithe "to be granted to his Majesty, to be paid to Doctor Edward Jenner, for promulgating the discovery of the Vaccine Inoculation," Mr. Courteney of the House of Commons noted that 10,000 lives had been saved by the discovery. Taking into consideration that every British life was "allowed to be worth 51 [pounds] per annum," that would accrue to the revenue a saving or income of £200,000. Under those circumstances, and the fact the inventor sacrificed his considerable private practice and had spent no less than £6,000 in maturing his system, the vote was 59 for and 56 against, making a majority of 3.[4]

In October 1802, Jenner received, by the hands of Lord St. Helens, a present of a most valuable diamond ring from the dowager empress of Russia. Accompanying the gift was a letter from her imperial majesty, announcing her introduction of the "vaccine inoculation" into the charitable establishments under her care.[5] (Arm-to-arm vaccination had begun in 1801, at the St. Petersburg Foundling Hospital after the empress obtained lymph from Jenner and was continued until 1867, when vaccine from cows was utilized. During the years 1826–

1846, there were 17 epidemics of smallpox: out of approximately 15,000 foundlings vaccinated, only 34 developed smallpox, with only one fatality.)[6]

The first annual festival of the Governors and Friends of the Royal Jennerian Society for the Extermination of Small Pox held a meeting on May 17, 1803, at the Crown and Anchor, in the Strand. The day being chosen in honor of Dr. Jenner's birthday, the Earl of Egremont chaired the event that attracted between 500 and 600 attendees. This illustrious society had as its patron the king, and as its patroness the queen. Vice patrons included their royal highnesses the Prince of Wales and the Dukes of York, Clarence, Cumberland, Sussex, Cambridge and Gloucester, with the Duke of Bedford standing as president.

At the 1805 meeting, it was stated that 12,011 persons had been inoculated by the society and 16,236 charges of vaccine matter had been furnished free of expense over the past year: "This gratuitous diffusion of Vaccine Virus has been a principal means of spreading the Vaccine Inoculation throughout the British Empire, and the World."[7]

The city of London voted Jenner the freedom of the city in 1803. The honor was presented in a gold box valued at 100 guineas, "as a token of their sense of his skill and perseverance in bringing into general use the inoculation for the cow pox."[8] An

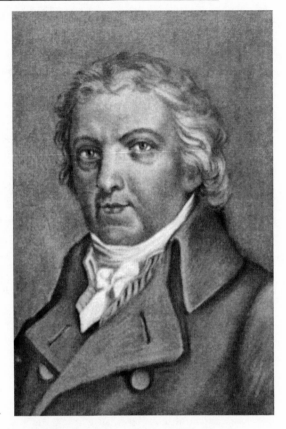

Dr. Edward Jenner, who immortalized himself by introducing the method of inserting cowpox matter under the skin as a means of providing protection from smallpox, was equally revered for offering his discovery to the world free of charge so that vaccination might not be deprived to those who could not afford it. This card, in the authors' collection, is undated.

even greater reward came from Parliament, in 1806, when that body voted Dr. Jenner an additional £20,000 as a reward for his investigative work and personal sacrifices.

In January 1814, Dr. Jenner received the degree of doctor in medicine from the University of Oxford[9] and in July of the same year, England's most famous physician was introduced to "the whole of the Royal Families of Russia and Prussia previous to their departure from England," where the emperor of Russia offered to bestow on him the Russian order of nobility.[10]

As a reflection of his professional success, it was reported that the population of Great Britain and Ireland, "not withstanding the long and bloody wars in which we have been engaged," had rapidly increased over the past thirty years, "in great measure owing to an important discovery of VACCINATION, which has nearly exterminated that horrid and dreadful disease the *Small Pox,* and has, as was well observed by an eloquent Preacher, '*Blotted out* one of the *blackest pages* from our Book of *Nosology*'"[11] (Nosology: The doctrine of the names of diseases; the arrangement of diseases into classes, orders, genera, species, etc.).[12]

Sir Henry Halford, president of the Vaccine Establishment in England, summarized to Lord Sidmouth that although there may have been rare instances (8 cases out of 67,000) where smallpox was contracted after vaccination, on the whole, "this controlling power of vaccination must be admitted as next in importance to its preventive influence; and surely justifies our high estimation of the value of this great discovery."[13]

Other nations around the world reported even more impressive results using Jenner's research. According to one American authority writing to the editor of the *Baltimore Federal Gazette* in 1818, "since the introduction of vaccination into the kingdom of Denmark, not a single instance of death by smallpox occurred; when, for fifty years prior to this, or from the years 1749 to 1798, 2,100,000 persons are calculated to have died of natural or inoculated small-pox-saving to the state, in this short period, and at a fair estimate, a population of 73,000 souls. We are informed by the same authority that not less than 22,500 persons have been vaccinated during the year 1818 in Denmark."

The author goes on to report that in a late work by Dr. Migliatta, he stated that in the previous ten years 280,038 had been vaccinated in the small kingdom of Naples, from which number he calculated 47,480 to have been spared to the population." Dr. DeCarro, the first to extend the benefits of vaccination not only to his native country but also to Asia, informed the author that "he has seen not one instance to weaken that confidence he has always maintained in vaccination — And that in the condensed population of Vienna, small-pox has occurred among such of the poor only who have, by concealment, evaded those salutary laws which enforce vaccination."[14]

Canada established the Bureau of Vaccine in Quebec in 1821, based on a grant to promote Jenner's system.[15] By 1822, vaccination had also reached the colony of Sierra Leone on the western African coast. After several years of repeated failures obtaining viable vaccine from England, Dr. Barry, surgeon to the "Forces," received a shipment in April. He immediately introduced the disease among some of the local children, "and by the speedy extension of vaccination, the progress of the small pox, which had at that period commenced its ravages in several of the Negro villages, and particularly at Hastings, has been happily arrested." Between April and early July, upwards of 2,000 persons were vaccinated within the peninsula.

Dr. Barry also sent lymph to the Isles de Loss, the Gambia and the Gold Coast, and every measure was taken to induce the natives of the interior to partake of its advantages. An article dated July 6, 1822, from the *Sierra Leone Royal Gazette* observed that the variolous disease had completely disappeared, not one instance lately having come within the writer's knowledge, who concluded, "Dr. Barry has therefore by his success, conferred a most important benefit on the Colony, for which every individual interested in the welfare of Africa must feel grateful."[16]

More honors for Dr. Jenner were to come. In 1821, a festival attended by the faculty of Berlin, together with the most eminent individuals in the kingdom, was held. At the close of the banquet, the counsellor of state, M. Hufeland, presented a list of children vaccinated in Prussia during the year 1819. The number reached upwards of 400,000.[17]

Not everyone chose to honor Jenner, however. He was refused entry into the College of Physicians, London, until he should first pass a test on the theories of Hippocrates and Galen. Jenner refused to accede to their demands, observing that his accomplishments in conquering smallpox should have qualified him for election. He was never elected to the college.[18]

Jenner returned to his home, where he maintained a letter-writing campaign, answering questions from practitioners around the world and sending quantities of cowpox matter preserved in glass tubes. On September 13, 1815, his wife, Catherine, died of tuberculosis. To occupy his mind, he devoted himself to other interests, including fossil hunting, bird watching and gardening. He became an expert at propagating fruit bushes and in 1818 introduced young grapevines from the famous stock at Hampton Court. (Interestingly, he had also had a fascination with hot air balloons from the time of the first flight of the Montgolfier brothers. Jenner's close friend Dr. Caleb Hillier Parry was one of the first people to fly a hydrogen balloon from the Crescent in Bath, on January 10, 1784. Jenner requested a length of silk and created his own balloon, launching it from Berkeley Castle on September 2, 1784.[19])

In 1817, well aware of the scarcity of cowpox from which to obtain fresh material, Jenner experimented with "equination" vaccination (taken from horse "grease") and stocks of virus from cases of horsepox were sent to the National Vaccine Establishment and widely distributed. Although the majority of vaccine still came from cowpox, horsepox vaccine was extensively and successfully employed in France, supported by the Animal Vaccine Station at Bordeaux, where it was successfully renewed from equine sources.[20]

On January 29, 1823, the London *Times* reported:

> With unfeigned sorrow we have to announce the death of our distinguished countryman, Dr. Jenner, the discoverer of vaccination. He died yesterday morning (Sunday, the 26th inst.) after a very short illness, at his house at Berkeley, in the 74th year of his age. An event so awful from its suddenness, and so impressive and mournful from the eminent qualities of him who has thus been removed from among us, demands an ampler notice than we can now give; but we cannot refrain from expressing our ardent hope, that due and ample honor will be paid to the memory of an individual, not less worthy of love for his private virtues than of esteem and admiration as one of the greatest benefactors of mankind.

The chancellor of the Exchequer promptly acknowledged the important services of Dr. Jenner, and Mr. Peel announced there was every disposition on the part of the government to have given Dr. Jenner a public funeral and a tomb in Westminster Abbey, but that the relations of the deceased wished the funeral to be private.[21]

Five months later, a meeting of Medical Gentlemen gathered at "Glocester" [*sic*] for the purpose of raising a subscription for a monument "to perpetuate the memory of that great benefactor to mankind, the late Dr. Jenner." Among letters read in praise of the physician was a communication from the medical public in America, "where his name and character were always held in the highest veneration."[22] In 1858, a statue to Dr. Jenner, executed by W.C. Marshall, was placed in Trafalgar Square.

Perhaps the greatest testimony to Dr. Jenner came from the fact that until smallpox was eradicated, smallpox vaccination was the most widespread immunization procedure in the world.[23]

Early Development of Quarantine for Contagious Fevers

By 1815, the smallpox hospital at King's Cross, established in 1746, was replaced by the London Fever Hospital, which had transferred from its original site in Gray's Inn Lane. In turn, the smallpox hospital was moved to Highgate, where it remained until 1896, when it was removed again to Clare Hall, Barnet. In 1848, when the ground was required for the Great Northern Railway, the London Fever Hospital was removed to Islington.[24]

Well aware that epidemic fevers were contagious, the "Institution for the Cure and Prevention of Contagious Fever in the Metropolis" was created in 1821. Established in London, this charity aimed to guard against the introduction of infection from abroad and to diminish the mortality of contagious malignant fevers by a speedy removal of infected persons into the House of Recovery. Paramount to the plan was purifying the apartments of patients by whitewashing and fumigation. With amazing foresight, the institution differed from the ordinary regulation of public charities by expediting admissions through the elimination of "formalities of recommendation," thus receiving patients without delay.

Second, they offered assistance beyond the walls of the hospital by reaching into the infected dwellings of the sick in an effort to preserve their families and make the rooms safe and habitable upon return. The means adopted were:

1. All poor persons and domestic servants laboring under contagious fevers residing within the metropolis and neighborhood were considered proper objects of the charity.
2. On application to the House of Recovery, the patient was to be inspected by the resident apothecary. Once an order was signed by him or a certificate obtained from any physician or surgeon that the fever was of a contagious nature, the sufferer was entitled to admission.
3. A vehicle, provided with a moveable lining, was kept at the house in which all persons admitted as patients were transferred, at the expense of the Institution.
4. Once the patient had been removed to the House of Recovery, his apartment was cleaned for the purpose of checking the disease and preventing its renewal. All infected bedclothes and apparel were purified or destroyed.

The cooperation of medical practitioners, overseers and parish officers was solicited to report cases of infectious disease. The nineteenth annual report, for 1820, stated that most contagious fevers originated where poverty created overcrowding, leading to generally small, filthy and badly ventilated apartments, thus exacerbating the physical wants and moral anxieties of inhabitants.

As it was conceded that in the congested areas of Essex Street and Whitechapel it was impossible to inculcate cleanliness, as the people had not the means, timely removal of the sick was viewed as the primary method of preventing the diffusion of disease. In that view and conceding the need for finances, all ranks of society were asked to unite in a common cause of supporting the institution, which "embraces the relief of individual suffering, and *the safety of the community at large.*"[25]

The rules set down by this charitable organization would, in various forms, be presented, debated and in some instances, adopted by cities around the world, but the issue of quarantine would never be completely resolved. Funding always remained scarce, bitter quarrels arose over the placement of such "pesthouses" (the common 19th century reference for a quarantine area, typically spelled as one word but occasionally hyphenated or broken into two words), political support peaked at times of epidemic and dissipated during lulls; and economic factors weighed heavily in favor of business, while public cooperation vacillated between compliance and disregard. Debate over "the safety of the community at large" would result in a long and arduous struggle.

Compulsory Vaccination

The Sheffield (England) wiseacres consider the right to have the small-pox one of the privileges guaranteed them under the English constitution. They have accordingly got up an indignation meeting to protest the act making vaccination compulsory.[1]

Dr. Jenner's work went on, progressing throughout the world in the hope "the small-pox would be known by name only; and every nation on earth would have cause to rejoice at this happy discovery."[2] Four recurring problems, however, remained an impediment to complete success: quantity and quality of vaccine, fear, religious intolerance to vaccination, and, last, the issue of revaccination.

In 1835, Dr. George Gregory of the College of Physicians, London, read a paper on the diminishing quality of vaccine, observing it appeared to have "lost much of its virtue from having passed through the system of too many persons," smallpox then being increasingly prevalent. He suggested that fresh matter be procured from its original source.[3] The following year, physician Edward Ballard made the same observation, suggesting new strains of cowpox be created by reintroducing the pustule matter back into cows to increase its potency.[4]

During the severe epidemic in France in 1828, the *Societe Roy de Medicine* published a report on the number of deaths from smallpox in relation to the vaccinated and nonvaccinated population:

Total population from 1 year to 30, susceptible:	*40,000 cases*
Cases of smallpox	6,020
Deaths by smallpox	1,024
Numbers protected by previous smallpox	2,000
Cases of smallpox	20
Deaths by smallpox	4
Number protected by vaccination	30,000
Cases of smallpox	2,000
Deaths by smallpox	20
Number unprotected	8,000
Cases of smallpox	4,000
Deaths by smallpox	1,000[5]

The situation had not improved by 1830, when it was reported that "owing to the hostility of the ignorant classes of the people in Paris to vaccination, it appears that the most frightful mortality is occurring from small pox in the Hospital des Enfans Malades. Nor is that the limitation of the evil; children leaving that hospital full of the variolous poison, spread the infection throughout the city."[6] There was better vaccination acceptance in Genova, as evidenced by a traveling physician who reported that of 2,000 persons who had been felled by the smallpox there was "not one that had been previously vaccinated."[7]

Nor was superstition eradicated by the introduction of vaccination. In 1830, a British officer wrote of witnessing a "Hindoo" ceremony of walking on fire. This particular instance "was in the middle of the Holy feast, and, I understood, the particular ceremony was in honour of the small pox deity, Mariamah, to whom they sacrifice a cock, before they venture into the furnace."[8]

Since its inception, the Royal Jennerian and London Vaccine Institution had been concerned with smallpox epidemics around he globe, and "the universal diffusion of the practice of Vaccination through the agency of this Institution." At their January 1828 meeting, a history of vaccination in the New World was read, beginning with the statement that before the introduction of vaccination, "100,000 Indians were destroyed by the Small Pox in one year in the single Province of Quito." This dreadful mortality was effectually abated by the work of missionaries, but their vaccine matter soon "became effete, through the excessive heat." With one-third of the infant population perishing from the disease, appeal was made to England. The Vaccine Institution responded by transmitting new supplies monthly to the Brazilian ambassador, Viscount de Itabayana, who distributed them throughout the 17 provinces of the Brazilian Empire.

The Vaccine Institution not failing in its duty to the United Kingdom, furnished a total of 658,405 charges of vaccine matter to 153,395 applicants, 54,388 of which had been dispensed in 1827.[9]

Realizing one of Dr. Jenner's fondest hopes, in 1840 the Royal Jennerian and London Vaccine Institution announced the increased facility of distributing vaccine matter among the poor throughout the United Kingdom. Although lower than the previous year, the number of persons vaccinated by the institution in London for 1839 amounted to 6,538. They also continued the spread of benefits to the colonies. By supplying vaccine virus to naval officers, eight ships bound for Australia were spared a great loss of life after a virulent epidemic of smallpox broke out. Mr. Sullivan, one of the ship's surgeons, was able to promptly inoculate the emigrants and not one died of the disease.[10]

Less fortunate were the people of Central America, where an epidemic of smallpox decimated the city of Panama in 1840, the population reportedly being reduced by upwards of 20,000 to less than one half. Almost every family in the city suffered from it, "and the inhabitants had no knowledge of any means to stop its progress."[11] The disease would strike Panama again during the second half of 1863, where reports indicated nearly one-fifth of the entire population perished from smallpox. Churches and cathedrals were without pastors, forcing victims to be buried without religious ceremony and marriages to be performed by civil authorities, consuls or by the chaplains of warships.[12]

Based on statistical returns, attention was directed toward the observation that a single vaccination did not offer a lifetime of protection. An Edinburgh newspaper of July 22, 1829, warned that as smallpox was extremely prevalent among the higher classes of society (presumably those who had previously undergone the operation), "it has now been thoroughly ascertained that the prevailing quality of vaccination wears out in seven or eight years."[13] This subject would be much debated over the following decades. Eradication of smallpox proved elusive at home and abroad, but numbers indicated an improvement.

Partial List of Disease and Casualties (London)
December 12, 1837 to December 11, 1838

Consumption	2,236	Drowned	77
Age and debility	1,826	Suicides	27
Convulsions	1,397	Worms	16
Fever (ague, scarlet, typhus)	1,340	Excessive Drinking	5
Small-Pox	788		

Four causes of death now ranked above smallpox. "Teeth" and "Executed" fell off the list; new entries included such causes as "Insanity," 210; and "Died by visitation of God," 58. A total of 19,833 persons were christened, while 18,266 were buried.[14]

With public and professional awareness acutely high in the United Kingdom, efforts were finally successful in creating what was to be the first vaccination act, passed in 1840:

Vaccination Act of 1840

1. Acknowledging the dangers of variolation, the law made the operation illegal.
2. Vaccination was offered free of charge.

At this point, the vaccination of children remained optional, with enough reports of sudden death to frighten parents. In 1843, for instance, an inquest was made into the death of a three-year-old child who had been taken to the London Hospital to be vaccinated. After the vaccine was introduced in the usual way into both arms, the child sickened and died within a two-minute span. A postmortem revealed distension of the vessels of the brain, "the probable result of nervous excitement, jointly caused by vaccination and teething." Verdict: Natural death.[15]

By 1845, a frightful increase of smallpox appeared in England, requiring a more thorough legislative look at how to prevent further epidemics. The Vaccine Institution attributed the outbreak to the inefficiency of the Vaccination Act, "as, through the ignorance of many practitioners, vaccine matter was used which was not pure, thus rendering the patient, by it being inoperative, liable to the attack of the small-pox." To prove their point, the report stated that one medical gentleman used vaccine matter that had lost its virtue on account of being carried in his pocket, thus causing it to decompose.[16]

The incidence of smallpox in 1845 led the Royal Jennerian and London Vaccine Institution to report that during the past year, there had been an increase in the number of persons vaccinated over all preceding years:

Year	Number Vaccinated
1843–1844	5,889
1844–1845	6,717

The jump was attributed to "the high and increasing estimation in which the institution was held."[17]

In 1844, a table of smallpox deaths revealed:

Years of Age	Died
0–5	6,926
10–30	1,013
40–70	117
75–95	16[18]

This bore out statistics that smallpox killed the very young at alarming rates while indicating more work needed to be done by the medical community. In the second week of June 1848, death from smallpox (nearly all of them children) was twice the normal number. Fifteen of the number had never been vaccinated — a sin chargeable to the parents, since the poorest were offered vaccination free of charge.[19]

Partial List of Disease and Casualties (London)
January 8, 1848 to December 30, 1848

Zymotic diseases (epidemic and contagious)	18,117
Tubercular diseases	9,253
Lung diseases	7,892
Diseases of the brain and nerves	6,121
Dropsy, cancer	2,257
Age	2,148
Violence, privation and intemperance	1,713
Heart disease	1,691

The weekly average of deaths for this time period was 1,113, or 159 per day, or 6.6 per hour. The fewest deaths occurred from April to July; July was the worst month for epidemic diseases. Total deaths for the year were 57,899, of which 29,550 were males. Total births for the same period were 71,003, of which 36,131 were males. Broken down by age, the statistics follow:

Age	Number of Deaths
0–15 years	28,423
15–60	18,663
60 and up	10,385

The average age at which the gentry died in Liverpool was given as 43.[20]

By 1850, current thinking dictated that a child should be vaccinated within the first few months of life, but at puberty, when the system underwent a change, revaccination was considered necessary.[21] During the decade of the 1850s, the concept of revaccination received considerable attention. An investigation of many thousands of cases led to the following conclusions:

1. The protective power of vaccination was absolute and general for the first 5–6 years, up to the 12th year.
2. After this, a number of vaccinated persons become "liable" to contract smallpox.
3. The greater number of those vaccinated probably remain completely protected during their entire lives.

Statistics from European committees investigating the matter determined that children were seldom attacked with smallpox before the 9th year after vaccination; and smallpox attacked, in preference, persons who had been vaccinated 15, 20, 30 and even 35 years previously. The general consensus held that in ordinary times, revaccination should be practiced after 14 years, but sooner during an epidemic. The Academy of Medicine at Paris stated, "Re-vaccination is the only method of proof which science possesses of distinguishing persons who have been definitely protected by vaccination from those who are only so in various degrees." Dr. Condie of Philadelphia added his concurrence, stating, "The facts upon record afford conclusive evidence of the necessity and importance of re-vaccination, in all cases in which persons are liable to be exposed to the infection of small pox."

Equally pertinent was the question of whether vaccine communicated other diseases. On this point, it was widely held that matter taken from patients suffering from scrofula, itch or related afflictions caused these diseases in those receiving the vaccine. To put the theory to the test, the French physician M. Tanpin vaccinated a large number of patients at the Children's Hospital in Paris with virus taken from various subjects affected with itch, scarlatina, varioloid and variola, scrofula, tubercles and chronic eruption. In no cases were the preexisting diseases transmitted to the vaccine recipients. It was noted, however, that in persons in whom these diseases had lain dormant it was possible to awaken them, "but for this virus cannot be blamed." That noted, it was concluded that a physician would scarcely be justified in using virus from a diseased person.[22]

By 1853, a regard for public welfare in England dictated that a "Vaccination Extension Bill" be introduced, and on April 12, 1853, Lord Lyttheton presented it for consideration. The data used was based upon a study entitled "Report on the State of Smallpox in England and Wales and other Countries and on Compulsory Vaccination," issued by the Epidemiological Society, among whom were Sir Benjamin Brodie, Dr. Bright and Dr. Southwood Smith. Also participating were J.F. Marson, physician to the London Smallpox Hospital, and Edward C. Seaton. The report was forwarded to the Home secretary who ordered it printed by the House of Lords on June 27.[23]

The primary difference between the Vaccination Extension Bill and previous legislation centered on the concept of compulsory vaccination. Sir John Pakington of the House of Lords spoke for the necessity of the new act. "The object was to prevent a fearful disease by timely foresight and precaution, and the classes most in need of this protection were the poorest and most ignorant — those least likely, by their own impulse, to adopt precautions."

Sir G. Strickland objected to the compulsory principal. The best course, in his opinion, was to allow vaccination to be voluntary, "and education would in a short time overcome prejudice."[24] Further debate followed. The *Medical Times and Gazette* stated that the proportion of deaths from smallpox in London was three times, and in Glasgow, six times what it was in Brussels, Berlin, or Copenhagen. Of each thousand persons who died in England and Wales, 22 were from smallpox; in Ireland, the ratio was 1,000 to 49, while in Lombardy, where vaccination was required, the ratio was 1,000 to 2.[25] With those statistics at hand, the act was made into law. The Vaccination Act of 1853 required:

1. That every child, whose health permits, be vaccinated within three, or in the case of orphanage, within four months of birth, by the public vaccinator of the district, or by some other medical practitioner;
2. That notice of this requirement, and information as to the local arrangements for public vaccination, shall, whenever a birth is registered, be given by the registrar of births to the parents or guardians of the child;
3. That every medical practitioner who, whether in public or private practice, successfully vaccinates a child shall send to the local registrar of births a certificate that he has done so; and the registrar shall keep a minute of all the notices given, and an account of all the certificates thus received;
4. That parents or guardians who, without sufficient reason, after having duly received the registrar's notice of the requirement of Vaccination, either omit to have a child duly vaccinated, or, this being done, omit to have it inspected as to the results of Vaccination, shall be liable to a penalty of £1; and all penalties shall be recoverable under Jervis's Act, and shall be paid toward the local poor-rate.[26]

Although the act of 1853 was, to a considerable extent, experimental, and "largely imperfect in its provisions," Seaton, in his 1875 report, "The Recent Epidemic of Smallpox in the United Kingdom, in Its Relation to Vaccination and the Vaccination Laws," cited evidence of its overall effectiveness. During the year after the enactment of the 1853 law, the number of infantile vaccinations more than doubled, with over 300,000 vaccinations over the age of 1 year also performed.[27]

The idea of compulsory vaccination did not sit well with everyone. In a series of letters ignored by the *Critic* but published in the *London Nonconformist*, August 30, 1854, the author of a pamphlet entitled "Our Medical Liberties" defended his position as an anti-vaccinationist by accusing defenders, including the Epidemiological Society, of collecting data "with a determination to find matter to support a foregone conclusion." He reasserted that many persons were manifestly unsusceptible to smallpox; that not every case was a "centre of contagion," nor was every unvaccinated or imperfectly vaccinated person "a nidus for the disease."

The writer further argued that "frequent" cases of death from smallpox occurred among the vaccinated, compulsory vaccinators flew to a practice "as deceitful as it is disgusting," and the entire act usurped the rights of individuals. From the following tables, he drew the conclusion that mortality was higher in "lands compulsorily protected (?) [*sic*] by vaccination."

Mortality from All Causes in Various Parts of Great Britain and Ireland, Vaccination Being Voluntary

Town or Country	Year	Population	Deaths from All Causes	Deaths per Thousand
London	1851	2,373,799	55,254	23.3
England and Wales	"	17,922,768	395,933	22
Liverpool	1850	258,236	7,500	29
Manchester	"	228,433	6,680	29
Dublin	1851	258,361	6,931	26.8
Cork	"	85,745	2,002	23.3

Mortality from All Causes in Various Parts of the Austrian Empire, Vaccination Being Compulsory

Town or Country	Year	Population	Deaths from All Causes	Deaths per Thousand
Lower Austria	1850	1,538,047	54,970	35.7
Upper Austria	"	852,323	23,646	27.7
Styria	"	1,006,971	30,534	30.3
Illyria	"	738,180	34,630	44.2
Bohemia	"	4,409,900	170,432	38.6
Silesia	"	438,586	12,123	27.4
Lombardy	"	2,725,740	92,550	33.9
Venice	"	2,281,732	76,150	33.3
Military Frontiers (without the Boroughs)	"	1,009,109	44,610	44.2

As with those he criticized, the author neglected to make any direct correlation of deaths to the prevalence of smallpox outbreaks or to other causes/diseases/sanitation issues that might have accounted for the discrepancies.

Two years after the initiation of the second act, the Royal Jennerian Society gave the legislative effort poor grades, deprecating what it considered interference by stating the vaccine could be spread only "by the conviction of its excellence," meaning that no government "could give the supervision necessary to ensure a continuance of genuine vaccine; that such supervision can only be secured by the agency of the voluntary effort of those engaged by their duty and by their necessity to present the public with a pure vaccine." In other words, they felt physicians, by training and integrity, were better able to police themselves and the entire vaccination operation than if the process were to be controlled by government regulation. The report added that all the good generated by the Society had been done by voluntary contributions at an expense of under £250, but that considering the smallness of the sum, it still "laboured under a debt."[28]

A year later, the idea of compulsory vaccination was revisited, this time in an expanded version. The new "Vaccination Bill" proposed to widen the scope of the Act of 1853:

The Proposed Vaccination Act of 1856

1. All persons under the age of 13 years, as well as all emigrants and crews of emigrant ships were required to be vaccinated.
2. All scholars in schools receiving aid from government grants, and all inmates of workhouses, lunatic asylums, and prisons were to be vaccinated.
3. Provision was made for appointing public vaccinators and vaccination establishments. All vaccinators were to be furnished with a proper license to perform vaccination. The fee for vaccinators would increase from 1s 6d to 2s 6d.
4. In the case of the infection not taking, the process was to be repeated again and again, at stated intervals, until it did, or until the public vaccinator gave a "certificate of insusceptibility to vaccine disease, which would be available for a twelvemonth only" after which the same round of vaccination and revaccination was to be repeated.
5. Penalty for "refusing or neglecting to comply with any requirement of this act" was 20 shillings, with 5 shillings a day additional after notice.
6. In the case of death from smallpox of persons under 13 years of age, a coroner's inquest was to be held, and was to inquire whether the provisions of the act had been complied with. In case they had not been, the guardians of the poor would be instructed to enforce the penalties against the parents.
7. Whenever smallpox was prevalent in any part of England, regulations were to be issued to restrain its progress "by re-vaccination or otherwise," with a penalty for resisting their authority set at 5*l* (pounds).[29]

Unfortunately, the bill aroused public and private sentiment not only against the proposed act, but also in opposition to compulsory vaccination and in some cases, arguments against the efficacy of smallpox vaccination altogether. Editorials argued that sanitary legislation was being carried too far when it unnecessarily "infringed upon the liberty of the subject in his individual character, and domestic relations, and invests the healing process with the terrors of penal obligation."

Those disputing the act claimed that "vaccination tends both to the moral and physical deterioration of the human race ... checking the free elimination of the humours of the human body [by propagating] all sorts of hereditary and accidental diseases formed in the various subjects through which the lymph [pustule matter] passes." While these arguments might be in dispute, it was considered a pity that, except in the face of a very strong and pressing necessity, individual feelings should be violated and parental authority and responsibility superceded.[30]

Before a second reading of the Vaccination Bill in the House of Commons, it was agreed by lawmakers that all eminent medical men believed that vaccination, when properly performed, "was a guarantee, generally speaking, against small-pox." Legislators summarized that the first year after its introduction into England, deaths by smallpox were reduced from 16,000 to 6,338 and deaths in 1856 were calculated annually to be 5,000–6,000. The argument was made, however, that deaths in the United Kingdom were more numerous than in continental countries in which the system of vaccination was more completely carried into effect. (Over the course of the next several decades, this fact was often used against vaccination in the United Kingdom, frequently with little or no follow-up as to why it was true or providing any serious public investigation into the superior techniques adopted in France and other nations.)

Further arguments against the proposed law came from parents who claimed eruptions had broken out on their children after they had been vaccinated. Despite the fact that this likely stemmed from incompetent administrators, it was questioned how more skillful men might be solicited to work for a "paltry fee of 1s 6d." Dr. Mitchell stated the people of England would not tolerate the measure as written and believed the bill was "nothing but a scheme to keep up the Medical Board of Health." (In fact, the law was not to be under the auspices of the Medical Board of Health.) Even more disturbing, Dr. George Gregory (College of Physicians) who, for 50 years had superintendence of the Small-pox Hospital, doubted the usefulness of vaccination, claiming it "very often produced death."

Edward Miall, echoing the sentiments of the Jennerian Society, where he stood as chair, likewise argued against the bill, but on very different grounds. He believed vaccination was a most useful prophylactic, but "making it compulsory had led to a carelessness in its use, resulting in a deterioration in the lymph used and in consequence, an increase in deaths from smallpox." If the principal of the proposed law were to be carried out, he concluded, "we should be having a department set up for the purpose of inquiring into the health of every person every morning, and of prescribing what medicine he should take during the day."[31] The unfortunate exaggeration elicited laughter. The bill did not pass. Pitting the idea of public welfare and government regulations against individual determination continues to be played out on large stages to this day. The predominance of one argument over the other tends to be cyclic.

The Royal Jennerian Institution continued to speak out against compulsory vaccination, reiterating their belief that "vaccination being a good, will spread of its own goodness." They criticized hasty legislation that created "interested parties" performing services for payment rather than "wise benevolence," and pressed for a repeal of the Act of 1853. To promote their beliefs, they asked for a commission to vaccinate six children each, then have them exposed to the disease at the Small-Pox Hospital. When the children proved immune, the fact, widely diffused throughout Great Britain and Ireland, was suggested to do more good than any act of Parliament.[32]

While arguments continued, an interesting article appeared in the *Medical Times* (1858), recounting a discovery by Professor Beka. He stated that since 1856 he had vaccinated hundreds of children by first placing the vaccine on the tip of a magnetized needle. A single magnetization served for many vaccinations, greatly increasing the rapidity with which the vaccine was absorbed. By this technique, he had scarcely any failures.[33] During the same decade, Nelaton of Paris revived the old practice of drawing into *naevi materni* (body of matter) threads saturated with vaccine virus. The thread was introduced into the tumor through the skin, enclosed in a cannula to prevent the virus from catching on the skin.[34]

No matter the technique, Dr. Greenhow's report to the board of health reaffirmed that smallpox was avoidable, affirming his belief that "if vaccination were universally performed in the best-known manner, deaths by smallpox would be among the rarest entries in the register."[35]

Dr. Letheby's report in 1863 stated that 36 percent of nonvaccinated persons died after contracting the disease. He reaffirmed that mortality was entirely dependent on the original vaccination, offering specific guidelines by which to assert the efficacy of the operation. If one cicatrix (scar) remained on the arm, deaths from smallpox were 7.57 percent; two scars lowered mortality to 4.13 percent; three scars resulted in a 1.15 percent chance of dying and if there were four scars or more, not one in one hundred died, mortality being 0.74 percent.[36]

Nonvaccination and improper technique (failure to use active lymph or contamination with smallpox matter) continued to add to mortality statistics, as the table for 1858–1859 revealed:

The Causes of Death in England
Partial List from the Registrar-General's Report for 1858

Zymotic diseases (epidemic and contagious)	90,414
(In the ratio of 22 in every 100)	
Tubercular diseases	65,762
Pulmonary diseases	58,320
Cardiac diseases	14,784
Smallpox (separate from zymotic diseases)	nearly 4,000
(an increase of 1,659 from previous year)	
Drowning (exclusive of cases at sea)	2,807
Poison	428

Deaths from smallpox were explained by imperfections of the Vaccination Act and the want of a more compulsory system.[37] Further research presented by Dr. Moore of Dublin, entitled "Statistics of Small-pox and Vaccination in the United Kingdom," revealed that, according to the Registrar's Report ending December 1858, there were 376,798 vaccination certificates, although they registered the births of 655,697 children. He set down the deaths in England and Wales for smallpox annually at 4,000, of which 3,990 could have been saved by vaccination.[38]

Statistics from around the world also supported vaccination. Dr. Simon, physician to the board of health, Birmingham, England, provided a history of its adoption in various countries. In Sweden, deaths from smallpox before vaccination was introduced averaged 2,050 annually to each million of the population; by 1857, deaths had decreased to 158 per annum. In Westphalia, deaths decreased from 2,643 to 114, and in Bohemia, Moravia and Austrian Silesia, from 4,000 to 200.

Dr. Simon calculated that during the 18th century, the yearly smallpox death rate of London ranged from 3,000 to 5,000. For the years 1841–1853, the average death rate from smallpox was only 304; in 1854, only 149; and in 1855, only 132. The same decreases held true for the English army and navy. In a paper attached to Dr. Simon's report written by Dr. Balfour, it was determined that after vaccination, mortality in the navy was not a third and in the army not a fourth of the London rates. At the Royal Military Asylum during the previous 48 years, only 4 deaths from smallpox occurred among 5,774 boys, and those children were unvaccinated. These reports were substantiated by 359 of the most eminent physicians and surgeons in the United Kingdom.[39]

The thesis "Vaccination," read to the graduating class of Harvard, 1860, by Frank D. Beers of Charlestown, Prince Edward Island, gave supporting statistics for the procedure. He stated that smallpox in Copenhagen was an eleventh of what it had been before vaccination; in Sweden, a little over 13 percent; in Berlin and large parts of Austria, a twentieth, and in Westphalia, the occurrence of the disease was only 25 percent. From observations made for 21 years on 40,000 persons in Bohemia, death for those vaccinated, if they happened to catch smallpox, was calculated to be 5½ to 100, but the risk of death to nonvaccinated persons contracting smallpox occurred at the rate of 29⅘ for every 100 patients. Concurrent testimony from London, Vienna and Milan demonstrated that out of nearly 26,000 cases, if a previously vaccinated person contracted smallpox it was but ⅕–⅙ as dangerous as the natural disease. As to the suggestion that re-vaccination was necessary, "if it confers no benefit, at all events does no harm."[40]

To put a face to the dry numbers, a case was reported of a poor woman working hard to keep her family from the workhouse. Her husband had lost the use of his legs and required nursing and attendance. Her daughter was "modest and industrious," while her 16-year-old son was just starting to be of assistance to the family. Unfortunately, he contracted smallpox; his mother applied for and obtained an order for the parish doctor to visit the youth.

The physician attended the boy and demanded why he had not been admitted to the Smallpox Hospital. She replied that she did not know how to set about it "and timidly requested some information as to how she was to get him there." He replied, "The best way you can," and departed. As the parent had no patronage to bestow or fee to give, the parish doctor announced that he would return in three days to pronounce the boy dead. Unable to accept the news, the mother begged a neighboring surgeon to examine him. Finding that the spark of life yet burned, he treated the patient on a daily basis and sent medicine. Ultimately, the boy survived and eventually returned to work.

The article concluded, "We have no reason to doubt our correspondent, but if his statement is true, the attention of the Poor Law Board ought to be drawn to the fact. We are well aware that the life of a parish doctor is one of continual worry and discomfort, but when a professional man seeks and obtains an appointment of trust, it is generally understood that he will carry out his duties in a manner creditable to a christian [sic] and a gentleman."[41] Perhaps the editor suspected the feel-good story was too good to be true; nevertheless, it poses a slice of life of the impoverished of 19th century England — one as grim as it was tragic.

In a separate case demonstrating unqualified practitioners, a coroner's jury investigated the death of a 13-year-old named Anne M'Carthy, who died after being treated by a chemist for measles. Their verdict read, "That the deceased child not having been vaccinated died from small pox; and the jury censures the parents for not having the deceased to be vaccinated, in accordance with the terms of the act of parliament, and also for not having taken the deceased when ill to a medical man instead of to a chemist."[42] Being censured had little effect on the overall numbers seeking vaccination. Nor were pecuniary measures effective. In 1865, although fined 15 shillings for refusing to have his child vaccinated, Dr. Spencer Hall remained obstinate, citing his own bad experience with the operation.[43]

In light of this, a comparison of deaths in London and the United States are chilling. In 1861, the *New York Times* published a report indicating that a mortality of 40 persons to 1,000 was present in the larger American cities, noting that the numbers were "a very great excess; it is little short of murder, indeed!" The statistics for London were strikingly lower. In the first half of 1861, the number of deaths were 16:1000. In both examples, nearly half of those who perished were children under the age of five years.[44]

Reworking the Laws

Containing and ultimately eliminating deaths from smallpox continued to be a priority of the British government.

THE VACCINATION AMENDMENT ACT OF 1861

Failing to widen the Act of 1853, Parliament addressed the issue again in the Vaccination Amendment Act of 1861. Just as they had eight years earlier, proponents faced an uphill battle. This time, however, a formidable enemy appeared from the liberal ranks of the House of Commons: Mr. T. Duncombe. Taking the offense against Duncombe, an editorialist for the *Penny Newsman and Sunday Morning Mail and Telegraph* of July 14, 1861, written entirely in italics, proclaimed, "The political and the medical opinions expressed by Mr. Duncombe equally astonish us." The writer not only deprecated compulsory legislation "on the ridiculously strained plea that it is an act of indefensible tyranny to compel a parent to have a harmless operation performed which increases the chances of the life of his child, and prevents that child becoming a contamination to the country," he also expressed doubts contrary to every principal of public policy and opposed all medical men on efficacy of the preventive.

On one subject the newspaper did agree: the notorious use of lymph matter less than requisite strength, and in many cases, over forty years old. The cure, the protagonist argued, was "simple in the extreme." Britain should copy the example of France, where a government establishment kept cows suffering from the pock. Large draughts of the virus were annually made from them and circulated throughout the country, "fresh, strong, and healthy" (see chapter 23 for a discussion of "Vaccination Farms").

During debate in the House, Mr. Lowe countered Duncombe's objections by citing the number of deaths in Great Britain from smallpox:

Year	Deaths
1856	2,227
1857	3,336
1858	6,460
1859	3,840

Further discussions centered on proposed amendments, the first relative to costs. It was suggested that payment for vaccination be taken from the common fund of the union rather than paid out of parish funds. This was rejected by a vote of 70 to 44. Next, Duncombe objected to parents being held responsible until their children reached their majority; he proposed a limit of between three to five years. Mr. Lowe did not feel a parent became more entitled to a consideration because he had neglected his duty for a great number of years. The clause was agreed to. The third proposal dealt with a payment to informers. Mr. Henley objected, stating he could not conceive a greater curse than such a practice. The wording was struck from the clause.[45]

12

The Health and Well-Being
of the General Populace

We are concerned to state, that this alarming disease is at present in Tarborough,
and that it has been introduced there by the very means taken to prevent it.[1]

The move to promote vaccine institutions in the United States originated from a
very early period in the nation's history. As mentioned in chapter 8, Dr. Benjamin Waterhouse began his efforts in Boston but was rebuffed by the medical elite. In 1802, the
New York Kine-Pock Institution was formed during a gathering of physicians at the
Tontine Coffee-House and operated out of a Lower East Side apartment before being
absorbed by the New York Public Dispensary.[2] Dr. James Smith, a contemporary of Waterhouse, established a vaccine institution in Baltimore with better success and far-reaching
effects.

In the summer of 1800, Dr. John Crawford was one of two early inoculators in Baltimore. The following year, Dr. Smith, attending physician at the Baltimore Alms House,
received cowpox matter from an American merchant who had obtained it in Europe.[3] Smith
immediately recognized its significance and began vaccinating in the spring of 1801. Like
Waterhouse, he performed the operation on his two sons and members of his family as
proof of his faith in the procedure and as a test of its efficacy. Unlike Waterhouse's reception
from the medical community, "the profession of Baltimore, including almost the entire faculty, gave public and early expression of their approval."[4] As testimony to the high regard
in which he was held, the mayor appointed Smith to the Committee of Physicians in 1822
during a threatened smallpox epidemic.

Smith was fortunate in his choice of residence, as the citizens of Baltimore were leaders
in medical innovation and public health. Their support helped propel him into the public
eye at a time when acceptance of vaccination was far from established in the fledgling nation.
Skeptical authorities continued testing the new procedure. Similar to those in Boston in
1802, an experiment at Randolph, Vermont, exposed 75 inoculated persons to pustules of
smallpox victims; not one was found to be susceptible to the disease. Not content with the
results, the authorities subjected an infant to kine-pox vaccination and its mother to smallpox. She developed the disease but continued to suckle the baby. The child survived as
though it had not been nursed by a mother suffering from the disease.[5]

It became Crawford and Smith's dream to create an arena by which the technique of
vaccination could be performed. More important, their goal was to maintain an unadul-
terated supply of vaccine that could not only be used for the people of Baltimore but also
shipped throughout the country for vaccine inoculation. They created the Vaccine Institution

in Baltimore in 1802, the same year such an institution was founded in New York City, making these two municipalities the only ones with such forethought.

The importance of preserving a large supply of pure, viable lymph was obvious to those espousing the cause of vaccination. It was discovered very early in the era of vaccination that improperly obtained matter offered the veneer of protection rather than actual immunity. Believing they were safe, individuals later exposed to the disease often contracted smallpox. (This became one of the main arguments used by antivaccinationists.) Second, little care was taken by uninformed physicians when performing the arm-to-arm transfer; without obtaining an accurate history and physical of the donor, it was believed doctors inadvertently passed along communicable diseases such as syphilis to the recipient. Third, improperly preserved smallpox matter often became weak and ineffective when sent through the mail, the most common method of distribution. In any case, matter did not retain efficacy longer than several months, making fresh supplies an absolute requisite.

In 1803, when King Charles IV of Spain desired to introduce vaccination into his colonies, it was felt the best way to maintain a fresh supply was to keep the smallpox virus alive by introducing it into pairs of children during the voyage. By staggering the inoculations, it was hoped by the time they reached their destination at least two boys would have fresh pustules from which to take lymph.

It is almost inexplicable that the technique of maintaining a fresh

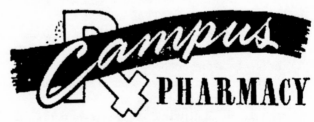
This Historical Medical Highlight pictures a cow (where Dr. Jenner first obtained his cowpox matter), a syringe for vaccination and a dairymaid, who was instrumental in Jenner's first studies. To reassure the public, the Campus RX Pharmacy reassured its customers that it supplied scientifically prepared vaccines, serums and biological preparations (from the *Greeley Daily Tribune* [CO], June 1, 1951).

supply of cowpox virus by propagating the disease among cows did not become a major source of lymph for nearly two-thirds of the 19th century. Instead, physicians relied almost exclusively on taking live virus from infected people. One reason would seem to be the popular sentiment against injecting animal disease directly into humans. The visualization of two-headed men or people depicted with deformities resulting from such transfers was common fodder for satirists and political cartoonists of the age. The National Vaccine Establishment in England also adopted a tone of almost paternalistic defense of Dr. Jenner's original stock of vaccine matter taken from milkmaids, defeating efforts in 1839 to extract vaccine directly from the cow. (See a discussion of the degeneration of vaccine matter in chapter 13.)

More pointedly, during epidemics when matter was scarce, the medical community often resorted to variolation, injecting live smallpox into patients in the hope of inducing a mild case of the disease. This was particularly evident in the western territories of the United States when repeated calls for vaccine went unanswered, forcing physicians to adopt variolation as the only means available to protect individuals. Less excusable was the abandonment of vaccination by some practitioners during the Tarboro Incident of 1821–1822, when the efficacy of the procedure was brought into question (see below).

Although most enlightened nations punished such inoculators with the severest penalties by the second decade of 1800 (except Great Britain, where it was a misdemeanor until 1840, when inoculation was outlawed), engrafting was practiced in the United States far into the 19th century.

Dr. James Smith and His Appeal to the States

The solution to all these problems was the national vaccine center that Smith and Crawford envisioned. There was already talk of such establishments in England and France; by 1808, England created the National Vaccine Establishment, assuming control from local municipalities and providing supplies of uncontaminated vaccine. The concept was also adopted in France, where vaccination was attributed to increasing the life expectancy of its citizens from 23 to 38 years for men and from 27 to 41 years for women, this occurring between the years of 1795 and 1817.

In fact, precedence had already been established in the United States, albeit on a small scale. In July 1809, when smallpox struck Boston, the neighboring town of Milton organized the first government-sponsored vaccination clinic. Charged only 25 cents, 337 people (one quarter of the town) were vaccinated in three days. Milton's selectmen were so successful that fourteen adjacent towns followed suit. Realizing that vaccination on a wider scale was required, in January 1810 the selectmen petitioned the governor and legislature of Massachusetts for funds to establish a statewide vaccination program that included a mandate for local municipalities to provide vaccination clinics. In what would become a repeating pattern, evidenced on both state and federal levels, the electorate of Massachusetts passed an act sanctioning vaccination as an accepted means of personal protection, granted permission for towns to raise money, but refused to allocate state funds for the purpose.[6]

The same year the Milton selectmen were establishing their clinic in Massachusetts, James Smith sought to widen the scope of his Baltimore vaccination institution by approaching the legislatures of Maryland, Pennsylvania and Virginia. In return for providing free vaccine throughout their states, he asked a $1,000 allotment. The request passed the Maryland house but was rejected in the senate as too expensive.[7] In the next session, Smith expanded his time frame, asking $1,000 for three years but adding a request enabling him to operate a lottery to raise money for his institution. Direct funds from the state treasury were again denied, but Dr. Smith did receive the lottery privilege, allowing him to operate a $30,000 game of chance. (In contemporary numbers this would equate to roughly $300,000.)[8] The money raised was expected to cover the cost of free vaccination in Maryland for six years, whether or not the lottery raised the anticipated funds.

In colonial America and the early years of the republic, lotteries were common means by which states and licensed individuals raised money. George Washington, Benjamin Franklin, John Hancock and other important figures sponsored the idea of using lotteries to support public institutions. Their success, so closely tied to patriotism that it was almost a civic duty to buy a chance, helped establish Harvard, Yale and Princeton universities. Commonly referred to as a "scheme," the lotteries typically offered one large prize and numerous small ones. An example from 1828 for the Union Canal lured buyers to take a chance on one top prize of $10,000; on the low end of the scale, 4446 winners would receive $5.[9]

The right to run such a scheme was not easily obtained and Smith's privilege was quite a coup for him. Had it achieved the sum anticipated, the ultimate outcome of the Vaccine Institution would have been significantly altered. As it was, during the same session, the Maryland legislators authorized a $100,000 lottery to raise money for the Washington Monument, with a greater top prize.[10] Nearly desperate to make his lottery succeed, Smith was forced to mortgage his own property to insure the scheme and eventually gained $12,797.20 to put toward his work.

In 1809, the same year he approached Maryland, Smith traveled to Lancaster, Pennsylvania, initially seeking only to sell his lottery tickets in that state[11] but then expanding his request by asking for an annual $1,000 to disperse free vaccination in the commonwealth. A committee reported on the petition:

> [S]hall we refuse to supply our citizens, with the simple, cheap and invaluable means of preservation, from a most loathsome and destructive disease?... [N]othing else seems to be necessary than a supply of pure and genuine Vaccine Matter.... Dr. Smith's plan appears to be the most competent, to attain the great object of a general security from Small Pox, of any which has been yet suggested.[12]

Several plans were discussed, but after passing in the house, every proposal was defeated in the senate, 14 to 12. The plan for widening the scope of his institution also failed in North Carolina, although private citizens did petition the state government to enter into a contract with the Baltimore doctor, paying his costs to distribute free vaccine to citizens of the state. Sadly, Smith received the all-too-familiar rejection that, "taking into consideration the low state of our financial affairs," it was deemed impossible to spend public funds in that manner.[13]

The Commonwealth of Virginia took a different approach. In 1813, the governing body agreed to provide Dr. Smith $600 a year for the same proposal offered in Maryland, Pennsylvania and North Carolina, making it the only state willing to expend government money. Unfortunately, the stipulation that Smith present himself in Richmond every six months to collect a $300 payment and once a year to renew his contract proved onerous. Over the next four years, he missed several appointments, apparently not able to collect back payments on his next visit; by 1818, Smith abandoned the project, having received only $1,500 for his efforts.[14]

It is clear from a study of Smith's efforts that in the first twenty years of 1800 the value of vaccination in America was not in question. Despite the fact there were naysayers in the United States and Great Britain, state governments unanimously agreed that vaccination was tantamount to public good and would save countless lives. In every case except Virginia, his offer to supply gratuitous vaccine was rejected on the sole merit of money, and even that state placed prohibitive restrictions on his collection of revenue.

In his thesis, "Missed Opportunities," Rohit Singla offers a depressing analysis of why state governments, by and large, refused to allocate funds for vaccine, even though the finances requested were extremely low when balanced against overwhelming public welfare. He argued that "no special interest group was favored; no interest group was willing to trade votes or elections funds for an appropriation. There were no drug companies who might benefit from quality controls on vaccine or subsidies for vaccine production. It is even possible, that such legislation was against the interests of physicians. Only Dr. Smith was specifically interested in subsidies for vaccination, and he did not have the resources to offer the state legislatures any inducements. He was not even a resident of most of the states concerned." The observation is damning. But for a too brief period, not without its own nasty controversies, the federal government stepped up to take its place as a protector of the poor and the needy.

The (National) Vaccine Institution

Dr. James Smith's long and lonely journey to promote vaccination would take him from relative obscurity to the national stage and then nearly destroy him. His story is representative not only of one individual heroically attempting to alter the course of a deadly disease but also one of politics, constitutional interpretation, the power of special interests, economics, the perceptions of medicine in the 19th century and, tragically, human error.

Smith's goal was both altruistic and noble: he wished to provide all Americans a ready source of uncontaminated smallpox vaccine, free of charge. A firm believer that a well-informed person was just as capable as a physician of administering the vaccine, he envisioned a center where a ready supply of matter could be drawn upon and mailed to anyone requesting it; to reach a wider audience, he advocated a staff traveling across the country, distributing vaccine and vaccinating people by the thousands. If he were to succeed, it was not improbable that the dread scourge of smallpox could be eradicated in the country and ultimately around the world. In addition, he claimed that by tracing the requests for vaccine he could follow the progress of the disease and respond proactively by mailing lymph to postmasters in the areas of spreading disease.[15] The pity is, given continued support and financial aid from the Congress, he might have done all he proposed and more.

During repeated failures to negotiate on the state level he was prompted to seek authorization from the federal government. His efforts initiated what became the first federal involvement in overall public health. Prior to this, the only time the federal government had intervened in public health was by establishing rules protecting seamen. In 1798, the Marine Hospital System was created to collect a nominal sum from the wages of sailors. This money went into a general fund for establishing and operating hospitals providing them free care. The Marine Hospital Act was extended in 1802, requiring captains of rafts and barges working the Mississippi to collect fees from their crews, thus entitling them to the free health care at the marine hospitals. The Act of 1798 was extended again in 1830 to include steamboat crews along the interior waterways, and in 1837 Congress provided funds for a number of new seamen's hospitals.[16]

The most obvious benefit to a national Vaccine Institution was the power and authority of the federal government. This prestige granted immediate widespread respectability and trust, something individual physicians or even state-run operations lacked.

Another persuasive argument dealt with the need for a constant and adequate supply of vaccine matter. Since epidemics were impossible to predict, large quantities of vaccine were required at any given moment. Maintaining this supply was expensive and could not be operated on a profit-driven basis unless vaccination was made mandatory. In that case, lymph would be required year-round, supplying distributors with an ever-present market. The political climate in the early years of the republic would not permit the levying of such a law impinging on personal freedom, although the same argument was presented in England and overcome on the grounds of national welfare. It could also be argued that the federal government did not have the means or the structure to enforce a mandatory vaccination act.

In periods between epidemics, Americans tended to ignore the threat of smallpox, creating low demand for vaccine. When the disease struck, the high demand would not be great enough to cover losses accrued during lean years. As discussed in his paper, "Missed Opportunities: The Vaccine Act of 1813," Rohit K. Singla argues that "private enterprises would face perverse incentives to maximize business by ensuring that smallpox remained epidemic. The extermination of smallpox would obviously not be in the best interest of a profit-maximizing vaccine provider ... [who] would want regular epidemics to encourage the sale of vaccine."

In 1811, Dr. Smith solicited Congress for assistance in establishing vaccination in the District of Columbia. His petition was referred to a select committee on January 30 but never acted upon. Undeterred, the following year he lobbied Congress for an appointment as the country's "National Vaccine Agent," presenting petitions from people in Pennsylvania and Virginia espousing his cause. (Interestingly, the petitions were printed with a blank space where the name of the state would be inserted, indicating Smith hoped to add petitions from many states.) The petitions were passed to the House Committee on Post Offices and Post Roads on January 14, 1813. Smith followed this by sending a letter to the committee, promising to provide vaccine free of charge if he were granted a franking privilege (the ability to send mail without charge) and a small annual stipend for operating costs. Asking nothing for himself (well aware of how scarce money was during the War of 1812), he volunteered to maintain a continuous supply of genuine vaccine and regularly test its efficacy

Without established precedent and little adversity, Congress passed the Vaccine Act of 1813. Endorsed and signed by President Madison on February 27, barely a month after its introduction, the act established a de facto national vaccine institution by legally mandating Dr. Smith to provide genuine, uncontaminated vaccine to any citizen upon request. Smith was to receive no money for his services but was granted the franking privilege (free postage to or from the agent, up to one-half ounce, of material related to vaccination), a not inconsequential subsidy traditionally reserved for executive positions, members of Congress, former presidents and their widows. The codicil to this was that if Smith were convicted of abusing the franking privilege, he would be subject to forfeit and required to pay a fine of $50.

Smith immediately went about publicizing his new position and the importance of his Baltimore Vaccine Institution, but he was not without critics, who complained that Congress had granted him a monopoly, a very serious charge in the early 1800s. Even Dr. Waterhouse argued against giving one individual a monopoly on vaccine. He was viewed as a person with a favored position, something the Jacksonians railed against. Although he received no salary, Smith was assailed by others who accused him of making money on the venture, a charge hardly substantiated by fact.

In yet another vindication of Lady Mary Montagu's 1717 prediction that physicians would resist any procedure that deprived them of income, among Smith's harshest critics were doctors who envisioned substantial loss of revenue from their private practices. Smith considered such opposition pure greed and advocated lay vaccination. He not only provided the means for ordinary persons to perform such operations free of charge but went two steps further, offering to examine vaccine scabs sent to him and issuing free certificates of successful vaccination. In so doing, he not only cut into doctors' earnings but also diminished their prestige, creating powerful enemies.

Aside from providing vaccine by mail, Smith assigned a number of agents to go into the field and perform mass vaccinations, reportedly treating hundreds of individuals at a time. He observed this gratuitous service had "often given great offense to many practitioners of selfish & contracted views, who complain, that we thus take a business from them; which they think themselves privileged to turn to their own particular advantage ... [and] indulge a hope that some day might come when they would derive a little profit from vaccination or reap perhaps an abundant harvest from such a loathsome and fatal plague as the Small Pox."[17]

While Smith battled his critics, cities attempted to address local concerns. During the smallpox epidemic of 1815, the New York Vaccine Institute was awarded $1,000 to vaccinate the poor of the city.[18] The following year, a bill was introduced into the New York legislature to establish a Vaccine Institute in Albany, allocating $1,000 a year to serve the poor, maintain a ready supply of vaccine and distribute lymph matter to physicians outside of the capital free of charge. In Albany, however, one provision stated that vaccination was to be performed solely by agents of the institution, giving them a monopoly over local doctors. Innovatively, the bill required the proposed institution to build a medical library, laboratory, and museum, and award prizes for the best annual dissection. Despite the fact the state was one of the wealthiest in the Union and in the middle of an epidemic, the act failed to pass. In 1817, it was reintroduced with a smaller allocation and failed a second time.[19]

Financing the Vaccine Institution

The Act of 1813 did not provide James Smith with any funding for the maintenance of the vaccine, for his own service or for field agents. It is debatable whether Congress actually believed Smith was a monopolist capable of turning a profit on the venture by charging for vaccine, but ultimately they dismissed the subject of funding the institution out of a lack of capital (the War of 1812 was draining national coffers); or, legislators may have believed they did not have the power to authorize funds. In any case, their lack of foresight became a recipe for disaster.

Although he did not ask for a salary or an allotment of funds during the 1813 debate on the Vaccine Bill, it soon became apparent that Smith could not continue to support the project on his own or with the means obtained from his lottery scheme. This finally compelled him to petition the 14th Congress in January 1816. With the war with England successfully concluded, he likely felt safer to state that it had always been his intent to receive some financial aid from the government.[20] When that did not happen, he proposed a small federal tax on every vaccination performed by a doctor. Although he asked for mere pennies per operation, Smith offered to accept less "if and when vaccination became more universal."[21]

The proposal was as impracticable as it was untenable, as direct federal taxes were almost unheard of at the time, and the government had no practical means of enforcing such a tax.[22] Perhaps more to the point, private physicians would most certainly have looked upon the idea of placing them below the status of the vaccine agent and resent the demand. In rejecting the tax, Congress, surprisingly, devised a plan of its own whereby the vaccine agent (in this case, Dr. Smith) would receive $1,500 for his services. For this sum, the agent would agree to forego any payment from the states or local governments, provide free vaccine and supply postmasters with at least five parcels of fresh vaccine every three months. The bill also required that Smith report regularly to Congress and also mandated compulsory military vaccination.[23]

The proposed legislation was stunningly progressive both in appeal and breadth. Not only would it have ensured fresh vaccine matter to every part of the country, thus severely limiting the loss of life from smallpox epidemics, it might, with the active superintendence of the postmasters (whose positions were clearly advanced), have also ultimately all but eliminated the disease from the United States. Implementation of this national health care plan would have placed the country on a status equal to or greater than any other nation, making the United States a world leader in disease eradication. A project on such a scale would also have, by necessity, firmly established one vaccine center, or several, where pure vaccine was attainable year round. By including the clause concerning mandatory military vaccination, this law might even have become so acceptable to the citizenry that eventually it could have been expanded to the nonmilitary population.

Initial debate was favorable but serious consideration was not taken up until April, near the end of the session. After initial approval and an extension from three to seven years' duration, the bill was ultimately tabled by a vote of 49 to 48. Leading the opposition was Daniel Webster of New Hampshire and Representative Pickering of Massachusetts, perhaps ingenuously claiming a lack of time to properly consider ramifications of the proposal.[24]

Having come so close, Dr. Smith renewed his petition at the start of the new congressional session in December 1816. This time he slightly altered his emphasis by stressing the military need for vaccine. Representative Condict, serving as one of Smith's greatest advocates, then proposed a bill similar to the one abandoned in April. This time Representative Atherton led the opposition and it was defeated 87 to 55, ostensibly on the argument that Congress lacked authority to pay for vaccine. (One side note to this bill was the stipulation that Smith continue in private practice while serving as vaccine agent, making it plain that the proposed $1,500 was not to cover his personal expenses.)

Atherton's 1817 argument against passage was directed against the proposition of lay people performing vaccination rather than being a bill to promote vaccination in general.[25] It is interesting to conjecture whether physician groups sponsored his opposition, as they would well remember Smith's proposal of a tax on their performance of vaccination. In the same vein, the eradication of smallpox would have a direct influence on their livelihoods. Singla notes, "Had any of the proposals been enacted, it would have been an unparalleled milestone in Federal support for the public welfare." As it was, it did not pass and the visionary doctor was left to his own devices.

Upon his appointment in 1813, Smith had expended a considerable amount of effort and money on providing vaccine for the military during the War of 1812 and well beyond.[26] It is significant to note here that the army made vaccination mandatory in 1818; a year earlier, a navy surgeon had traveled to ports with orders to vaccinate all seamen. By the 1820s, however, the navy discontinued the practice, believing smallpox did not significantly affect sailors. This proved erroneous, however, when smallpox ravished navy ships in the 1830s, converting them into smallpox hospitals.[27] Regulations in the army grew lax and the mandate fell into disuse. This would have tragic consequences during the Civil War when large numbers of volunteers, brought together from outlying towns, were exposed to smallpox for the first time. Disease quickly spread through both armies, killing great numbers.

In January 1818, seeing an opportunity to ply a different tactic, Smith proposed a $1,500 annual compensation for supplying the military, along with civilians in Washington, DC, and the federal territories — areas indisputably under congressional control. Peculiarly, the House committee determined that military surgeons could carry out vaccinations without Smith's involvement or the money he requested, apparently unaware that it was Smith's Baltimore Institution that supplied the vaccine. Without addressing the other two beneficiaries — those in Washington and the territories — Congress refused his request. Responding in anger, Smith threatened to stop supplying the army with vaccine. The surgeon general of the army, under the authority of the secretary of war, took matters into his own hands by paying Dr. Smith the $1,500 he requested.[28]

The year 1818 would prove to be a complex one for James Smith. Five years after the Vaccination Act passed, growing opposition prompted the introduction of a bill into the House. This legislation suggested that each state appoint its own vaccine agent and that the franking privilege be extended to these agents. The bill passed the House but was rejected by the Senate by a vote of 17 to 12 on the grounds of its being "unnecessary, bad precedent, and subject in itself to abuse."[29] Coupled with a prompt denial of his request for funds, Dr. Smith took the latest action as a personal assault and he condemned "attempts ... by some, who are professedly hostile to every National Establishment, to take the Management of this Plan out of my hands, to give it to others who would be under the immediate direction and control of the State Authorities."[30] Interestingly, but not surprisingly, 1818 was the first year that Smith designated his operation as the "*National* Vaccine Institution."[31]

Realizing he was on his own, Smith sought revenue from a source previously dismissed by announcing that he would charge the public $5 for a supply of vaccine.[32] It is likely Smith knew this plan would not work, as he was well aware the public erroneously considered him a government employee paid by Congress and would resent being charged. Worse, soliciting money hurt Smith's pride, placing him "on the degrading level with every advertising Quack or Imposter, who expects to enrich himself upon the suffering of his fellow creatures."[33]

In addition to the above, he decided to reach out to physicians favoring his cause by raising private charitable capital. In the spring of 1818, he published "Prospectus of a Permanent National Vaccine Institution," offering $10 memberships to doctors; a subscription would guarantee them up to five years of unlimited vaccine with the money used for continuing projects of the national institution. He calculated that with 500 subscriptions and sundry donations he could build a vaccine center in Washington.[34]

It is interesting to note that one demand placed on subscribers was that they not share the vaccine received from him with nonmember physicians.[35] Like Dr. Waterhouse before him (who was severely criticized for demanding a share of the profits from vaccination by physicians to whom he supplied vaccine), the attempt was likely both one of quality control and of monetary survival, with an emphasis on the latter. When discussing lives, it is easy to overlook the fact that even charitable institutions required financing to continue operations. Asking for a small remuneration hardly constituted the desire to create a monopoly (a charge leveled against both men) or to enrich one's self at others' expense. The idea of moving the center from Baltimore to the nation's capitol was astute, in that his work might be more closely observed and appreciated by legislators. In order to garner approval for his prospectus, Smith posted a $40,000 bond payable to the president as a pledge that he would return all memberships and donations if his plan did not come to fruition.

By 1819, Smith had procured vaccine agents to visit various states, perform mass vaccinations and collect memberships. By January 1821, he estimated his team had performed 100,000 vaccinations in Pennsylvania, Delaware, Maryland, Virginia, Kentucky and North Carolina during the two previous years. It is interesting to speculate on such scenes where "the young and the old, the rich and the poor" were gathered by the hundreds to listen to these agents promote the benefits of vaccination in what must have looked like a revival meeting. No doubt the agents gave a hearty endorsement, for they were empowered to keep 20 percent of the proceeds for themselves.

The same year, Dr. Waterhouse released new findings on vaccination. He reported that if a person were infected with smallpox in the casual, or "natural way" (by exposure to a person suffering from the disease as opposed to vaccination), and had eruptions, "if within an hour or two, or even four hours after, and perhaps still longer, you vaccinate him by *twenty* or *thirty*—or if you please *forty* punctures in his arms, legs, thighs, and on his body," the effects of smallpox might be mitigated and "arrest the progress of a threatening calamity."[36]

Smith reported on January 1, 1821, that he had received pledges of $23,125 in subscriptions and $12,509 in straight donations; but as was typical with fundraisers, he managed to collect only $14,460 out of a possible $35,634. Smith was disappointed in the effort, having to cover out of his own money the expenses of twenty-one agents (eleven of whom were still active in 1821) that included horses, stationery and vaccine.[37] (In 1822, Smith claimed that he spent more money on printing instructions for lay vaccination "than all the fees I ever received for vaccine matter since ... 1813."[38]

Raising money was critical, but the ultimate success of James Smith's institution would be its continuity during and after his lifetime. To ensure this, the doctor petitioned Congress in 1820 to incorporate the Vaccine Institution. (Congressional approval for incorporation was needed until the Jacksonian Era.) Federal authorization would have deepened the association between the institution and the national government, but also ensure that future funds went for the intended purpose. Lacking such status, on Smith's death his financial bond with the president expired and all monies belonging to the Vaccine Institution would revert to his heirs.[39]

The January 1820 bill was laid over until the next session, when myriad arguments were presented. Considering the rather selflessness of the request, even Smith could not comprehend its failure to immediately pass, complaining he did not understand "why intelligent men, who represent a Numerous & enlightened people should feel themselves constrained to oppose this institution & indulge in the most pointed disapprobation of our views."[40] Smith's February 16, 1821, report to Congress was introduced, but no further action was taken, possibly stemming from the fact no smallpox epidemics were raging at the time, lessening the urgency of the matter. This proved extremely unfortunate as subsequent events discredited Smith, bringing down the Vaccine Institution thus inextricably tied to his name.

"Down with the Vaccine Agency"

In 1821, Dr. Smith received a request for vaccine to be sent to Plymouth, North Carolina, where an outbreak of smallpox had been identified; by November, the disease had spread to Tarboro (also spelled "Tarborough"), a town less than 50 miles away. On November 1, Smith sent a letter to Dr. John F. Ward at Tarboro. He meant to enclose glass slides of cowpox lymph, but through some inexplicable mistake, his paper flyer, postmarked November 9, actually contained live smallpox scabs, kept on hand to test the efficacy of his vaccine. (This eight-day gap would later be called into question concerning the possibility of sabotage; see chapter 13.) Although clearly labeled "Variol" in Smith's handwriting, Dr. Ward apparently assumed he had received matter for vaccination and inoculated his patients, actually performing variolation rather than vaccination. The patients developed mild cases of smallpox but as a too-common complication of engrafting, they spread the disease to surrounding counties. By late winter of 1821–1822, sixty people were infected, and ten perished.[41]

On December 29, 1821, Dr. Ward wrote Smith that "the vaccine matter, sent to him from this Institution, about the first day of November last, had a different effect upon those he vaccinated than could have been expected!! Twelve persons, he says, out of fifteen in whose vaccinations he used this matter had a crop of pustules." It was later confirmed the persons so vaccinated contracted the natural smallpox.[42]

Upon hearing the results of Dr. Ward's vaccinations, Smith first presumed the matter had "transmuted in shipment" into a new form of the disease called "varioloid," recently identified in Europe. Smith's reference to a potentially mutant disease called "varioloid" originated in England, where smallpox had been comparatively dormant until 1818, "when it suddenly burst forth and presented in its career some abnormalities, which for a while shook the confidence of some of the first men in the preventive character of vaccination." In a published letter by Patrick Macaulay, from Baltimore, 2 February 1822, he described varioloid: "It is not a new disease; but the phenomena presented to us from the contagion of small-pox operating on systems in which some change has previously been produced by vaccination." He added that varioloid has, "so far as we have observed, been unattended by dangerous symptoms, and leaves no disfiguration."[43]

Upon review of a letter written to him from Dr. Hunter at Tarboro (quoting the exact words Smith had written on the paper, including the notation "Variol"), Smith realized that "small-pox scabs and marked as such, was put up in Dr. Ward's letter by some mistake or inadvertence, instead of the glasses of vaccine matter which I intended to send to him, and which, from his letter to me, I supposed he had received and used." He immediately dispatched an agent to Tarboro to supply genuine vaccine and guidance.[44]

In a published letter dated January 24, 1822, Dr. Smith described the "accident, such as never occurred before, and there is no danger that the like will ever occur again." In it he stated that about October 4, 1821, he removed some smallpox scabs from a person named Whitefield; placing them on a paper, he wrote, "carefully, to avoid accidents, that it contained the variolous or small-pox matter." The paper was mislaid and he presumed it to have been "swept out of my office with other waste papers."

After despairing that petty impositions arising from artifice, prejudice, ignorance and interest forced him to frequently address memorials (petitions) "to the national and state legislatures without receiving any proper or effectual assistance from them," Smith warned that if he found it beyond his power to preserve vaccination in a pure state, he would cease to furnish that which he had "any reason to fear has become adulterated." In defense, he informed the American people that his supply of matter for the last six weeks had been taken from places that were free from any epidemic disease and were as genuine as any he had ever used.

In addition, he vowed never to send any vaccine supply unless the recipient first complied with the established and fair regulations of the institution. Smith defended this action by declaring that the directions he sent Dr. Ward, as was "too frequently the case," were "entirely neglected." He charged that if Ward had used the matter in proper time and sent him the crusts it produced, he "would have been able to answer all his questions, and would likewise have prevented all the mischief which I fear has happened."

Quickly chastised by the community as being incompetent enough not to properly decipher the abbreviated Latin word "Variol" (for "variolous" or smallpox) and being unable to differentiate between smallpox and cowpox pustules, Dr. Ward published a letter demanding that "those, who, with the vilest prejudice, have heaped upon me much personal abuse," to desist, since the original mistake was Smith's.[45] In a subsequent letter dated February 21, 1821, Ward altered his original claim by stating that there were no markings on the package from Dr. Smith.[46]

Although Dr. Ward was an auxiliary vaccine agent, the designation does not necessarily signify that he was versed in Latin or that he had the experience to identify smallpox from kine-pox. Ward reported that a mere 1 percent of the area surrounding Tarboro had been vaccinated, indicating he may have had little experience in the operation. Furthermore, the title of "doctor" was widely conferred upon individuals without proper medical training and he may simply have been an apprentice who completed training with another country practitioner and hung out his shingle. That said, retracting his statement that the pustules had been labeled "Variol" was ingenuous at best and libelous at worst. Dr. Hunter's letter (cited above) easily disproved Ward's retraction.

More damning was a further attack by Ward, unfairly questioning Smith's competence in that he had failed to eradicate smallpox from Baltimore. Adding fuel to the fire, Ward raised the suggestion of an unknown strain of the virus occurring in Baltimore. Presumably Smith himself gave Ward the idea by first suggesting a mutant type of "varioloid" might have caused the spread of smallpox in Tarboro. Ward's charge was completely unsubstantiated, but it created further doubt as to Smith's credibility, leaving open the interpretation that he might have been at fault for creating an entirely new and deadly contagion infecting people in Maryland and North Carolina.[47]

The situation was destined to deteriorate rapidly. In January 1822, Dr. Smith issued a circular "To the Citizens of the United States," promising that all facts would be fully and freely made known to all concerned. Acknowledging any mistakes he may have committed "either from ignorance or through carelessness," he expressed no wish "to be spared from the rod of correction." At this point, having no definitive explanation for the outbreak, Smith's open communication touched on three possibilities: that he had made an error and sent smallpox rather than vaccine; that the vaccine had somehow deteriorated during transit; or the disease they were trying to combat had mutated into a form of varioloid. Later, the fourth possibility of an untoward event would raise far more disturbing questions.

Smith's circular greatly exacerbated an already critical situation, causing doctors and patients severe distress and actually leading to the speculation that Smith purposely tried to start an epidemic in order to sell more vaccine. This necessarily led critics to question the value of both the institution and vaccine in general. Dr. Ward realized that matters were taking a wrong turn. While desiring to place blame on James Smith, he did not wish to see the entire vaccination program destroyed, writing, "It is, however, my serious wish, that the National Vaccine Institution, as proposed by him [Smith], may be carried into effective operation, and that the citizens of the United States will not suffer it to languish in the consequence of one fatal mistake."[48]

However strong defenders were, once politicians realized the "plum" they had been given anti-vaccinationists became formidable enemies. Leading the pack was Representative Hutchins Gordon Burton of North Carolina, who claimed his constituents had been "slaughtered with indifference" by Dr. Smith. Burton became the leading figure in the House debate over repealing the 1813 Vaccination Act. Calling the Institution "a nuisance of the most dangerous kind" ("nuisance" was typically used in reference to infectious diseases; here, it is used sarcastically as a play on words), he indulged in character assassination, charging Smith with collecting over $45,000 from different parts of the Union and implying the act was "taxing people at large for the profit of the agent of vaccination." He also raised Ward's charge of James Smith's incompetence by spuriously charging that the city of Baltimore suffered from smallpox to a larger degree than any other part of the country.

In refuting this charge, Smith wrote:

By steadily persevering in the practice of vaccination for many years, we had completely banished the small-pox from this city, and many began to imagine we would never again be visited by it. Our fancied security however, served to create the same neglect of the kine-pox as is common in other places until we had many subjects fit to be preyed upon by the variolous contagion — and in this situation we were found suddenly exposed to great danger by the arrival of the *Pallas*, Captain Otis, on the 14th August, 59 days from Liverpool with a few passengers having among them the small-pox.

He then provided an extract from the bills of mortality, showing the progress of the disease since then:

Deaths by Small-pox in Baltimore

In October	2
November	2
December, 1st week	6
December, 2nd week	2
December, 3rd week	4
December, 4th week	9
January, 1st week	6
January, 2nd week	16
	47 deaths[49]

Lastly, Burton raised the incendiary flag by charging that the agent had introduced smallpox into the interior of the United States, "where, in all probability, it would not have found its way for forty years."[50] Obviously the latter charge flew in the fact of facts, as smallpox had appeared at Plymouth, North Carolina, and spread to Tarboro, but the accusation served its purpose.

On January 20, 1822, Burton called for a select committee to investigate Smith's negligence. This committee, comprising Baltimore physicians, was to determine the facts and advise whether the Act of 1813 should be repealed. Preparatory to the final report, Patrick Macaulay published a letter on February 2:

We, in common with our fellow citizens, deplore the unhappy events which have taken place in the state of North Carolina, by the introduction of the small-pox from matter sent by the vaccine institution established in this city; but we protest, for the good of our common country, against its being attributed to any other than an accidental cause.... We would protect that which should be a national blessing, and instead of repealing the existing laws, new acts have become necessary for its preservation.

Dr. Macaulay concluded by referencing Dr. Smith's letter, where he stated that in light of a loss of confidence in vaccination, Dr. Davidge and Dr. Potter of the University of Maryland had recommended and were then practicing "the old inoculation for small pox." (Dr. Potter had, by this time, denied his involvement in inoculation.) Macaulay summarized the opinion of the medical brethren of the city emphatically: "Legislators! Citizens! I beseech you, if you would preserve your country from an ever-during pestilence, to stand forth, and by wise laws, and the force of enlightened opinion, *prohibit the inoculation for small pox; encourage and protect vaccination.*"[51]

On February 22, the committee reaffirmed that the tragedy at Tarboro had been an accident and concluded the benefits of vaccination were too great to repeal the act, not only recommending its continuance, but also advising no changes to it.

In a clear example of abuse of power, Burton (who envisioned great political gain and actually worked the tragedy into a governorship) claimed "the present agency was not only a nuisance, but a nuisance of the most dangerous kind" and demanded that a second committee reinvestigate the facts. The North Carolina legislator appointed the members and actually wrote its report. Presented on April 13, the findings were harshly critical of Dr. Smith and called for the repeal of the 1813 Act.[52]

Smith, likely reacting from his personal exposure to physicians, credited the medical society as being more onerous than either Dr. Ward or Representative Burton, charging that they opposed lay vaccination and the issuance of free certificates of vaccination, adding that "down with the vaccine agency" was the popular cry of these economic interests.[53] A case in point came from a letter published in the *Torch Light & Public Advertiser* (Maryland), February 19, 1822. In arguing for vaccination, the author attributed failures "to the carelessness & negligence with which it has been practiced." He observed that epidemics raged in those states where least attention was paid to vaccination "and [was] completely banished from such where the practice has been enforced by legal enactments, and confined to regular practitioners."

He contrasted Great Britain, where "quacks, farriers, *old* women and young," performed vaccination, little or no attention was paid to the quality of the lymph or the disease afterward. In countries "where vaccination is performed by the *regular practitioner only,* and is under the surveillance of the police, where all are compelled, under a heavy penalty, or imprisonment to submit, we shall find the small-pox has been completely expelled [from] these countries." Although the author's intent was to promote vaccination by "regular practitioners only" (clearly opposing Smith's policies), he wrote as one individual.

In a separate letter dated February 5, 1822, Dr. Nathaniel Potter, professor of surgery and anatomy at the University of Maryland, questioned how Dr. Smith could issue certificates of vaccination by examining dried pustules sent to him by mail. He argued, "If there has been any criterion discovered by which we can pronounce a subject completely guaranteed against the invasion of the small pox from vaccination, it is to be found in that insensibility to the vaccine virus which is the result of repeated vaccination, 'till not even a local vaccine inflammation can be excited."[54]

Significantly, Singla found no records in the congressional or National Archives from physician groups complaining about the Vaccine Act of 1813. Rather, the rhetoric came from the House, where Burton's group argued against it on antimonopoly grounds and as an inappropriate exercise of federal power. In what would remain a continuing thread throughout American governance to the present day, Burton argued such legislation was "not properly within the province of this Government but of the several States" and "professional men possessing the confidence of the community."[55]

Newspapers were filled with news of the Tarboro incident, many people picking up details from North Carolina papers and private correspondence. The *Ohio Repository* of February 14 reported on the death of Joseph Phillips, who "has fallen a sacrifice" to Dr. Smith's error. The same day, the *National Intelligencer* added that smallpox continued to spread, "and that several have died of the disease." Articles typically contained paragraphs similar to the one at the head of this chapter; others noted, "What heightens the calamity, and necessarily increases the fears of the citizens, is the extraordinary fact that vaccination is found to be a very uncertain preventive of the disease."[56]

Reacting to Dr. Smith's circular, "To the Citizens of the United States," editors were quick to address the supposed new disease — "varioloid" — appearing "under modifications differing from the old small pox." Just as quickly, other newspapers picked up "investigations," describing varioloid as "chicken-pox" that was seen after vaccination as well as after smallpox, fortunately reporting that "vaccination remains what its illustrious discoverer pronounced it, a shield against the pestiferous effects of the small-pox."

Statistics on Varioloid

	Vaccinated (80 persons)	Unvaccinated (41 persons)
Died	0	13
Sickened	6	Many dangerously ill; much pitting and deformity after recovery[57]

Dr. James Smith offered to resign as a means of saving the National Vaccine Institution, but the momentum had shifted against him. President Monroe revoked his commission in April "as a consequence of the violent prejudices against him." That same month the Repeal Act quickly passed the House and on May 2, 1822, the Senate concurred. Although several attempts were made to reinstitute the Vaccine Institution, first in 1824 with a plan to restore Smith's appointment and franking privilege and later in 1838 and 1882, Congress failed in its duty to protect the public health.

13

The Vaccine Institution
and Beyond

One or two physicians of that city [New Orleans] are endeavoring against the opposition "of certain persons," to prevail on all inhabitants to accept the aid of the vaccination.[1]

Dr. James Smith refused to admit defeat and continued in his labors against smallpox. Barely a week after Congress repealed its authorization of the National Vaccine Institution, Smith published a letter, attempting to explain the situation:

VACCINATION.
To the Citizens of the United States

An erroneous idea has been taken up, in consequence of the repeal of the law relative to vaccination; and many persons have been induced to believe that this Institution was thereby broken up and abandoned. "But this is not the case." The law which has been repealed never granted any money, or made any other provision to encourage vaccination except to permit all letters to and from me on the subject, to be carried free of postage.

It must be evident, then, that the Vaccine Institution can be continued as well without the aid of this law as with it. The repeal of the law, indeed, renders an Institution of this kind doubly necessary; and clearly proves that the public good requires it should be permanently fixed upon some sure foundation. It should not be liable to be affected at any time by personal caprice, private interests, or vulgar prejudices, of any kind.

I will continue my exertions, therefore, to establish the Institution on the plan proposed, in opposition to every difficulty that may be presented, and I hope that a discerning public will give it such encouragement as they must perceive it merits.

The auxiliary agencies already established, shall be continued; and other agents shall be appointed, to whom this remedy will be forwarded occasionally for distribution. If these agents should not want it at the time I may send it, they need not pay postage or receive it. My letters containing the vaccine matter will, in this case, remain in the hands of the postmasters, to be returned as dead letters to the General Post Office.

After all that has transpired under my observation, after an experience of twenty one years, (and particularly since the natural small pox has been prevalent in this city,) I can assure the public, that when perfect kine pock matter is used, and the vaccine process is suffered to terminate without interruption, Vaccination is a sure preventive of the small pox.

Those interested, who may wish for further information on this subject, may address me through the medium of the post office, postage paid.

JAMES SMITH
Late Agent of Vaccination for the United States
Vaccine Institution, Balt. May 10, 1822[2]

This almost sad letter was virtually an unintended epitaph for the Vaccine Institution. Dr. Smith never regained the public's confidence and although he made a concerted effort to explain the Tarboro tragedy and defend his work, going so far as to publish five issues of the *Vaccine Inquirer* between 1822 and 1824, his efforts were futile. In 1824, desperately short of money, he was forced to scale back his work.[3]

Perhaps to ignite a spark of enthusiasm, or at the very least defend his reputation, Smith publicly alleged there had been a "Small Pox Plot" behind the Tarboro affair.[4] He suggested that the tragedy was not an accident but a malicious act of some unknown conspiracy.[5] One of his strongest points was the eight-day gap between his letter to Dr. Ward enclosing what turned out to be smallpox virus (November 1, 1821) and the postmark on the letter (November 9, 1821). Since Smith was habitually punctual in answering his mail, the implication held that the letter might have been tampered with. He also claimed that during the subsequent congressional investigation, a considerable amount of paperwork, relating entirely to the Vaccine Institution, was stolen.

Congress authorized an investigational committee to look into Smith's charges. The process required three years to complete, during which time a bill was introduced in 1824 to reinstate his appointment and franking privileges. No significant action was taken on the bill, but the final congressional report credited much of Smith's account.[6] Interestingly, Dr. Ward refused to testify, despite repeated requests for him to do so.

In retrospect, Smith's arguments seem compelling. The charges leveled against him — that he purposely started a smallpox epidemic at Tarboro to sell more vaccine; that he desired a monopoly on vaccine (a serious accusation during the Jacksonian Era); that his efforts at lay vaccination deprived physicians of their livelihood; that his authority as the Federal Vaccine Agent gave him considerable power to influence congressional action; his passion for public health; and, just as significant, a vulnerability to becoming a public scapegoat and thus a target for publicity and power-seeking individuals — paint a very disturbing picture.

The mysterious loss of documents pertaining to the Vaccine Institution and Dr. Ward's refusal to testify before Congress lend strength to a conspiracy theory. There was much to gain by bringing Smith and his institution down: Representative Burton rode the scandal into the governor's chair of North Carolina and without a recognized source supplying pure (or any) vaccine, smallpox epidemics provided countless patients for practicing physicians. If even part of this were true, it is indeed a black mark on American history.

The year 1827 marked the final time James Smith's name appeared in congressional records. To the shame of the nation, he died in 1841, a largely forgotten figure. Except for the events at Tarboro, North Carolina, his tireless efforts to eradicate smallpox might have placed his name at the top of American medical heroes.

The Benign Friend of the Human Race

Although Dr. Smith's influence was seriously curtailed after his dismissal as vaccine agent, American confidence in vaccination remained strong. Quoting an extremely laudatory (and, incidentally, nonaccusatory) notice from the *National Intelligencer,* the *Republican Compiler* of March 20, 1822, reported that the latest accounts from Tarboro made it appear general vaccination, "with the aid of other precautionary measures," had almost entirely eradicated the smallpox. With only one case remaining in town, the newspaper expressed "renewed cause for confidence in that benign friend of the human race."

Confidence was one thing; actually compelling people to become vaccinated on a large scale was another. Without a National Vaccine Institution, responsibility again fell to the states and individual practitioners. A sampling of reports from the 1820s presents a consistent theme of smallpox "making an appearance" in one place or another. During one mild outbreak, the *York Gazette* (PA), February 12, 1822, advised "all such as have neither had the small pox nor been vaccinated, to resort to the safe and simple preventive."

As an example of how the disease was considered within the scope of daily living, a single article from the October 10, 1825, edition of the *Adams Sentinel* (PA) contained information that favorable weather increased the prospect of escaping an epidemic, noting, "The small pox was prevalent but excited little alarm." (Immediately following was a report on the discovery of some "*Great Bones*" that elicited keen interest until they were identified as belonging to a "*Whale.*" The good news in this case was that the discoverer of the relics made a handsome profit from their exhibition.)

As testimony to how misinformation spread, an article entitled "Interesting Facts" appeared in the August 5, 1823, edition of the *Torch Light & Public Advertiser*, where it was stated "by a gentleman of respectability" that no instance was known of smallpox having been taken (contracted) west of the Ohio River; and that although emigrants from the East had been dispersed throughout every quarter of the country, "while laboring under the dire effects of the disease, & although many of them have actually died" under its influence, no case was ever *communicated* west of the Ohio. The same authority also avowed that not one case of hydrophobia had ever been reported in Ohio. Strangely, the editor chose to comment: "In truth, if these things are so (and we are not prepared to controvert them) they are truly interesting facts, and worthy of notice."[7]

As "truly interesting" as the observations may have been, they were hardly accurate. In a report that might have been taken from any newspaper across the United States and its territories, a January 11, 1826, notice from the *Adams Centinel* (PA) informed the public that smallpox was making frightful ravages in New Orleans. "One or two physicians of that city are endeavoring against the opposition 'of certain ignorant persons,' to prevail on all inhabitants to accept the aid of the vaccination."

The decade of the 1830s presented more of the same, with isolated deaths still considered newsworthy enough to make the dailies. For example, on June 29, 1830, the *Gettysburg Republican Compiler* announced the death of Mrs. Friedline, aged between 18 and 19 years of age. She caught the disease while visiting a cousin in Somerset County; accompanying the young mother was her four-month-old infant. The child was vaccinated as soon as the attending physician diagnosed smallpox; the baby contracted kine-pox as anticipated and was expected to do well. A contrasting case occurred in New York where a father and his six children contracted smallpox, notwithstanding the fact he had been inoculated and the children had the kine pox in infancy and had been revaccinated for it without effect a few months earlier.[8]

The presence of smallpox usually served as a deterrent to businesses, and men often resorted to newspapers as a means of protecting their establishments. On April 8, 1830, Hugh C. Raney published a card denying that two families suffering from the disease resided at his house, adding he believed the report was put in circulation with a view of injuring him in his calling. He probably regretted his action, for the editor's note following the text sarcastically confirmed Raney's denial, adding, "There exists but *one* case of Small Pox in this place at the present time."[9] Conversely, smallpox occasionally offered the opportunity for a quick profit. One "strolling chap" set up practice as a vaccine doctor in Winchester and offered his services for half the going rate. Obtaining what he thought was a vaccine scab he began his work, only to discover his patients had not developed kine pox "but a less salutary infection, known, of old, by the name of the *Scotch fiddle*" (a vulgar term typically referencing "the itch" of the genitals).[10]

Instances of persons contracting smallpox after having been vaccinated would be a recurring theme throughout the 1800s. The *Bangor Daily Whig and Courier*, June 9, 1838, reported on the death of the Reverend Mr. Knowles, who had vaccinated himself in his youth. "The bad quality of the matter employed, or the bungling manner in which the operation is sometimes performed" prevented the desired effect. This may have been one reason the city council of Bangor passed an order that the health committee would operate a vaccination clinic with a physician in attendance from 9:00 A.M. to noon and from 2:00 P.M. to 5:00 P.M. every day, Sundays excepted. The city government offered the procedure free of charge and it was hoped this opportunity would not be neglected.[11]

Another issue that would come to a head in the next several decades concerned the introduction of smallpox into the United States by immigrants. A report by the *New York Journal of Commerce* in 1830 announced the arrival of the British ship *Brunswick* from London. It was quarantined on arrival with 112 out of 209 passengers suffering from the disease, including 5 who had died on the voyage. Of the total, only 68 had been vaccinated and 29 inoculated or had taken it by contagion. Of the 68, not one contracted smallpox on the voyage.[12] Not only was the threat of introducing smallpox into the city a very real one, bitter debate on where the sick were to be kept and who was to pay for their treatment would also later dominate headlines.

Nor was that the only portent. The day before Christmas 1830, a one-sentence notice preceded by the word "Horrible," read: "A female slave, suffering with the small pox in Nashville, was confined in the third story of a lonely house at some distance from Nashville, when some one communicated fire to the building, and burnt it and the helpless creature within to ashes."[13]

Degeneration of the Vaccine Lymph

Epidemics continued to rage throughout the world, at times appearing unchecked by mass vaccinations. During a particularly virulent outbreak in England during 1838 and 1839, a Bristol physician named Estlin determined that the vaccine strain currently in use had deteriorated to the point of being ineffective. This prompted him to speculate that matter obtained directly from the cow would provide a more effective strain for vaccination. At a dairy in Gloucestershire he found proof of kine pox in a young woman who had contracted the disease while milking. On August 11, 1838, he used lymph taken from an infected cow to vaccinate a child, who subsequently developed a perfect case of kine-pox.

GENERATIONAL LYMPH

Matter taken directly from the cow and given to an individual in the form of vaccination was considered first generational. All matter taken from that individual and used for vaccinating others became known as the second generation and so on. In this manner, numerous generations stemmed from the original inoculation.

In its earliest transmissions, "unhumanized lymph" produced extreme local irritations, exactly as described by Dr. Jenner. Research at the time indicated the skin irritations were so extensive as to endanger, and in some cases actually prove fatal to, the patient being vaccinated. After several transmissions (generations), the virulence abated. Estlin and others who used his fresh strain regarded it as superior to the multigenerational lymph then available. Estlin distributed his new strain extensively throughout the west of England and the United States.[14] Vaccine taken from the tenth generation was sent to Dr. Jackson, of Boston. Along with Dr. Putnam, the two extensively used and confirmed the success of vaccination with this new strain, making available to other doctors the eleventh and twelfth generations from the cow.[15]

The reception of Estlin's strain was not as well received in London. Many physicians decried Estlin's basic premise that the lymph matter then in use had deteriorated, countering with the argument that vaccine used at the best public stations produced perfect results, "not failing once in a 170 times." Comparisons by Mr. Aikin between Estlin's cow lymph and Jenner's original stock did prove very little difference between the two. To go one step further, Mr. Gilham, of the National Vaccine Establishment, tested a number of children with Estlin's lymph, reporting that it produced severe local effects. He afterward tested the children by variolous inoculation and for comparison inoculated with variola an equal number of children who had been vaccinated by him with Jenner's old stock. Both series equally resisted the variolous infection. The conclusion, therefore, indicated that after the first or second transmission, results of cow lymph "do not differ from those of ordinary vaccination, either in respect of the progress or character of the vesicle."[16]

Estlin induced the National Vaccine Board to employ his new vaccine on the grounds it produced better marked and developed vesicles, "attended with more constitutional disturbance" than those produced by the old (and in his opinion effete) stock of lymph. Ultimately, the board expressed their complete satisfaction with the lymph currently resulting from their own successful vaccinations.

After regretting that any anxiety should have occurred, their official statement read, "We have the opportunity of bearing our most ample testimony to the continuance of the efficiency of the original vaccine lymph introduced by Dr. Jenner, through nearly a million of subjects successfully, of whom many thousands have been exposed, with entire impunity to small-pox in its most malignant form."

Estlin was less than pleased with the response. In a magnificently crafted and wildly sarcastic response, he stated:

> Now it is only forty years since the introduction of vaccination and however numerous may be the subjects that have been vaccinated at one time from the same individual, the stock of matter at present employed at the National Vaccine Establishment, can only have passed through 2080 subjects, even supposing that lymph for subsequent vaccination has been taken every seven days from a fresh subject, without any interruption, from the time when Dr. Jenner first sent it to London.
>
> In order that it should pass through a million subjects, the lapse of 19,230 years and ten months would be required.
>
> In periods of general alarm, to what extent it may be justified to have recourse to the *pious fraud* of strong and not very accurate statements, for the purpose of calming the public mind, I am not casuist enough to determine; my preference, however, is for truth and correctness at all times; and I cannot but think it a matter of regret, on the present occasion, that an official document should have emanated from the National Vaccine Establishment of England, attested by the name of the learned President of the Royal College of Physicians, and destined to be circulated, not only throughout our own Kingdom, but in countries where great attention is paid to the

accuracy of medical statistics, so expressed, as to refer the origin of vaccination to such a remote period as thirteen thousand years before the beginning of the world.[17]

In a further comparison, researchers determined that all primary stocks were not identical in their local action on the human subject (referring to skin irritation) but that there was nothing beyond this to indicate a difference in the protection provided. After three years of study, Mr. Ceely announced in 1841 that he had observed and tested more than fifteen different stocks of vaccine lymph, either taken directly from the cow or from the hands of milkers and artificially produced in the cow. His conclusions substantiated earlier studies by determining that the different stocks "all varied in their effects, both locally and constitutionally, but none lacked the essential qualities and properties, nor had any possessed them in a superior degree to those indicated by Jenner."[18] Ultimately, English authorities concluded that, while the old stock Estlin used before turning to vaccine taken directly from the cow may have been inferior, his was an isolated case and they saw no reason to abandon the stock established by Dr. Jenner.

The question of vaccine degeneration was to reappear numerous times during the 19th century. In the United States during the early 1850s, various authorities discussed the topic through the medium of the newspapers. One individual who signed his name "Matuchen" agreed with his English counterparts with a codicil, declaring, "Lymph that has passed through a great number of subjects, and used from Jenner's time to this day, does not *necessarily* become *deteriorated,* and therefore does not require to be '*rediscovered.*' This, however, can only be said when unceasing attention is paid to every successive transmission, for if a deviation commences, it may be perpetuated, and afford a gradual decreasing protection."[19]

Smallpox at Mid-Century

Although vaccination had been proven a successful preventive for smallpox, no one stepped up to take Dr. James Smith's place and the practice assumed a more or less catch-as-catch-can place in American lives. Those living in large cities tended to be more aware of the procedure, taking care that their children were protected. Those living in more rural towns and in the territories probably had little knowledge and less inclination to become vaccinated.

What held true for the population at large also applied to doctors. Those having regular recourse with vaccination understood the necessity of testing the efficacy of the operation, while those less familiar performed vaccination with questionable results. Thus, throughout the period leading up to the Civil War, the disease continued to make inroads while numerous articles appeared in circulation, both promoting and questioning the value of inoculation. To make matters more complicated, other diseases such as chicken pox confused physicians as to proper diagnosis and treatment.

In 1844, an epidemic broke out in Longueuil, a town near Montreal, Canada. The *Aurora* reported that the disease (either smallpox or chicken pox) appeared "with a virulence and a fatality resembling what is recorded of its ravages in the middle ages." Scarcely a family member, young or old, escaped the infection. More distressing was the observation that "more than five hundred persons, of whom a large portion have been vaccinated, have been more or less affected." The inhabitants of Montreal, needless to say, were very much alarmed lest the disease expand its ravages to that city.[20] The smallpox appeared just at the time when an influx of emigrants was expected, causing people to hope that "for both humanity and the material interests of the country" the authorities would drain the swamps that had been allowed to stagnate and putrefy, and vaccination of the young would be attended to. Dr. Walker's theory (which he gave as president of the National Vaccine Institution, England) of preserving the efficacy of vaccination by renewing it every six or seven years was touched upon, with the consensus that no one could be certain of full protection unless tested with the insertion of fresh vaccine matter.[21]

Such outbreaks, of course, were good for those in the business. It was not uncommon to see advertisements, such as this one appearing in 1846:

> GENUINE VACCINE VIRUS procured of Doct J V Z Smith, resident Surgeon and Physician of the port of Boston for sale by CUNNINGHAM, Druggist.[22]

The interesting thing about this notice was that it ran in a Wisconsin newspaper. The danger in purchasing vaccine from a stranger meant the buyer had no way of ascertaining its pureness. Without the National Vaccine Institution to guarantee purity, a case in the county of Huron, Ohio, proved the rule rather than the exception. A physician purchased vaccine matter from Cincinnati but upon using it a number of his patients died. It was subsequently determined that the vaccine matter had been taken from a patient having erysipelas (an infection of the skin, usually caused by streptococci, characterized by a bright red, sharply defined rash on the face or legs, accompanied by fever, chills, swelling and tenderness; without the use of antibiotics, which were unknown at the time, nephritis, abscesses and septicemia were likely to develop.)[23] The vaccine proved so dangerous it was discontinued, with the warning that too much care could not be expended in selecting matter for use.[24]

In a similar instance, Dr. William P. Richardson of New Kent County, Virginia, charged a vaccine agent of the state with having furnished him with "genuine vaccine matter" that proved impure. After he used it on 80 patients, all of them fell sick with smallpox, in some instances with critical outcomes. The subject was sent to the legislature for investigation.[25] On an equally disturbing but no less surprising note, the *Janesville Gazette* (WI), June 16, 1855, reported under the heading "Important If True" that Dr. Tinsley, of Cuba, claimed to have discovered that vaccine, "after passing through the system of a [N]egro, is valueless to the white race."

Nor did the passage of time improve the situation. In 1857, "Alphonzo" lamented that smallpox had broken out in the vicinity of Galveston, Texas, but unlike every other city in the Union the size and importance of Galveston, that city had no regularly appointed physician to perform vaccinations. Such treatments were left in the hands of "midwifes and barbers," who, instead of preventing the disorder, might actually create it. "Shall the poor suffer and die because they have not the almighty dollar to protect themselves and their offspring?" he demanded. "They suffer enough here already now from want of a *Dispensary* where they could get their medicine gratis, as it is in every large city, and I think the evils might easily be removed by appointing a physician who could and would answer all these purposes."[26]

The *concept* and *technique* of vaccination provided the American imagination with an amalgamation of wonder and science, easily transferred to other methods purporting equally astonishing cures. In 1857, F. Coggswell offered for sale his "Antiphlogistic Salt," an anti-inflammatory that supposedly equalized the fluid of the body, "the want of an equilibrium in which, is the sole cause of inflammation." It exerted, "like the vaccine matter, an extraordinary influence over the circulation.... Such is its potency, that like the virus just mentioned, it requires merely what adheres to the point of a quill dipped into a solution of it, to affect the entire system but must be instantly used to prevent decomposition and secure its full virtue."

The salt was so effective its discoverer expected to suffer the fate of Jenner, who, after announcing his discovery to the world, was declared a "Quack," "Imposter" and "Humbug." Fortunately, Coggswell still humbly believed his salt, "like all inventions and discoveries, is the mere development of what always had existence in the mind of the Great Infinite."[27] As with any good huckster, Coggswell learned to employ key names and words associated with reputable science to promote his "cure." Likely the use of words like "Jenner," "vaccine," "decomposition" and the identical method of introduction into the body served him well in his collection of $2 per dram.

Antiphlogistic salts were not the only sure cures. The *Atlanta Intelligencer* published a conversation with Dr. Alexander of that city, in which he stated that during the late smallpox panic he vaccinated over two hundred children and found that vaccination was "a certain and speedy cure for the whooping cough." The newspaper noted that if the observation were founded on a principle of fact, it deserved the attention of medical men.[28]

14

The American Indian Vaccination Act

These unfortunate beings have been fast disappearing before our advances, and Providence has at last threatened to sweep them from the earth, leaving nothing but their graves, as mementos of their former existence. Our country abounds with evidence of having once been occupied by another race, and may they not as these have fallen victims to some such scourge. The ways of Heaven are just, yet mysterious, and nations must bow before its will, as the reed before the storm.[1]

"Americans"— those first, second and third generation European immigrants who called themselves Americans, as opposed to American Indians, who called themselves by names with spellings Europeans imposed— looked at the "Red Man" with a mixture of fear and awe. Those with an eye for compassion wished to aid their brethren during the horrific outbreaks of disease introduced by their ancestors; others less inclined toward charity looked upon them as inferiors, often grouping Indians and Negroes into the same slave category. The rest, composing the majority, shared a little of each sentiment.

Newspapers, serving as the voice of the people during the 1800s, tended to pander to their readership: those published in areas of high disease tended to be more compassionate, while editors in states and territories where Indians represented a threat were either derogatory or cold. Those in the middle published reports from outlying states covering the gamut from graphic descriptions of suffering to unemotional statistics.

Representing what might be considered a detached view of middle ground, the *Wilmingtonian and Delaware Advertiser*, May 11, 1826, ran two paragraphs under the heading "Foreign and Domestic Gleanings":

The Small-Pox has made its appearance among the Choctaw Indians, and has carried off great numbers. It was introduced into that nation from New-Orleans.

At the date of the last advices from New-Orleans, April 10, a report was in circulation in New-Orleans that the small-pox was making dreadful ravages among the slaves in the valley of the Mississippi.

As representatives of the people in a political sense, the United States government acted on reports of the smallpox epidemic of 1831–1832 that had affected Indian communities across the Great Plains. On April 4, 1832, the Senate considered a bill making appropriations for vaccination among the Indians as a preventive of smallpox. After discussion, it was postponed. During the same session, a bill for the relief of the surviving officers and soldiers of the Revolution was taken up. Mr. Wilkins moved an amendment expending provisions of the bill to "Indian Spies." After discussion, the bill was tabled. In the House of Representatives, the bill providing for vaccination of Indians was amended and ordered to be engrossed for a third reading. The House passed the bill April 10.[2]

J. Diane Pearson's study, "Lewis Cass and the Politics of Disease,"[3] presents a fascinating look at the ulterior motives behind this act. She noted that passage in the Senate proved more difficult, as nine Southerners argued against the bill on the spurious point that there was no precedent for the legislation. Additionally, they argued against the cost, demanding the proposed appropriation be whittled from $12,000 to $6,000 and surgeons' fees be reduced from $6/day to $4/day. They also insisted the secretary of war should not be given discretionary spending authority.

Among the most viciously outspoken was Senator Buckner of Missouri, who stated that he did not wish to cherish his natural enemies who had "so frequently snatched the infant from the nipple of its mother's breast, and dashed its brains out against a tree."[4] Ultimately, ten senators voted against the bill, nine from pro–Indian removal states, including Alabama, Indiana, Missouri, Louisiana, South Carolina, North Carolina and Virginia. The tenth senator was from New Jersey.[5]

The bill ultimately passed on May 5, 1832, with the original allocations intact, becoming the first federal legislation directly addressing the health needs of Native Americans. Concerned exclusively with vaccination, secretary of war Lewis Cass, an appointee of President Andrew Jackson, issued a general circular on May 10. This outlined the general plan for vaccination.[6] A day earlier, Cass had written a private letter to Indian agent John Dougherty, ordering him to "limit vaccinations to tribes located in the Lower Missouri River Valley," adding, "I will state to you, however, my general views, in relation to the Indians upon the Missouri River.... Under any circumstances, no effort will be made to send a Surgeon higher up the Missouri than the Mandans, and I think not higher than the Aricaras."[7]

While the intent of the legislation was to provide the preventive to Native Americans, the actual politics behind this act were somewhat less than humane. At this period, the government was actively arranging for the removal of Indians off southern lands, transporting them further and further west. Since smallpox epidemics were frequent in these areas, promising vaccination appealed not only to those suffering forced deportation but also had the added benefit of positive press. While there were always some who felt "the only good Indian was a dead Indian" (a paraphrasing of

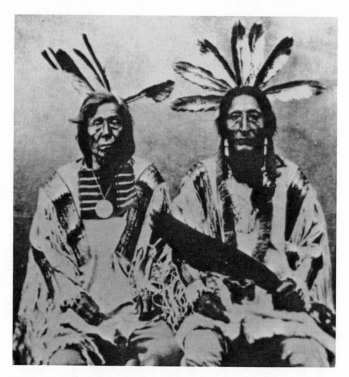

This daguerreotype shows two Indians of the Mandan tribe who survived the smallpox epidemic of 1872. The photo is from the Provincial Archives of Manitoba, published by Panarizon Publishing Corp. (from the authors' collection).

General William T. Sherman, who replied to the statement, "Me good Indian," with, "The only good Indians I ever saw were dead," January 1869),[8] the majority of whites did not want to think they were sending susceptible tribes to their deaths.

Cass's order to Dougherty to deny Mandans, Hidatsas and other Upper Missouri River tribes, including the Arikaras, Cree, Blackfeet and Assiniboine vaccination, also appears to have been economically motivated. The lands they inhabited had lost considerable importance as trading areas; in contrast, the Sioux, who supplied valuable beaver pelts, were heavily vaccinated. Just as significantly, no tribes known or suspected to be hostile to whites were vaccinated, Cass regarding them as "beyond the concerns of the United States."[9]

Removal tribes receiving vaccination were the Choctaws, Shawnees, Kickapoos, Cherokees, Creeks, Seminoles, the Indians of Ohio, and the Lewistown Senecas. Those slated for reservation reduction and removal who received vaccination included the Potawatomies, Miamis, Indians of Illinois and those located immediately west of the Mississippi: the Osages, Chippewas (Ojibwas), Ottawas, Menominees, Chippewas of Lake Superior, and groups of Wyandots, Munsees, Shawnees, Winnebagos and Christian Indians.

Interestingly, of the $4,795.50 spent on vaccination in 1832, $800 of it went to finance Henry Schoolcraft's expedition to discover the source of the Mississippi. While officially to "proceed into the country upon the heads of the Mississippi, and visit as many of the Indians in that, and the intermediate region, as circumstances will permit," vaccinating the natives as he went, Schoolcraft, a geologist, and Cass were old friends. In 1820, they had explored the region, mistakenly identifying what became known as Cass Lake as the source of the river.[10] The vaccination assignment gave Schoolcraft not only an excuse but also the finances to continue the quest. The expedition physician, Dr. Houghton, apparently vaccinated 2,070 people, but he was dissatisfied with Schoolcraft's lack of involvement. In his report to Congress, Schoolcraft emphasized the maps, surveys and census data he had gathered over vaccination data.[11]

During the years 1837 and 1838, a smallpox epidemic swept across the United States. Due to the fact many whites and Native Americans had been vaccinated, the death toll was not as high as it might have been. The same could not be said for the tribes purposely left off Cass' list: the Mandans, Hidatsas, Arikaras, Crees, Assiniboines and Blackfeet. Newspaper accounts as early as 1836 reported that smallpox was raging at Fort Winnebago, with the Ottawas, Menominees and Potawatomies suffering severe losses. The writer "supposed [the smallpox] would have the effect of repressing their hostile dances."[12]

According to the *St. Louis Bulletin,* the epidemic started at the end of April 1837, when Messrs. Pratte and Choteau and company left that city on the steamboat *St. Peters* with supplies for various trading posts on the Upper Missouri, with the ultimate destination being Fort Union, a 2,000-mile trip. Among the cargo were annuity goods from the government to a number of tribes along the river. When the boat arrived at Black Snake Hills, a trading post 60 miles from Fort Leavenworth and 500 from St. Louis, a mulatto man became infected with what was thought to be measles. By the time the boat reached the agency at Council Bluffs, where the annuities were to be delivered, the nature of the disease had become apparent and all aboard had been contaminated by smallpox. Finding it impracticable to deny Indians their goods, many were exposed to the disease and smallpox soon spread throughout the river communities.[13]

A letter dated November 30, 1837, stated, "All our prospects on the Upper Missouri are completely prostrated, the trade is ruined, if not forever, at least for years to come." On the author's arrival at Fort Union on October 10, he found smallpox as far away as the most distant part of the Assiniboine country, where the "poor Indians were dying by fifties and hundreds a day." After complaining of pains in the head and loins, they fell down dead, bodies turning black almost immediately. For many weeks, his men collected the dead and buried them, but after the ground froze, corpses were consigned to a watery grave. He concluded, "I should have been more or less than man, if I could have beheld the misery and wretchedness around me with indifference. And sir, I am not ashamed to acknowledge that I have shed tears of bitter anguish over the dying and the dead."

By March 3, 1838, a further report noted that a boat arriving with supplies contained smallpox victims. Although the Blackfeet were warned away, they went too close and became infected, resulting in the death of thousands of individuals. Pine Stem, a chief of great influence, blamed himself for the calamity. On his deathbed he lamented not following good advice and ordering his people to stay away, as the traders were his friends and they spoke truth. Significantly, the same newspaper reported that smallpox had not spread to the Sioux, "as many of them had been vaccinated."

By March 1838, it became apparent that the Federal Vaccination Program had failed, at least in regard to tribes on the Upper Missouri, and public indignation was aroused. The Mandans, a once-great nation reduced to 1,600 souls living in permanent villages about 1,600 miles above St. Louis, were reduced by smallpox to 31 individuals; the 1,000 Minatarees of Gros Vontres, living near the Mandans were reduced by one half, with the disease still raging; 3,000 Arickarees (also known as the Ricaras) who had lately abandoned a wandering life and joined the Mandans, suffered in the same proportion; the Assiniboines, 9,000 strong who lived entirely by the chase, ranging north of the Missouri in the plains below the Rocky Mountains down toward the Hudson Bay Company on the North Red River, were "literally annihilated." Their principal trade was at Fort Union at the mouth of the Yellowstone River. The Crees, numbering 3,000 and living in the same region, were all destroyed; the Blackfeet, who wandered and lived by the chase, divided into bands of Piegans, Gres Vontres, Blood Indians and Blackfeet, amounting to 50,000–60,000, also deeply suffered. One thousand lodges (the average number in a lodge being from 6–8 persons) were destroyed, with smallpox still active among them. The disease was expected to travel to all the tribes on the Columbia River and, in all probability, from the tribes south of the Missouri to the Mexican settlements.[14]

The above summary appears to have been taken, almost literally, from a letter written by Major Pilcher, from St. Louis, February 27, 1838, and sent for publication by General William Clark, superintendent of Indian Affairs at St. Louis. Joshua Pilcher was a Sioux agent with a reputation of advocating violence against the Indians. He was once reported as saying the only way to deal with the Arikaras was to "kill them off."[15] Pilcher's observation that "the small-pox among most of the Indian tribes of the Upper Missouri surpass all former scourges, and that the country through which it has passed is literally depopulated, and converted into *one great graveyard*" did not mention Cass's order to omit those tribes from benefits of the act, nor did Clark make any mention of that fact. The *Republican Compiler* (PA), March 20, 1838, which reran the original letter, offered information, that in consequence of the above, "funds for vaccinating the Indians were immediately remitted, with authority to employ the necessary agents." In fact, an additional $1,000 was added to the fund by March 6 but was forwarded to Pilcher for gifts and vaccinations for the Sioux bands located within his agency.

In what must be viewed as an announcement of economic interest ignoring the fact of contagion, when the steamboat *Antelope* arrived at St. Louis on July 18, 1838, it carried

"1,000 packs, chiefly Buffalo robes; and more valuable furs are on their way in Mackanaw Boats."[16]

The new secretary of war, C.A. Harris, professed no knowledge of the tragedies and it was not until six months after the epidemic that he requested a written report about the deaths. Clark replied that he had not known of the smallpox epidemics until after the fact and expressed the opinion nothing could have stopped it. He exonerated himself and Pilcher, casting blame on an absent Mandan subagent, William N. Fulkerson, who reportedly rarely, if ever, visited his post. Harris immediately sent funds for a new vaccination campaign.

After repeated requests from the military and Indian agents, in 1838, the Commissioner of Indian Affairs, in conjunction with the Department of the Interior, agreed to provide special agents for vaccination. These doctors were to receive $1,000/year; the salary was increased in 1862 to $1,200/year. In addition, the following year, $5,000 was appropriated for vaccinations. Internal unrest during the Civil War ultimately forced special agents Dr. Joseph C.R. Clark and Dr. H.T. Ketcham to resign from federal service. In 1839, Congress appropriated an additional $5,000 for the federal program. Eventually, Clark and Pilcher were freed from blame and nothing was ever made of Cass's order denying vaccination to the Upper Missouri tribes.

While the Indian Vaccination Act was the largest program of its kind in the United States and did succeed in protecting some Native Americans, the program was designed and implemented without consulting the Indians. It ultimately served to facilitate Indian removal off their lands and expedited white westward expansion. For his part in excluding hostile tribes, Lewis Cass was appointed minister to France. He returned in 1842 and lost a bid for the presidency in 1844; the following year, he was elected a United States senator from Michigan.[17]

The Mormon Colonization and Interaction with American Indians

In a study relative to the Mormon colonization of "Zion," author Richard W. Stoffle wrote that the sect introduced/reintroduced over half a dozen epidemic or endemic diseases to the Numic-speaking people between 1847 and 1853. Among those diseases were measles, cholera and malaria in 1849; tuberculosis (1850); scarlet fever and whooping cough (1853); typhoid fever and intestinal parasites (1854). By the end of this six-year period, Brigham Young remarked that he had watched some Indian bands shrink from 150 to 35 warriors and estimates place the mortality rate exceeding 77 percent. The first reports of smallpox appeared in 1856.

By August 1875, smallpox broke out among members of an emigrant wagon train near Salt Lake City. Brigham Young, Heber C. Kimball and Jedediah M. Grant failed in efforts to convince the Mormons to quarantine the area and the virus quickly spread to 30 inhabitants of the valley. By December, the town of Nephi on the Mormon corridor toward Fillmore reported fresh cases of smallpox.

Mormon immigrants, not dissimilar from any Euro-American group, unknowingly contaminated local water supplies, leaving typhoid and intestinal parasites in their wake. Not only did this affect the natives, it also resulted in high infant mortality rates among Mormon children at St. George during the city's formative years. From 1862 to 1881, a total of 324 Mormon children under 5 years perished, 57 children between the ages of 5 and 15 and 125 people older than 15 years.

For indigenous populations, particularly those in the southwestern portion of the Americas, smallpox proved devastating. The disease also traveled rapidly, and from the Mexican pandemic of 1520–1524, outbreaks occurred in 1564, 1695–1699, 1704, 1719, 1738, 1748, 1759, 1780–1781, 1799–1800, 1816 and 1837.

When not directly the result of exposure to Europeans, cross-contamination between tribes provided a nearly inexhaustible supply of smallpox germs. Contamination tended to follow established trade routes, with one trading partner infecting another. In 1853, for example, Southern Paiutes and Utes traded with the Hopis. That December, when a railway expedition sent Zuni guides to recruit Hopi scouts for a westward trip, the Zuni discovered that smallpox had killed nearly every adult male in the Black Mesa pueblos. Unable to bury the bodies, survivors merely shoved the dead down slopes. In June of the following year, one eyewitness visited the Hopis and observed "the whitened bones lay thickly strewed around," which he attributed to smallpox. Newspaper reports indicated that smallpox was "said to be sweeping off the Indians in Utah, by the thousands."[18]

Stoffle concluded that the virus "spread from the Rio Grande Valley Hispanic-Pueblo population to the Zunis, from them to the Hopis, and probably from Oraibi tribes to Southern Paiutes."

Their Melancholy Destiny

Despite attempts to vaccinate American Indian tribes, nothing could have totally arrested the spread of smallpox. Bands were too scattered and those living in permanent settlements had little access to vaccine. Other tribes were suspicious or outright hostile to the concept. And, like their European-American counterparts, in times of relative quiet thoughts of preventive were put aside until the appearance of a new epidemic.

By 1847, the newspapers were filled with accounts of what was considered a hopeless "melancholy destiny" of the Indians. The earliest reports cited the disease among the Cherokee and the Chippewa near Fort Winnebago. By 1850, the Sioux near Fort Laramie were so infected they "burned those who were taken with it." In May the following year, Major Barry, United States Indian agent at St. Louis, warned that along the Upper Missouri in the vicinity of Fort Pierre and Medicine Creek, several hundred Sioux had died. As the disease worked its ravages downriver, the Iowas, Sacs and Foxes also experienced severe outbreaks, although newspapers indicated that it was not known how the disease was communicated to them. By mid–June, a dire combination of cholera and smallpox had destroyed 4,000 Sioux. While carrying this news, the steamer *Durere* from Council Bluffs also reported a full cargo of robes and furs in its possession. No connection between "robes and furs" and the spread of disease was made.

This disconnect would only widen. Information gleaned from Rocky Mountain pioneers stated that smallpox and cholera had made fearful inroads among the Sioux during the winter of 1850–1851 and midway through 1851. They supposed that 3,000–4,000 deaths occurred by the introduction of both diseases by emigrants passing through to Oregon and California. Against logic if not outright fact, newspapers tended to discredit this idea, one noting that among the "more credulous of the red men" was the belief that introduction of smallpox and cholera came from the large California emigration that had crossed the Plains since 1819. The article concluded, "The agents of the American Fur Company have done much, however, to remove the erroneous impression from the minds of these children of nature."

In the same article, the *Adams Sentinel* (PA), July 5, 1851, reported that the St. Louis papers of June 20 credited traders from the American Fur Company for saving many lives by providing medicine and vaccine matter. By July, an eyewitness from St. Ange, 200 miles above the mouth of the Yellowstone, stated that not fewer than 6,000 Indians of the northwestern tribes had died that season from smallpox.[19]

In March 1854, smallpox raged with great violence among the Chippewa along the south shore of Lake Superior and on the headwaters of the Chippewa River. A month later, the governor of the territory sent Dr. T.T. Mann to vaccinate the Indians of Minnesota: "He found them almost frantic with dread of the pestilence. As soon as one is attacked by it his companions desert him; and thus it proves fatal in almost every instance."[20]

As proof that nothing ever changes, the *Illinois State Chronicle,* of April 21, 1855, published the following: "A captain of the U.S. army, in view of the anticipated troubles with the Indians in Nebraska, suggests that blankets taken from small pox hospitals be freely distributed among the different tribes. This, in his opinion, will do more towards effecting an extermination than the six new regiments. Very humane, indeed."

More depressing news followed. A trader reported that smallpox was killing off the Osage to an alarming extent. During the space of two weeks he saw almost 200 perish, noting that when they contracted the disease, they "immediately get into the water, and there lie until death ends their lives." Isolated news articles placed smallpox among the Indians at the mouth of the Yellowstone in 1856; 60 deaths at Pembina in 1857; and smallpox among the Flathead and Nez Perce, the most powerful tribes in Oregon. A less-than-generous report from 1859 provided the news that smallpox was among the Menominee at Lake Shawano: "being so careless and unguarded in their habits, many of them die of the fearful pestilence."[21]

If anything contributed to how Americans of the 19th century viewed the Indians — and passed their perspectives on to the generation who followed, some of whom transferred such tales into novels and screenplays of the "American West" — the following serves as a prime example:

> *Horrible Massacre of a Missionary Family.* — The Rev. Mr. Klifman, a Methodist missionary who has been preaching for the Indians of Oregon since 1838, was murdered, with his family, not long since, under singular and appalling circumstances. The small-pox having broke out among the savages, while the missionary's family was not attacked, the former thought that the pestilence had been introduced by the whites with the intention of exterminating the red race. Acting upon this horrible suspicion, their next step was revenge. A bold chief was selected for the deed, who stole into the chamber of the sleeping family, and buried his tomahawk in the brains of the missionary and that of his wife, and then the other Indians rushed in and helpless children, male and female employees, were butchered, the house razed to the ground, fences destroyed, and every vestige of a once happy home disappeared.[22]

Thus, on the eve of "the great bloodletting known as the Civil War" (Rod Serling, opening narration to *The Loner* television series, 1966), where soldiers fighting white-on-white, brother-on-brother slaughtered more men than in all other American wars combined excluding the Vietnam War, reports of Native Americans murdering the innocent and United States officers suggesting murder-by-smallpox filled the newspapers. Not inconsequentially, for the next five years, reporters would discover the disease would take center stage in a new and unlooked for arena.

15

Quarantines and Death Statistics

A good story is told of a well known physician, of the old foggy style, in this city, who went to a drugstore to purchase some vaccine virus. The article was handed to him, enclosed in a covering of beeswax, shaped like a bird's egg and about the same size. This is the latest style of putting up the article — entirely new to Dr. Foggy. A few days afterwards, the doctor returned to the store and handed back the vaccine, stating that it was not fit for use, as he had tried it on a large number of patients, without success. The druggist quietly explained to the doctor that he had not used the vaccine in the centre of the wax ball, but had been scratching the wax into the flesh of his patients. Dr. Foggy, not being a pious man, swore a terrible oath, denouncing in set terms all the new fangled notions of the day and left the store a sadder and wiser man than when he entered.[1]

With a neglect of vaccine or improper techniques providing little or no protection, epidemics continued to plague the expanding country. The greatest weapon in the arsenal possessed by local municipalities continued to be quarantine. A series of orders issued for the town of Viroqua, County of Badax, Wisconsin, represent a common defense at mid-century.

1. All persons who were exposed, or who were in danger of being exposed to the "Small Pox," as determined by a board-appointed physician as health officer, were required to absent themselves from the company of others who had not been so exposed.
2. Those persons not exposed were to absent themselves from persons or dwellings where the infection was present. Infected persons were to be taken from their homes by the sheriff and placed in an area for the care of persons infected with "Small Pox."
3. The owner or occupant of any dwelling place where the contagion was known to be present was obliged to give notice to all persons who might pass that way by putting up a board in a conspicuous place, with the words "Small Pox here."[2]

When an individual did contract smallpox, as in the cases above, there were certain prescribed methods of treatment. The following is taken from a medical text published in 1842:

Treatment of the Smallpox Patient

The treatment of smallpox begins by taking away a moderate quantity of blood; the exhibition of an emetic is generally advised, the bowels cleaned, diaphoretics employed and the antiphlogistic system strictly enforced. It is useful, particularly during the eruptive fever to expose the patient freely to cold air. After the eruption has come out, symptoms are usually so much mitigated that little medical interference is necessary.

Confluent smallpox requires more management: after evacuating the *primae viae,* and employing other means to moderate the fever, several remedies adapted to support the strength and counteract the septic tendency must be resorted to as the disease advances with techniques similar to the treatment of typhus. The chief points of difference are that bark may be more freely given to promote the process of suppuration, and opium to relieve the irritation in the skin. When the eruptions come out, it may be generally proper to direct a full dose of this remedy every night to procure rest, using proper precautions to obviate confining the bowels, or determining to the head. When alarming convulsions occur, opium is the medicine chiefly to be relied upon. Sometimes the tepid bath may be relied upon when the skin is pale and cold and the pulse weak. When a more advanced period the pustules flatten and alarming symptoms follow, the most powerful cordial and antispasmodic remedies must be tried, as the confectio opii, aether, wine &c. To prevent the eyes being injured, a cooling lotion may be applied, and blisters behind the ears or even leeches to the temples.[3]

The spread of disease from one country to another, from city to town, and person to person, was greatly exacerbated with the advances in transportation. Colonization, commerce and leisure travel opened borders previously closed or inaccessible, leading to an international movement of individuals on an unprecedented scale. As noted above, the creation and expansion of mass migration presented serious health risks to native populations. In order to combat the influx of sickness, regulations on both a national and local level attempted to prevent epidemics by quarantine, the only controllable preventive. In an era of extreme nationalism, however, this led to vastly varying regulations that not only differed from country to country, but from state to state and from one municipality to another.

Those residing in port cities were always faced with the dangers of immigrants importing the disease. Notices like the following appeared with some frequency:

A vessel arrived at Baltimore on Wednesday last from Bremen, which contained thirteen cases of small pox on board. The ship was ordered [to anchor] off the new hospital-ground by the health officer, where she will remain until the passengers, 242 in number, are vaccinated, and those down with the disease are cured. The vessel will then be purified. Here is another strong proof, says the *American,* that this loathsome disease is brought to our shores by foreigners.[4]

Yet not everyone approved of quarantine regulations, particularly those established in New York, which were far stricter than those of Boston and Quebec. Due to careless techniques practiced the world over (Russia alone perhaps excepted), vessels arriving in the city carrying smallpox victims required vaccination/revaccination of all passengers and crew, followed by 5–7 days of detention within quarantine enclosures on Staten Island. The weeklong detention was determined to be a safe waiting period for the variolous disease to fully develop and pass through the system. Those so detained were urged to accept the law with the understanding that the shipowners were required to foot the bill for their "week of leisure," while the ounce of prevention spared the "greater annoyance" of carrying the loathsome disease into the bosom of one's family.

In the early 1850s, some latitude did exist as port authorities made a clear distinction between ships arriving from what were generally considered "healthy" and "unhealthy" ports of origin. In 1854, a passenger and emigrant ship arriving at Staten Island from the former reported little sickness aboard, with the notable exception of "a few cases of smallpox brought from Havre." These passengers were allowed to disembark. On the other hand, vessels from the latter ports, particularly Havana, were assumed to carry yellow fever and other sicknesses with regularity. Diseased persons on such vessels were sent to the Marine Hospital. Typical statistics there indicated that out of 225 patients, a large portion suffered from typhus, while 50 were treated for smallpox. Such quarantine was not always advantageous to patients.

In a particularly telling report, an instance where the "afflictions to which patients of constitutional sensibility are necessarily more or less exposed in Hospitals" was furnished. A young German woman was admitted in April 1854, with typhus fever; she recovered and was discharged. A few days later she was brought back, having contracted mumps; before getting better, she had a second attack of fever, followed by cholera. As if that were not enough, she was scarcely convalescent when smallpox appeared.[5]

In 1859, the New York Chamber of Commerce was summoned to address the issue of quarantine. To clarify the theory upon which legislation was founded and laws administered, they began with this: "The definition of Quarantine, as given by McCullough, who has long been regarded as authority on commercial subjects, is, "a regulation by which all communication with individuals, ships or goods, arriving from *places infected with the plague or other contagious disorders,* or supposed to be peculiarly liable to such infection, is interdicted for a certain definite period."[6] In detailing the history of quarantine, the chamber acknowledged the wildly disparate interests of merchants and men of science. Noting that "quarantines were originally the result of fear and ignorance," they traced the idea back to the first centuries of plague, where both heathen and Christian nations believed disease to be a divine punishment or predestined event that was impossible to avoid. The former stoically submitted to their fate while the latter relied on prayer and fasting. By the 14th century, however, the Italians deemed it possible to guard against infection by imposing a 40-day quarantine.

When the Turks introduced plague into the Levant, it was attributed to "their filthy personal habits, their unhealthy manner of life, and their ill-ventilated dwellings." Although finding it difficult to trace contagion into dwellings of local populations suffering from the same conditions, quarantine was introduced "to produce the desired result [of containment] by a rigid enforcement of sanitary rules on all those who came within the reach of public control." From there, infected persons were often isolated and the idea of purification of clothing and personal items became the rule.[7]

Sanitary Commissions

Over the following centuries, quarantine rules became unnecessarily complex, frustrating those attempting to follow or enforce them. In order to address these complex and occasionally irksome laws, a call went out for an entire revision of the laws of quarantine. In July 1851, the first International Sanitary Conference (*Conference Sanitaire*) was assembled at Paris. Recognized as the first international public health assembly, twelve governments were represented: Austria, France, Great Britain, Greece, the Papal States, Portugal, Russia, Sardinia, the two Sicilies, Spain, the Sublime Porte (Turkey) and Tuscany.[8]

The French minister of agriculture and trade assumed the original initiative for the conference, with each government represented by two delegates—a diplomat and a physician. During a six-month period, 48 plenary sessions and numerous committee meetings were held before the close on January 19, 1852.[9] With its primary purpose "to harmonize and reduce the numerous quarantine requirements of different European countries," discussions centered around the importation of plague with an emphasis on minimizing the spread of cholera, plague and yellow fever.[10]

The delegates composed the text of international sanitary regulations containing 137 articles and signed a draft on December 19, 1851, with an amended draft signed January 16,

1852. This did not commit their governments to following the recommendations, however, and four months later only France, Portugal, Sardinia, the Sublime Porte and Tuscany had ratified the regulations. Ultimately, the several governments failed to agree and the drafts never developed into international law.

The United States had not been part of the European conference. Although roundly criticized as antiquated and cumbersome, its quarantine laws were left to individual states and municipalities. Taking matters into their own hands, some shipping lines began stocking surgeon's medical chests with smallpox vaccination in order to avoid disasters at sea. The directors of the company operating the mail steamship USS *Eldorado* luckily possessed that foresight. In April 1853, two days out from the port of New York, destined for Aspinwall under the command of Lieutenant Griffin, USN, it was discovered a carpenter had a virulent form of smallpox. The commander immediately isolated the victim in a stateroom and prevented all contact with him. He then offered vaccination to all who wished it; 132 passengers took him up on the offer. In this number, the surgeon included himself. Having recently passed through a severe attack of fever, he questioned whether a change in constitution might have left him susceptible.

After the insertion of the virus, the doctor developed a very sore arm but not the disease. The doctor having determined he himself was not immune, the care of the sick man was designated to a passenger. The carpenter survived until the boat reached Aspinwall, when the hot tropical climate proved too much for him and he died. Three of the crew who had previously passed through the disease wrapped the body in a flag, rowed ten miles to sea, affixed heavy weights to the body and consigned it to a watery grave. No other reports of passengers contracting the disease are known.[11]

The issue of local, national and international quarantine continued to be a major topic of discussion. Proponents of unified regulations in the United States closely tracked the proceedings of the European conference, observing that in England, where the matter of external health laws had been minutely investigated, the Paris decree had been entirely abrogated. From their standpoint, in 1857, the Philadelphia Board of Health noted:

> No one who has made himself familiar with the exciting system of existing segregation as set forth in the antiquated Quarantine laws which, with few exceptions, prevail throughout the United States, or has other directly or indirectly been made the unfortunate victim of their overbearing interdictions, but must admit that in many of their leading features, insufficiency, oppressiveness, and inconsistency far outweigh the benefits which a well ordered code of regulations would confer upon any community.... The enforcement of an indeterminate quarantine in one State is calculated to operate with serious embarrassment upon another, recognizing and acting under principles at variance with the former, and it is in vain we can expect any change in the policy of quarantine restrictions at present adopted and enforced by the different sea-board cities, for the purpose of establishing a uniformity of laws, unless by a simultaneous movement of the several municipal corporations or Boards of Health, indorsed by legislative enactments.

With an eye toward commerce, the board further clarified its stance by acknowledging that existing quarantine laws had not kept pace with the rapid strides made in the science of public hygiene and that those laws were "singularly burdensome by clogging the wheels of a foreign trade wherever and whenever enforced." Desiring to create a code of laws, "uniform under all circumstances if possible," the Board of Health of Philadelphia appointed a committee, to correspond with the boards of health of New York, Boston, Baltimore and New Orleans, on the propriety of calling a quarantine convention.[12] The date was set for 15 May, 1857, and was to be held in Philadelphia.[13]

The National Quarantine Convention at Philadelphia began May 13, 1857, having for its object the framing of a uniform system of quarantine laws for ports in the United States. The results were expected to exert an important influence upon the public.[14] The proceedings opened with a paper submitted by Dr. J.W. Starling, formerly of the marine hospital, Staten Island, setting forth the utility of quarantine and reviewing the manner in which typhus fever, Asiatic cholera and yellow fever exhibited themselves, together with remarks as to their course and influence. The document concluded with Starling's opinion that "cleaning foul ships, prohibiting the landing of damaged cargoes, or rotten fruits, or rotting clothing, into our city, or in any populous town ... and you have seemed most of all the good that can be derived from mere quarantine. Beyond these, quarantines are an intolerable burden, annoying to the traveler, frequently distressing to the sick, oppressive to the merchant, and injurious to the trade, beneficial only to *attaches,* and to seaports where they do not exist. In short, without domestic sanitary measures ... quarantines are but of little use...."

Six proposals were drafted the first day of the convention:

1. Certain diseases perhaps could be introduced into a community by foul vessels and cargoes, and diseased crew and passengers.
2. The diseases were small pox, and under certain conditions, typhus fever, cholera and yellow fever.
3. When these diseases were introduced in this manner, their action was limited to individuals coming within their immediate influence and could scarcely be expected to become epidemic unless there existed in the community circumstances which were calculated to produce the disease, independent of the importation.
4. That local circumstances were the collection of decomposing substances in a season marked by certain meteorological conditions.
5. That efficient sanitary measures including quarantine would, in most cases, prevent the introduction of these diseases, or disarm them of their virulence.
6. That quarantine measures as they stood in most States were inefficient as a preventive and were prejudicial to the interests of the community.

On the second day, a letter from Dr. Thompson, physician to the Marine Hospital at Quarantine Station, New York, was read. He stated his opinion that the New York system of quarantine was the most perfect that could be desired, "and that he viewed all opposition to it as nothing more that the effort of a visionary brain."

The Committee on Business then reported their findings on how disease was introduced:

1. By a foul vessel, especially when bilge water was allowed to stagnate; or from water-soaked sugar or molasses, coffee or other cargoes allowed to remain beneath the timbers of the ship;
2. By cargoes of rags, cotton or other porous substances, shipped from ports where malignant disease was present;
3. By the filthy bedding, baggage and clothing of emigrant passengers, particularly when they were crowded together in uncomfortable quarters, when the passengers themselves might be free from disease;
4. By the air that had been confined during the voyage in closely sealed and unventilated holds;

5. By squalid and diseased passengers landed and crowded together in unhealthy neighborhoods, or small, unventilated dwellings;
6. By infected passengers and crews and their bedding, clothing and baggage.

The report concluded:

1. To prevent the introduction of disease, careful inspection of all vessels should be made immediately upon arrival. No passengers or cargoes should be unloaded until the hold was fully and freely ventilated by opening the hatches and the introduction of wind sails, nor until the bilge water was entirely removed and the run effectually cleansed and purified.
2. All cargo, baggage and passengers judged capable of generating or communicating disease should be unloaded and purified before their admission into the city.
3. Provisions should be provided for the immediate landing of all infected persons on board as they arrived and comfortable quarters provided for their treatment until they could be properly taken care of by friends.
4. In the case of a shipload of squalid passengers, their clothing, beds, and other effects should be subjected to ventilation and purification and measures adopted to prevent them crowding together in unhealthy dwellings.
5. When a vessel arrived in a foul condition or when disease had been present, the passengers and crew should be removed and the vessel undergo a thorough process of cleaning and purification. In this case it would perhaps be necessary to discharge cargo at a safe distance from the city, and to allow only such portions of it that incapable of creating disease. Passengers and crew were subject to vaccination.
6. The carrying out of these provisions were to be entrusted to a single officer with assistance as required.
7. This officer should be a regular physician of unquestionable talents and experience.
8. His compensation should be sufficiently ample to allow him to devote his entire attention to his duties.
9. This officer should have sole and entire decision making authority concerning these general provisions.
10. In every community a board of health should watch over sanitary conditions and prevent and remove all domestic sources of disease.

In addition, the committee stated that yellow fever was "not contagious, *per se*," and that it was propagated only in a foul or infectious atmosphere. They added that "quarantine measures *alone* can never protect a community, either from the introduction or propagation of disease, however rigid they may be," that emigrants be vaccinated if not so protected, and that public records be kept and published monthly.[15]

On the third and final day of deliberation, the Southern delegates strenuously objected to the resolutions in relation to yellow fever (the disease being found primarily in hot climates, thus directly and negatively affecting them) and they were removed. The final adoption of the resolutions, as amended, passed with only two delegates voting against it; the New Orleans delegates were divided. Before winding up with an entertainment at the Lazaretto, the title of the convention was changed to the "National Sanitary and Quarantine Convention" and another meeting was scheduled for April 1858, at Baltimore.[16]

Smallpox and New York City Mortality

A review of mortality rates from New York City provides an insight into the general health of the population (not surprisingly, those diseases proving fatal did not differ significantly from those given for London during a similar time frame):

Partial List of New York City Mortality
(for the week ending January 29, 1853)

Cause of Death	Number of Deaths
Consumption	63
Convulsions	32
Dropsy	6
" head	18
Fevers, scarlet	22
" puerperal	1
" typhoid	1
" typhus	7
" unidentified	2
Heart, disease of	9
Inflammation of the brain	10
" lungs	28
Killed or murdered	2
Marasmus*	10
Old age	2
Small pox	10

*Marasmus: Emaciation, or a generalized wasting of the body caused by malnutrition.[17]

Of these deaths, 62 were men, 77 women. Deaths among children amounted to 113 boys and 112 girls, of which 146 were two years of age or younger. The total deaths for the week was 364; the week previous, the death total had been 360. Places of nativity included United States, 256; Ireland, 71; England, 6; Scotland, 3; Germany, 21; France, 1; China, 1; British Possessions in North America, 2; Unknown, 2. For the same week, deaths in the city of Brooklyn amounted to 56, of which 25 were male, 31 female, with 35 classified as children. The greatest killer was consumption with 9; smallpox claimed 1 victim.[18]

Four hundred and eighty one persons died in New York City in the first week of 1854, one fewer than the preceding week, or "about the expected average for the season." Of these, consumption was the number one killer, claiming 63 lives. (Interestingly, the newspaper observed that the word "consumption" was vague in its application, including "all sorts of diseases upon which a cough attends, which the physician fails to cure.") Following consumption came smallpox, moving up the list from number seven to number two. The *New York Daily Times* noted, somewhat caustically, that

> [Smallpox] is coming to be one of our institutions. It has no business here at all, but our people fancy it. It is very prevalent just now in the City, but there are hundreds of children here yet unvaccinated. People don't mind riding in stages or the Third-avenue cars up to Sixty first-street, with one or two on board who are just breaking out with small pox, and can take no other means of reaching the miserable shanty that they call the "Small Pox Hospital" on Blackwell's Island. They shudder at the thought of exposing their little ones, but they care too little about it to have their little ones vaccinated. And so they died and were buried, as victims jointly of this loathsome pest, which we ought to have banished before now, and the gross carelessness of parents and

guardians in this City, for the last week, 43 persons. The small pox is fairly entitled to the succession, and if consumption ever loses its position as prime minister to Death, it must stand first in the list of fatal diseases.

Partial List of New York City Mortality
(for the week of January 1–7, 1854)

Cause of Death	Number of Deaths
Consumption	63
Smallpox	—
Convulsions	36
Stillborn children	35
Inflammation of the lungs	32
Croup	26
Dropsy, head	23
Scarlet fever	20
Marasmus	17

As the times reflected, the *Daily Times* considered "the health of the City is good but it ought to be better. Instead of 481 burials there should not certainly have been more than 438, and if some female Brutus would thrust the dagger into the neck of the tyrant Fashion, doubtless 400 would outnumber those that would remain on the list."[19]

Three years later, smallpox had dropped to number 8 on the list. For the period January 24 through January 31, 1857, there were 491 deaths in New York City and New York County, of which 80 were men, 73 were women, 171 boys and 167 girls, an increase of 18 from the previous week.

Partial List of New York City Mortality
(for the week of January 24–31, 1857)

Cause of Death	Number of Deaths
Consumption	52
Scarlet fever	46
Convulsions	44
Stillborn	35
Croup	31
Inflammation of lungs	29
Marasmus	2
Small-pox	18
Dropsy, head	18

In order of nationality, the bulk of deaths occurred to those born in the United States, 388; followed by Ireland, 56; Germany, 21; England, 8; Scotland, 4; Switzerland, 3; France, 3; British America, 2; Holland, 2; East Indies, 1; Spain, 1; Sweden, 1; West Indies, 1; Unknown, 1.[20]

As conditions worsened and regulations were more strictly enforced, the New York City health officer was "very roundly abused" for his adherence to the law, but he defended himself by arguing that "stringent quarantine ha[s] alone saved us from rotting with smallpox." During the months September 1857–May 1858, ten vessels with an aggregate of 3,328 passengers were detained in quarantine on account of the disease. The number of cases on board at the time of arrival was 81, with 83 fresh cases breaking out among passengers after they were placed in quarantine.

Although the city averaged a dozen deaths from smallpox weekly, quarantine was credited with the singular fact that not a single case was attributable to vessels arriving from abroad. On the contrary, emigrants traveling by carriage or railroad from Boston and Canada were blamed for fresh outbreaks. Dr. Walser, of the Marine Hospital at Staten Island, compiled the following table from July 1857 to May 25, 1858. The fifth column exhibits the number of cases active on arrival and the sixth the number of cases that broke out during detention at Quarantine.

Date of Arrival at New York	Name of Vessels	Port of Clearance	Number Psgr Cases	Number Active on Arrival	Number in Quar
July 14	Ellen Austin	Liverpool	497	21	39
July 16	Albert Gallatin	Liverpool	581	16	28
Aug. 4	Amalia	Bremen	143	4	2
Aug. 11	Carolina	Bremen	165	2	—
Sept. 1	Reinhart	Bremen	337	16	3
May 10	Universe	Liverpool	239	2	—
May 21	Haroest	Havre	256	5	3
May 21	Dewitt Clinton	Liverpool	437	5	2
May 22	Alberto	Bremen	377	3	5
May 25	American Union	Liverpool	296	7	1
		Totals	**3,328**	**81**	**83**[21]

Clearly the rationale and the numbers spoke for themselves, but they were to prove tragically inadequate, as subsequent events proved.

16

The Quarantine Wars

Never was demolition more complete: never was a sadder wreck. An acre of ground is covered with the debris of what but the same day were buildings devoted to humanitarian purposes and the cure of the sick.[1]

The lead to an article under the heading "Opposition to Quarantine" read: "The quarantine war has begun in earnest—and the opening act of aggression is a conflagration at Sequine's Point [Staten Island], in which all the buildings there have been consumed." Being over 150 years distant from these events, it is difficult for people today to imagine how opposition to quarantine laws could incite men to arson. But the issue was of paramount importance to those living in the middle years of the 19th century, and the "war" that began on May 6, 1857, would not end until wanton destruction finally led to unspeakable acts of mayhem and death.

The principal issue pitted those in favor of strict public health regulations against the commercial interest of importers, who chaffed at what they considered unnecessary delays in obtaining goods brought in by ship, and passengers aboard those ships who decried regulations demanding their segregation until any threat of disease had run its course. Violent protest appealed to the more radical opposition members and a Vigilance Committee was appointed at the quarantine meeting held in Richmond, New York, on April 29, 1857. On Wednesday, May 6, a second meeting was held, followed by a public gathering. It was believed that at this meeting a determination to burn the estate of T.R. Lush (also known as Wolfe's farm) was fixed.

Out of Lush's 132-acre property, 50 acres had been sold to the quarantine commissioners for $23,000, with the deed transferred to the state, together with the insurance policies worth $12,000. Having sold the property at a very low figure, Lush expected to realize a profit by the sale of houselots from the remainder.

About midnight on May 6, some twenty persons dressed in ordinary clothes and, making no effort to disguise themselves except that they spoke not a word throughout, forcibly entered the estate house by breaking down the doors. After indiscriminately breaking furniture (owned by Wolfe), doors and moveables, the house was set on fire without regard for the three servants sleeping upstairs. These three—Samuel Fitzpatrick, 18 years old, James Murray, a boy, and Mary Atrinson, a woman of color—were forced to jump from a second-story window to save their lives.

From the estate house, the arsonists proceeded to a nearby farm owned by Mr. Morrison. Without giving a word of warning, the mob set the place on fire, then torched all the outbuildings, reducing them to ruins. During this destruction, the three servants arrived, finding Morrison, his wife, son and daughter standing outside. Fitzpatrick helped get two horses out of the stable and then attempted to save possessions from the house, with little success.

Former alderman Benson, one of the commissioners, departed the following evening for Albany to convey the facts to Governor King. He also intended to ask for the state to provide a suitable armed force to guard against future depredations and a reward for the arrest of the perpetrators. In this he failed, for although several arsonists were recognized island inhabitants shielded the villains from arrest.

Ironically, for all the violence and destruction committed by the group that came to be known as the Prince's Bay Incendiaries, the vandalism ultimately achieved little more than the financial destruction of Morrison, the unfortunate farmer, and forced the insurance company to pay on the $12,000 policy on the estate house. Considering it was too elaborate for the purposes of the Quarantine Committee, the money received provided well over the $10,000 estimated to construct three new hospitals, docks and the placement of four buoys in the lower bay for the anchorage of infected vessels. In the meantime, a large, two-story building opposite the entrance to the grounds was offered as a residence for the Marine physician. It was estimated that by May 14, when proposals for construction were due, work on the new quarantine hospitals would begin, with a finish date set at June 1.[2]

Matters concerning the arsonists remained unsettled as the Quarantine Commission moved forward with the construction of the necessary buildings at Sequine's Point (Staten Island). Taking a cue from the Princes' Bay Incendiaries, who succeeded in burning "with impunity," inhabitants at the other end of the island threatened to do the same at Tompkinsville, where the hospitals and physicians' houses at the old Quarantine stood.

The general feeling among locals held that the Princes' Bay rioters had a shadow of right on their side, inasmuch as the proposed quarantine buildings had been arranged contrary to their wishes. No such latitude was granted the residents living by the old Quarantine, as they were "voluntary occupants of the land," all of them having purchased lots and built homes, "knowing the perils they encountered in settling in such close proximity to the Hospital grounds." The Quarantine had been in its present location over fifty years and every home within a dangerous distance of it had been constructed within that time. The *New York Daily Times* of May 16, 1857, warned that if those residents "should imitate the incendiary example of the lawless ruffians at Wolfe's farm, they must not expect the same degree of sympathy to be extended to them that has shielded the former from arrest."

At the same time, a proposal was made to relocate the new quarantine to Coney Island, "with the concurrence of joint owners on the water-front, and to an extent covering all the land and water necessary to the public health and for commercial purposes." The idea was hailed with enthusiasm and it was hoped prompt action would be taken, thus exonerating the commissioners of Quarantine, whose character had been "somewhat compromised by their unsatisfactory selection of Sequine's Point, and to allay the irritation of the citizens of Richmond County."[3]

The Staten Island Arson

If the opening aggression in the Quarantine War started May 6, 1857, then it culminated September 1, 1858, with the near-total destruction of the quarantine buildings on Staten Island. The simmering anger over having the station so close to the city had lingered for years, with the arson at Sequin's Point exacerbating local feeling but doing nothing to solve the problem. On a more fundamental level, it should also be noted that the citizens of Stapleton, who had built extensive shoreline properties on the island, were angry at what they considered a "nuisance" that deprived them of the patronage derived from the city's wealthier population making pleasure excursions to the island.

In August 1858, several fatal cases of yellow fever in the neighborhood of the Quarantine landing led to the spread of that disease among the resident population outside the quarantine enclosure. In consequence, "it was well understood by those in the secret, that the Quarantine buildings, hospitals, physician's residences, and, in short, every edifice and shanty connected with them, were to disappear." In fact, a handbill containing an extract from the minutes of the board of health of the town of Castleton, Richmond County, was posted and widely distributed, one actually being placed on the wall where the arsonists first broke through:

> *Resolved,* That the whole Quarantine establishment located as it is in the midst of a dense population, has become a pest and a nuisance of the most odious character, bringing death and desolation to the very doors of the people of the towns of Castleton and Southfield.
> *Resolved,* That it is a nuisance too intolerable to be borne by the citizens of these towns any longer.
> *Resolved,* That this Board recommend the citizens of this county to protect themselves by abating this abominable nuisance without delay.
> A.W. BOYCE, Sec'y. R. CHRISTOPHER, Chairman.
> Sept. 1, 1858.

Tragically, the authorities took no special precautions and on Wednesday night, while the city was celebrating the laying of the Atlantic cable, a well-organized mob "who did not care to disguise themselves or to disavow their intent" commenced their attack.

As early as 9:30 P.M., Dr. R.H. Thompson, the health officer, and Dr. D.H. Bissell were informed mischief was afoot, and in less than a quarter of an hour alarm bells sounded. The wall of the hospital cemetery was broken and the mob rushed through, first setting fire to a large row of buildings known as the "small-pox shanties." Several patients undergoing treatment there, some in the last stages of the disease, were in the buildings and it was only by the utmost exertion they were removed before the stiff breeze destroyed the compound. They were left on the ground, wrapped in blankets.

The stevedores, boatmen and others working at the quarantine facility joined Dr. Bissell, but they were unable to stop the marauders. A stevedore named Hegeman, a Swede, was shot in the back and taken to the New York Hospital where he subsequently died, while the doctor was beaten with the butt of his own musket. Another physician, Dr. Walser, who had charge of the yellow fever patients, also resisted the mob and was nearly shot for his efforts. Although fifteen members of the harbor police had been on duty at Quarantine since April 1858, their efforts at assistance proved ineffectual.

Reports from the time make it evident that the attack not only received the support of most residents of Stapleton, but also that the authorities were "apathetic" in their duties, some police not only encouraging the mob but participating in the arson, while the fire companies, after breaking open the main gates into the Quarantine, offered little help because their hose had been cut — "a calamity which they did not seem much to lament." When Mr. Tallmadge, the general superintendent of city police, was informed of the attack around 2:00 A.M. and asked for assistance, he refused to do it on the grounds that Staten Island was not included within the limits of New York City. Additionally, the cost of rowing several hundred men over in small boats and having them exposed to infectious diseases did not seem prudent. When Dr. Thompson reached the mayor at 11:00 A.M. the following day, he asked for and was promised a squad of 50 men to protect what was left, yet these officers did not make an appearance.

The yellow fever and smallpox shanties were the first burned, followed by the smallpox hospital known as the "Saint Nicholas," a large brick building with a wooden sailor atop. As the floors gave way, approximately one hundred iron bedsteads from the Saint Nicholas fell to the ground, twisted and ruined. What made the devastation all the more heinous was the total disregard for human life, as deliberate attempts were made to murder innocent victims lying in their sick beds. Many were too ill to save themselves and had to be dragged out, left exposed to the heavy smoke from the smoldering coal, the flying embers and the elements.

A particular target of the arsonists was the house of Dr. Thompson. The doctor, in his official capacity as health officer, had become an unpopular figure with the citizens of Stapleton, and the incendiaries destroyed his property "in a very deliberate and particularly cruel way. 'Let us save the Doctor's house,' they cried, and immediately it was set on fire in five or six different places," everything being spoken in opposites. Mrs. Thompson, an invalid, had to be hurried away by servants, while the physician fled for his life. In lieu of perpetrating violence on him, the arsonists threw his valuable collection of books into the fire, scattered his personal papers and manuscripts and reveled in champagne found in his wine and liquor store. Thompson's loss was estimated at $5,000–$6,000. Although the Women's Hospital was set on fire it was saved, and by daylight it remained the only building still standing. This was used to house as many of the patients as possible, with the rest lying on the grass with only the stevedores to attend them. By 5:00 P.M., a ship was moored at the Public Store Dock for the purpose of being transformed into a floating hospital.

Many of the locals claiming a hand in the destruction were men of wealth and influence, including a justice of the peace and the owner of a prominent livery stable, who claimed that during the height of the yellow fever "mania," the Quarantine establishment deprived him of $300 per week by keeping away tourists. Hotel keepers joined the cry of denouncing the hospitals for economic reasons, citing the *rumor* that cases of yellow fever had driven away all lodgers from a large boardinghouse at the southeast end of the island, while "respectable persons also, or those whose wealth had secured their influence and standing, were not backward in upholding the mob who had taken this summary way to dispose of Quarantine." Indeed, a man said to be the former health officer, who had grown wealthy by that station, declared that the citizens of the island had been "persecuted, and were the immense losers by the Quarantine establishment," rendered so impoverished by its presence "they could not even pay their taxes, to such a low state had property fallen." The September 3, 1858, report from the *New York Times* concluded: "In such cases as the present grievance the public had always approved of taking the remedy into their own hands. With such sentiments from respectable persons it is easy to guess what the feelings and opinions of the more ignorant are."

The September 4, 1858, issue of *New York Times* ran a itemized description of the destroyed buildings, which gives a thorough picture of the extensive quarantine compound.

1. The "Small Pox Hospital": a brick building, 30 by 60 feet, two stories high with two piazzas. It stood on a hill behind the doctor's residence. There were no patients in the building when it was burned as it had been under repair at the time.
2. Five shanties, 200 feet long set on brick pillars about two feet from the ground and

filled in with brick. They were all of one story; some contained cooking stoves and ranges.

3. Three shanties, 120 by 25 feet, the same height as the others. One held smallpox patients, one yellow fever patients and those with various other diseases; the third was used as sleeping quarters for the stevedores and nurses. They were filled with iron bedsteads, crockery and hospital furniture.

4. Various outbuildings and four large piles of coal equaling 150 tons.

5. The "Saint Nicholas," a large building used for the accommodation of passengers in quarantine. It measured 60 by 130 feet, was 3 stories high, and was built of heavy brick walls with porticos at each end, with a stoop and pillars of brown stone. A piazza was placed on the east side.

6. Two large brick outhouses; even the pumps were burned.

7. The fences surrounding the compound were set on fire in more than 20 places. Two large breaches were made in the west wall.

8. The "dead-house" (also known as the coffin-house), containing 20–30 empty coffins and one body — that of the engineer from the *Philadelphia,* who had recently died from yellow fever. Also the dissecting room.

9. A barn, 30 by 50 feet, two stories high and filled with hay; two horses and a quantity of hogs were in the barn. The animals were driven out and saved. Also burned was a sick wagon, a cart and a light wagon.

10. Carriage house and coal house containing 600 tons of coal. A large lot of steam-heating apparatus, a brass six-pound cannon and an icehouse were destroyed. Also the wood-house and henhouse.

11. A baggage house for emigrants, also used as a fire-engine house, 25 by 60 feet. The engine, 250 feet of hose and three dozen water buckets were burned, along with considerable unclaimed baggage belonging to deceased persons, together with some belongings of people living on the grounds.

12. The health officer's house, occupied by Dr. Thompson, was of wood, three stories high, filled in with brick; it also included a wing.

13. The revenue office was burned but the fire went out from lack of air. Mr. Locke, the inspector, was notified to remove his goods from the office and storehouse before they were burned (Locke was a supporter of the arsonists).

14. The Women's Hospital, a large, two-story brick structure fronting the bay, with two corridors extending the whole length, supported by round brick columns.

15. The U.S. Inspector's Office, belonging to the Quarantine. It was a small building of two stories, one of the oldest wooden structures on the ground.

16. The washhouse, a large, squat building on the extreme end of the second pier. The whole wharf on which it stood, together with the bathhouse was also destroyed.

17. The warden's building, situated on the end of the pier, and its lantern and illuminating tower for the benefit of shipping. It was used as a lookout by the watchmen and as a storage area.

18. The entire wooden pier, including the dock used by the health officer and the U.S. Barge officers as a landing.

19. The gatekeeper's lodge, a brick building a story-and-a-half high.

20. The cookhouse, a long, narrow brick building, 80 feet in length, divided into three compartments where food for 1,400 patients was prepared.

During the melee, a ringleader named O'Hara, who incidentally was a member of the No. 4 Fire Engine Company, was arrested, along with two of the harbor police, one of them being Officer Boodle. Ray Tompkins, chief of the fire police and an influential man on the island, was present during the burnings and, after concluding a statement of involvement, acknowledged that he expected to be arrested that day for his complicity.

On Thursday, the weekly meeting of the Commissioners of Emigration was held. A letter from Dr. Bissell was read giving details of the fire; it was "ordered on file," and a motion was made to have the walls of the Quarantine repaired. Acknowledging that the Castleton Board of Health had passed resolutions "tantamount to the declaration that the Quarantine establishment is a nuisance," the matter was referred to committee to confer with counsel and call in the attorney general, if necessary.

On September 2, a meeting of the citizens of Richmond County was held at Nautilus Hall, Tompkinsville, "to celebrate the burning of the Shanties and Hospitals at the Quarantine ground," with Ray Tompkins the chair. A number of resolutions were passed, among them the complaint that they had to "bear the burdens of harboring all the pestilential diseases of the world which have concentrated at the port of New-York for over half a century," spreading death and destruction among them. They passed thanks to the Castleton Board of Health "for authorizing the citizens of this county to abate the nuisance without delay," and cheerfully recommended "to the Commissioners of Health and Emigration to secure the Battery for the purpose of locating a Quarantine establishment there, that it may be under their immediate supervision." The Battery, a former promenade at the tip of the island enjoyed by the wealthy, had, by the mid–1850s, fallen on hard times and become little better than an open slum that harbored New York's first emigrant depot, at Castle Garden. Described as an area of decay where "freshly arrived foreigners, ragged, tattered, and drunken men and women sit under old trees," it was considered as unsafe a place as any in the city.[4]

On Thursday night, September 2, the same group of arsonists under the control of Ray Tompkins and Tom Garrett returned to the Quarantine, and entered the block of cottages occupied by the doctor's boatmen. Piling hay and loose material around and inside the cottages, they set the buildings on fire, adding camphene to increase the heat. Amid approving shouts and laughter, they next moved to an adjoining house, where the process was repeated. The houses of Dr. Walser, deputy health officer, and Dr. Bissell were also burned. Once the fire bell was rung, firemen arrived who busied themselves aiding the work of destruction. One reporter noted, "While this is going on, mock calls are made for water, the firemen rushes up and down the street, making hoarse outcries which nobody understands or cares to. The whole scene is one of the most horrible farces which it has ever been my fortune to witness."

The federal buildings occupied by the inspectors were left intact as there were sixty marines to protect them. Of note, this property was considered worthless; when applied to for help in preventing the destruction of the Quarantine, the soldiers replied "that they had been sent down with instructions from Washington to protect the United States property and nothing else." Without their intervention and the failure of Governor King to send armed men to protect the enclosure, the result became inevitable. The reporter's eyewitness account concluded:

> The Hospital is now on fire, (12:10 o'clock,) and the flames are bursting through the roof.
>
> What is being done to preserve the lives of the helpless sick within its walls, I do not know. God preserve them.

P. S.—12:30 A.M.— The sick have been taken from the Hospital, and are left on the ground in the angle formed by the wall and Dr. Bissell's fence. Unless removed from here, I fear they will perish when the Hospital is fully on fire. The flames are now bursting through the roof.

As a final act of wanton inhumanity, two vessels arrived at the lower Quarantine, the schooner *Laura Gertrude,* from Charleston, and the bark *Charles Brewer,* from Havana. Both had crew sick from yellow fever, the latter craft having lost its captain to the disease. The sick were unable to be removed as there were no accommodations for them.[5]

The Aftermath of Terrorism

With the final destruction of the Women's Hospital, the patients, in every stage of suffering, some delirious with fever and others dying from their afflictions, were taken outside and placed on open ground where they were subjected to the fall of burning embers from the fire. Many ran around piteously crying, "Will they burn us? Will they burn us?" The *New York Times* reporter described it: "The roar of the flames, the clouds of dense smoke rolling upward, the furious outcries of the mob, crazy with their infernal work, all formed a scene most horrible and impressive."

Forty-four male and female patients were placed in the ironically named boat, *Cinderella,* anchored at the wharf. Of those, twenty were yellow fever victims, three or four suffered from smallpox and the rest were afflicted with generic "ship fever." Doctors Bissell and Walser had charge of them, the two men having gone sleepless since the first fires on September 1. The Castleton Board of Health desired the patients to be removed to an old bark adjacent, but as the true health care professionals considered that incarceration "certain death," the victims remained where they were. Houseless, unsheltered and lacking even the common utensils for cooking, these unfortunate people surveyed a scene hardly befit "a community which is called 'civilized.'"

The curious from the island and those who had come across for a peek at the conflagration stated at the patients, apparently content to see they were alive; none inquired how the afflicted were to be provided for afterwards. Mr. Locke, head of the United States inspectors, openly applauded the destruction, triumphantly declaring, "Now we shall have a road through these grounds all around the Island. All the State has to do is to take Coney Island and set up the Quarantine there." When it was suggested the state did not own that property, Locke retorted that it could be seized by the right of eminent domain. To complicate matters, the project of burning the infected shipping in the harbor and the houses of the infected district of Tomkinsville was a controversial topic.

The complicit Castleton Board of Health issued eight resolutions and a series of orders pertaining to the Quarantine. They dictated that those shore men working on infectious vessels, along with the crew and passengers, were prohibited from coming into town for a period of ten days; nor should they be permitted to take the ferry from Staten Island to New York City. The same held true for their baggage. They were also prohibited from throwing anything overboard.

The same rules held for those within the Quarantine, including physicians, the health officer and the boarding officer, with an end purpose of stopping all intercourse between the inside and the outside. Anyone having knowledge of violations was required to report to the board or suffer criminal prosecution. If convicted, the guilty party could suffer imprisonment of up to three years or fines not to exceed $1,000. The document, posted in lettering half as large as a man's hand, was signed by R. Christopher, chairman and A.W. Boyce, clerk.

Of only slightly more use was the meeting of the Commissioners of Emigration, including Governor King, Mayor Powell of Brooklyn and the health officer. After tabling an offer from Charles McNeil, who offered the west end of Coney Island and the Pavilion for the sick, all the dignitaries could agree upon were to provide tents from the arsenal and to send out one hundred policemen.[6]

In November 1858, Judge Metcalf of the New York Supreme Court ruled in the case of Ray Tompkins and C.J. Thompson, charged with having set fire to the Quarantine buildings. He decided that "the quarantine was a nuisance, and that private citizens had a right to abate it."[7] Debate over their punishment, or lack of punishment, would continue for years, while an editorial in the *New York Times* (March 18, 1859) best summed up the quarantine controversy: "The great problem of the age seems to be, to establish a Quarantine without having it located anywhere.... Somebody must be put to inconvenience by them [quarantine laws]. And if the State is quietly to stand one side and allow itself to be overborne by the individuals whom its action may aggrieve, it can never have any public establishments of any kind."

The terrorism perpetrated on the Quarantine at Staten Island and the wanton celebration of the murderers was an unparalleled and shocking event staining American history. Even arguing that the arsonists were frustrated by having their fears of contagion ignored by the authorities, the preponderance of evidence pointed toward economic motives. The citizens of the island wanted to make it the playground of the rich and famous, thus increasing property values and bringing in revenue for shopkeepers, tavern owners and stable owners. Nor should merchants, shippers and travelers be absolved: goods delayed from being unloaded, the urgency of captains to sell their cargoes and passengers complaining of long delays due to quarantine laws all played a significant role in the uprising.

Using the erstwhile "Board of Health" as their cover, men of influence and position willingly and inhumanly sacrificed innocent victims for their own ends. Just as greedy individuals seeking political power destroyed the National Vaccine Institution, health care and the public good were sacrificed on the altar of the Almighty Dollar. While none of those associated with either tragedy were likely affected by another series of incidents, it bears a direct correlation to the above acts:

> SMALL POX.—It is stated that in the thirty years prior to 1837, only thirty-seven persons died of small pox in Boston, and most of these were seamen and emigrants who died at Rainsford Island. In 1837, all laws relating to small pox were repealed, placing it on the same footing with any other disease, and in the succeeding twelve years 538 persons died from small pox in Boston alone, and the increase in other parts of the State was about in the same proportion.[8]

(Interestingly, in 1887, during excavation work on Boylston Street, Boston, a large collection of bones was discovered. The interred were buried in their clothes and without coffins, leading to the supposition these had been smallpox victims from this period.)[9]

Debate on the culpability and punishment (or lack thereof) of the arsonists during the riot on Staten Island (September 1858) would continue for years. Numerous commissions made reports, lawyers argued for and against the accused and contradictory judgments were issued by judges and courts. By August 1860, the total amount of damage done to federal, state and personal property was set at $129,714.37.[10] Collecting it from taxes assessed on citizens of Richmond County or from the perpetrators was problematic.

The Quarantine Question was equally debated in England. During a meeting of the "Public Health" department, a paper was read by the Rev. Charles Kingsley, entitled, "The

Influence of our Elective System on Sanitary Improvement." He argued that elective systems were a great hindrance to sanitary improvement and that local boards made up of self-serving merchants had an eye toward status quo rather than public health. At the same meeting, a paper submitted by Florence Nightingale entitled "Notes on the Health of Hospitals" provided insight into deficient ventilation and overcrowding in hospitals.

Discussion centered around contagion and infection, the argument being "contagion had always resulted from the want of sanitary arrangements. It has been the groundwork of almost every false reasoning, and the excuse for the superstition of the quarantine law and the general neglect of sanitary law." Miss Nightingale stated there was no such thing as "inevitable infection," as it actually stemmed from carelessness and ignorance. She insisted on the importance of building large hospitals to alleviate overcrowding that caused so many deaths at Scutari and to provide fresh air and light. Dr. Farr and Mr. Rawlinson expressed astonishment at her insight; Dr. Milroy, a sanitary commissioner, thought she had done a "great injustice" to the army medical men.[11]

The "Great Botch"

By June 1860, New Yorkers proclaimed the city had never been healthier and attributed the fact to the board of health. The mayor, controller, select aldermen and councilmen, and two salaried officers — a physician and a clerk — comprised this board, whose power was described as "absolute," there being no appeal from its decisions. The ordinances and by-laws passed by this body included the sale of meats, ordering the disposition of bone-boiling establishments and cow stables, directing the cleansing of streets and tenements and providing places for the sick and those suffering from contagious diseases. Except in cases of pestilence, the board seldom went beyond the ordinary requirements of law and at the first meeting in April the membership resolved to hold their sessions behind closed doors. Peculiarly, no complaints arose from this decision, presumably because "for years, the board has had as little to do."

In addition to the board of health there were the commissioners of health, comprising the mayor (as presiding officer), the health officer of the port, a resident physician, a special health commissioner, the city inspector, the physician to the Marine Hospital, inspector of vessels and presidents respectively of the board of aldermen and councilmen. Except for the mayor, health officer and city inspector, the others were paid for their attendance at meetings, the presidents of the two municipal legislative boards receiving the extremely lucrative sum of $500 annually.

The special province of the health commissioner was to guard against the introduction of epidemical diseases through vessels arriving from foreign ports. The captains of such vessels were required to report their arrival and the ports from which they sailed. Much had changed since the burning of the Quarantine in 1858: instead of rigorous laws dictating quarantine, the commissioners determined which ships should be allowed to come directly into the city or be detained at Quarantine; the health officer also determined the time of detention, fumigation and lighting of cargoes.

By June, only two vessels had been detained at the lower quarantine anchorage — the schooners *Oscilla* and *Montrose*—and those for yellow fever. Several others, not exceeding a dozen, were detained a few days for observation, which meant "holding them in waiting long enough for any pestilential disease to make its appearance among the crew, if it exists on board, through the vessels having touched at infected ports." Harbor pilots, under heavy penalty, were required to detain in the lower bay all vessels coming from ports where infectious diseases prevailed, until boarded by the health officer.

In 1860, the New York health officer of the port was Dr. A.H. Gunn. He became the first health officer to require a captain to sign an affidavit before coming up to the city:

> Quarantine, _____ 1860
>
> The undersigned, captain of _____, from _____, being duly sworn, deposes and says the ports of _____, from which he sailed were, to the best of his knowledge and belief, perfectly healthy, being free from all malignant, contagious, and infectious diseases; that no such disease existed among the shipping in said ports at the time of his departure, and that no cases of sickness or death from such disease have occurred on board his vessel while in port, or on the passage homeward.
>
> Sworn before me this _____ day of _____, 1860

In accordance with a law passed after the Staten Island Quarantine Arson, all cases of smallpox and noncontagious diseases arriving on shipboard were removed to the smallpox hospital on Blackwell's Island. There, the commissioners of emigration paid the expense of their care. In June 1860, there were six smallpox patients and fifteen others ordered there by the health officer. The bark *Pilgrim,* a craft measuring 140 feet long and 40 feet wide, was used to convey those in shore quarantine to the island.

Not surprisingly, the new quarantine *regime* was based on economics. Prior to September 1858, on average a hundred vessels were kept at quarantine anchorage, running up "enormous bills for extra towing, lighterage [lighters were small boats used to transport passengers to and from a ship], stevedoring, and fumigation." This frequently caused shipowners to put into nearby Connecticut ports to unload their cargo, thereby saving a considerable sum. Under the system enacted after the quarantine uprising, shipowners experienced a savings of hundreds of thousands of dollars. Instead of having a fleet anchored off quarantine, only two or three were to be seen at any one time. Without a mention of public safety, this was considered the elimination of "wholesale robbery."[12]

As an alternative to land-based quarantine, in 1859, an old steamer called *Falcon* (renamed the *Florence Nightingale*) was "got up" as a floating hospital, familiarly referred to as the "dead-house afloat." She was originally located in Gravesend Bay, but at the commencement of quarantine season (typically when the weather turned warm) the citizens of Staten Island and Long Island refused to have it anchored off their coast, with Utrecht and Bay Ridge residents raising "such a storm of indignation" she was removed to an area about five miles off Sandy Hook. Annoyingly for New York, Sandy Hook belonged to New Jersey and discussions between the respective state legislators, much of it seemingly conducted through the newspapers, quickly reached the ludicrous stage

In better days, the *Falcon* had transported gold-seekers to California, returning with hides and precious metals. As the gold craze died down, later return trips saw her hold filled with men of broken spirits, so it was perhaps ironic she would be purchased and outfitted by the Quarantine commissioners for a sum of $15,000.

Measuring 224 feet in length and 70 feet in breadth, the boat was of 1,500 tons burden. Moored with two anchors weighing 4,000 pounds, a superadded deck provided no more of a view than the upper halves of her masts. The main deck was partitioned off into forty wards averaging 8 feet wide by 10 feet long by 8 feet high. The lower deck was left open at the ends and was to serve as one long ward filled with iron bedsteads. Accommodation was for over 200 patients suffering from yellow fever and cholera.

Not surprisingly, the question of lightering at Quarantine quickly arose, for the business was large and lucrative. When the health officer, who had control over persons engaged to conduct the business, gave exclusive privileges of lightering to Captain A.H. Schultz and that of stevedoring to Messrs. Ryan and VanValkenburg, charges of political cronyism quickly surfaced. Dr. Gunn was forced to reconsider his appointments and "show more respect for his position and the public."[13]

By 1859, the subject of quarantine was broken into three distinct groups. The first comprised those who believed in a stringent quarantine (the "old contagionists") and who required vessels from infected ports be isolated, well ventilated, fumigated and cleaned, with their cargo and passengers detained. The second group contained the "noncontagionists," who believed that typhus and yellow fever could not be transmitted from one person to another, that only goods and vessels passed disease. They argued that passengers and crew, whether healthy or sick, should be permitted to depart their ship after having cleaned themselves and their clothes. The third group, "sanitationists," believed in stringent quarantine but felt the best way to keep epidemics from the city was to clean, ventilate and light the domiciles of the population and thus by sanitary measures prevent its spread.

In the third quarter of the 1800s, it had not been established whether yellow fever was contagious or not; depending on individual belief, men debated, at times with sarcasm and at others with acrimony, the benefits of quarantine. During the 1850s and 1860s, concern over the spread of yellow fever occupied civil and legislative leaders; there was less argument over quarantine for smallpox. Smallpox was generally held to be a contagious disease capable of being passed from one person to the next. The debate in this case centered on the approach to containment. The most reasonable answer was to compel vaccination at home, while making all sailors and passengers display their vaccine scars before entering port.[14] Toward that end, for the year 1859, a total of 13,657 persons were vaccinated, many of them emigrants in Quarantine, while 2,207 persons were revaccinated by various institutions in New York.[15]

Commenting on the inaction of politicians at Albany, one sage summed up the situation: "Did you ever know a greater botch than we have made of this whole business of removing Quarantine? I don't think there was ever anything to compare with it. I mean to write its history some day, and sell a million or two copies, under the belief it is 'a sensation story.' And I don't know, then, as I could be very severely dealt by, for false pretences."[16]

Of the Promotion of Health

One of the most stirring observations on the health of New York came from a report contrasting mortality rates between that city and London. For the years 1859 and 1860, deaths in New York revealed a staggering increase of 1,065; London, on the other hand, notwithstanding the far greater increase of population, demonstrated "the most remarkable absolute decrease." In each successive quarter of the same year, deaths decreased over the previous period. In the quarter ending September 29, 1860, deaths in London were less, by 3,094, than in the corresponding period for the past ten years. In the last quarter of 1860, deaths decreased by 1,109. The editorialist in the *New York Times* observed, "This remarkable diminution, too, is attributable to no other cause than the scientific labors of the health officers." Consequently, 4,203 persons who might otherwise have perished survived due to sanitary measures by which the causes of death were removed.

Total deaths in New York for 1860 were reported at 22,710, or a ratio of 28 to every

1,000 of the population. In London, the ratio was only 20:1000. The awful results in New York were attributed to "the total *want* of anything like sanitary science in our health department," and embarrassingly debunked the city inspector, who had previously announced that official data of the mortality of London for 1860 did not marginally differ from that of the city.[17]

Regardless of whether the authorities of New York City considered the city "healthy," other municipalities, including those in the Empire State, were not so fortunate. A sampling of reported cases indicate that in Berkshire County, Massachusetts, a panic occurred in February 1860, while in Springfield, 325 cases of smallpox were reported in the year 1859–1860. As a testimony to lax public health laws, the newspaper reported, "The authorities can do nothing but give advice; they cannot compel vaccination nor force people who have the disease to keep themselves and their families from contact with neighbors and the public at large." Significantly, it was added:

> A Law is passing through the legislature to give the local boards of health power to restrain free intercourse by persons sick with this contagious disease, which is now the principal cause of its spread and continuance. Flagrant cases of carelessness, some thoughtless and others willful, have lately occurred here among families having the disease, and show how necessary is the proposed legislation.[18]

Also in February 1860, six cases of smallpox were reported in Lansinburgh [*sic*], New York. By July, smallpox appeared in Chicago in a form more virulent than usual and in quarters of the city ordinarily unvisited by it; authorities advised everyone to be vaccinated. Also in July, smallpox raged in Bristol, Wisconsin, where it was supposed the epidemic had been brought in by Norwegian emigrants who landed at Sun Prairie. Local boards of health put up notices forbidding people to collect in numbers for public worship and dismissed schools.[19]

In September 1860, cases of smallpox drastically increased in Jersey City, forcing the common council to appropriate $500 for the erection of a temporary smallpox hospital. By November, it was noted, "small pox is prevailing to an alarming extent in New Jersey."[20] The disease also raged in Olivetown, Clinton County, Iowa,[21] and ran the course of the railroad in Wisconsin, prompting the board of health in Baraboo, Sauk County, to call for vaccination and an avoidance of all suspected persons.[22]

One step ahead of Massachusetts, the threat of contagious disease in 1860 prompted the city of Madison, Wisconsin, to publish ordinances concerning the promotion of public health. The mayor was to appoint one alderman from each ward to serve a one-year term on the board of health. Their duty was to oversee and "make diligent enquiry with respect to all matters affecting the health of the city." In these regulations, "every person practicing medicine" (as opposed to limiting the mandate solely to physicians) was required to report any patient suffering from malignant fever, smallpox or any other pestilential disease to the authorities; neglecting to do so was a misdemeanor, punishable by a fine not less than $5 nor more than $50. The superintendent of streets or the chief of police was to inspect the building or apartment identified and the number of persons living therein; they were also to inspect the cellars, privies, cesspools and drains and cause "the abatement and removal of such nuisances." Infected individuals were to be removed to the city hospital or another place as directed by the board. Citizens were warned that it was unlawful for them to "resist or molest" officials in performance of their duty.[23]

The Contagion of Smallpox

Jenner's experience had taught him that in [the past] almost every other man had at one time in his life been taken with smallpox, but that those who got well almost unexceptionally remained free from the disease for all future time. It became, therefore, a custom to purposely infect children with a mild type of smallpox by bringing them in contact with those stricken with this malady. This was called "buying pocks."[1]

The frequency of smallpox and weekly newspaper reports on "The Health of London" ensured the disease maintained a high profile. One particular fear was the insidious method of contracting it. While most citizens knew that it could be spread by breathing contaminated air or by touching clothing of sufferers, a new scare appeared in 1863, when a woman was reputed to have come down with smallpox by riding in a cab. An investigation attributed the spread of disease to the state of the vehicle, which had likely been contaminated by transporting victims. With the public greatly agitated, authorities attempted to reassure them by stating a specific cab was kept at the workhouse exclusively for patients. That fact, however, was not generally known and consequently seldom called upon. It was determined, therefore, to house the vehicle at a more convenient location and to make its presence better known.[2] The Metropolitan Association of Medical Officers of Health followed up this and similar reports, quickly identifying three major concerns: the all-too-frequent problem of infected persons exposing others in the same dwelling; a lack of quarantine, allowing victims to expose those in the streets, public conveyances or in waiting rooms of hospitals; and the absence of adequate means of isolation.

Although problems were easy to identify, they proved harder to correct. Being refused admittance to the Smallpox Hospital for sundry reasons, infected persons were forced to apply to general hospitals for treatment. As smallpox patients were not accepted at these institutions, sufferers were sent back home, "and thus became the means of aggravating the evil." The Metropolitan Association recommended that during the epidemic, temporary buildings be erected at places distant from inhabited houses where smallpox patients could be maintained.[3] At least in one instance, a wing of the workhouse was appropriated for such a purpose.[4]

Schools became an equally dangerous site for the spread of smallpox that would ultimately prove more difficult to contain. Although the Act of 1853 called on infants to be vaccinated and children to be revaccinated at the time they entered school, this precaution was often neglected, resulting in a quick spread of the disease among the non-vaccinated. In such cases, local medical authorities were called in to vaccinate those who had not received the prophylactic treatment as infants, while the others were revaccinated as a precaution. In those districts situated in confined, ill-drained neighborhoods, the bodies of children who died from smallpox were sent to the coroner's office for autopsy. If it were discovered the child had not been vaccinated, due punishment was meted out to the parents.[5]

Problems of a similar nature affected English tourists. In 1861, smallpox broke out in Nassau, where the "devilish rich" had been vacationing. Four years later, an English tourist in Chambry, Switzerland, was sued for 10,000 francs in damages for introducing the smallpox into a hotel at which she had stopped. Mr. Harris, the British ambassador at Bern, protested on her behalf but the local authorities had already dismissed the suit.[6]

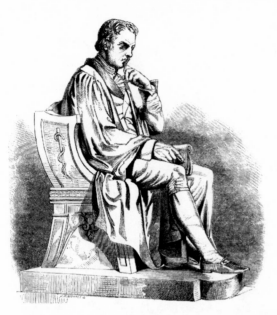

The text accompanying this line illustration of the statue of Edward Jenner reads, in part, "Taken all in all, perhaps no disease is more generally dreaded than small-pox.... Notwithstanding that the great discovery of Jenner has not accomplished quite all that he and his later contemporaries expected of it, nevertheless it is a great fact, and can hardly be overrated as to its importance" (taken from *The Leisure Hour*, London, December 23, 1858, in the authors' collection).

The annual meeting of the Royal Jennerian and London Vaccine Institution, 1863, reported that during the past year, it had supplied the means of protection from smallpox to 1,388 and supplied vaccine lymph to almost every part of the globe. In consequence, the institution was still in debt to the amount of 221*l*.[7]

In 1864, Sir Charles Hastings made a bold statement at the Social Science Congress at York: "The time will assuredly come when the laws of health will be generally known and obeyed throughout the community. None of us are likely to reach that day, but we may hasten its coming for a future generation, and even now we may see it and rejoice." His optimism was tempered, however, when it came to the lamentable state of eliminating smallpox. More than 60 years after Jenner's "brilliant yet simple discovery," there remained six chief obstacles to total success:

1. The carelessness and want of foresight by a population who seldom think of providing against the evils of a future day;
2. The prejudices of a few who persist in believing vaccination is injurious;
3. The insufficient payment of public vaccinators under the Poor Law Act;
4. The want of a duly authorized medical officer to see that the provisions of the Vaccination Act are properly carried out;
5. The want of a more complete registration of births;
6. A general aversion on the part of the public to legislation in a matter which they believe to involve interference with their natural rights.

In a telling conclusion to his talk on smallpox, Hastings chastised those who claimed the "so-called liberty" of refusing vaccination, remarking that the law did not permit parents to starve, ill-use or overwork a child, but compelled from them proper care and maintenance. It was just as criminal to defy the law regarding vaccination as to set fire to a barn or hayrick. That said, he admitted, "in such matters, the law must always be less powerful than public opinion," and it was the duty of social science societies to disseminate proper and positive information on the operation.[8]

Alternative Smallpox Vaccinations and Home Remedies

Throughout the course of the 19th century, various methods of protection from smallpox were attempted. One came from Dr. R. Landell of Porte Alegre, Brazil. After he and his son, Dr. John Landell, found success with the technique, the former transmitted the idea to the consul of the United States at the Rio Grande de Sul, Brazil. He, in turn, gave it to the secretary of state, who submitted it to the *American Journal of Medical Sciences,* where it was published in October 1857 on page 55.

The idea came to Dr. Landell during a smallpox epidemic in 1837, but he first administered it in 1842. His procedure called for dissolving the 4–5 drops of vaccine contained in a capillary tube in four or six ounces of cold water and administering a tablespoonful by mouth every 2–3 hours. The advantage of this system was that it "mitigates the symptoms, modifies the species, and cures the small-pox." Under its use, Dr. Landell claimed that fever, delirium, hoarseness, diarrhea, pneumonia, cerebral congestion and, finally, the secondary fever disappeared. In order to keep the bowels loose, castor oil was given to adults and calomel to children, as well as gargles of nitrate of silver and "chlorurate" [sic] of lime. Dr. Landell also claimed that administering the vaccine inwardly was a therapeutic remedy for whooping cough.[9]

Although death from smallpox was high, people often survived, albeit with permanent and disfiguring facial scars. One of the early techniques for lessening scars was publicized by a prominent physician in 1858, after a 14-year trial by Dr. J.W. Starling, senior surgeon for diseases of the skin at Guney Hospital, New York. He applied cantharides (derived from dried insects, usually Spanish flies, and used as a counterirritant) or any vesicant (causing or forming blisters) fluids by means of a camel hair brush to the apex of each pustule on all exposed areas of the body until blistering was evident by the whiteness of the skin in the parts subjected to the application. The fluid produced was then washed off with water or thin arrowroot gruel. The pain attending the application of the vesicating fluid was said to be slight and transient.[10]

By 1863, Dr. Smart, of the Royal Infirmary, was using a technique he developed to eliminate scarring. His treatment consisted of using a facial mask (also covering the neck in women) when the eruptions were fully developed, consisting of a solution made of India-rubber dissolved in chloroform. (India-rubber was far from soluble in chloroform and had to be cut in small pieces and added slowly until dissolved.) Guttapercha (a tough plastic substance from the latex of several Malaysian trees that resembled but contained more resin than rubber) was also tried, as it was very soluble in chloroform, but it had a tendency to tear into ribbons whenever muscles of the mouth were used.

After application, the chloroform dissolved, leaving a thin elastic film of India-rubber over the face. Patients discovered the mask to be "rather comfortable than otherwise," as it alleviated the disagreeable itchiness commonly associated with eruptions. The mask was pliable, allowing free use of the mouth without tearing. When finally removed, faces were free from "pitting," although untreated arms and other parts of the body were covered with small scars.[11]

A less complex method to prevent pitting originated, albeit unintentionally, in one of the prisons in New Orleans. After contracting smallpox, prisoners lodged in the lower and darker cells suffered from a more virulent form of the disease; yet upon recovery they, sustained few, if any, pitts. Those incarcerated in the upper, lighter cells experienced a comparatively milder form of the disease; yet on recovery, their pitts were observed to be very large and numerous. When the writer covering that story contracted smallpox years later in

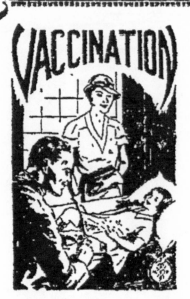

Against Marring Her BEAUTY

"A vaccination scar is a mark of good judgment, because statistics prove that in communities where vaccination is neglected, SMALL-POX sooner or later finds its way in, and leaves a trail of scarred and disfigured human beings, suffering and death

—*Bower*

SMALLPOX has practically disappeared where vaccination is adequately put into effect, but there are great areas in the United States where the population is largely unvaccinated. Arizona, Utah, North Dakota and Minnesota have no form of compulsory vaccination, and with their combined population of 3,817,555, developed 46,130 cases of smallpox from 1919 to 1928. Massachusetts, with compulsory vaccination, and a population of 3,852,356, accumulated only 408 cases in the same period. ONE HUNDRED AND THIRTEEN TIMES AS MANY CASES in the unprotected area.

In only nine States out of forty-eight is vaccination compulsory, and in several others there are various local regulations. In these days of crowds, moving populations and wide travel, and with vaccination so simple a matter, it is wholly unnecessary to run the risk of contracting smallpox.

Not only school children should be immunized, but adults also should co-operate in stamping out this disease.

Warren Drug Store
A. NEWTON McCAUSLAND, Prop.
233-LIBERTY ST. • WARREN, PA.

FILLING PRESCRIPTIONS IS THE MOST IMPORTANT PART OF OUR BUSINESS

"Telling the Public About the Doctor" appears weekly in this paper.

The Warren Drugstore advised readers, "A vaccination scar is a mark of good judgment, because statistics prove that in communities where vaccination is neglected, small-pox sooner or later finds its way in, and leaves a trail of scarred and disfigured human beings, suffering and death." In its well written and effective notice, the company shied away from directly promoting its business, leaving adults to draw conclusions from the cited statistics (from the *Warren Times-Mirror* [PA], November 10, 1941).

Philadelphia, his physicians kept him confined to a dark, shuttered room. Although he was quite sick, his hands and face being literally covered with pustules, he recovered with few scars, and those were nearly indistinct.[12]

Dr. Rendle of Park Hill, Iowa, subsequently supported this idea in 1871. After observing that smallpox scars were never found above the hairline, he deduced that darkness might offer a protecting influence. He therefore washed his patients' faces with collodion (a glue-like substance) and then applied a thin layer of fine wool that adhered to the adhesive. After it dried he brushed the wool with a solution of starch of gum to prevent any movement. Upon the doctor's removing the material, his trial patients were left without a vestige of marks.[13]

Less appealing was the "pomade of Baudeloque," made of 6 parts pitch (pix nigra), 10 parts yellow wax

This illustration from Jenner's *An Inquiry into the Causes and Effects of Variolae Vaccinae*, p. 40A, represents the pustule taken from Hannah Excell, a healthy girl of 7 years. She was inoculated from the arm of William Pead on April 5, receiving an injection under the cuticle of the arm in three different points. "The pustules which arose in consequence, so much resembled, on the 12th day, those appearing from the infection of variolous matter, that an experienced Inoculator would scarcely have discovered a shade of difference at that period." Three of seven children and adults receiving inoculation at the same time developed an extensive erysipelatous inflammation. Jenner treated them with mercurial ointment to the inflamed parts ("a treatment recommended under similar circumstances in the inoculated Small-pox") and the complaint subsided.

and 24 parts mercurial ointment. It was to be used warm and spread over all parts of the skin, being kept covered for four days. This was said to reduce spotting without leaving any marks behind.[14] For those with more expensive tastes, an article from the *Select Medical Library of Philadelphia* described the practice of Egyptians and Arabs, who prevented unseemly scars by the application of gold leaf as soon as eruptions made their appearance. The treatment was to continue morning and evening for the duration of the fever, the gold leaf made to adhere by means of gumwater. If mercury or gold leaf did not appeal to the sufferer, the same beneficial results might be achieved by anointing the face with almond oil.[15]

Following the trail of "revolutions" in the healing arts is almost as interesting as the prescriptions. On January 7, 1860, a letter writer signed "A.H." submitted a "recipe for that prevalent disease, the small pox," to the *Boston Journal*. The article had originally been printed some 20 years earlier when it came into the hands of "A.H." The article itself began, "A merchant and shipowner of this city has the following recipe sent him from England, where it was furnished by Mr. L. Larkin, member of the Royal College of Surgeons." Eventually, the *Boston Journal* reprint was picked up and printed by the *South Western Local* (WI), April 27, 1860.

Mr. Larkin advised that at the first appearance of fever the patient should take a mixture of one grain each of powdered foxglove or digitalis (the plant being valuable in the ratio of its greenness — the dark should be rejected) and one of sulphate of zinc (commonly known as "white vitriol"). They should be rubbed together in a mortar with 4–5 drops of water. This done, a noggin (or about four ounces) of water mixed with syrup or sugar should be added. One tablespoon for an adult or two teaspoonfuls for a child were to be given every second hour until symptoms of the disease vanished. The medical man concluded, "Thus conducted, convalescence, as if by magic, will result. The rapidity of an event so auspicious will equally delight and astonish." The *methodus medendi* was explained by stating the antifebrile qualities of the herb "lays hold at once of the fever, the prolific source of woe, which it immediately strangles, while the zinc acts the part of tonic, instantly restoring the equilibrium."

If the bowels became obstructed by the treatment, the doctor prescribed a dram of the compound powder of jalap (two parts cream of tartar with one part of jalap) and one grain of digitalis, treated as above and mixed with syrup or sugar, one tablespoon for an adult and half that for a child, to resolve the complication. Larkin concluded, "No emigrant or government vessel should hereafter be allowed to put to sea without a few pence worth of these protectors; and it is further ardently hoped that as the dearest interests of our common humanity are so vitally involved in this discovery, the press of all countries will give publicity to this announcement." As noted above, he achieved at least part of his hope by having his recipe published in at least two newspapers in the United States. Use of such treatments were encouraged by anti-vaccinationists at it seemed to eliminate the need for vaccination. As Larkin observed, "This simple medicine shuts out every other form or article whatever, as totally unnecessary, if not pernicious."

There were, finally, the supporters of onions, supporters who proclaimed that when onions were placed in the room with smallpox patients, blisters appeared on the onion skins as the vegetable decayed. From this, it was concluded that onions retained and communicated the virus for many weeks and that they prevented the disease by absorbing the virus.[16]

One of the more interesting discussions on the prevention of smallpox came from the *St. John's Morning News* (WI) in 1860. That newspaper published an article from "a gentleman of intelligence and observation," who noted that there were no cases of the disease in houses where gas was burnt. "The Gas," he supposed, acted as "a powerful disinfectant, and hence there is no contagion within the circle of its influence." If a person contracted smallpox while traveling abroad and took it home with him, it would not be communicated to anyone in a home burning gas.[17]

The continuing increase in smallpox cases drove people back to folk remedies; and in 1863, the attention of Bishop Berkeley's treatise, "Sivis," written in 1744, suggested tar as a legitimate cure. Citing an epidemic of the disease in Cloyne, Ireland, where tar water was used to good effect, the anti-zymotic, depuvative (presumably an agent that acts to cleanse the body by evacuation) and antiseptic properties were also stated to be an antidote to scarlet fever and typhus. Considering that tar water was unpalatable, J. Wetherfield, M.R.C.S., suggested making it into a pill by covering the substance with flour. In that way, it could be swallowed "without offending either the palate or the stomach."[18]

The Blue, the Gray and
the Speckled

The Small-Pox in Columbia [South Carolina]: To a New Yorker who at home is accustomed to blandly read in the weekly summary of deaths of ten or a dozen cases of the above mentioned disease, the panic which has recently beset the good people of Columbia on that head, seems altogether unaccountable.[1]

It is, perhaps, not inappropriate that on the eve of the Civil War, Southern delegates meeting at Columbia, South Carolina, were beset by the appearance of smallpox. To a hardened New Yorker looking on the scene (and reporting to the *World*), the panic over the disease seemed unaccountable. Somewhat tongue-in-cheek, he wrote that country people visiting the city "rushed precipitately" home, townspeople closed their doors and looked upon passersby as "lepers." He added, "as per time-honored custom," the myrmidons fought royal battles at the railroad station, whispering that those hotels in competition with theirs were "perfect hospitals, and that the people were dying off there like sheep."

On the doors of the state house where the secessionists met was pasted a notice ordering "all persons visiting the sick with small pox are most respectfully requested to keep from the halls of the State house." Newspapers around the country reported "the small pox panic is intense among the citizens and strangers" of Columbia and "there is hardly a doubt about the small pox epidemic here. It is also at Camden." Finally, the proprietors of Institute Hall, Charleston, offered its use to the state legislature or convention, "in case the small pox in Columbia should increase."[2] Panic of a different sort appeared in the *Columbia South Carolinian*:

Charleston Police Look Out!

Mr. Editor:— By a letter from New York there is reason to apprehend that the Lincoln men have been gathering up all the rags they can find from the small-pox hospital, and intend an incursion in the South, to chase the secession conventions and legislatures from place to place until they are made powerless.[3]

Whether or not this was a legitimate threat, war did come, and smallpox followed in its wake. While vaccination of all soldiers had been performed in the period around the War of 1812, the procedure had fallen into disuse. An examination of volunteers for the army revealed that a very large percentage of them had never been vaccinated. Of those who were, a still larger number had not developed the proper protective sore, indicating ineffective matter or technique.[4] Thus when men gathered in large groups, the spread of disease often became epidemic. Waves of smallpox, measles and mumps became the killer without face, nationality or mercy, striking soldiers on both sides with impunity. Ultimately, the visitation of the Grim Reaper in the form of disease came to represent death without honor, and twice as many soldiers died of disease than of actual wounds sustained in battle. Lack of sanitation, poor food, contaminated water, exposure to the elements, inexperienced and overwrought doctors, a dearth of medicines and, more significant, even casual contact with the sick, extracted a terrible toll.

In September 1861, Dorothea L. Dix, the general superintendent of the nursing department of the federal army, arrived in Chicago from Washington, en route to Missouri, where she was to see to hospital and nurse arrangements. Reporting that the Union army was in "splendid condition," she stated her belief that "the rebels are badly organized, demoralized and full of the small pox, typhoid fever and the measles."[5] Patriotic hyperbole aside, the South had already established Chimborazo Hospital in Richmond, Virginia. During the two-year period November 1, 1861–1863, a total of 47,176 patients were admitted. Of this number, 17,384 were transferred, 17,845 returned to duty, 4,378 were furloughed, 635 were discharged, 846 deserted and 3,031 died. A mortality of slightly greater than 6 percent represented an outstanding success rate.

On the opposite side, soldiers enduring the winter campaign in western Virginia suffered from weather-related pneumonia, typhoid fever, smallpox and measles. Union doctors isolated the smallpox cases but not those suffering from other contagions, increasing the spread of those diseases and compounding efforts to contain them.[6] Other physicians were not as careful in isolating smallpox patients, raising public ire. On December 9, 1861, a report from the *World's Dispatch* noted, "The small pox is getting prevalent by the carelessness of the surgeon general, in allowing cases of this disease to be in the same hospital with other patients."[7]

The transfer of disease from one side to the other was not uncommon, usually occurring when infected prisoners were taken. In the Revolutionary War, such "humanitarian" gestures as exchanging prisoners were often a double-edged sword, particularly when those returned (as with escaped slaves) were diseased. During the Civil War, tactics that could be considered germ warfare were not unknown. In June 1862, for example, some "spicy correspondence" occurred in the Western Theatre between Generals Pierre G.T. Beauregard, CSA, and Henry Halleck, USA, over the former's charge that Halleck sent him some Confederate prisoners infected with smallpox, "with a view to breeding pestilence in the rebel army." Needless to say, Halleck denied the accusation.[8]

Nor did it take prolonged contact for contagion to spread; even brief encounters could prove fatal. One such example happened in November 1861. While on picket duty with the army near Munson's Hill, Virginia, William S. Conrow of Delaware arrested a Confederate spy infected with smallpox. Conrow contracted the disease from him and died at age 23, leaving a wife and two children. The disease spread quickly and twenty-seven others in the regiment also contracted smallpox.[9]

As a response to the large numbers of soldiers who had never been vaccinated, efforts both North and South were begun and continued throughout the war to provide effective lymph matter. This became a special concern when troops were to be transferred into areas where a high prevalence of disease persisted. In October 1861, for instance, all the Federal troops of the Second Wisconsin Regiment were vaccinated — not because of a present danger but stemming from the fact the men were to be sent to the Gulf of Mexico, where it was proposed to winter some part of the army.[10]

Writing of his efforts to contain smallpox, Charles S. Tripler, the director of the Army of the Potomac, described his actions:

Not satisfied with what had been done, I asked for, and obtained, another order ... requiring division and other commanders to cause the brigade surgeons to again inspect all the men, vaccinating such as were still unprotected, and to report the results to me. At this late period, most of the brigades were found to have some men unprotected; in a few, the number was serious. In Slocum's brigade, there were fifteen hundred, in Blenker's, twelve hundred and fifty, and in Sickle's, seven hundred and fifty. Crusts were furnished, and the vaccination completed. As a result, smallpox, though rife in the community, never gained a foothold in the army.

Depending on the definition of "foothold," disease and injury played a staggering role in decimating the ranks. During the months of October–December 1861, as many as 3,930 men were discharged from the Army of the Potomac upon certificates of disability; that December, General Johnston, CSA, reported that of an assigned strength of 91,988, only 54,004 were present for duty, the remaining 37,984 being absent with sickness.[11]

Kalorama Small Pox Hospital

One of the most important of "Uncle Sam's" institutions in Washington was the Kalorama Small Pox Hospital, where thousands of soldiers received treatment. The Kalorama estate was located on Rock Creek, near Georgetown, about two miles from the capitol. At one time it had been a magnificent private residence, built by Joel Barlow before he became minister to France. At one time, it had been occupied by Robert Fulton, who made experiments with steamboat models in the nearby waters of Rock Creek, and by Commodore Decatur, who went from there to a duel with Commodore Barron, only to be brought back a corpse.[12]

On May 3, 1861, the United States Eruptive Fever Hospital was organized under the supervision of Dr. R.I. Thomas, surgeon, USA, late of Dubuque, Iowa. The grounds were located on 1st Street between B and C streets, Capitol Hill, where it remained until August 22, 1861. At that time, the smallpox patients were removed to Kalorama (for the use of which the government paid $6,000 per year). It was used as a general eruptive facility until December 10, 1861, when, under orders from the surgeon general, the hospital admitted only smallpox patients. From May 3 until December 1, 1863, the patients were entirely under the treatment of the surgeon in charge; after that date, two assistant surgeons, Dr. R.B. Lanley and A. Thomas, were added, completing the medical staff. Assisting them were two stewards, one apothecary, five clerks and one general ward master.

The corps of nurses and attendants comprised men who had all had smallpox "and fully understood the duties devolved upon them." Dr. Thomas acted upon the principle that "cleanliness is next to godliness" and placed an emphasis on ventilation.

In addition to the general hospital, another building contained three wards for the use of employees — teamsters and other assistants in the Quartermaster's Department, who were also under the charge of surgeon Thomas. After January 1864, five new wards were constructed, three to accommodate soldiers and two for male and female contrabands. Measuring 150 × 30 feet, each ward was supplied with water from Rock Creek, a stream flowing through the estate. The water was forced by steam power through pipes at a distance of 600 yards into a tank and from there conveyed through other pipes. Hot and cold baths were available at all hours of the day. Similar to the soldiers' wards, those occupied by contrabands were thoroughly cleansed and purified, with all patients receiving the same care and attention. The cooking and culinary departments afforded ample facility for preparing diets required by the infirm.

Statistics from Kalorama,
May 3, 1861–December 31, 1862

Patients admitted	2,351
Returned to duty	1,730
Deserted	11
Discharged	47
Transferred	75
Furloughed	35
Died	453

There were 157 patients in the hospital as of January 1, 1864.

During the first four months of 1864, smallpox prevailed throughout the District of Columbia and the army in Virginia to such an alarming extent that the city government became seriously alarmed, making recommendations for sanitary measures to be enforced throughout the area. During this period, Kalorama received an average of 20 cases a day, the majority of which were of a virulent type. In February alone, upwards of 700 beds were occupied, most by severe cases of the disease.

A reporter who visited the hospital, known as the "Pesthouse of the Nation," armed himself with bottles of eau de cologne, flasks of whisky and a dozen cigars to ward off the horrific smells. At the outer gate, a guard asked him, "Have you had the small pox?" Answering in the affirmative, he was allowed to pass. While traversing the halls, he reported there was "but very little inconvenience from the bad odor arising from the mass of human corruption which the eye beholds." That said, attendants coming in close contact got "the full benefit of the loathsome smell arising from a bad case." In all, the hospital was considered a model of efficiency and care.[13] Kalorama was destroyed in January 1865.

The Sanitary Commission

With masses of men being assembled in Washington, trained and then shipped out as part of the Union preparation for war, the concept of sanitation took on great importance. Not limited to latrines and washing, the word "sanitation" encompassed disease and pestilence prevention, clean, spacious and well-ventilated hospitals; field units for immediate treatment of the wounded; prompt burial details; nutritious food, proper cooking techniques and storage; clean drinking water; trash removal; and even comfort, including blankets and spirits.

Because of the dire warnings published before the Crimean War and the consequences of ignoring those warnings — the death of an estimated one-quarter of the British army from disease — calls went out for the United States to appoint a "distinct and sufficiently powerful body of sanitary officers, and also of workmen to carry out their instructions." While acknowledging that the number of soldiers who died from disease was always immense in comparison to those who fell in battle, the idea of losing 24 out of every 100 Federal troops without aiding the actual object of success struck the nation as horrific.

Authorities "knowing that" the opinions of army surgeons were not met with sufficient consideration, and moreover that their attention during a campaign left them little time for additional duties," a Sanitary Commission was felt to be the best way to preserve the lives of the volunteer soldiers.[14]

Although early reports of epidemics were scarce, there were widespread incidents of disease. In June 1861, intermittent fever and diarrhea were found at Cairo, Illinois (between April 21 and June 7, there were 614 cases of dysentery, 113 cases of fever and ague, rheumatism, pneumonia and "miscellaneous" treated at the Brigade Hospital). Measles were found among New Englanders at Fort Monroe, scurvy among the Marines at Fort Pickens and isolated cases of smallpox in nearly every camp. Yellow fever infected troops at Santa Rosa Island and an epidemic raged in New Orleans. With the heat of the summer months upon them, authorities feared greater outbreaks of yellow fever and other contagious diseases in troops stationed in the southern states. While many of the sick were "discharged cured," as the phrase went, the dreaded "miasmatic exhalations" that poisoned the atmosphere were to be found in every direction.

While "sudden changes in climate, malarial exhalations, atmospheric vicissitudes, and exposure" were the unavoidable lot of the soldier, avoidable causes were considered an "imperfect commissariat, and inefficient medical and hygienic regimen generally." The government responded by authorizing the Sanitary Commission for the volunteer army. Also approved by the Medical Bureau, this body comprised a corps of eminent scientific authorities who volunteered to aid in advising, planning and carrying out measures aimed at reducing the "avoidable causes" of distress and danger.[15]

The commission was divided into two branches, one of inquiry and the other of advice. The first branch observed the real condition and wants of the various bodies of troops, consulted with officers, surgeons, chaplains and soldiers and suggested to the public authorities whatever improvements intelligence and science might suggest. Members were to visit camps, quarters, tents and hospitals, investigate theoretical and practical solutions on diet and cooking and address the economizing, changing or exchanging of rations, clothing and body gear. They were also to approach methods of containing malaria and contagions by ventilation and vaccination in camps and hospital sites. Their perspective was to stem from addressing "questions from the highest ground, with the newest light of science, and the latest teachings of experience in the great continental wars."

The second branch had the responsibility of attending to the practical execution of the various plans suggested after first obtaining approval from the Medical Bureau and the government. Once that was achieved, this body would, "by inspection, urgency and explanation, by influence and all proper methods," enforce "upon careless or ignorant officials" the various regulations adopted. In instances of failure, the agents were to report to the department incidents of disobedience, sloth or neglect. If that were not enough, the Sanitary Commission was to secure uniformity of plans and harmony of action between the states, look after necessary ways and means, solicit donations from state treasuries or private beneficence, and methodize and reduce to serviceableness "the vague, disproportioned and haphazard benevolence of the public."

Although assembled on a larger scale, the Sanitation Commission had much in common with the ill-fated vaccination officer: those involved were volunteers, their authority to make change tenuous, and no money was authorized. Not surprisingly, agents of the Sanitary Commission were furnished nothing from the government "except its general countenance and aid, and a central office at Washington." The editorialist for the *New York Times* (June 25, 1861) added to the above: "Fifty thousand dollars placed immediately in the hands of this Commission would probably save tens of millions to the Government, while its value in preventing and providing against suffering, and in saving human life, can only be estimated by those who know how the epidemics from which sanitary science can furnish an absolute immunity, now imperil our gallant fellow-soldiers in the camp and at the seat of war." An appeal to the public for money (as opposed to the government) appeared in another column of the newspaper.

The Sanitary Commission, housed at the Treasury Building, Washington, was composed of the following men:

Henry W. Bellows, Unitarian Minister	President
Prof. A.D. Bache	Vice-President
Elisha Harris, M.D.	Corresponding Secretary
George W. Cullum	U.S. Army
Alexander E. Shiras	U.S. Army
Robert C. Wood, M.D.	U.S. Army
William H. Van Buren, M.D.	
Wolcott Gibbs, M.D.	
Samuel G. Howe, M.D.	
Cornelius R. Agnew, M.D.	
J.S. Newberry, M.D.	
George T. Strong	Treasurer
Frederick Law Olmsted	Resident Secretary[16]

Immediately, calls went out for ice "by the cargo," wine and pure spirits, sheets and sheeting, flannel and toweling, mosquito netting and articles which could not be provided by the government, including loose drawers, soft slippers, dressing gowns, handkerchiefs and abdominal or body bandages. The Adams Express Company offered to convey such necessaries at half price.

It did not take long for the rosy picture of camp health and hospitals to turn gloomy. On July 8, 1861, Mr. Russell, special correspondent of the *London Times,* reviewed field camps, on a pass from General Scott, writing, "The visitors most formidable to camps are diseases, and although this army is not very sickly there are certain signs in some of the corps that care will be required to prevent the spread of epidemics and diarrhea, scurvy and dysentery." After questioning the qualifications of members Reverend Bellows and F.L. Olmstead ("the zealous author of the works on slavery") to serve on the commission, the reporter pointed out that the mission of the Sanitary Commission was not popular among commanding officers and that members of the commission already complained of a want of authority.[17]

The first major conflict of the war, fought at Bull Run, Virginia, on July 21, 1861, resulted in a resounding Union defeat; by August 5, the Sanitary Commission reported that camps near Washington were in very bad condition as regarded healthfulness.[18] The loss brought a sense of urgency to health care relief, and groups such as the Woman's Central Relief Association urged the public to respond with generous contributions of money and supplies. In this case, bundles collected at the Cooper Institute, New York, were transported to Washington free of charge by the Adams Express Company.[19]

By August, the situation looked worse:

> To the medical men in charge of the troops little thanks are due, for in the first place there has been too great a proportion of "scalliwags" among them, quack pill dealers, dissipated apothecaries, and "last year graduates;" secondly, the medical men of the army have nothing to say or to do, efficiently and practically, till the soldier is actually sick.... So too with the Sanitary Committee.... Practically, so far as the past is concerned, this body has done nothing.[20]

Clearly opinions differed: over the names "A. Lincoln and Winfield Scott" ran the following statement.

The Sanitary Commission is doing a work of great humanity, and of direct practical value to the nation, in this time of its trial. It is entitled to the gratitude and the confidence of the people, and I trust it will be generally supported. There is no agency through which voluntary offerings of patriotism can be more effectively made.[21]

By November, the Sanitary Commission had received and expended $200,000; during November, it spent $1,000 per day procuring necessities for invalids, while employing twenty-five inspectors.[22]

In a bit of flag-waving, one reporter added that while the health of the Union army remained generally good, such was not the case with the Rebel army, where measles, variola and other diseases were very prevalent. This was explained by their "habits," including whisky, which "flowed too freely" among them.[23] In a different type of distortion common in warfare, the *Cleveland Ledger* reported that a Dr. S.W. Tolhurst, under the auspices of the "United States Humane Society," was collecting funds for medical supplies by consent of the government. There proved to be no such person and his "base and cowardly attempt to swindle the patriotic public" was roundly denounced.[24]

During a smallpox epidemic in the fall of 1861, the Medical Bureau became short of vaccine, requiring the Sanitary Commission to provide vaccination for over 20,000 men. Nor was the bureau responsive to the threat of an anticipated attack on the capital, informing the Sanitary Commission there would be "time enough to order hospital supplies after the battle had occurred." After a skirmish in September, the Medical Bureau was obliged to seek medical supplies from the commission.[25]

By February 1862, a slight abatement of smallpox in Washington was reported, although there continued to be "daily proofs of the criminal negligence of the medical department of the army in its dealings with this loathsome disease." Through the efforts of the Sanitary Commission, a bill on medical reform was presented to Congress.[26]

As with all large agencies handling an influx of money, charges of graft and appropriation of funds were leveled against those of the Sanitary Commission throughout the war. Charges of army officials "gobbling up" delicacies sent by the Sanitary Commission for sick soldiers impaired confidence in both the army staff and the Commission.[27] State fairs held to raise money for the commission and appropriations from cities often went unrecorded, leading to suspicions of theft.[28] Yet there was no denying the benefits the commission provided to soldiers in the field as it maintained depots and agents at military centers from Washington to the Rio Grande.

George T. Strong, treasurer of the commission, stated that thousands of men needing "special relief" were daily cared for in its "homes," while steamboats and wagon trains followed the armies. At Fortress Monroe in Virginia, for example, the steamer *Daniel Webster* was fitted out as a floating hospital,[29] while reports of the humane treatment of the wounded by Commission employees were judged to be far in excess of army surgeons, "to whom we would not entrust the life of a favorite cat."[30] By August, the commission appealed to the president on behalf of new recruits, asking they undergo the strictest kind of medical examination and that none but healthy, sound men be accepted.[31]

This raised an important issue, as the influx of emigrants into the Northern states vastly increased during the war years. The effectiveness of the Union blockade deprived British manufacturing and textile districts of Southern cotton, forcing many laborers to seek employment elsewhere. By the first three months of 1863, the number of emigrants doubled from the same period in preceding years: In 1861, the numbers were 38,000; in 1862, they were 83,290. Of these, 56,000 went to the United States, 40,000 of whom were

Irish. Augmented by the zeal of Federal agents recruiting soldiers in Ireland, many entered the army upon arrival.[32] Of those who enlisted, a proportion likely suffered from contagious diseases or had not been vaccinated, making them susceptible to smallpox.

The Western Sanitary Commission, headquartered in St. Louis, reported in June 1863 that the whole number of patients admitted into their fifteen hospitals were 19,467, of which 1,400 died; additionally, 162 died on their floating hospitals. Of the remainder, 15,717 were furloughed, discharged or returned to their regiments, with 3,750 remaining.[33] Additionally, the Women's Central Association of Relief for the Army and Navy, a branch of the United States Sanitary Commission established in April 1861, provided 106,899 articles of clothing, 81,267 of bedding, 35,458 towels and handkerchiefs, bandages, groceries, jellies, dried fruit, wine and syrups. Their total expenditures for correspondence and supplies amounted to $4,031.49, of which only $654 went to wages. Ninety-one nurses were educated and placed in the field at a cost of $1,332.15. Needless to add, the association was in debt and appealed to the public for funds.[34] Sanitary and hospital inspections, hospital directories and transportation of the sick and wounded required a monthly cost of "not less than forty-five thousand dollars per month," while an expenditure of $70,000 after Gettysburg and an equal amount after the battles at Chattanooga were spent in humane pursuits.[35]

After Gettysburg, two agents of the Sanitary Commission were captured and sent to Libby Prison in Richmond. Ascertaining their identity, a number of Confederate surgeons sent a petition to General Robert E. Lee, asking for the release of the agents. In their letter (mentioning four agents) they praised the Sanitary Commission, stating:

> Through its kind provisions *our* hospitals are supplied with many comforts which are of inestimable value to our wounded and suffering men.... We respectfully submit, that as these men were taken without arms, and while in the employ of their charitable office as almoners of the Sanitary Commission to the wounded soldiers of either party, they be released from restraint and permitted to return to their work of benevolence and good will to all.[36]

A follow-up, dated September 24, special dispatch from the *Chicago Tribune*, advised that Dr. Alexander McDougal and the Rev. Mr. Schandling of the Sanitary Commission were released as prisoners of war and arrived in Washington that day.[37] Clandestine agents, supposed to be members of the Confederate Sanitary Commission, had a different experience in August 1863. Being overly solicitous of three trunks they were transporting through Louisville, the police thought it best to "assist" them. When opened, the trucks were found to contain $1,600 worth of quinine, "doubtless destined to do service among the 'shakers' in Dixie." The two agents disappeared too suddenly to be arrested.[38]

Revisiting Quarantine and Compulsory Vaccination

During the first winter of war, the passage of large numbers of soldiers and civilians through major cities increased the prevalence of disease, demanding civil authorities to take another look at various forms of quarantine. In January 1862, smallpox prevailed to such an extent in the Wilmington, Delaware, area that the mayor was compelled to issue a proclamation, forbidding any infected persons to come within one mile of city limits under heavy penalty.[39] In Washington, the city council countenanced a report stating that 500–600 cases of smallpox were presently in the city. Statistics from the Eruptive Fever Hospital seemingly disputed those numbers, showing but two deaths from that disease and a limited number of others suffering from a nonvirulent form.[40]

The threat, if not the actual numbers, remained palpable, however, and fear levels in the capital remained high. A February report noted there was "a slight abatement of small pox in this city, though there are daily proofs of the criminal negligence of the medical department of the army in its dealings with this loathsome disease." There was hope that Congress would deal with the matter in an effective manner, "and even at this late date beneficial results may be obtained. Great credit is due to the sanitary commission, who have perfected a bill for this much needed medical reform."[41]

In May 1862, fugitives from Fortress Monroe, Virginia, reported that smallpox and "black measles" were prevailing to a considerable extent in Richmond, many cases proving fatal. The National Hotel, the Episcopal church and the city hall were filled with Confederate soldiers "dying off like sheep." Many private citizens fled to the interior to escape the epidemic, leaving grass to grow in the streets. None but army business was conducted and most of the stores were closed. Eyewitness accounts stated that over 1,000 soldiers were buried within a ten-day period, the principal sufferers being from the interior of Virginia, Tennessee and Alabama. Hearses and funeral processions were considered "as common as drays," with the presence of typhoid fever adding to the misery of those left behind.[42]

As times changed, the city of New York revisited the old quarantine arguments and regulations. In March 1862, a bill introduced into the state legislature designated ship fever, smallpox, cholera and yellow fever as the only diseases requiring quarantine. The floating hospital was set aside for yellow fever and cholera victims, the hospital at Blackwell's Island for smallpox sufferers and Ward's Island for ship fever. The commissioner of emigration was to collect an unspecified amount from shipowners to cover the costs of patients arriving by sea; the cities of New York and Brooklyn were responsible for paying for the care of those sent from their municipalities.

Further details required the commissioner of quarantine to locate a quarantine buoy in the lower bay not less than three miles from the nearest land, with a circle of one mile from the buoy being considered quarantine ground. The bill provided for the sale of the Quarantine grounds at Castleton and appropriated the insufficient sum of $5,000 for the immediate use of quarantine. Additionally, charge of the floating hospital was awarded to the health officer.[43] Politics reared its ugly head when the Health Bill was presented at the state capital of Albany. Mayor Opdyke and David Dudley Field opposed it on the grounds the mayor was not made a member of the board of health. Argument against the mayor's position was succinct:

> For many years now, the most intelligent portion of our citizens, without distinction of party, have been striving to secure for New-York, what every considerable commercial city in the world has enjoyed — a Board of Health under the control of medical men. The absolute necessity for such a Board has long been made manifest by the extraordinary mortality of the City, by the unchecked establishment in the very heart of our population of the causes of pestilence, by the filthiness of the streets, the deaths of thousands of children every Summer from causes directly traceable to official neglect, and by the dissemination to other cities every year of small-pox and other contagious scourges of the human race.

The argument continued by declaring that nothing would cure the evil except the same remedy which proved efficient elsewhere — the establishment of a uniform sanitary system over all the waters of the harbor and the neighboring shores, "and the execution of that system by a Board of *Medical* men." Echoing sentiments eschewed several years earlier, it was further argued that to be effective, a sanitary system had to be metropolitan in character, "because measures against contagion in one city are of no value whatever unless aided and made effectual by similar measures in the other."[44]

Equally important, the New York commissioners of health met in February 1862, "for the purpose of considering and acting upon the subject of vaccination." Dr. Lewis A. Sayes presented a report showing the absolute necessity of general vaccination in large cities, leading to "the conclusion that if people will not be vaccinated when the authorities are willing to cause it to be done free of charge, the law should, for the preservation of the general health, compel them to be vaccinated."

Sayes' statistics showed that out of one million persons, the lives of 52,000 were saved by vaccination. Furthermore, before vaccination, mortality in armies was enormous, while at the present day, with strict attention to vaccination, "mortality was trifling." A draft of a law based on these facts was approved and sent to Albany.[45]

In support of legislative action, W. Argyle Watson, M.D., from the United States steamer *Cuyler,* wrote to the health commissioners on May 20, 1862, offering a firsthand account of the value of compulsory vaccination. He stated that the day after his ship left port, a seaman who had never been vaccinated developed a full-blown case of smallpox that proved fatal at the end of ten days. During that period, Dr. Watson vaccinated all hands, only to discover one case developed among the crew. It turned out that the individual had "skulked away" from the lancet from prejudice against the operation, thus depriving himself of protection. The doctor concluded, "This man now lives to exhibit the marks of his folly on a deeply scarred face, the result of a most fearful attack of small pox."[46]

The act did not become law. In February 1863, a more comprehensive bill entitled "An Act to Prevent Small-pox" was proposed. It required that every person in New York who had not already had smallpox or varioloid be vaccinated. Noncompliant persons who developed smallpox were to be removed to any hospital or place designated by the board of supervisors. Hotel and boardinghouse keepers were required to notify authorities of smallpox cases; violators were to be penalized. Furthermore, unvaccinated children were not allowed to attend public school; those who were vaccinated were required to have the operation repeated every five years until the age of 21.[47]

On the War Front

General George B. McClellan received a report from the surgeon general of the army in January 1863, citing the familiar refrain that the health of the army "left little [much] to be desired." The statistics presented covered the past nine months. Of 247,700 cases of disease and injury reported, 40,000 were for diarrhea and dysentery; over 10,000 cases of typhoid fever (both the result of improper sanitation and contamination by human feces); nearly 6,000 cases of measles; and close to 47,000 instances of catarrh and bronchitis. The plague of armies everywhere, syphilis (3,545 cases) and gonorrhea (4,100), were probably underreported. Measles, mumps, smallpox and chicken pox made up a portion of the remaining numbers.[48]

Despite an ongoing vaccination program initiated in the Army of Northern Virginia and the large number of Confederate hospitals in that state (39 by the end of 1863), smallpox remained an omnipotent threat. At the Receiving Hospital at Gordonsville, Virginia, a pesthouse was created out of a shanty, eventually growing into a much larger structure. Reserved exclusively for smallpox patients, it was attended by Dr. E.A. Craighill, who had, at one time, as many as 84 patients in various stages of illness. The only surgeon who would care for these sick soldiers, he wrote about his experience:

> No one can know how horrible it is unless they experience what I did, not the least being the disgusting and unmistakable odor that attends particularly bad cases, and I had some of the worst. I had no dread of the disease, but vaccinated myself every morning and thought I was protected.... Of course, I always changed my outer garments when I went to the hospital, and when I left, keeping my smallpox clothes in the woods in the open air when not in service.[49]

Civilians, of course, were not exempt from debilitating diseases and with troops from both sides stationed around the Richmond, Virginia, area, it was not surprising that reports of smallpox epidemics appeared. On December 12, 1862, the *Richmond Examiner* published a report that smallpox prevailed in that city as an epidemic.[50] Aiding the spread of smallpox were people traveling throughout the state and into neighboring states. A month after the Richmond report, the disease appeared in North Carolina to such an extent that the authorities were prompted to offer vaccination at the office of the surgeon general.[51]

During periods where high instances of smallpox prevailed, the question of self-vaccination usually reappeared. In North Carolina, one justice bragged that "every man, woman, and little boy or girl in Union county know how to vaccinate as well as the M.D.'s, and are doing it." An astonished local sarcastically wrote of this claim: "A progress in medical society so surprising that were it not for the present desolating war, now over the land, that Union county would become the Mecca of the medical pilgrim, in the pursuit of the invaluable information there to be gained."

Citing smallpox statistics from around the world gleaned from contemporary publications, he concluded that four reasons currently existed for an increase in smallpox:

1. Unqualified persons performing vaccination
2. Cow pox matter tended to deteriorate by descent*
3. Demand had exhausted the best quality matter
4. No government requirement of mandatory vaccination

*Discussed in chapter 13. Interestingly, the author blamed the National Vaccine Establishment in England for not renewing the lymph and being unable to supply that of the best existing quality. He made no mention of the National Vaccine Institution in Washington or its untimely demise, possibly because Dr. Smith was brought down by the efforts of a politician from North Carolina, the same state in which the writer resided.[52]

Treatments and comfort to the afflicted varied by state with at least one "Common Council" in Oregon protesting that the expenditure of seventy-five cents per pound for sugar and a charge for whisky for the nurse (which was ordered by the physician) was "very good, but it may cost too much." In an aside, the paper noted that $4,520.77 had been donated to the Sanitary Fund from Washington Territory.[53]

At Camp Douglas, a holding area for Confederate prisoners in 1863, many prisoners were found to be sick, requiring that upwards of one thousand prescriptions be written daily. The prevailing diseases were colds, fevers, pneumonia and some cases of smallpox. Deaths among the men were frequent, 21 having died in less than one week. To accommodate those with contagious diseases, the pesthouse was removed from inside the prison enclosure to outside "for sanitary reasons." Hence, a large building formerly used by a cavalry regiment was remodeled to accommodate 50 sufferers, while the chapel was converted into a hospital with a capacity of one hundred. Not incidentally, a new prison was also constructed, measuring 30 × 50 feet.[54]

Interestingly, in an advertisement for blacksmith work placed in the *Hornellsville Tribune* (NY), February 5, 1863, the proprietor, B.S. Freeman, reminded prospective patrons "The 'Small Pox' Scare Played Out!" He added "no danger from small pox, if competitors do say so, that's played out." This was a reference to the commonly held belief that "horse grease" originating in the hooves was both a contaminant of smallpox and a protector, much in the same way cowpox was spread to dairymaids.

Contrabands who had gathered at Washington fell under the charge of James S. Wadsworth, the military governor. When their numbers became too great, he moved a large group of African Americans from the Old Capitol Prison where they had been housed to the nearby houses of Duff Green's Row. In July 1862, smallpox broke out among the residents; the sick were left there and the remainder were transferred to the camp on North Twelfth Street.

While awaiting the Day of Jubilee, the number of blacks in Washington swelled. The camp on North Twelfth Street became so crowded tents had to be erected. Its smallpox hospital also overflowed, with loud and angry complaints from whites about careless burials in the graveyard on Boundary Street.[55]

On January 1, 1863, President Abraham Lincoln signed one of the most significant documents in American history. The Emancipation Proclamation promised that "all persons held as slaves within said designated States, and parts of States, are, and henceforth shall be free." For the newly emancipated African Americans, however, problems abounded. The February 10, 1863, edition of the *Tri-Weekly News* (TX) reported that smallpox was prevailing in almost every neighborhood in Washington City. Three weeks later, a letter writer from that city informed his Southern friends that "the [N]egroes in the city have increased 50 per cent since the emancipation Act, which, it was thought, would drive them out. Southern people would not hire them unless they were slaves, and they could not get work. The small pox is raging amongst them, and they were dying at the rate of twenty per day."[56]

It would not get any easier for those remaining under the yoke of slavery. By December of that year, D.W. Hand, a surgeon at New Bern, North Carolina, reported that smallpox prevailed extensively among the refugees and Negroes in and around that city. Every effort, he wrote, was made to vaccinate the soldiers, but 27 had variola or varioloid and six died. He added, "*Sarracenia purpurea* was at this time extensively used in the treatment of smallpox, but without any beneficial result."[57] (*Sarracenia purpura* was a plant known familiarly as Ladies' Saddle or Water Cup, the root of which was the remedial part. When made into a tea it was believed to cure smallpox. The medical term "purpura" was described in 1842 as a disease of uncertain origin consisting of distinct purple specks and patches, attended with general debility, with or without fever, believed to occur as a *sequaela,* a condition following and resulting from smallpox and measles.[58] Vaccination derived from resulting pustules would not have been an effective preventive of smallpox.)

Disease continued to strike indiscriminately. In the early months of 1863, soldiers of the Army of the Mississippi, stationed five miles below Vicksburg, complained bitterly that they were overcrowded, without sufficient protection from the rain and cold, and lacked hospitals and medicines. Furthermore, the sick and well were indiscriminately mixed together and all were exposed to smallpox: "The sequel of all this shows a sick list appalling, almost, and we have the small pox developing itself daily." The correspondent added: "If the mistreatment and fearful sacrifice of British soldiers, on the altar of red tape, Generalship and doctorship in the Crimean campaign, called out from the press and public of England, an investigation of Parliament, and a remedy, surely some one ought to call for an investigation of the treatment of part, or all of the sick of this Army."[59]

The correct diagnosis of smallpox continued to be problematic, with the *Dodge County Citizen* (WI), February 26, 1863, complaining that, "out of many rumors and conflicting opinions," it was determined that probably three cases of "varioloid" occurred in the city, probably not true smallpox as the patients recovered in a short time without being "pitted." Other cases which rumor magnified into smallpox may have been chicken pox, or "erysypilas" [erysipelas], but, as the doctors disagreed, it was decided to call the affliction "unctuous itch, and let it go at that." Worse was the affair of Professor Lyon, of Milwaukee, who contracted smallpox and died. In his case, ordinary medical assistance was not employed; rather, he and his friends relied upon the treatment prescribed by spiritual mediums. Unable to find a more severe charge, city authorities arrested the two parties who had charge of Professor Lyon, citing them for failure to give notice of a contagious disease.[60] Of wider implication, after the fatal appearance of smallpox in Ripon, Wisconsin, the newspaper observed how little alarm was felt in the city regarding the presence of smallpox, adding that a few years since, a single case would have closed business for "a month of Sundays."[61] Within the year, the Common Council of Milwaukee, facing a growing population of smallpox victims, called for the creation of a pesthouse.[62]

By October 1863, Lieutenant Colonel William S. Pierson, commanding the Federal prison camp at Johnson's Island, Ohio, notified Colonel William Hoffman of the Federal Commissary-General of Prisoners that in three separate instances smallpox had been brought to the island by incoming Confederate prisoners, twice from the prison at Alton, Illinois. He further advised that the disease caused somewhat of a panic among the prisoners, although those so stricken were quarantined in the pesthouse. The same month, Brigadier General Gilman Marston, commanding the prison at Point Lookout, Maryland, notified Hoffman that among every lot of prisoners sent from Fort Delaware there were cases of smallpox, the latest consignment containing 26 infected men. He added, "So many cases create alarm here among the troops and the citizen employees of the Government. I trust no more will be sent here."[63]

The smallpox did not abate at the prison in Alton, situated across the Mississippi from St. Louis. During the unusually severe winter of 1863–1864 when the river froze, Rebels infected with the disease were removed from general confinement and taken across the ice to the "smallpox island," where the hospital consisted of cloth tents. There, patients were issued two blankets and fed on milk and cornmeal mush. D.C. Thomas, a Texas cavalryman sent there in November 1863, in writing of his confinement bitterly observed, "All day and all night, day after day, night after night, the groans and prayers of the poor, suffering prisoners could be heard piteously begging for water or for some trivial attention from the cold-hearted nurses."[64]

In December 1863, learning of smallpox epidemics among Federal prisoners held at Belle Island in Richmond and at Lynchburg, Virginia, Major General Benjamin F. Butler, commanding the Union Department of Virginia and North Carolina, wrote to Robert Ould, Confederate commissioner of exchange at the capital. He included a package of vaccine matter, "sufficient, as my medical director informs me, to vaccinate six thousand persons. May I ask that it shall be applied under the direction of the proper medical officer to the use intended." Butler added that more vaccine would be furnished if necessary. Major Mulford, assistant agent of exchange, delivered the package. Ould courteously responded:

Sir: The package of vaccine matter has been received and will be faithfully devoted to the purposes indicated in your letter. Permit me in response to the friendly tone of your letter to assure you that it is my most anxious desire and will be my constant effort to do everything in my power to alleviate the miseries that spring out of this terrible war.[65]

What horrific causalities were to come, no one could have guessed. Nor would it be in anyone's power to alleviate the miseries that sprang out of this terrible war.

19

The Last Full Measure
of Devotion

Now, every reader of this should at once be vaccinated, and should remember that every person in this country who had the small pox, had it because he was ignorant of vaccination or despised it, or only because he put off vaccination day by day, "till a more convenient season." And this very reflection has made the sufferings of the disease more unbearable, and the death which probably ended them, the more unwelcome.[1]

On November 19, 1863, President Abraham Lincoln spoke at Gettysburg, Pennsylvania, before 15,000 spectators. In ten short sentences, he immortalized not only the dead of that conflict, but also the birth and eventually the rebirth of the nation. The unbearable fact that Abraham Lincoln became what is traditionally honored as the last casualty of the Civil War underscores how close the divided country, the world and history came to losing the 12th president less than six months earlier.

It had long been speculated that Lincoln suffered from smallpox at the time he gave his dedication at Gettysburg. Within a week after returning to Washington, the president became weak and feverish and kept to his bed. Physicians attending him made the diagnosis of varioloid, leading Lincoln to characteristically quip that now he had something he could give to everybody.[2]

A contemporary article published in the *World* (New York), January 5, 1864, provided Americans with an explanation for the president's health problems:

The illness of President Lincoln is, we have reason to believe, a much more serious matter than has generally been suspected. At first it was supposed to be a cold; next, a touch of bilious fever; a rash then appeared upon his body, and the disease was pronounced scarlatina; but recently it has leaked out that the real complaint he labors under is small pox. For some time past the President has received no visitors; even members of the cabinet and personal friends have been excluded from his apartment. The excuse was that he was writing his message and could not be interrupted.

We believe, that we but echo the feeling of the whole country without distinction of party, in sincerely hoping that the President will soon be restored to health and strength. Men of his habit of body are not usually long lived, and the small-pox to a man of his age, even when the health is usually good, is a very serious matter. His death at this time would be a real calamity to the country, and would tend to prolong the war.

The symptoms and length of time he suffered would tend to confirm the diagnosis of smallpox as presented by the *World;* the suggestion of "varioloid" by Lincoln's physicians was more likely politically motivated than actual fact. It is not known whether Mr. Lincoln was ever vaccinated for smallpox; certainly, there was precedent in the United States for high elected office holders to have undergone the procedure. With the disease so prevalent, it is surprising he would have avoided such a commonly accepted preventive. It is interesting to speculate whether he had been vaccinated at some prior time and the operation failed due to poor technique or ineffective lymph matter or that he may have felt himself immune from past exposure.

Smallpox was epidemic in Washington through the final months of 1863 and while the citizens in the nation's capital celebrated the holidays, many also fled in terror at any sign of a mottled complexion. Soldiers were carried to Kalorama Hospital but there existed no systematic program of isolation. Negroes trudged through the streets and died where they fell; the smallpox hospital at the abandoned contraband camp on Twelfth Street was torched as a precautionary measure. Senator Bowden of West Virginia died of smallpox and when it was discovered that a House reporter had visited Kalorama "pesthouse," Speaker Colfax asked him to leave.[3] (This is the same reporter who detailed Kalorama Hospital cited above.)

As an example of the correlation/confusion between smallpox and scarlatina (scarlet fever), cases of both diseases were said to be raging to a serious extent in Toledo, Ohio, during December 1863.[4] It is also interesting to find a study around the same time from the *Eclectic Journal,* published around the time of the *World* article, admonishing physicians not to make a hasty opinion on disruptive disorders until they followed the proper diagnostic system. These authorities recommended that as soon as eruptions appeared, pressure with the point of a finger should be applied to them, feeling for the presence of a hard substance similar to that of small, fine shot placed under the outside of the skin. The presence of this hard material was attributed only to smallpox, making this test the "unfailing diagnostic system" for proper identification.[5]

At the same time, a letter first published in the *McKinney Messenger* from J.P. Barnett, a post surgeon, stated his concern over poisonous vaccine matter originating from an Indian regiment. Within 24 hours of vaccination, the lymph caused inflammation of the arm. Four days later, a small scab or crust formed, followed by simple erysipelas that formed a red ring between 1½ and 2 inches round. A soft, irregularly shaped (as opposed to round) scab continued to form but was easily broken up, discharging pus every day. The patient's "exillary" (axillary: armpit) became so swollen, the arm could not be brought down to the side. If the scab was removed, it left an indolent ulcer. After four weeks, soldiers showed no signs of healing and several suffered considerable fever. The physician noted that the effects were not as severe in children as adults but that both sexes suffered equally. Since those already vaccinated contracted the disease it became obvious this particular lymph offered no protective power against smallpox.

Dr. Barnett concluded by offering the remedy he employed against the poisonous matter: mercurial ointment, applied morning and night. He had not had time to ascertain the benefits of this treatment but believed it would prove beneficial. (Mercury was commonly used to cure venereal and eruptive diseases and as a laxative, primarily under the name "calomel." When mercury was used to excess, mercury poisoning was a frequent side effect.) An addendum to the letter relayed the fact it was feared some men from Colonel Brown's command who had undergone vaccination with the tainted matter would be compelled to have their arms amputated.[6]

In another instance of contaminated vaccine, nearly 1,000 exchanged Union prisoners from the Red River country arrived at Cairo, Illinois, on July 25, 1864, the majority belonging to Iowa (the 26th and 19th) and Indiana regiments. According to the *True Delta,* these men, who had been held in confinement between 12 and 16 months, presented a pitiable appearance, being hatless and shoeless and many without sufficient clothing to cover their nakedness. They were described as being "animated skeletons, whose feet left bloody marks in their tracks." They represented the first installment from the Prison Pen in Tyler, Texas, where 4,000–6,000 others were imprisoned in the stockade fort at the ratio of 1,000 to an acre of land.

At this prison, many officers were held in chains and all suffered from lack of food, medication and clothing. Two hundred were vaccinated, but instead of acting as a preventive of the loathsome disease, smallpox was communicated to them. Agents from the Western Branch Sanitary Commission and the state agents of Iowa and Indiana were immediately dispatched to alleviate their condition.[7] During the same month of August 1864, a large number of patients who had been improperly vaccinated due to improper harvesting technique or contamination arrived at Chimborazo Hospital, Richmond.[8]

The war was drawing to a protracted close, but deaths from smallpox continued unabated. The year 1864 proved especially deadly. In the early part of the year, 387 Confederate prisoners perished in one month at Camp Douglas, Illinois.[9] A year earlier, this same camp had attempted to initiate sanitary measures for the prevention of disease, but there was no way to protect men from the influx of new arrivals. Consequently, contact with the sick quickly spread smallpox with devastating results. One particularly striking story tells of a soldier from Company F, 59th Indiana Volunteers, who was taken with smallpox and apparently died. Five coffins were piled on him and the body lay unburied for two days, until he woke up with a suffocating sensation. His screams finally brought help and he was freed from his terrible confinement. He afterwards said he never lost consciousness and that his mind floated through a series of "surpassing beauty, amid strains of delicious music," such as he had never heard before. He survived smallpox and the war, eventually working as a clerk in the Pension Bureau, Washington.[10]

With the fall of Fort Fisher in January 1865, General Sheridan, then headquartered at Winchester, Virginia, broke up the last of the Confederate hospitals and sent the sick and wounded north. Union hospitals in Winchester were also closed with the exception of the Taylor Hotel, Lutheran church and the Methodist Episcopal church. Of the Union soldiers treated there, it is worthy to note that none suffered from smallpox.[11]

In a particularly interesting adjunct to history, in 1866, Treasurer Spinner received from a Federal surgeon at Bowling Green, Kentucky, the sum of $199 in United States currency, property of smallpox patients from the military hospital there. Deeming the money injudicious to be returned to circulation, the infected currency was securely sealed and burned by the treasurer, who, on his own responsibility, forwarded the same amount in new greenbacks to the Bowling Green Hospital.[12]

Statistics published by the Surgeon-General's Office in 1943 stated that with 2½ million men under arms, the number of reported cases of smallpox was nearly 19,000, a rate of 7.97 per 1,000.[13]

Sure Cures and Pesthouses

The use of vaccination was not even mentioned in an article from the *Palmer Journal* (Massachusetts) in its report of sixty cases of smallpox and varioloid being treated at the state alms house during the period May–July 1864. The remedy, said to have been used successfully on all but one victim, was a tea made from the *sarracenia purpura* plant.[14] Dr. Frederic W. Morris, resident physician of the Halifax Visiting Dispensary, used the same tea as a remedy. The "Indian cup," being native to Nova Scotia, was said to cure smallpox "in all its forms 12 hours after taking the medicine," very seldom leaving scars in its wake. When vaccine matter was washed with an infusion of *sarracenia purpura*, it was reputed to be deprived of its contagious properties and of so mild a flavor that when mixed with tea or coffee not even a connoisseur would be aware of the admixture.[15] As this plant was not a cure for the disease, the question of misdiagnosis arises.

The use of "home remedies" continued to prevail throughout the 19th century. Another such "cure" for smallpox was a "popular, simple, and almost infallible remedy" used by English physicians. It consisted of cream of tartar, ¼ ounce; rhubarb, 12 grains; and 1 pint of cold water, well stirred or shaken immediately before administration. The dose was from a quarter to a half pint. Additionally, in severe cases characterized by delirium, bottles of hot water were placed at the feet. Fresh air was important and an outdoor airing at the earliest practicable period was recommended. It was purported that if the remedy was given at the earliest stages, the eruptions were arrested and suppuration prevented without injurious results.[16]

If cream of tartar did not cure smallpox, the *Eastport Sentinel* (ME) had a different prescription. They suggested giving the patient 2 tablespoonfuls of a mixture of hop yeast and water, sweetened with molasses so as to make it palatable, three times a day, decreasing the dose to 2 teaspoonfuls a day for children under 12 years. In addition, a diet of boiled rice and milk, toasted bread moistened with water and without butter was to be offered; the patient was to eat no meat. For thirst, catnip tea was the preferred beverage. When the patient was convalescent, broiled beefsteak might be sparingly offered; to offset constipation, physics were to be administered when necessary. If this regimen was strictly followed, it was claimed no marks of smallpox would remain.[17]

Opting for home remedies led down the path to disaster and reports of smallpox outbreaks continued to appear. Notices appeared such as "the small pox is so prevalent in N. Orleans, that people are cautioned against riding in the street cars"[18]; "the small pox is raging [at Horicon, WI] to such a serious extent there are some thirty or forty cases, and several places of business have been closed on account of it[19]; "the Small Pox is spreading with fearful rapidity over our State [Iowa].... There is no safety in neglecting [vaccination]. Any day may bring one into contact with a victim of the disease."[20] Perhaps not atypically, a report from Delaware stated that due to a lack of pesthouses, a farmer's wife died of the disease and her husband found it impossible to get anyone to bury her. He was finally compelled to put the corpse on a sled, dig a hole and put her in it. He then went home and died of the disease himself. It seemed to some people that this case seemed "too barbarous to have occurred in a professedly christian community" and humanity dictated that a smallpox hospital be placed on the corner of some large farm. Men of influence were solicited to hurry its speedy erection.[21] The board of health in Jackson, Michigan, was also directed to provide a suitable pesthouse to treat smallpox cases in that city.[22]

City death statistics continued along the same pattern as prewar fatalities. During the month of May 1864, medical and surgical services, vaccination and medicine were afforded gratuitously to 17,897 persons from the six dispensaries of New York. Of this number, 2,575 were treated in their homes, and 15,322 at the dispensaries, and 5,700 were vaccinated. A total of 19,602 prescriptions were filled free of charge.[23]

Brooklyn City Mortality
Week of April 11, 1864

Consumption	20
Scarlet fever	10
Inflammation of the lungs	10
Dropsy	8
Disease of heart	4
Convulsions	7
Typhoid fever	3
Smallpox	1

The total number of deaths for the week was 131: 26 men, 36 women, 43 boys and 26 girls. Ninety-six were natives of the United States, 22 were Irish, 5 were English, 5 were German and 3 were other nationalities.[24]

The commissioners of Public Charities and Corrections reported on the condition of those who survived in the abstract of the 5th Annual Report for the Year 1864. They reported that the Small-Pox Hospital was "filled to overflowing, under circumstances hardly to have been anticipated." In a less-than-charitable tone, the report complained of having forced upon them an entire class of patients who should have been cared for by the commissioners of Emigration.[25]

In what might have served as a defense, the 1864 report by the New York Emigration Society stated that in the course of the year, 222,338 passengers arrived from abroad, of whom 39,422 were American citizens and 182,916 were aliens, an increase of 27,072 from 1863. Breaking down foreigners, there were 89,766 Irish, 23,871 English and 57,572 German. The commission provided employment, food, lodging or transportation for 28,957 and cared for 7,363 in the refuge and hospital of the commission and for 235 in its smallpox hospital. Of these numbers, 978 died and were buried.[26]

The report by the commissioners of Public Charities also complained that they were called upon to care for and medically treat patients from the army and navy, adding "an extra call upon their resources." Those who occupied the Island and Fever Hospitals fell into their own class, where it was stated, "Although the victims of their own folly and imprudence, yet they are entitled to all the consideration which poor, unfortunate and erring creatures can lay claim to."[27]

New York City Mortality
Week of January 23, 1865

Consumption	78
Inflammation of the lungs	50
Small-pox	26
Scarlet fever	16
Typhoid fever	13

The total number of deaths for the week totaled 496: 101 men, 108 women, 167 boys and 120 girls. This represented an increase of 28 from the previous week and a decrease of 2 from the corresponding week of 1864. Deaths from smallpox were the same as the previous week.[28]

Although tuberculosis remained the number one cause of death in 1864 and 1865, New York suffered an alarming increase in deaths related to smallpox. Even without the Quarantine at Staten Island, serious outbreaks of the disease occurred in every town in Richmond County. Steps were taken to secure a general vaccination.[29]

Pandora's Box

As the "loathsome disease" became epidemic in New York City, inspectors found 644 cases during a two-day search; in two weeks, the number skyrocketed to almost 1,200, and it was estimated that only half the cases had been discovered. In many of the large tenant houses, between six and eight victims were found at the same time. And if further proof were needed, smallpox was found under every conceivable condition, tending to promote its communicability. The presence of the disease was in streetcars and hacks, on stages, ferryboats, in junk shops, cigar stores and candy shops. Furthermore, the disease was found in public and private charities and the families of tailors and seamstresses who made clothing for wholesale stores.

An investigative report from the *New York Times* (March 16, 1865) traced the spread of smallpox on the local level, discovering that bedding from a fatal case was sold to a ragman; infected clerks sold candy and daily papers; a woman cared for her sick husband and then tended bar; a girl making cigars had scabs falling off her skin; a seamstress making shirts for a Broadway store had carelessly thrown one over the cradle of a child sick with smallpox; sick children of tailors making clothing for soldiers ran around the shops, wrapping themselves in the garments; a woman selling vegetables had scabs falling off her face onto the produce.

The inspector of the Fourth Ward (NY) stated that he found infected tailors at work in the best clothing establishments; the uniforms they made brought disease and death not only to the wearer, but also had the potential to infect whole regiments. Contaminated clothing also infected the occupants of entire tenant houses and from there spread throughout the neighborhood, endangering the health of the entire community. Smallpox epidemics in rural areas also owed their origins to the transfer of disease by clothing and public transport. Even "in the remote solitude of the ocean the seaman opens the chest in which he has deposited such obnoxious apparel, and from this Pandora's box scatters the seeds of pestilence among his comrades, which, ripening, shall spread its germs to distant ports."

The inspector of the Fifth Ward (NY) reported that the largest wholesale establishments for the sale of dry goods on the American side of the Atlantic were in immediate contact with tenant houses harboring the worst cases of smallpox and typhus fever. Two freight depots and the principal passenger depot of the Railway Company were also in close proximity to these "nests of infection." Through them passed millions of travelers who carried this contamination through Broadway and other major streets, right to the doors of their homes. Perhaps worse, several large livery stables in the area were well known to illegally hire their conveyances to carry persons suffering from contagious diseases to hospitals or to attend funerals. The inspector concluded, "Is it any cause of surprise that cases of these diseases are here contracted, to be carried to distant sections of the country, there to develop themselves, to the surprise and alarm of whole neighborhoods?"

Facts, figures and lack of hygiene were well publicized throughout the mid–1860s, but the New York Sanitary Report of 1865, prepared by the Hygienic Council of Citizens' Association, added shocking details to the life of the inner city working class. Information gleaned from the report included an example of a "tenant-house" in the Fifteenth Ward, covering the region between Bowery and Sixth Avenue and Fourteenth Street and Houston. There, a family of seven persons lived in a cellar 18 feet square and 7 feet high; of these, two died of typhus, two of smallpox and one of erysipelas.

Many private residences in the same ward contained a living space of 20 × 40 feet, housing one family, or eight persons; in contrast, a tenant house typically contained 20 ×

25 feet of space, housing eight families, or forty persons. The former had an average air space of 4,000 cubic feet to each person, the latter 400. Private dwellings contained a ground area of 100 square feet while the multifamily dwelling had but 15. The rooms of the private home were light and dry; those of the other dark and damp.

Considering that 19th century sanitary standards recommended a minimum of 1,000 cubic feet of air space for each person, it was not difficult to draw the conclusion that pestilence and disease thrived in the poorer quarters. In the Fifteenth Ward alone, 4,940 persons lived in tenant houses and 234 in cellars.

In the First Ward, the custom was to erect a front house 25 × 50 feet and a rear house 25 × 25 feet on a lot 25 × 100 feet. The court between them measured 25 × 25 feet and contained the hydrant, cesspool and privy. Each building typically contained 24 families, with an average family of six individuals, leaving them a little over 10 square feet of ground and 480 cubic feet of air space, while dormitories contained a scant 89 feet to each. Inspectors described these double-houses in Washington Street as "a perpetual fever-nest." Typhus, smallpox, measles, diarrhea and cholera-infantum raged within all year round. The report added that miserable women seeking the stimulus which fresh air and sun did not provide found solace "in poisoned liquors at the drinking-shops, of which there are two to every tenant-house." The report provided formidable evidence of overcrowding and the existence of centers of pestilence throughout all New York City's wards and called for "legislation restraining the greed and the cruelty of those who derive vast profits from this packing of the poor in crowded rooms."[30]

The graphic descriptions are chilling. Taken with the plea of the *New York Evening Post* cited above, it is hard to fathom why sanitation and mandatory vaccination did not become the major health issues of the times. Yet there was no adequate legal power to prevent the spread of disease. Public transportation carried those infected and travelers filled hotel rooms that the night before were occupied by smallpox patients. Sick children were put to bed with healthy siblings and stricken adults continued to work in jobs where they had wide public exposure. Legislation and enforcement were indeed part of the answer, but it was not forthcoming. On the third reading of a bill presented by Dr. Richardson making vaccination compulsory, the New York Assembly defeated it.[31] Views contrary to the public good were often supported by well-educated individuals fearful of a "tyrannical law as a bonus to doctors," as well as an infringement on personal liberty.

In January 1865, the legislature of Maryland passed a law requiring children desiring to enroll in primary schools to be vaccinated before being permitted to enter. An educator who had been teaching for 15 years decried this as haughty and unnecessary, demanding to know if a child who did not have the means of vaccination deserved no education. Without broaching the idea of free public vaccination (England was only two years away from strengthening existing law providing for free vaccination and demanding mandatory vaccination for infants), this educator wrote that "our miserable legislators" placed one more obstacle in the way of education. He added this: "Suppose A's children are vaccinated, and B's are not, well then if vaccination prevents Small-pox, what have A's children to fear, if B's do take the Small-pox? What more right has A to dictate to B, than B has to A? Would not A, as a gentleman, better tend to his own family, and let B decide for himself? The entire law is nothing but a trampling on individual rights, without producing a public good." He likened the law to "slavery where we are the *Slaves*," making it "as obnoxious to us as [N]egro-slavery; or they may have ignorantly supposed themselves our absolute guardians, instead of our representatives."[32] The man who signed himself "A Teacher" failed to take into consideration the fact that "B's" children had a wider acquaintanceship than the classroom. Just as it was possible to take data obtained by the New York ward inspectors and hypothetically trace contagion from candy sellers to children and from children to tailors and from them to customers who traveled throughout the city, state and ultimately the world, so, too, would "B" and his family expose countless people. Using the teacher's own argument that some families were unable to afford vaccination, "B's" personal freedom would thus spread smallpox to innocent victims. Disagreement over this point, among others, would prevent the eradication of smallpox for another one hundred years.

Smallpox in the city of Washington, DC, was always a concern, not least because it housed the seat of national government. It also contained thousands of military personnel. In January 1864, when smallpox became epidemic, Mr. Lovejoy of Massachusetts, a member of the House of Representatives and the Committee of the District of Columbia, reported on sanitary measures being taken to prevent the spread of that disease. Communications from the mayor of Washington, the acting surgeon general and others were read, detailing provisions for the care of all persons suffering from smallpox and also on the progress of vaccination. Afterward, Lovejoy reported a resolution that passed, making it advisable (as opposed to mandatory) that the cities of Georgetown and Washington furnish vaccination at the residences of citizens.[33]

BUTTE NEWS

IS A THING OF THE PAST

The Smallpox Epidemic Is at Last Entirely Eradicated.

PEST HOUSE IS CLOSED

List Cases Discharged Yesterday and Dr. Sullivan Returns to the City. Treated 174 Cases—His Experiences.

Smallpox "Is a Thing of the Past," reads a headline published in the *Anaconda Standard* (MT), July 12, 1900. The story detailed the work of Dr. T.J. Sullivan, describing the "dead line" or quarantine area of smallpox patients isolated from the community. The issue of whether or not smallpox was contagious continued into the 20th century, creating a bitter divide between business interests and the medical profession.

Germ Warfare—Again

Of all the alleged atrocities committed during the Civil War few equaled the charges of germ warfare. After testimony during the "great Assassination trial" touched upon the subject that Rebels had sent clothing infected with smallpox and yellow fever throughout the North, suspicious behavior in Neenah, Wisconsin, was reevaluated. It seems that in 1864, certain peddlers sold bundles containing broadcloth for the price of $40. As these men were unnaturally heedless of collecting money for their wares it was later supposed they were part of "Mudd's Small Pox Spreaders." If the suspicion were true, the newspaper warned, "there is danger ahead, as Small Pox virus does not lose its infecting qualities for years, if indeed at all."[34]

Like charges were leveled against the Rev. Dr. Stuart Robinson, a leader of the Southern Presbyterian Church. Those "not friendly" to him charged that while sojourning in Canada he aided and abetted an effort to send the loathsome disease into Southern prisons where Union soldiers were confined. When Robinson contracted smallpox in 1872, some believed it was retribution for his alleged murderous designs.[35]

By 1879, the Democratic Party of Kentucky appointed Dr. Luke P. Blackburn as governor. This immediately aroused the indignation of Union men, who considered him "the notorious wretch who attempted to destroy the Northern people, during the war, by smuggling into the Northern cities a vast quantity of rags and clothing infected with yellow fever and small pox." Blackburn won the election despite the confession of a man named McKeogh, who kept a hotel in Montreal used as a headquarters for "traitors and Confederates." McKeogh positively identified Blackburn as part of that group but expressed his belief in the man's innocence concerning the smallpox plot. Those who believed there was enough evidence to convict him "by any but a Mississippi jury" ignored McKeogh's avowals.[36]

The Aftermath of War

Before the last shots were fired, soldiers and civilians anticipated the end of the bloody conflict. They could rebuild their homes and try to gather about them a sense of normalcy, but what they could not do was protect themselves from the continuing ravages of disease. Those who suffered the most had the least: the freedmen of the torn and scarred nation.

A report from the *Daily Milwaukee News,* January 4, 1865, is typical of the times: "Small pox is raging among the [N]egroes at Mobile. They stumble through the streets and fall down and die. Many families are compelled to resort to force to keep dying [N]egroes from staggering into their houses to expire."

In order to counteract the problem of smallpox in Petersburg, Virginia, Lieutenant Colonel Stephen Baker issued Special Orders No. 9, on July 14, 1865, ordering all destitute persons of the city to appear at the district assistant provost marshal's office for the purpose of free vaccination.[37]

Other reports continued in the same vein, smallpox "raging among the [N]egroes in and around Macon, Ga.," and "the small-pox is raging with great violence both among the whites and Blacks in Arkansas." The surgeon having charge of freedmen in North Carolina reported that during the prior three years, yellow fever and smallpox had greatly decimated blacks in the area. The mortality at Fort Anderson, one of the largest colonies in the state, was unprecedented during the spring of 1865, during which fever killed over 2,000 in less than two months. By December, however, the surgeon was able to report the sanitary condition of the sufferers was "constantly improving."[38]

The passage into a new year saw little improvement. As the Southern states adjusted to the new era without slavery, they found a great deficiency of labor. Many freed slaves fled north, while others sought to escape the fields by moving into towns. Those who remained behind to till the cotton crops suffered terribly from smallpox, particularly in Mississippi and Alabama. It was observed that the Freemen's Bureau "could do as much good in seeing to the vaccination of the blacks as in any other way." That disease was not the only cause of death, however, for the Union commandant in Alabama who had charge from about September to December 1865 reported that he had buried over 170 Negroes with no epidemics prevailing.[39]

In March 1866, the *Charleston Courier* reported that it was "hardly possible to imagine the extent to which the small pox prevails" throughout the South. According to a gentleman who had recently toured the various states, all the large Southern cities were more or less infected: in some places, freedmen were the only victims, while in others the white population also suffered. None of the infected, he said, were bid to stay within doors, and they walked the streets "in the most indifferent and unconcerned manner." In two or three towns, one house in three had the red symbol of smallpox displayed. The sickness also prevailed at Charleston, but not as heavily as some other Gulf cities.[40]

Nor had conditions significantly improved in Washington. By late April 1866, citizens began realizing the disease existed to a greater degree than was generally acknowledged. Several schools were affected and individual cases appeared throughout the city. Senator Fessenden contracted varioloid and was "more seriously sick than has been generally known."[41]

In the decades following the Civil War, little improvement would be made in the eradication of the "loathsome disease."

The Non-Eradication of Smallpox in England

From Pestilence! It is an unfortunate fact that people with infectious diseases must be either left or put somewhere. The poet quoted by Pope, who preferred the modest prayer —

> "Ye gods annihilate both Space and Time,
> And make two lovers happy,"

could scarce expect to behold the end of what German philosophers call the two great "institutions à priori," nor can even Space be altogether done away with by an entreaty when we have got patients with fever, cholera, and small-pox, whose neighborhood everybody dreads.[1]

With the American Civil War drawing to a close, English cotton markets slowly reopened. New business was expected to put unemployed factory workers, textile merchants, tailors and exporters of fine linens and clothing back to work. If a new prosperity lay on the horizon, however, it did not include a general advancement of public health. Death rates in London for the week of June 24–30, 1866, were 1,295, or 87 beyond the estimated mortality. Smallpox demonstrated an increase, with 45 deaths registered during that time. Nor was that the only disease on the rise: there were 69 fatal cases of measles, 43 deadly cases of diarrhea (increased due to summer heat) and one death from cholera. In contrast, 1,943 births were registered.[2]

For the week of November 18–24, 1866, the registrar-general reported 3,070 deaths in London and other large towns in the United Kingdom; deaths in London alone were 1,435, or 173 less than the anticipated number. Significantly, due to strict measures taken to combat the spring cholera epidemic, only 8 deaths were recorded. That represented a considerable drop in mortality from cholera, as the numbers of fatalities for the past seven weeks were 207, 144, 112, 73, 67 and 32, while weekly deaths from diarrhea fell from 47 to 26 in the same period.

Annual Percent of Mortality Rate for the Week November 18–24, 1866
Per 1,000 individuals

London	24	Salford	18
Edinburgh	30	Sheffield	22
Dublin	31	Leeds	29
Bristol	22	Hull	26
Birmingham	24	Newcastle-upon-Tyne	32
Liverpool	31	Glasgow	29
Manchester	30		

The mortality rate in Vienna was 30:1,000 during the week ending November 10, 1866, with an average temperature 6°F lower than the same week in London, where mortality stood at 23:1,000.[3]

During 1867, two important incidents regarding smallpox occurred. In France, the minister of the interior charged Dr. Danet to investigate and report on smallpox and vaccination. Danet's report to the Academy of Medicine detailed research that included vaccinating 8,500 persons and 40 animals:

1. Smallpox and cow-pox are two distinct diseases;
2. Vaccination does not predispose to other maladies;
3. After a certain time, vaccination loses the power of preserving from smallpox;
4. Vaccine matter, preserved in any way, has need of being renewed;
5. Predisposition to smallpox is greater in the young and the aged;
6. Revaccination is an absolute necessity;
7. Even those who had smallpox ought to be revaccinated;
8. Vaccine matter in passing through the human body borrows from its constitutional principles; it may, therefore, often be dangerous to vaccinate with vaccine matter from arm to arm*;
9. The cow is refractory to the syphilitic virus;
10. The revaccination from cow to man is the only one which presents all the guarantees of success and security;
11. A febrile condition is, in general, a cause of failure;
12. Injection of preserved vaccine matter and the multiplicity of scarifications, in general, was the best means of success;
13. Preserved vaccine matter ought to be revivified by transplantation to the heifer;
14. Vaccine matter ought not to be used but from the 4th to the end of the 6th day and never later.

*The Academy of Medicine had already decided that so far as regarded syphilitic affection, arm-to-arm transfer was dangerous only when blood was contaminated with the matter.

Danet concluded that of 8,395 persons of all ages vaccinated, it "took" on 2,826 patients, of which 40 percent had matter taken from the heifer and 26 percent had matter passed from arm to arm.[4]

The Process of Revaccination

When it became evident that vaccination did not offer a lifetime of protection, revaccination at varying intervals was recommended. This posed a problem, however, as interpreting reactions was often difficult. Four possible outcomes presented themselves, all of which were dependent on the balance between the potency of the vaccine and residual immunity:

1. No reaction: Although believed to mean the person was fully protected, it actually indicated that the vaccine used was of low potency;
2. Immediate reaction: This was a classic case of delayed hypersensitivity and might occur in highly immune persons or those with little or no immunity who were given inactive (dead) vaccine;

3. Accelerated reaction: Persons with some immunity developed erythema (redness on the skin) and the development of a vesicle and sometimes a pustule which evolved more rapidly than in primary vaccination;

4. Major reaction: If a long period had elapsed between vaccination and revaccination, the result was similar to that of primary vaccination.[5]

The question of proper diagnosis and treatment affected not only humans but also cattle. During this period, a terrible cattle plague affected Europe. Seeking answers and identification, Dr. Parsons wrote to the *London Observer* that he believed it to be a form of smallpox in that the pustules were seen under the skin as opposed to being merely a topical disease. He recommended vaccination as a preventive. In response, Secretary McCulloch in Washington directed customs officials to deny the landing of all hides from foreign ports into the United States unless given permission by the Treasury Department.[6] The question remained in dispute, however, as Dr. Murchison, writing to the *London Times*, argued that although the "rinderpest and smallpox are very striking, vaccination is no protection against the deadly distemper." He argued that rigid isolation and the suspension of all movement of living cattle be implemented, and he urged Parliament to devise some measure for grappling with the pest that attacked more than 10,000 cattle a week and continued to spread in spite of Orders in Council and local enactments.[7]

For the week of April 14–20, 1867, the registrar-general reported 2,725 deaths in London and the other large towns in the United Kingdom with an annual rate of mortality of 23 percent. Deaths in London registered 1,223; corrected for population growth, the average number of deaths per week was set at 1,429. The present return represented 206 fewer deaths than estimated, with mortality in the metropolis lower than any week in the present or preceding year.

Annual Percent of Mortality Rate for the Week April 14–20, 1867
Per 1,000 individuals

London	21	Salford	24
Edinburgh	30	Sheffield	22
Dublin	25	Leeds	29
Bristol	24	Hull	28
Birmingham	18	Newcastle-upon-Tyne	27
Liverpool	27	Glasgow	29
Manchester	22		

The mortality rate in Vienna was 33 percent during the week ending April 13, when the mean temperature was 7°F lower than in the same week in London, where the rate was 23 percent.

In the "Land of Jenner," however, efforts to eradicate smallpox were complicated and haphazard, as exemplified by a sad death in Soho. An inquest was held April 1, 1867, on the death of Remi Charboniere, a 19-year-old. The coroner's report detailed that the youth's mother was not against vaccination but the father was; in consequence of the boy being sickly, vaccination was never performed. Mr. Bennett, parochial surgeon, added that in St. Giles's parish there was no means of knowing whether children were vaccinated or not. Bennett testified that he had already encountered three more cases of smallpox that morning and within the prior six months the local infirmary treated 109 cases with 22 admitted to hospitals, 8 lodged in common lodging houses (having been turned out from hospitals) and the remaining 78 "taken casually into the house." Out of 98 cases where vaccination had been performed, only one died and out of 30 not vaccinated, 16 perished. The jury recommended a verdict of "death from small-pox, accelerated by want of vaccination," and recommended that the parish authorities of St. Giles institute an immediate visitation from house to house for the purpose of vaccinating those who had never undergone the procedure. They also suggested a provision to replace clothes and property destroyed for the preservation of public health.

On the same day, a special meeting was held in Marylebone to act on a request by the board of guardians for the immediate use of the iron-house in the stone-yard for the reception of smallpox cases, as there was no accommodation either in the workhouse or smallpox hospital. Acknowledging the necessity for increased smallpox and fever hospitals, the application was granted.[8]

In early 1866, published letters by Sir MacDonald Stephenson and Dr. Horace Jeaffreson appeared in the *London Times,* directing the public's attention to risks associated with street-cabs being employed to transport smallpox patients to hospitals. By January 1867, having collected 850£, the Hospital Carriage Fund had built six ambulances at an individual cost of 100£. In appearance, the vehicles looked like ordinary long-bodied carriages. The interiors were coated with hard paint, capable of being washed. Vulcanized India rubber air mattresses and cushions were fashioned for the stretchers.

Two ambulances were placed at the London Fever Hospital and could be used by either smallpox or fever patients willing to pay the necessary horse-hire. The other four were offered to five mainly unendowed hospitals if they would provide a coach-house. Four immediately responded and the London, St. George's, St. Mary's and Middlesex hospitals were furnished with an ambulance. However, authorities of the Small-pox Hospital refused on the grounds of expense incidental to acceptance.

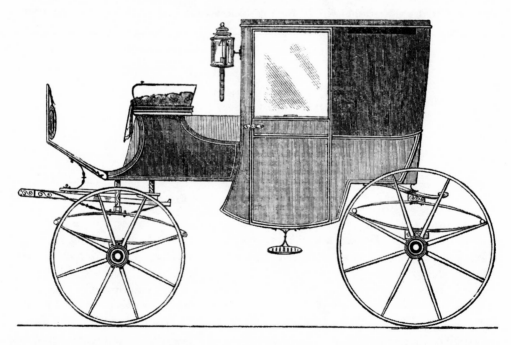

This line drawing from the *Illustrated London News* (February 23, 1867), depicts the outside of a model hospital carriage used to convey fever and smallpox patients. Conveyances such as this were designed to replace public transportation in an effort to limit contagion and to provide a more comfortable ride for victims. The concept was well-meaning but the expense limited production and public transportation remained the principal means of transporting patients.

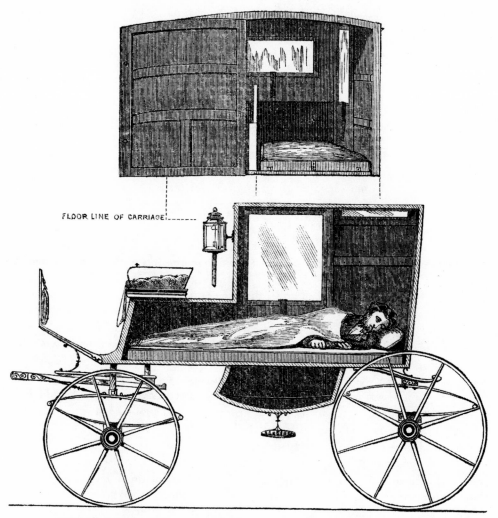

FLOOR LINE OF CARRIAGE

HOSPITAL CARRIAGE FOR THE CONVEYANCE OF FEVER AND SMALLPOX PATIENTS.

This illustration, also from the *Illustrated London News* (February 23, 1867), reveals the interior of the hospital ambulance. Designed by Messrs. John Woodall and Son, the carriage resembled a brougham drawn by one horse, with a back that opened on hinges to provide easy access.

To obviate this objection, the fund offered to construct a coach-house at the Smallpox Hospital and to pay all expenses of horse-hire in connection with the ambulance. Cooperation was peremptorily refused on the grounds the hospital had nothing to do with the way patients arrived; they were only bound to treat them once admitted.

Supporting the fund, the *British Medical Journal* hoped that ambulances would be provided other hospitals, making street-cabs as pest-vehicles "as practically unnecessary as it is now illegal." The publication hoped the more wealthy hospitals, including Guy's, St. Bartholomew's and St. Thomas's, would obtain their own ambulances without waiting for one to be bestowed upon them as a donation. Not coincidentally, deaths in London for the week of January 6–12, 1867, were 1,891, exceeding the average by 171.[9]

In order to address the continued presence of smallpox, the British government revised the Vaccination Act. Although not significantly different from the preceding law, the revision reinforced its provisions. The Vaccination Act of 1867 stipulated the following:

1. Vaccination districts were to be formed out of parishes and overseen by poor-law guardians, whose job it was to pay vaccinators 1–3 shillings per child vaccinated, the rate determined by the distance traveled by the practitioner;
2. Within 7 days of a registered birth, the registrar was to deliver a notice of vaccination. If the infant was not vaccinated within three months or brought for confirmation of its success, the parents or guardians were liable to a summary conviction and fined 20 shillings;
3. Any unauthorized person producing vaccine or inoculating another for smallpox was liable to be imprisoned for the term of one month.

The appointment of vaccination officers by the Boards of Guardians was made compulsory in another act in 1871.[10]

In acknowledging the 1867 London smallpox epidemic that began the previous year, Dr. Lankester, coroner of Central Middlesex, considered neglect of vaccination a potential crime. Using a provision of the Vaccination Act as his guide, he questioned whether parents who failed to vaccinate children fell under the spirit of the manslaughter law and conducted inquiries into the deaths of children who died without benefit of protection.[11]

Despite (or because of) the extraordinary fact that the Cork guardians declared that smallpox had ceased to exist in Ireland,[12] public health took a giant leap forward when University College and King's College instituted chairs devoted to the teaching of "State Medicine." Dr. W.A. Guy was appointed to the latter post and proposed to commence his course January 31, 1870. His prospectus consisted of eight lectures concerning the social and political consequences of fatal diseases, including the history of hygiene; of mental epidemics; of the plagues of the 16th and 17th centuries; of the third sanitary epoch from the fire of London to the end of the 18th century; of jail-fever; and of smallpox.[13]

The February 10, 1870, editorial in the *London Echo* cited J.S. Mill's essay on Liberty, which maintained that even error might have its use in stimulating a more active belief in those who held the truth. Thus, the heresy of anti-vaccinationists drew attention to the proofs in favor of the practice. Simultaneously with the announcement that smallpox had been eradicated in Ireland due to enforcement of vaccination, notice was brought to the Mile-end Guardians of the progressive mortality from smallpox. Side-by-side was the fact that in the district births numbered 1,715, while there followed only 731 vaccinations. The writer concluded, "These are hard nuts for the opponents of vaccination to crack."

21

The Franco-Prussian War and the Smallpox Pandemic of 1870–1874

Mr. Bloxam, the lecturer on chemistry to the department of artillery studies, has made a suggestion, which, if taken seriously, would be as ingeniously diabolical as the Powers of Darkness could wish. His proposal is, that abandoning gun cotton, we should collect in cotton wool the germs of smallpox and other malignant diseases, and load shells with them. In this way typhus and Asiatic cholera might be scattered broadcast among the enemy, whose army would melt away as

"The angel of Death spread his wings on the blast,
And breathed in the face of the foe as he passed."[1]

In point of fact, smallpox did not need to be used as a biological warfare weapon, as the natural occurrence of the contagion proved that it required little assistance.

The Franco-Prussian War (July 1870–January 1871) officially began July 17, 1870, when France declared war on Prussia. Stemming from complex political issues concerning ascendancy to the vacant Spanish throne and France's fear for the security of its borders (Prussia extended from France, Belgium and Holland in the west to the Baltic Sea and Poland in the east), the conflict would exacerbate a smallpox epidemic that would ultimately destroy 500,000 soldiers and civilians throughout Europe.[2]

During the pre-war period of January 1860–November 1869, smallpox deaths in Paris were always below 100 except in October 1861, when they reached 113, and during the winter of 1865–1866, when they ranged between 111 and 148.

The actual beginnings of the smallpox epidemic were present during the latter part of 1869, when the disease was prevalent in Brittany, Aisne and Pas de Calais and Gers, Ariege and Pyrenees Orientales. In 1869, the death toll for October was 39; by November, however, it had risen to 93 and by December to 113. By early 1870, Orleans, Bordeaux, Lyons and Bourg suffered under the disease and by June and July, 9–10 persons in Bordeaux were dying per day. The death toll eventually reached 4,164.[3] By 1870, smallpox was so common that it became the latest "touch" in Paris, spawning *robbery a la petite verole,* or robbery by the help of smallpox. Rogues confronted suffering patients alone in bed and demanded to be told where their money and jewels were kept. The victim was warned not to become excited or he would have a relapse: "Don't try and get out of bed or you'll catch cold." Of course the person yielded and the robber made away with his treasure.[4]

On May 31, 1870, the London newspaper *Echo* reported that Prince de Latour d'Auvergne and the Duke de Caumont la Force had both contracted smallpox. Furthermore, M.

Jules Ferry reported on its alarming spread, stating that in the week before it had killed 209 persons. He demanded a system of gratuitous vaccinations, the removal of smallpox patients from the hospitals in Paris to the country, and a congress of medical men to consider means of arresting the epidemic. M. Chevandier de Valdrome replied that the government was "anxiously studying the question," and on May 25, a conference was called to examine the escalating problem.

A month before the declaration of war, the health of Paris seemed to be improving, with official returns showing a diminution in the number of new cases. While the number of dead from the previous week reached 165, the current number reflected 8 fewer cases than the past seven days. Physicians credited vaccination as the major preventive, having verified it by actual observation.[5] Unfortunately, hope proved premature, as 1,940 fatal instances of smallpox were recorded in Paris in 20 weeks, exclusive of deaths in hospitals, indicating approximately 23,000 cases during that time frame.[6] By September, notwithstanding the reduced population of Paris owing to the removal of troops and the migration of foreigners, 187 deaths from smallpox were recorded in the week ending August 25.[7] News out of Paris carried by the "balloon post" (mail was flown out of occupied Paris by aeronauts and also attached to pigeons) for the week ending November 5, 1870, indicated 1,800 deaths and the following week 1,900, with ravages from smallpox being very severe.[8]

Despite vaccination's proven success, the majority of countries in the 1870s had low vaccination rates and of those people who had been vaccinated, the procedure was often ineffectual, resulting in little or no actual protection. During 1860–1869, only 59 percent of infants born in France had received vaccination and by July 1870, nearly one-third of the population remained unvaccinated. Out of 10,331 smallpox deaths in Paris during the war, 213 occurred to infants one month old or younger; 151 in the first to second month, 107 in the second to third month, 290 between 3 and 6 months, 397 between 6 and 12 months, equaling 1,158 deaths. The total number of smallpox deaths in Paris for all ages was estimated at 60,000–89,954.[9]

Prior to the war, there had been a gradual increase in smallpox cases in the French army, with vaccination and revaccination being poorly administered. Although the French War Office ordered the vaccination of all recruits in 1859, during the years 1866–1869, only 37–49 percent of primary vaccinations and 32–35 percent of revaccinations were successful. Because of this, by 1868, the number of smallpox cases in the army was three times what it had been. Worse, due to the urgency of the situation, at the outbreak of war vaccinations were omitted altogether. As regular soldiers died, these unprotected recruits comprised the bulk of the fighting force. Ultimately, among the 600,000 soldiers mobilized, 125,000 men contracted smallpox, resulting in 23,470 fatalities.

Florence Nightingale was an early believer that smallpox need not be brought into an army by a contagious person. Given conditions favorable to its development, she felt the disease would appear spontaneously. It was her opinion that in crowded, ill-ventilated hospitals and in army camps, smallpox could be seen and smelt "while it was growing" and before the victim had a thought of his danger. Because disease was often observed in armies a long time actively engaged, she and others inferred that epidemics followed great battles and continual wars, and was, in fact, endemic to them without outside contagion.[10]

Most physicians, however, felt the transfer of smallpox into Prussia was attributable to the massive number of infected French soldiers incarcerated there in prisoner of war camps. As early as August 7, 1870, prisoners were moved into camps in eastern Prussia; eight days later, the first case appeared at Konigsberg. By the end of September, smallpox appeared in camps covering the entire Prussian territory.[11] By October, the *Medical Times and Gazette* warned that smallpox was endangering the health of central Europe:

> German troops are entering France in large numbers, and for months past there have been two hundred deaths weekly in Paris from this cause. All troops who have entered France have been revaccinated. The recruits for the reserve battalions are also revaccinated; but those medical officers who have neglected to supply themselves with the glycerine lymph (namely, virus dissolved in glycerine, now much in use in the army,) have had to contend with many difficulties and delays. At the present time the danger lies in the small pox slipping into Prussia by means of the numerous prisoners who are daily arriving.[12]

Matters would get worse for the beleaguered country. A correspondent for the *Lancet* (England), in describing conditions at Orleans, wrote that "nothing could have exceeded the utter disorganization" in the hospitals there. It required days after major battles for medical supplies to arrive, while "overcrowding, dirt, foul smells, want of the commonest things, and an absence of all administration, prevailed on every side." In visiting a large number of hospitals, he saw upwards of 700 cases of smallpox and typhoid fever. The mortality rate was, upon average, two daily.[13]

Before the war, Prussia had been relatively free of smallpox. Unlike its army, however, civilians were very inadequately protected from smallpox. Prussia and Saxony had no compulsory vaccination laws, while Bavaria, Hesse, Baden and Wurtemburg had such laws but revaccination was not made mandatory until the Imperial Vaccination Law of 1874. Contact with prisoners, either from a humanitarian or business nature, exposed local populations, who, in turn, spread the disease across the empire.

Deaths from Smallpox

	1860	*1870*	*1871*	*1872*	*1873*
Prussia	4,655	4,200	59,839	16,660	8,932
Bavaria	456	516	5,070	2,992	869
Saxony	unknown	unknown	9,935	5,863	1,772
Wurtemburg	133	529	2,050	1,164	55
Baden	67	343	3,176	511	unk
Hesse	20	248	1,028	167	3
Hamburg	20	83	3,647	323	3[14]

Bavaria, regarded as the best-vaccinated country in Europe, had a population of 5 million and suffered 9,174 smallpox deaths between 1870 and 1874, while Berlin, with a population of 900,000, suffered 66,538 deaths during the same period. Significantly, in Leipzig, where anti-vaccinationists were especially active, smallpox mortality was only 4.25 percent in 18 years prior to the war, but rose dramatically to 14.7 percent during 1871–1872.

The question of vaccination's value was broached again in 1873, when Dr. Papilland read a paper before the French Scientific Congress, maintaining that while vaccination alone afforded sufficient immunity from sporadic smallpox, it was of little value during epidemics. His theory was to first employ the vaccine and then follow with inoculation, the purpose of the vaccination being to remove the danger that might otherwise attend the introduction of the smallpox virus.[15]

The cases of smallpox seen during the Franco-Prussian War were generally of the malignant hemorrhagic type, adding to the staggering death tolls. The epidemic outlasted the war, not ending until 1874, after causing more than 170,000 deaths throughout the empire.

This ultimately led to the passage of a law in April 1874, compelling every child to be vaccinated within two years of birth and revaccinated at age twelve. Strict compliance led to a drastic reduction in smallpox cases. Between 1874 and 1880, Prussia's death rate per 100,000 of the population never reached above 4 percent. After compulsory vaccination was enacted in Austria in 1884, similar results were achieved.

In contrast to civilian losses, the German army was well vaccinated due to regulations mandating compulsory vaccination and revaccination begun in 1835. Between that date and the beginning of armed conflict, only 77 deaths were recorded. During the entire war epidemic, the total number of smallpox cases amounted to 8,463 and 459 deaths, or a fatality of 5.43 percent. In contrast, during 1866–1869, when vaccination was carelessly performed, 380 French soldiers died. Despite these numbers, it was not until 1902 that vaccination in France became compulsory in the first year of life and revaccination at ages 11 and 21 years.

The Smallpox Pandemic Outside the Seat of War

The failure of compulsory vaccination laws throughout Europe during the period of the Franco-Prussian War was the principal cause of the spread of smallpox and the shockingly high number of casualties. Although its preventive powers were widely known and acknowledged, communities, towns, cities, states and countries either failed to pass appropriate laws or grew lax in enforcement. Careless providers of vaccine and sloppy technique or follow-through added to the unnecessary death tolls. Lacking any international standards or even agreement within the confines of individual nations, the world of the early 1870s became vulnerable to a monstrous loss of life far and above that witnessed on the battlefield.

Vaccination was not compulsory in Belgium and consequently its citizens suffered greatly when the influx of refugees after the invasion of France crossed into its borders. Additionally, more than 100,000 French soldiers were imprisoned in the Beverloo camp and citadel of Antwerp after the Battle of Sedan. Disease spread quickly, resulting in a total death count of 35,931 between the years 1870 and 1873.

As in neighboring countries, vaccination was not compulsory in Switzerland, and that country suffered from an epidemic of smallpox around the same time as Belgium and for the same reasons. The towns most affected were Zurich, Basel, Bern and Geneva.

Smallpox became epidemic in Holland in November 1870, with the provinces of North Holland, South Holland and Utrecht most affected, the towns of Utrecht, Rotterdam, Amsterdam and The Hague registering the highest fatalities. Vaccination was not compulsory until children were admitted to public schools, resulting in vaccination of children in the first years of life being "shamefully neglected."

Utrecht formed the center of the epidemic, where the inhabitants succumbed by low vaccination rates and improper care. In the Rijks Hospital, smallpox patients were not isolated but housed in general wards, while reports indicated they were often discharged early and sent back into the community where they spread contagion.

Italy was another country lacking a vaccination law and did not put one into effect until the 1880s, when infant vaccination and revaccination when entering school were made compulsory.[16] The country was already suffering from smallpox before the war, and a substantial increase was seen after the return of Garibaldi's troops. These volunteers, fighting for the French, had been infected in the Cote D'Or. Smallpox deaths in Rome between October 10 and December 31, 1871, totaled 325; 721 were counted in 1872.

The progress of smallpox through Austria was slow and did not peak until 1872, lasting another two years before finally ending. In Vienna, there were 52.7 percent of deaths per 10,000; in 1872 in Prague, the death rate from smallpox reached 39.7 percent. During 1870–1874, there were 155,335 deaths from smallpox, of which 141,088 occurred in the last three years. These nearly incomprehensible numbers were attributed to seriously deficient vaccination and revaccinations that continued almost unaltered after the pandemic, with no more than a vaccination certificate required for admission to school.

Smallpox did not become widespread in Denmark until 1872, when 1,220 cases and subsequently 86 deaths were registered between January and April. The total number of deaths in 1872 reached 108, and 381 the following year. The situation was slightly different in Sweden and Norway, where smallpox had been epidemic between 1865 and 1869. By December 1873, smallpox made a significant comeback, causing an additional 4,063 deaths, of which 1,206 occurred in Stockholm.

As testimony to the fact that laws were of no use if not enforced, compulsory vaccination had been on the books in Sweden for 70 years, but 49 percent of children in Stockholm went unvaccinated. During 1873–1875, a total of 7,204 deaths were recorded in Sweden. During the epidemic of 1865–1868, Norway suffered 6,620 cases with 445 deaths; the reappearance of smallpox in the war years was less severe than in Sweden, with 2,235 cases reported compared to 275 deaths.

Finland had an epidemic of smallpox in 1868, but sustained low mortality rates for 1870 (1.3 percent per 10,000), 1 percent in 1871, and 3.4 percent in 1872. However, during 1873–1874 the number rose to 45.6 percent, dropping in 1875 to 8.6 percent. Deaths in St. Petersburg between the onset of epidemic in April 1872 through June 1873, reached 1,850.[17]

In Melbourne, smallpox was believed to have been brought ashore from the ship *Avon Vale* in 1869. Although the leading medical men debated the diagnosis, questioning whether cases were smallpox or chicken pox, the colony was treated as being "suspect" by the adjoining British colonies, who had quarantine enforced upon vessels arriving in their ports from Melbourne.[18]

Smallpox on the west coast of Africa made terrible inroads in 1871, where a contemporary described conditions of the people as "dying off from small pox like rotten sheep," with a death rate of 20 percent of those afflicted. He added that "the Ju Jumen priests are very busy instilling into the minds of the ignorant natives that the disease is a judgment of their Ju Ju, or God, on the people for so many of them embracing christianity."[19]

The Smallpox Pandemic in England and Wales

Just as French soldiers infected with smallpox spread the disease through prison camps and from there into the civilian population, so, too, did refugees unwittingly introduce contagion into other European nations. Although England remained relatively free from epidemic until the latter part of 1870, there was never a time when the kingdom was entirely free from disease. Munk and Marson, on the staff of Highgate Smallpox Hospital, presented figures from August 1869, when only sporadic cases were reported. In each subsequent quarter, however, until October 1870, the numbers rapidly increased:

Smallpox Cases at Highgate Hospital, England

Quarter	Number of Cases
October–December 1869	93
January–March 1870	182
April–June	222
July–September	337
October–December	341[20]

In the beginning, the epidemic was confined to London and Liverpool, where 879 of the 1,229 deaths in England for the last quarter of 1870 were recorded. The mining districts of North England and South Wales followed, with smaller outbreaks attributed to these four areas. By 1871, nearly every one of the eleven registration districts in the United Kingdom were affected. The high point of smallpox was reached in the first quarter of 1872, when 7,720 fatal cases were registered in England and Wales.[21]

While these death statistics are staggering, they represent a considerable improvement over the pre-vaccination era, which was three times as great. The estimated smallpox death rate in 18th century England was 3,000 per million, while the mean annual death rate of the 1871–1872 epidemic averaged 928 per million, or 1,024 per million in 1871 and 833 per million in 1872. In comparison to the last great epidemic of 1837–1840, the years 1870–1873 represented a decline of two-thirds mortality. In comparison to other countries, the death rate in Prussia was more than twice as great, while in Holland the rate was three times as great.[22]

At the time of the 1870 epidemic, there were no public hospitals for smallpox patients. Although the London Smallpox Hospital and the London Fever Hospital were charitable institutions, payment was required from patients, though the guardians did defer payment for a certain number. The Metropolitan Poor Act of 1867 had provided for fever and smallpox cases, but hospitals at Hampstead, Homerton and Stockwell were not yet complete. The principal hospital for smallpox was the Highgate, but it contained only 100 beds and those were soon filled. On December 1, 1870, the Hampstead Hospital (later known as the North Western Fever Hospital), which had first been used by the Metropolitan Asylums Board, reopened, with an added 150 beds. Within two months, 572 cases were admitted, with 97 deaths, a mortality rate of 16.67 percent.[23]

Seventy beds were added to the London Fever Hospital in January 1871; the Stockwell Hospital opened in January and the Homerton in February. An old battleship called the *Dreadnought* was moored off Greenwich and served as a convalescent hospital for 250 male patients between March 13 and October 14, 1871. For females, the workhouse at St. Mary's, Islington, accommodated 300 beds.[24] Altogether, 16,000 patients were admitted to the various hospitals, but it was estimated that number reflected only one-third of smallpox victims; the remainder were treated in their homes by Poor Law district medical officers or private physicians.[25] In the "Thirty-fourth Annual Report" of the registrar-general, 1873, numbers indicated that deaths of unvaccinated individuals in London hospitals reached 45 percent, double the mortality seen in private practice. Of the vaccinated patients admitted to the hospital, there was a 10 percent fatality as compared to 3 percent of cases treated in their own homes.

With the number of victims rising, local citizens became angered when their approval was not sought for the construction of smallpox hospitals near the vicinity of their homes. Just as riots occurred in 1857 on Staten Island, New York, over the smallpox facilities there, similar outbreaks occurred in England. In 1870, some 25–30 men, "some with their faces blackened and some with masks; some were armed with sticks, and others had pokers, and one had an axe," demolished the house of John Palmer at White Waltham on the grounds that a pesthouse was about to be erected "at their own doors, and they went to make a demonstration against a nuisance." At trial, the judge dismissed the case against the perpetrators on the ground they feared for the safety of their families.[26]

Letters to the editor of London newspapers complained of overcrowding, particularly at Stockwell, where 630 patients were located on grounds intended for less than half that number. This, it was argued, increased the threat of the disease's spread into the community. A typical day at Stockwell saw sociables and unlicensed vehicles bringing patients to the already filled hospital, while hearse-carts conveyed away the dead. The greatest consternation prevailed in the neighborhood. The site of land on which the hospital was constructed was close to the late Theobald's stud farm and contiguous to a main road leading from Brixton to Clapham. Public traffic was nearly suspended on account of the hospital. Nearby homes were deserted, making it appear "as if a siege had been made in the locality." The only people who dared approach the building were a few old paupers delivering letters to and from the hospital.

The City of London School for the reception of liverymen's orphans, comprising nearly 200 boys and girls, was within 200 yards of the hospital, while St. Andrew's Church, also a close neighbor, was all but deserted as a result of the dread of infection by the community. Not surprisingly, the question was asked, "Why should not these hospitals be under similar restrictions to gunpowder manufactories, and placed far from the haunts of man?"[27] Three important studies from the period offer contrary conclusions to that held by the public at large.

Correlation Between Smallpox Hospitals and Contamination in the Community

1. Dr. Stevenson, medical officer for St. Pancras, reported that he was unable to trace any connection between the presence of smallpox at Kentish Town and the Hampstead Hospital. He claimed the district was thoroughly infected with the disease before the hospital ever opened for smallpox cases. In fact, his data indicated a reverse correlation: smallpox in Kentish decreased as hospitalized patients increased, and increased when hospitalized patients decreased.[28]
2. Dr. A. Collie, medical superintendent of the Homerton Hospital, reported that during the period February–July 1871, no cases of smallpox occurred in the city of London Infirmary situated 90 feet from the western-most pavilion of the hospital. Also, from October 1, 1871, to December 1874, a total of 3,178 smallpox victims were treated at Homerton Hospital simultaneously with 2,611 cases of fever without any crossover.
3. A study made by Gairdner and Russell in 1872 found no correlation between the Parliamentary Road Smallpox Hospital, Glasgow and cases in the neighborhood.[29]

In spite of these studies, Sir Rowland Hill (whose house adjoined the North Western Hospital), and two other property owners brought suit against the Metropolitan Asylums District Board. On January 28, 1879, after an eleven-day trial, the special jury declared that "the hospital was *per se* a nuisance, and that in certain respects it was carried on negligently."

The board appealed, but the injunction restraining the defendants from carrying on an asylum remained in effect. Between May 1879 and November 1882, the hospital remained closed. The case was finally settled by the purchase of Hill's property in 1883.[30]

Mortality Rates in London and 19 Large Towns, 1870

May 15–21

22 deaths for every 1,000 persons;
London registered 2,277 births and 1,313 deaths;
Smallpox was more fatal than in any week since the first five months of 1868, when fatal cases ranged from 17–33/week.[31]

November 27–December 5

26 deaths for every 1,000 persons;
London registered 2,178 births and 1,482 deaths;
Smallpox accounted for 60 deaths, 11 of which came from the northern districts where the Smallpox Hospital was situated.[32]

December 11–17

29 deaths for every 1,000 persons;
London registered 2,111 births and 1,787 deaths;
Smallpox accounted for 44 deaths, 22 of which came from the eastern districts where the Hampstead Smallpox Hospital was situated.[33]

By February 1871, the epidemic had reached alarming heights in London. Deaths in the first week of January registered 79, but by the third week they soared to 188, comprising more than 10 percent of the entire mortality in London. Worse, deaths were not isolated to single areas. Dr. Grieve, medical officer of the Hampstead Smallpox Hospital stated, "The history of the epidemic during the past fortnight is marked by a great extension of the disease within the metropolitan area." While Shoreditch, Bethnal-green, Westminster and St. Saviour's suffered as severely as ever, the disease was found at Holborn Union, St. Pancras, Marylebone, Islington and Chelsea. The Medical Department of the Privy Council issued new orders for isolating the sick and made spot inspections at the smallpox hospitals at Homerton and Stockwell.[34] The last week in January the death toll from smallpox stood at 157. Of importance, the registrar-general suggested that when medical men certified the cause of death as smallpox, they should add "vaccinated" or "unvaccinated," as the case might be.

In Middlesex, the disease was so prevalent that the local vicar of a parish containing 10,000 people assisted the authorities in working with school administrators. On an appointed day two surgeons were taken into a classroom adjoining the infant room and examined the students. Those found to be unvaccinated were subjected to the operation. A "mob of anxious mothers, breathing out a hurricane of invectives" gathered outside but they were too late to stop the "*coup d'etat.*" From that time, the epidemic rapidly abated. It was noted, "Here was undoubted interference with the liberty of the subject, but it is well for the vicar that the parents of the unvaccinated had also broken the law."[35]

In another case of an individual's making a difference, Mrs. Gladstone, wife of the prime minister, offered two houses at Chapton for patients recovering from smallpox. In addition, she started a collection fund to meet the expenses of bedding, nourishment and physicians, beginning with Lord Overstone, who pledged £100.[36]

The numbers remained grim, with Dr. Curtis, a member of the Metropolitan Sick Asylum Board, stating that the smallpox epidemic raging in London "was, perhaps, one of the most virulent which had existed within the memory of any man living." There were 700 paupers suffering from the disease, and provision had been made for only 500. Of those dying, fully one-third were unvaccinated. The dead who had been vaccinated mostly comprised the elderly, who had partly lost the protection given them early in life. Fortunately, because the precaution of revaccinating nurses and physicians treating smallpox victims, scarcely any of them fell victim to the disease.[37]

On the subject of compulsory vaccination, a "Select Committee" was established to inquire into the efficacy of the Vaccination Act of 1867. After hearing the evidence of anti-vaccinationists, who considered vaccination useless and injurious and who therefore objected to the law, the committee reported that cow pox afforded if not an absolute yet a very great protection against death from the disease. They also found that with due precaution, it did not injure health.[38]

By April 1871, at a meeting of the Pancras Board of Guardians, it was reported that parochial vehicles had removed 97 cases of smallpox to various hospitals in less than two weeks; there was also read a communication from the Poor Law Board. Acting in conjunction with the Lords of her Majesty's Privy Council, they formed each parish into one district for the purpose of public vaccination. The Poor Law Board also added a deputy-vaccinator to act for the vaccinator-general in case of the latter's unavoidable absence.[39]

Additionally, during a meeting of the Wandsworth District Board of Works, it was decided that the inspector of nuisances should visit every home in which the disease had occurred to see what means were used for disinfecting. While directing that vaccination was to be applied under the Poor Law, Nuisance inspectors were to carry out proper "disinfectant," even if that meant the officer had to perform the operation himself and charge the cost to the various parties found wanting. The resolutions were passed despite Mr. Brown, "as a medical man," protesting against the inutility of the measure, he being a "non-believer in vaccination."[40]

Possibly, Mr. Brown would have preferred the method practiced by a surgeon in the British army in China whose mode of treatment dictated that when fever was at its height and just before eruptions appeared, the patient's chest was rubbed with croton oil and tartaric ointment. This was said to cause the whole of the eruption to appear on that part of the body to the relief of the rest, thus preventing smallpox from attacking the internal organs. It was "now the established mode of treatment in the English army in China, and is regarded as a perfect cure" for smallpox.[41] Croton oil was toxic to the skin; it may have altered the development of eruptions but would not have offered any protection from smallpox. (There was, however, one useful purpose for Croton oil. A convict in the Albany Penitentiary rubbed it on his face to give the appearance of smallpox and was immediately transferred to the smallpox hospital. From there, he easily escaped and went on to steal a set of valuable furs at Washington.)[42]

But nothing was ever perfect. In 1871 a great stir was caused in London when an embittered parent insisted that the inscription "died from the effects of vaccination" be chiseled on the tombstone of a child. The wording inspired so much rancor that it was not permitted.[43] More exciting was the escape of a smallpox patient from Hampstead Smallpox Hospital. Clad only in his nightdress, he managed to climb over the outer wall and was alternately followed by some convalescent patients and a police constable, all intent on his capture. He was ultimately arrested and returned to the hospital.[44]

Sparing the public from contamination remained the goal of authorities. In another small-scale effort, they fined a baker, Charles Jeffries, £10 for allowing his son, who was infected with smallpox, to assist in the manufacture of bread. They followed this by ordering the destruction of a large quantity of bread.[45]

On a wider scale with equal human import were the details encapsulated under the heading "How Smallpox Is Spread." Putting names and faces to an all-too-common occurrence, the story followed, a girl named Munday, who left William Lyall Atchison, her employer's service, on January 7, 1871, when infected with smallpox. Conveyed to her friends at Staines, she died on the 18th. On January 30, Jane Jennett, a 15-year-old girl, assumed Munday's position with the Atchisons and was given the same room in which to sleep. Jennett was taken ill on February 12, and sent by her master and mistress to Dr. Langston, of Broadway, Westminster. The following day, he diagnosed her condition as smallpox and directed another servant, named Whitton, who had been sent with her, to taker her home and keep her warm. Mrs. Atchison promptly redirected the girl, in the company of Whitton, to the servant's home in Egham. The pair took a cab to Waterloo station, where they remained one hour waiting for the train. After riding with five other passengers, the girl arrived home clearly bearing the marks of the disease on her face, neck and chest. She was ill for three weeks but recovered.

When the case became known to the authorities, nine summons were brought against Mr. Atchison and his wife, Priscilla, along with Ann Whitton, nurse, for sending a smallpox victim from their house without taking any precautions against spreading the contagious disorder. Not surprisingly, evidence given by the railroad company confirmed that had they known of Jennett's condition, they would have refused to carry her. None of the defendants contradicted the facts.[46]

Mortality Rates in London, 1871

Week	Smallpox Deaths	Week	Smallpox Deaths
January 1–7	79	June 11–17	240
January 8–14	135	June 18–24	232
January 15–21	188	June 25–July 1	235
January 22–28	157	July 2–8	164
January 29–February 4	196	July 9–15	133
February 5–11, 1871	211	July 16–22	135
February 19–25	227	September 17–23	57
February 26–March 4	213	September 17–23	89
March 5–11	194	September 24–30	51
(96 unvaccinated, 74 vaccinated,		October 1–7	72
1 inoculated, 23 not stated)		October 8–14	61
April 30–May 7	288	October 15–21	53
May 7–13	232	October 22–28	61
May 14–20	267	November 12–18	76
May 21–27	257	November 19–25	67
May 28–June 3	229	December 10–16	106
June 4–10	245	December 17–23	90[47]

Aside from the human toll, one consequence of the high death numbers was the reduction in the scale of payments by local burial societies.[48] Mortality rates slowly decreased until August 1872, when the epidemic was declared over after the duration of 93 weeks. Returns from the Metropolitan Asylums Board showed that for the years 1870–1872, death rates among males was 19.50 percent, compared to 17.64 percent among females, the difference being attributed to the harsher life and more irregular habits of men. In young people up to the age of 20, death rates were nearly identical.[49]

By September 1872, only eight smallpox deaths were registered, compared to 16 and

15 in the two previous weeks. Of the 8 who died, 6 were unvaccinated. Interestingly, as the numbers dwindled, the public was warned against circulating libraries, given that books loaned into infected houses were liable to infect new readers. People were asked not to use such conveniences until all supplies of reading material were thoroughly disinfected.[50]

Smallpox in Scotland and Ireland During the Pandemic

Scotland and Ireland fared better than their neighbors in England and Wales. In the report for 1868, the registrar-general for Scotland stated that in that year, 106,181 children were vaccinated, with only two recorded deaths. The report concluded that if it had not been for the success of vaccination, 500 of those children would have perished from the disease. In total, only 15 deaths for smallpox were registered for the entire year, making it the smallest number ever registered in Scotland in a year.[51]

The pandemic significantly changed those statistics, with the maximum number of causalities peaking in 1872, nearly a year after England's death rate reached its highest point. Smallpox deaths were greatest in Edinburgh, Leith, Glasgow and Dundee. In Scotland the statistics during the worldwide contagion were:

Number of Deaths from Smallpox in Scotland per 100,000 persons

1871	42
1872	71
1873	33
1874	37

In the period 1855–1857, when vaccination was optional, 89 percent of deaths from smallpox occurred among children under 10 years of age. In the period 1870–1872, six years after the Compulsory Vaccination Act in Scotland, where 85 percent of children were vaccinated, the proportion of deaths under 10 years fell dramatically, to 38 percent, and of those between birth and 5 years was demonstrated an even better ratio of 26 percent. On children born before vaccination became compulsory, the death toll rose from 4 percent to 12 percent.[52]

The smallpox epidemic reached Ireland around the third quarter of 1871, and persisted until the second quarter of 1873.[53] The total number of smallpox deaths in that country was 4,292, broken down as:

Mortality in Ireland

1871	665
1872	3,248
1873	379

The highest mortality was seen in Dublin and Cork. T.W. Grimshaw, senior physician to the Cork Street Fever Hospital, reported that at three Irish hospitals, Cork Street (21.6 percent) Hardwicke (Dublin) (20 percent) and Cork Hospital (22.5 percent), fatalities were higher than in London hospitals.[54]

22

Case Studies of Misdiagnosis

> The duties, responsibilities and labor of our physicians are onerous, and there are
> no class of our citizens who are more self-sacrificing and none to whom we are
> more indebted; and in justice to them, who are liable to be called at any moment,
> and meet disease in all its various forms, we should be careful not to let our minds
> be prejudiced against them by believing reports derogatory to their characters as
> men or physicians.[1]

The 1870s were pockmarked with isolated cases of smallpox and arguments — sometimes heated — concerning numbers and locales, but what stands out from the literature
and news reports is one glaring item: misdiagnosis. With the casual philosophy of "every
man his own doctor," men with college degrees vied with those who apprenticed in the
trade, who, in turn, competed with the common variety of physician, earning rights to the
title by no more than hanging out a shingle.

Throughout the third quarter of the century, perhaps nothing epitomized the state of
medicine in general and smallpox in particular better than a series of five letters written to
the editor of the *Waterloo Courier* (Iowa) between March 12 and April 2, 1868. They convey
a tale worth telling.

The background to this tale is that the citizen of the 19th century was a letter writer;
postage was inexpensive and service reasonably efficient. People wrote to relatives who had
migrated from their home states by marriage, business opportunity or adventure; travelers
wrote from foreign countries providing graphic details of ancient castles and meandering
waterways; homesick soldiers penned love letters to lonely fiancées; merchants reported on
sales in France or India; bankers sold bonds to overseas investors and everyone, it appears,
wanted to express their opinions on everything, from recipes to the newest invention, via
the newspapers. Perhaps the most intriguing thing about the latter class was their penchant
for writing *anonymous* letters. This left them free to express thoughts or criticize others
without suffering the consequences of having to defend their beliefs to the offended. Except,
of course, when those offended fought back with anonymous letters of their own. A titillating
war-of-words was gold for publishers hoping to sell papers to patrons eager to read of escalating scandals from one edition to the next.

Such was one series in Iowa that began March 12, 1868, when an unsigned writer
offered the editor "a statement of facts through the medium of your paper" concerning the
"grossly exaggerated" appearance of smallpox in their midst and the unjust reports attempting
to injure a worthy doctor. The Saga of the Iowa Smallpox Debate included three patients:
"a stranger," a laborer and the only child of a Mr. William Groves. While seemingly innocuous enough, the fourth sentence of Writer #1's initial letter included this statement: "The
first two cases were cared for, and through the exertion of our physicians the spread of the

disease was stopped, and the community owe their thanks to those of the number who at once gave warning, that the necessary precautions might be taken to prevent it becoming an epidemic."

The author continued in his praise of a physician (subsequently identified as Dr. Middleditch, who also happened to be Writer #1), who used "care and prudence" to prevent the spreading of the disease. When called upon to attend a stranger, Writer #1 diagnosed his condition as venereal disease and "accordingly treated him for that." He was later summoned to the house of Mr. Groves, his patient of long standing, to treat the man's son. Middleditch identified "the disease" (not naming it smallpox) and wishing to prevent its spread to

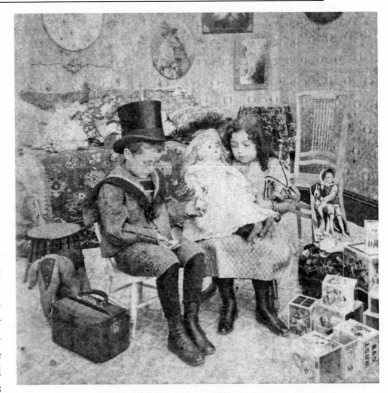

Daguerreotype of two children. The boy, dressed as a doctor, complete with top hat and black bag is preparing to vaccinate the girl's doll. The photograph was manufactured into cards that were captioned: "She has symptoms of small pox." On the back, the same statement is repeated in six different languages, indicating its international appeal. The card was sold by Underwood & Underwood, New York, London, Toronto and Ottawa, and published by Strohmeyer & Wyman, New York, New York (from the authors' collection).

his other numerous and needy patients, turned the case over to his partner, Dr. Eddy. This, Writer #1 (Middleditch) avowed, was satisfactory to all parties. "Under the circumstances," the author stated, writing of himself in the third person, "Doctor Middleditch done what any honest and conscientious physician would and should have done." He concluded by warning the public against minds being prejudiced by derogatory reports.

The following week, on March 19, a rebuttal appeared by a writer describing himself as a "friend to all the physicians of the town," later identified as Dr. Peabody. He wondered why the true facts of the averted epidemic had not caused the physician (Dr. Middleditch) to "suffer in medical reputation" in that he misdiagnosed the stranger (residing in the poor house) as having "a syphilitic eruption" rather than smallpox. Therefore, contrary to the first letter's assertion, Middleditch gave no alarm for smallpox.

Peabody then addressed the case of the laborer who contracted smallpox from the stranger at the poor house. Dr. Lichty attended this victim "through the preliminary stage of fever." Some three days later, eruptions were discovered; Dr. Lichty pronounced it smallpox and corroborated his opinion with Drs. Barber and Peabody (Peabody also referring to himself in the third person), who concurred and gave "first notice" to the public. Lichty and Peabody then hurriedly provided themselves with vaccine virus, "giving the people an opportunity of fortifying themselves against the much dreaded disease." Friends of Middleditch, Peabody wrote, immediately accused the pair of raising the alarm of smallpox as being "actuated only by pecuniary motives," and maintained their claim that both the stranger and the laborer suffered from syphilitic eruptions.

Writer #2 (Peabody) then went on to accuse Writer #1 (Middleditch) of misdiagnosing Mr. Grover's son (who eventually died) of having disease of the lung and then diphtheria until eruptions appeared, when he pronounced it scarlet fever "and so insisted for four days." By that time, hearing there was smallpox in town, Middleditch summoned the opinion of A.R. Whitney (not a physician) and "several soldiers," who declared the child had smallpox. At this critical juncture, Peabody asserted that Middleditch "discovered that his country patients required his undivided attention" and turned over the case to Dr. Lichty. Thus, Middleditch could hardly have given prompt warning as stated in his letter of March 12.

From the date smallpox was confirmed, Middleditch asked Dr. Eddy to handle the child's case, although not to the satisfaction of Mr. Groves, who summoned Dr. Noyes to attend his family in conjunction with Dr. Eddy. As an excuse for abandoning the family, Middleditch wrote Groves a letter in which he professed himself unacquainted with smallpox and stated his fear of transmitting the disease throughout his extensive practice. He also noted that his own child had not been vaccinated and he feared bringing the disease into his own house. Writer #2 (Peabody) finished by remarking that if a doctor took the proper precaution of changing his clothes after attending the child, there was no chance of his spreading the disease and accused him of either having a personal fear of smallpox, "or a still greater reason of losing a few dollars and cents."

Needless to say, this elicited the third letter in the series, published March 26. Abandoning his already-lost anonymity, "A. Middleditch and Eddy" signed the letter, but as it was written in the first person, undoubtedly the former penned it. After noting that Writer #2 (whom he correctly identified as Peabody) lied when he called himself a "friend" to all physicians in Waterloo (implying the writers were not friends), he introduced what the gladsome editor must have considered a bombshell by stating that the stranger (now identified as Thomas Wright) had *first* been treated by Dr. Peabody, who diagnosed his condition as "fever and ague," prescribing quinine for the condition. Afterward, when he (Middleditch) saw the patient, he concurred in the diagnosis of venereal disease.

After Wright was taken to the poor house (he having no money), Dr. Eddy examined him and observed "a good vaccination mark on his arm." Wright told the story that his mother said he had smallpox when a small boy and that while in the army, he had been detailed as a nurse to attend those suffering from the disease. Eddy declared the man suffered from varioloid and ordered his clothes destroyed. Afterward the doctor vaccinated all the inmates of the poor house, none of whom took either form of the disease.

With circumstances turned in his favor, it was now Middleditch's turn to question whether Peabody refused follow-up care to "the poor soldier" (Wright) because he had no money, because he feared to contract a contagious disease or because he did not recognize the nature of the disease. And if Peabody did believe Wright had smallpox, why did he not "sound the alarm" at that point? Had he done so, Middleditch charged, Mr. Groves' "sweet little babe" would then be alive. Speaking of the child, Middleditch defended Dr. Eddy's treatment, stating the latter immediately identified smallpox and ordered the children taken from school and warned the family not to admit anyone to the house. Denying Peabody's claim that Groves was dissatisfied with Dr. Eddy's treatment, he quoted the father as saying no more than if Dr. Eddy desired a second opinion, he was free to call whomever he chose.

Defending his own action regarding the child, Middleditch stated he first saw him on February 10 and found him suffering from congestion of the lower left lung (the same lung which once before had been so affected) and some fever, afterwards proving to be the primary fever of smallpox. He did not see the boy on the 11th, but went with Dr. Eddy on the 12th. They discovered a rash had just appeared and the throat was diphtheritic. (Here he cited *Flint's Practice,* page 862, which stated the throat may be so affected *"even in smallpox"),* reaffirming his diagnosis of diphtheria. On the 13th, both doctors determined the boy to be suffering from scarlet fever. The following day, the patient presented symptoms of small-pox; Middleditch asked Eddy to confirm the new diagnosis, which he did, pronouncing it "in its worst form."

Because his numerous patients would have abandoned him (and, by implication, proper medical care) if they knew him to be treating a smallpox patient, Middleditch turned over the case to Dr. Eddy. His letter included a quote from Mr. Groves, avowing, "After due explanation, I believe that Dr. Middleditch was justifiable in doing as he did in relation to small pox at my house."

Middleditch was not quite through. In self-defense for his delay in diagnosing the child's disease as smallpox, he did his research. In the first instance, he described Dr. John Swinburne, one of the first physicians of Albany, who, on October 23, 1855, diagnosed a young man as suffering from typhoid fever; when, on the 25th, an eruption appeared and he thought it measles. By the 27th, he changed his mind again and decided it to be smallpox in its worst form. No one, Middleditch claimed, censured "Dr. S. for the long time it took him to make out the case!"

Going back to *Flint's Practice,* page 865, Middleditch quoted that, of 1494 cases of smallpox admitted into the smallpox hospital on Blackwell's Island in 1860–1862, there were 48 cases proved not to be smallpox. Of these, 10 proved to be scarlet fever, 9 measles, 29 syphilitic and other affections. He then questioned whether "we have some professional giants out west here, who can throw them [eastern experts] in the shade."

That said, he addressed Peabody's sarcastic insinuation that he was afraid of smallpox by stating, again in the third person, "He has treated some of the contagious diseases quite extensively and believes he never has contracted any of them, and therefore small pox and the others have lost their terrors to him." In conclusion, he wrote (back to the first person), "I submit to the reader if that correspondent has not made much ado about nothing; and what object could have been in making such wrong representations — so personal and untrue, but to ruin, if he could, Drs. Middleditch and Eddy's reputation as men and as physicians?" Finally, he said, "In his quaint and truthful reflections on mankind, Josh Billings* thus expressed himself: 'The man who kant git ahed without pullin others back, iz a limited cuss.'"

Dr. Peabody's response on April 2 was directed pointedly to Dr. Middleditch: "You have commenced this controversy: whether for the purpose of relieving a guilty conscience, or for the more obvious reason of covering up some of your acts which you must have known looked, in the eyes of the community, inconsistent with your duties as a physician and as a man, is not for me to say." But Peabody had plenty more to say. He "'fessed up"

---

*Josh Billings was the pen name for the 19th century humorist, Henry Wheeler Shaw (1818–1885), who often wrote in slang and used phonetic spellings to accentuate his point.

to being at the City Hotel on January 4 "on business not connected with his profession," and was requested to see a stranger (Wright) residing there. Testimony from two men presumably associated with the hotel stated that "Dr. P" was informed beforehand the man had no money and that there were no eruptions on his body at the time, those not appearing until January 6. When Dr. Eddy saw Wright on the 9th, "the character [of the smallpox] must have been such that no intelligent physician could have mistaken the disease." He then challenged Middleditch's calculation that the disease must have passed through the different stages of smallpox in *four days,* when, "all works on practice will inform you that it takes from fourteen to twenty days."

Peabody then scoffed at Middleditch's defense of mistakes made by physicians at Blackwell's Island and nitpicked the quotation from *Flint's Practice* by pointing out that while "29 *syphilitic* and other affections" were among the cases misdiagnosed, the author did not say that "one single case proved to be *syphilitic*." Picking on what any foresighted reader could have seen coming, he questioned how the doctor could correctly quote "the buffoon, Josh Billings" but be ignorant of professional papers.

Equally obvious was Peabody's picking up on the statement Middleditch offered from Mr. Groves, who expressed his satisfaction, "'*after due explanation,*' implying there must have been a dissatisfaction *before* you made the explanation." Resuming the attack on Middleditch's defense of using the mistakes of others, Peabody calculated that at Blackwell's Island, the ratio was 48:1494, while the Waterloo doctor's stood at 2:2. As far as Middleditch's professed fearlessness of smallpox, Peabody cited a 4-year-old case where Middleditch abandoned Mrs. Wilder and family because they had the disease. He suggested that if it were not fear that prompted Middleditch's desertion, it stemmed from the fact there was scant chance of collecting a large bill, adding, "It comes with ill grace from you to charge me with neglect of a patient because he has no money [Wright], when you boast frequently that you refuse to attend to any calls except such as are able to pay.... You are entirely welcome to all of the sympathy of your patrons in this matter and you certainly need it, for the discontent that I am told you were obliged to make on your bill against Mr. Groves, places you in a *position new and very unpleasant, I am certain.*"

Dr. Middleditch began his rebuttal of April 2 by noting he did not propose to answer Dr. Peabody's article in detail and then proceeded to do so. After stating the letter of April 2 "mystified some points," he defended his statement that Wright's disease passed through the various stages in four days because the patient suffered from varioloid rather than smallpox because he "had the evidence on his arm that he was protected by vaccination against small pox," adding that "all authors" state varioloid may pass through its stages in four to five days. Concerning the word "syphilitic," from *Flint's,* he stated he "unintentionally misquoted in one single word" the text, but the mistake did not disprove his point.

As for his abandoning Mrs. Wilder (spelled here "Wildy"), he reported that the woman's anger was so great upon hearing the diagnosis that she told him not to come back, so it was no fault of his if she sent for another physician. In the case of fees, he included testimony stating that in a conversation between himself and Dr. Eddy the latter asked what he should charge Mr. Groves, the charges as they stood being $108. Dr. Middleditch suggested $90, "but be sure to charge little enough, and to have Mr. G. *perfectly satisfied* if it were not over $25."

The final letter in the series, dated April 16, contained the following:

Dr. Middleditch-Sir —:— I find nothing in your last article worthy of any notice from me whatever; I will just say to you, that the next time you find yourself guilty of such professional improprieties as I have proven to all disinterested parties to be true, do not undertake to vindicate yourself by commencing a newspaper controversy.— Your friends told you better, and it would have been much to your reputation had you been sufficiently wise to have heeded their advice.

Yours, O. Peabody

Fear and Fees

While the exchange of letters was amusing and at times bordering on the ludicrous, beneath it was a level of seriousness that touched on numerous complicated issues. Physician competence clearly ranks foremost and these incidents certainly were not isolated, as the participants acknowledged when citing statistics from *Flint's Practice*. In all fairness, the early stages of smallpox *were* difficult to diagnosis and many doctors from the major cities to "out west" were guilty of mistakes.

In 1870, the *Morning Oregonian* of November 12 started out an article, "NOT SMALL POX— Dr. Dickson publishes a card in relation to a case of sickness in this city which he is treating and which has been currently reported to be a case of small pox. He denies that it is small pox but says, 'I admit that there is foundation and color given to such report in eruptions of *Acne osacea* and *Lichen* which have appeared upon the surface, forehand, neck, etc. Medical gentlemen not having had practical experience would be likely to confound it with the small pox owing to the ... form which it assumes and the accompanying symptoms.'"

Two days later, the newspaper followed up with a report stating that there was still a difference of opinion among common people and physicians as to the proper identification of the disease. It was noted the mild form of the disease might be accounted for by an outbreak two years previously when everyone was alarmed and resorted to vaccination. There were, however, several small children who were not vaccinated and who all had symptoms of the genuine smallpox.[2]

Interestingly, in the Iowa cases, Dr. Middleditch used as a defense of his diagnosis that the patient Wright had an obvious vaccination scar that precluded the diagnosis of smallpox — a subject Dr. Peabody did not address.

Another, less obvious problem raised in the correspondence was the subject of spreading contagion. Both Middleditch and Peabody agreed that changing clothes after visiting smallpox patients precluded their spreading the disease to others, but in their carefully scripted letters they did not mention hand washing or cross-contamination from their shoes or medical bags that surely were not cleansed after leaving the premises. Their confidence in the obvious probably led them to overlook the subtle. The fact they were hardly alone in overlooking sanitary precautions explains one reason why epidemics began without traceable cause.

In their correspondence, the dueling doctors also touched upon fear, both in patients, who feared they would not receive proper treatment if so diagnosed, and by a mother, who outright denied the diagnosis and sought another opinion hoping to hear something less frightful. And certainly, it is unfair to discount the fear of health care professionals. Middleditch defended himself by stating he considered himself immune because he had treated numerous cases, although at the same time acknowledging he was unfamiliar with smallpox. In the 19th century, a diagnosis of smallpox realistically carried with it the potential for death, and even men who had sworn oaths to treat the sick were susceptible to fears for their own mortality.

Such fear should have been put to constructive use but was not. Middleditch stated he felt protected from exposure rather than vaccination, and confessed his own child had not been vaccinated. This prompts the question of why a prominent doctor neglected so vital a protective. If he had no faith in the technique, how could he prompt his patients to undergo it? Likely, he did not. While he could quote (and misquote) medical literature, he failed to follow standard medical practice. In fact, when Peabody and Lichty went out and procured vaccine, they were charged with acting out of pecuniary motives.

The subject of money then played out on three other levels: one doctor being apprehensive of losing well-paying patients, the questions both faced of refusing to treat a stranger without means and the excessive fees charged. While not every physician fell under these heavy accusations, those who did gave credence to the popular saying that every man ought to be his own doctor.

With that in mind, an article entitled "Doctor's on Strike," from 1867, fits in well with a typical and humorous view of the profession:

> The doctors of Galveston, Texas, are on a strike for higher wages. They have struck so high that they have probably excluded sickness from the city more effectually than they ever did by the use of their compounds, nostrums and prescriptions. In fact they demand such fees that no one but a millionaire can afford to be sick; and henceforth good health is necessary to any kind of economy. Sickness will now become a luxury for the patricians; good health is the distinguishing mark of the plebeian. The doctors have published their programme — and to use the printer's phrase, no "ratting" is to be allowed. For a day visit when a minute examination is required, ten dollars. For advice when such examination is required, fifteen dollars. For an opinion involving a question of law, twenty-five to a hundred dollars. For treatment in case of yellow fever, fifty to two hundred dollars. For a treatment of a case of small-pox, one hundred to two hundred dollars. This scale of prices is mild compared to the charges for surgery, which go up to five hundred dollars, and don't go much below it, with the usual scale of charges for all visits subsequently to the first.[3]

The question of financial reward played out on a larger stage in New York, with two newspapers, the *Herald* and the *Times*, taking opposite sides on the issue of Dr. Swinburne, health officer of the port. Acknowledging that no other port in the world served as a greater *entrepôt* for immigrants, the *Herald* argued that Swinburne paid more attention to the business of enriching himself and his confederates than to proper quarantine. An example of the steamer *Queen*, arriving from Liverpool on May 10, 1869, with 1,200 passengers, was offered. The quarantine doctor went aboard and, "to his intense delight," discovered two cases of smallpox, meaning that in an hour he could earn $1,200 by performing mandatory vaccination. When the two shipboard physicians asserted the cases were measles, the subject reached a threatening point, finally forcing the officer to back away.

New York law required only one case of smallpox aboard to merit ship-wide vaccination, and although the officer eventually conceded for "the first instance in a long time," multiplying the number of passengers by $1 proved a rough estimate of the profits derived from the procedure. The *Herald* sarcastically noted that it was as well that Christopher Columbus never ran into an official like Swinburne, or he would have had to hand over his loose change and submit to a dose of vaccination. The indignant *Times* argued that charges of corruption were meant to divert attention from the legitimate problem of infectious diseases entering the city.[4] On one point, however, there was no disagreement: smallpox drained the public coffers. In 1870, expenses at the Smallpox Hospital alone were $6,772,[5] explained by the fact that there were estimated to be 200,000 unvaccinated persons in the city.[6]

Smallpox: Variola,
Varioloid and Vaccinia

The Diseases as They Were, Incurable:
As They Are Now, Curable

Much as been said and written about the prevalence of smallpox in this city. Some
people look upon its existence as one of these terrible curses which Eugene Sue
made the deathless companion of the Wandering Jew.[1]

An article in the *New York Herald*, January 22, 1870, using the above as its opening
proclamation, began by stating that smallpox had always afflicted New York; there had not
been a week in the last ten years "when this evil has not prevailed in one stage or another."
Looked upon by the medical profession "as a disease, in its virulence, in its fatality and in
its obstinacy to medical treatment," science had advanced from an imperfect understanding
where treatment was violent and unsatisfactory into the modern era where the disease had
yielded "to the concentrated experience of the medical profession."

Instead of "heating and smothering a patient," the new regime favored soothing with
cooling drinks, purification with fresh air, so that the infected person did not "inhale the
products of his own contagion," and stimulating the system broken down by terrible fever.
Among the class suffering most from inattention or proper medical care were the prostitutes.
Not only were they carriers of the disease, those who recovered also remained scarred by
pox marks, shorn of their outward charms. Weakened by disease and unable to make a
living, they were driven into the streets, sinking lower and lower into deprivation and finally
death.

The epidemic the *Herald* addressed was believed to have reached the eastern seaboard
from dual sources. In the fall of 1868, smallpox struck California; soon after, the scourge
traveled east by both land and water. Simultaneously, the disease traveled westward from
Europe while the pandemic associated with the Franco-Prussian War was in its infancy.

Like many western cities, San Francisco found itself woefully unprepared for an epidemic of smallpox. During the early part of 1868, when it was feared the city was at risk
from cholera and smallpox then raging in Central America and the West Indies, Dr. Elliott
presented the new and elaborate Quarantine and Health Law to the state legislature.
Designed for the city but crafted to protect all interior towns, the proposal was submitted
for examination to eminent physicians and practical businessmen. The group declared it
superior to existing law, which "did not give adequate protection even in ordinary times."
Inexplicably, the measure was "talked dead" by a senator from San Francisco, who seriously
misjudged the potential for disaster.[2]

Once obtaining a foothold, smallpox spread quickly. Reports in November 1868 from

Mendocino in the northern portion of the state mentioned isolated deaths on Cold Creek that were "unaccountable," as no one living nearby had been exposed. At the same time, smallpox was reported in Monterey County, where eyewitnesses stated, "The Small Pox in its worst form prevails in San Juan [CA]," and added, "The town is rotten with Small Pox.... There have been some 40 died, and some 100 cases yet. Many of them only live two days. It is a most terrible type of Small Pox."[3]

Locals believed the disease was carried into San Juan by a man newly arrived from the grape-growing district of Sonoma County. As a precaution, the traveler had been vaccinated before leaving home, but within 24 hours his arm "swelled to the size of his body, and was covered with gangrenous sores. An examination by physicians resulted in the discovery of the fact that the man had actually been inoculated with the most malignant type of the small pox." Within 48 hours, he died, a "sickening mass of putrefaction," and was buried at midnight. The stranger's clothes and blankets were burned, but unfortunately some schoolchildren discovered the half-burned rags and caught the infection. In one week, a number of them died and ultimately, out of a population of 1,000, four hundred were taken ill and 160 perished.

From San Juan, smallpox reached Sacramento and rapidly crept into the "City by the Bay," where it found "those atmospheric conditions at San Francisco which are most favorable to the development of the most malignant type of the disease. It found the city wholly unprepared to combat it. There were no hospital provisions or worse than none. The pest-house very soon proved a frightful nuisance and to be taken to it was regarded as being doomed to the most horrible death."

According to a reporter from the *New York Sun* in correspondence dated January 12, 1869, San Francisco authorities were slow to react to the developing epidemic when it first reached the city in December. Nothing more than the "ordinary course of vaccination" was followed and the disease grew virulent, exacerbated by impure vaccine that not only failed to offer protection but also worsened symptoms. This finally brought the matter to public attention.

By mid–December, the San Francisco Board of Supervisors decided to enlarge the smallpox hospital "at once," and authorized the Building Committee to prepare additional sheds for the accommodation of patients. Ninety-four new cases were reported the week of December 6–12, and in a single day following, 30 more were confirmed. Death reports climbed to three times what they had been the previous year, leading to the consensus that "there are no means devised to stay its progress. It will probably be left to run its course and wear itself out for want of material to act upon. If the interior manages it no better than the metropolis has done we do not see any chance of getting rid of the pestilence for months. Its victims are already counted by the hundreds and it will be lamented by thousands unless we act promptly to arrest its spread and confine it to the present limits as much as possible."[4]

Most coverage of the disease was toned down to a moderate degree by city newspapers for fear of affecting the usual winter and spring tides of immigration: "People seem disposed to cover up the fearful ravages of the disease and to conceal its deadly character. The streets are filled with funerals, and the grave-digger has his hands and graves full. In some cases burials are made by night." The pest houses remained full and nearly everyone in the city lost a friend or relative. The Chinese suffered terribly, as "their native doctors have neither experience nor common sense in the treatment of the small-pox, and as a natural consequence three out of every five of their patients run into eternity."[5]

Less than helpfully, word began spreading from "an intelligent chinaman" that the disease raging along the Pacific coast was not smallpox but the black measles (a highly contagious viral infection marked by dark red papules), more fatal to adults than to children and brought from China on emigrant ships.[6] Worse, a physician from Stockton circulated a "panecea [sic] ... as enfailing [sic] as fate, and conquers in every instance ... also fail-proof for scarlet fever." His cure was a familiar one: sulphate of zinc, 1 grain; foxglove (digitalis), 1 grain; half a teaspoon of sugar, mixed with water. Either disease was promised to disappear in 12 hours. "If counties would compel their physicians to use this, there would be no need of pesthouses."[7]

Disinfectants were commonly believed to deter if not prevent smallpox, but medical authorities disputed these claims. A common reference work titled *Aitken's Science and Practice of Medicine* (1868) warned, "No dependence must be placed on vinegar, camphor, or other supposed preventives, which, without attention to cleanliness and admission of fresh air, are not only useless, but by their strong smells, render it impossible to perceive when the room is filled with bad air or noxious vapors." A further discussion stated that smallpox was "perpetuated by its

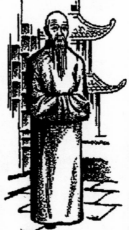

Chinese Proverb

"To understand the present, one should examine antiquity."

It is obvious that things would not be as they are now had it not been for discoveries made in the past. Smallpox, for example, was the first disease for which immunization was available. However, ignorance and prejudice often prevented health authorities from giving mass immunizations during the early years. Fortunately, this is no longer a problem under our present enlightened system of health care.

We always carry a complete stock of biologicals, which can be dispensed according to your physician's orders.

PORTS' DRUG STORE
— Walgreen Agency —

117 WEST MAIN ST.   PHONE 37

The Chinese proverb in this advertisement states, "To understand the present, one should examine antiquity." Port's Drugstore, a Walgreen Agency, observed that smallpox was the first disease for which immunization was available, but noted that ignorance and prejudice often prevented mass immunizations. "Fortunately, this is no longer a problem under our present enlightened system of health care" (from the *Press Gazette* [OH], June 15, 1956).

own specific poison, miasma, effluvium or virus, which spreads it about by the media of impalpable substances, technically called fomites, and which are capable of receiving, preserving and carrying germs of the disease." Since it was not determined at what period the poison of smallpox was first generated by the infected person, it was generally held to be most powerful when manifest to the sense of smell.[8]

That stated, as the disease spread throughout San Francisco, vaccination among many circles was pronounced a failure and the use of carbolic acid as a disinfectant was urged as a "very reliable preventive," as it killed the contagious atmosphere.[9] In Virginia City, disinfectants were taken a step further, as the *Territorial Enterprise,* December 11, 1868, noted that "men were going about the street with vials of carbonic acid and other diabolic distillations in their vest pockets, which they from time to time smell at, rub upon the palms of their hands or sprinkle upon their clothes. A smell of coal tar, camphor, creosote, chloride of lime, gin, garlic, asafetida, turpentine, muskrat, peppermint, and skunk, pervades the moving mass of humanity.... When half a dozen of these vials of wrath are uncorked, the effluvium for rods about is worse than the odor from a prosperous slaughterhouse in dog days." Not only did these "pestiferous pest disinfectant disseminators" hope to ward away smallpox from themselves, these "curb-stone doctors" took a "devilish delight" in disinfecting their friends on the sly.

Faith in vaccination continued to erode and other remedies were tried. Among them was the herb *Hydrastis canadenis.* Also known by the common names goldenseal, orange root, yellow root and yellow puccoon, it was used in both local and internal administration to modify smallpox by abolishing its symptoms, shortening its course, lessening the danger and greatly mitigating its consequences.[10] Orange root was a woodland plant of the northeastern region of the United States, primarily found in the Ohio Valley during the 19th century. The Cherokee used it for cancer and general debility and as a tonic for inflammations; the Iroquois used it for whooping cough, diarrhea and fever. In 1760, it was introduced into Great Britain, where it was known as "Warnera." By 1850, on the strength of its virtue as an astringent, anti-inflammatory, mild laxative and muscle stimulant, it became an important export from the United States to Europe.[11]

In another case where native plants were used in place of vaccination, the *Atlantic Medical and Surgical Journal* (April 1872) published a report from the Alabama State Medical Association stating that the use of a tea made from black snake root (*Cimicifuga,* also known as "black cohosh") was a preventive of smallpox so long as it was taken.[12]

San Francisco causalities for December 1868 ultimately reached 148,[13] aided by careless observance of sanitary measures. On January 8, 1869, the *San Francisco Chronicle* reported that a French laundry at No. 1,322 Kearney Street contained two persons confined with smallpox. Notwithstanding, the work of the laundry went on: clothes were gathered from various houses, washed in the infected premises and hung up to dry over the sick lying in bed. The clothes were then ironed and taken through a backyard to an adjoining laundry and from there distributed and delivered, "small pox and all, to the various owners."

By January, the entire state was infected, although it was reported that Sacramento, Marysville and Stockton had escaped the worst type of the disease. In Gilroy and Los Angeles, the disease was fatal beyond precedent, and in spite of every available prescription, some of those affected "appear[ed] to rot by inches." The *Sun* reporter graphically wrote, "In some cases vaccination seems to have entirely lost its power, and men, women and children with vaccine scars on their arms as large as twenty shilling pieces have fallen victims to the epidemic. Hospitals have been hastily furnished, and every effort has been made in these towns to stay the progress of the disease, but thus far with little effect."

If the statistics were grim, the result of autopsies presented an even worse picture. Those conducted by Dr. Howell, San Francisco health officer, and Dr. Johnson, resident physician of the smallpox hospital, found, on examination of the brain, that pustules, well filled with matter, "completely studded the coronal portion of the *dura mater,* the outer membrane of the brain." Further examination revealed pustules existed on the mucous membrane of the mouth, fauces, trachea and esophagus, as well as the bladder and lower portion of the intestines. They concluded, "In these cases, while the patient was living, he or she became insane from the absorption of pus (pyaemia)."

If numbers and autopsies do not put a "face" on the human agony of smallpox, individual histories often have that power. One San Francisco man, a strong, middle-aged worker, had been vaccinated in youth and revaccinated during the crisis with slight results. He was taken ill on a Friday morning with headache and back pain but worked all day and again on Saturday until noon, when extreme agony drove him back to his boardinghouse. His skin became dry and harsh and, after feeling no better, on Sunday a physician was called. The man was diagnosed as suffering from bilious fever. By Monday, he was covered with nearly black, livid spots; his lungs were congested and every breath caused him to spit blood. He was incontinent of bladder and bowel and stimulants failed to restore warmth to his extremities. The doctor being unable to save him, the man mercifully died within four hours of the doctor's arrival.

A second man, vaccinated in youth, decided to undergo revaccination "for the novelty of the thing." He was confined for several days afterwards and entirely recovered, having what physicians typically called a "splendid mark" as proof of successful vaccination. However, a month later, he contracted smallpox and died before he could be admitted to the hospital.[14] By March 1869, the epidemic had begun to abate with weekly totals registering only six deaths from smallpox and fifteen new cases admitted to hospitals.[15]

An Ounce of Prevention, a Pound of Cure

In 1868, Dr. Harris of the New York State Board of Health predicted that the smallpox epidemic then raging in the western part of the United States and the developing epidemic in Europe would reach the eastern coast of America within the year. Over 10,000 posters were displayed in public places, inviting the poor to be vaccinated free of charge and advising the wealthy to consult their family physicians.

Dr. Harris proved correct, and by May 1869, a corps of sixty doctors were appointed to increase the numbers vaccinated; by June, more than 30,000 persons underwent the procedure. Those who had it within their means underwent vaccinia (cowpox) vaccination as further protection.

New York City Statistics 1869

Before Vaccination		After Vaccination	
Cases in May	112	Cases in July	83
Cases in June	161	Cases in August	27
Cases in July	83	Cases in September	69
Cases in October	38		

The method devised by Dr. Harris to limit the spread of smallpox consisted of his reviewing the particulars of each new diagnosis. The sanitary inspector was then notified by telegraph to check the residence of each confirmed case and isolate the patient. Every resident on the block was then vaccinated and no one was allowed access to the patient except the nurse and physician. When possible, the afflicted was sent to the hospital; if the sick lived on a busy thoroughfare, he was removed "at the expense of life."

Needless to say, Dr. Harris' method represented a best-case scenario. Although over 50,000 individuals had been vaccinated since 1868, the numbers reflected the fact that too many remained unprotected. In the statistical year ending in October 1869, there were 593 cases reported, with 107 deaths, while in the first quarter of 1870, ending January 1, an exactly equal number of 593 cases were reported, with 109 deaths. Adding unreported cases to the total, it was estimated that smallpox affected 2,000 people.

Extracting data from the British registrar-general, Dr. Harris noted that during the 14 weeks ending January 1, 1870, there were 270 deaths from smallpox in Paris and 34 deaths in London. Although finding it consoling to know fresh breezes and cold temperatures provided one of the best antidotes to the contagion, his conclusion was hardly optimistic, as he noted, "Every opinion touching the future of smallpox in New York must rest to a great extent, on speculation."

While purposely meant to be amusing, the following scenario at the board of health is likely representative of life in any major city circa the 1870s:

> The engineer's office is room 47. His assistant arrived in due season yesterday morning, threw away the stump of a cigar, off with his overcoat, dropped his cane, stood his beaver hat on end and settled down to his desk. There were two other occupants of the room, people well advanced — Germans.
> "Are you waiting to see the engineer?"
> "No speak English," replied the woman.
> "What is the matter with him?" pointing to the man covered with pustules.
> "Smallpox!" Exit overcoat, beaver and cane with the late arrival. Another head is pushed into the room.
> "Thunder! Smallpox! A darned shame to bring it here." Again the door creaks on its hinges; a brief survey of the apartment is made, and another quick departure. Dr. Harris passes into the contagious presence, smiles a little, examines, gives a scientific wink and pronounces it a beautiful case. Meanwhile there is a pallor in many faces, caused, doubtless, by the feeling that these faces may some day be indented with a deeper pallor. The doctor, however, has the arms bare, and Dr. Post — a post deluvian — plays with a sharp-edged weapon upon susceptible flesh and the endangered are prepared for a brief turn at vaccina. That is all — so far.[16]

Doubtless, Dr. Harris would not have smiled at an article from the *Troy Times* (New York) that published a story relating the "common opinion among the people that the small pox, if it doesn't kill its victims, cleans out the system of all impurities. All other traces of disease disappear with it upon recovery." As proof, the newspaper cited a patient at the insane department of the Marshall Infirmary, who recovered his senses after a bout with the disease.[17] Even less amusing was a notation that the physicians in Salem, Massachusetts, had gotten a "corner" on smallpox by advancing the price of vaccination to $2 an arm.[18]

Pen-Pictures from Hell — "Man Aggravating the Evils Inflicted by Providence"

In July 1871, two important articles were published in the *New York Times* concerning the smallpox hospital at Blackwell's Island. They are chilling in nature, and it is tempting to say they more appropriately represent Dickens' London. They do not. Even over the span of nearly one hundred and fifty years, the horror and indignation remains as fresh to the 21st century reader as it likely was to a citizen of the 19th century. One brief sentence summaries the pesthouse: "Many thousands of souls, now the inmates of cemeteries, of poorhouses and houses of refuge, legions of widows and children dependent upon the cold hand of charity, may trace the date of their indigence and downfall to their entrance of that inferno, the denizens of which too truly leave all hope behind."

What was it like being on the outside, looking in? Once a person was committed to the hospital, they lost communication with loved ones beyond the confines of the island, as quarantine forbad the exportation of letters. That left friends and family to seek updates from the authorities. Those with means and at least a modicum of influence applied to the board of health; from one member, a note was obtained permitting access to the superintendent of the office of the Charities and Corrections Department at the corner of 11th Street and 3rd Avenue. Here, a gentleman with gold spectacles listened to "the monotonous stream of woes, ever varying in their details," issuing tickets for passage to the island, receiving parcels for the inmates and accepting letters of inquiry to be forwarded to the physician in charge. Three days of "hope deferred" left the anxious petitioner with no alternative but to seek information through personal application with the physician. That required a return trip to the office of the Charities to obtain a ticket for passage across the river in the steamer *Bellevue*.

For people unaccustomed to the slums of the wharf district, taking the cars to 26th Street was the beginning of a descent into the pit. Unable to determine the exact point of demarcation, as the street numbers on the corner street lamps were wholly or partially removed, the unwary often passed their destination, requiring a second trip on another car to reach the corner of Bellevue Hospital. Remarking, "The moments flew on leaden wings," this particular seeker finally found himself at the pier, destined to wait with a crowd comprising a cross section of New York: squalid women and children, dapper youths and groups of "expensively dressed, tolerably featured women" belonging to the band of sisters (prostitutes), transported that morning from the House of Corrections on the "Black Maria" wagon for incarceration at Blackwell Prison.

Following directions "given in the usual high tones of ignorant people when they talk to the simple, the deaf, or foreigners," the throng was pushed back "while wagons and buggies drive in and out, bringing prostrate patients, coffins (at which slight low wailings bursts forth here and there) and sporting-looking officials." Finally allowed to pay the 20 cent fare, visitors boarded the steamer and made the short trip, after which the "goats and sheep are separated," as prisoners were detailed to the areas of incarceration. The few coming to hear news of smallpox patients were passed through a very low gate, designed to prevent someone from running through in defiance of anti-contagion rules.

Most found the trip for naught, as information was spotty and sparse. Petitioners inquiring whether clothes had been delivered to a patient were informed inmates were not permitted to wear civilian dress; some asked about friends who had unknown to them, been released; other patients' conditions were unknown. Writing for most, one author succinctly summed up the experience by observing, "It is not a pleasant trip, will never be a pleasant memory."

If standing on the outside looking in was bad, the opposite proved hellacious. Blackwell's Island Smallpox establishment comprised two departments: the "Stone Building," for patients who could pay for their accommodations, and the pauper's ward. In the former (and clearly the better of the two), the unvarying menu consisted of two eggs, tea and bread and butter for breakfast; beefsteak, bread and beer (if ordered) for dinner; tea and bread and butter for supper. According to testimonies, the eggs were "positively rotten, the butter was disgustingly rancid, and the tea was simply a decoction of stalks and sediment, (alias sweepings,) without the slightest aroma or taste of tea."

Eyewitness statements described patients with eruptions being treated with great brutality; when lack of care forced them to ask other patients for help, one staff member turned off the lights at 9:00 P.M. with the sour comment that "he might go to bed and die if he couldn't attend to himself during the day time." Infrequent visits by physicians, badly cooked food and ventilation that permitted wind, rain and dampness to permeate wards was inhumane, but worse, inmates at the asylum were not all smallpox victims. As chronicled, proper diagnosis was often difficult (or, as the *Times* article noted, resulted from carelessness or ignorance) and many were sent to Blackwell actually suffering from typhus or nondescript fevers. The inevitable consequence was that they "died from erroneous treatment, neglect, or from contraction of the disease after admission."[19]

Vaccine Farms: Animal Versus Human Lymph

Although Dr. Jenner's brilliant discovery of vaccination had been in use less than half a century, questions on the efficacy of vaccine matter derived from human-to-human transfer were being raised by the mid–1830s. Due, in part, to numerous failed vaccinations, discussions pointed toward the supposition that the vaccine had passed through the system of too many persons to be trusted as total protection. The subject was raised before the College of Physicians, London, in 1835, where Dr. George Gregory suggested a return to the original source. The argument of animal versus human lymph would continue, prompting some to seek new sources of vaccine.

Suffering a scourge of smallpox in 1859, the city of Little Rock, Arkansas, applied to the celebrated physician Dr. Julius Gottschalk, of Druseldorf (Dusseldorf), Prussia, for advice and a quantity of virus. He forwarded the lymph via the ship *Asia,* together with a copy of the latest scientific studies.[20] By 1871, many considered the best lymph for vaccination to come from Germany, imported on quills.[21] Attitudes were about to change.

Spontaneous cases of genuine cowpox were rare, but in 1836, the disease was discovered at Passy, France. From this, a stock of lymph was obtained by transmission and for many years was carefully guarded and utilized to great advantage. In 1866, another case of cowpox occurred among a herd of cattle on the estate of the Marquis of Beaugency, on the Loire, situated not far from Paris. Dr. Constantine de Paul, chairman of the Committee on Vaccination in the Academy of Medicine, Paris, advanced 6,000 francs for the testing and preservation of the lymph obtained. It soon became one of the most important stocks in the world.

Dr. Walton, of the Cincinnati Clinic, summarized the argument for bovine vaccination by enumerating the following points:

1. Humanized virus procured immunity from smallpox for a number of years;
2. Humanized virus may convey syphilis*;
3. Humanized virus may convey other diseases*;
4. It is probable humanized virus degenerates;
5. Many persons oppose humanized vaccination;
6. It would not be right to compel vaccination with humanized virus;
7. Bovine virus procured immunity from smallpox for a number of years;
8. Bovine virus cannot convey syphilis;
9. It is not probable bovine lymph conveys any disease;

10. It is not probable bovine virus degenerates;
11. Very few persons oppose bovine vaccination;
12. It would be right to compel vaccination with bovine virus.

*The medical community did not support the idea that syphilis, scrofula or other skin diseases were spread through humanized vaccination, but as the lay population continued to harbor such beliefs, the idea of bovine vaccination was particularly appealing.

In 1870, Dr. Henry A. Martin, of Boston, procured lymph from Beaugency and introduced the virus into a heifer, the first time such a trial had been done in the United States. Two years later, the business of producing and dispensing vaccine matter derived from heifers became so extensive and lucrative that the doctor abandoned his medical practice to devote himself to the project. Eight hundred cows a year were used to obtain lymph.[22] Dr. Frank P. Foster, of New York, followed Martin's example with similar experiments and in November 1872, Dr. E.L. Griffin, of Fond du Lac, Wisconsin, president of the state board of health, opened a stable for the same purpose.

Dr. B. Rush Seusenoy, of Pennsylvania, secured a stock of animal vaccine from Beaugency in 1874, and opened the first large-scale vaccine farm in America, located in the Cumberland Valley, one mile from Chambersburg. The establishment was designed along the premise of the former National Vaccine Institute to provide a depot for a fresh and reliable supply of vaccine in any quantity desired. This, it was hoped, would eliminate panics during smallpox outbreaks. In addition, Seusenoy was not insensitive to the growing belief that the frequent failure of vaccination was due to the engrafting of impure humanized vaccine.

Dr. Seusenoy perpetuated his Beaugency strain of cowpox through an unbroken series of many hundreds of "full Alderny or grade heifers," this breed being preferred because of the thinness and delicacy of its skin, thus allowing and favoring a better maturation of the vaccine virus. The animals were stabled in large, warm and well-ventilated barns, in which a fire was kept burning in very cold weather. When lymph was to be transferred into an animal, it was taken to an "operating room," placed upon a cushioned rack and secured upon its back by a large strap passed around the body, each limb being securely fastened to an upright post. It was then washed around the udder and the hair shaved before being inoculated in ten or twelve places with the Beaugency virus.

The lymph obtained was advertised as being of pure Beaugency strain and entirely reliable, sold in four different forms: crusts, quills, ivory points and lymph tubes. For crusts, the heifer was carefully secured in a warm stall, well fed and kept constantly supplied with clean litter for 15–18 days, when the crusts were removed. When lymph was desired, the vesicles were pricked open on the 7th day and quills charged with fluid lymph upon the convex surface by dipping the point in and then turning it round, leaving the lymph on the outside surface. Ivory points were charged by dipping them into the virus, "much after the manner of an Indian charging his poisoned arrow." Both quills and points were then placed on racks to dry. Lymph tubes (very delicate small glass vials) were filled with lymph and the ends hermetically sealed.

Quills and ivory points were considered the most reliable of the various forms and were shipped from the Pennsylvania farm throughout the world. Among Seusenoy's clients were physicians in the Sandwich Islands, the Japanese dispensaries at Yokohama and Hong Kong. Desiring to price his vaccine within the reach of every doctor, Seusenoy charged 20 cents per whole quill and sold quill slips at 10 cents each. (Other propagators charged 50 cents for each quill and 25 cents per quill slip.) Large, double-charged ivory points went for $1.50 per dozen.

Like Dr. Seusenoy, Dr. E.L. Griffin opened a vaccination farm about three-quarters of a mile east of the business center of Fond du Lac, Wisconsin. Employing clean, well-appointed stables on a 15-acre farm of pastureland with a brook running through it, he maintained seven animals, ranging in age from four months to two years. This differed from farms in the East, which used only young calves for the purpose. The animals were vaccinated directly, one being always under treatment even when demand was light. His technique was similar to that of Seusenoy: after shaving the hair off the upper part of the thighs, the vaccination was made using numerous incisions. On the 7th or 8th day, the vesicles were ready for opening; when fair success attended the operation, one thousand or more points were obtained from one animal.

Great care was taken of the animals during their sickness, with particular attention paid to diet, which consisted of hay, bran mashes and other light food. The only departure from their normal conditions was a slight increase in temperature approximately 5 percent above normal. Heifers could be used only once, as subsequent vaccinations uniformly failed to "take," and no ill effects from the ordeal were reported. Griffin's stock was procured from neighboring farms, many farmers willingly loaning them for the purpose. Griffin used ivory points, crafted in Connecticut. During the smallpox scare in Chicago in 1877, he supplied many physicians there with his bovine lymph.

Two other early American proponents of a return to the bovine vaccination were Dr. Robbins and his associate, Dr. Lewis, of Brooklyn. Robbins went to France and brought back some of the Beaugency stock, upon which the two grafted the celebrated Vincennes stock. By 1880, they were engaged in large-scale production, using heifers of the Jersey breed from a few days old to a year or more, their tender age making the animals easier to handle. While it was noted the original stock was just as potent as ever, its power varied, "according to the constitution of the animal from which it was obtained."

Their method was to secure a small heifer, throw it upon its side on a table and secure its forefeet and head. Then, the hind legs were stretched apart and spots upon the belly 6–8 inches wide were shaved, "and if necessary the epidermis or skin is thinned down." After vaccination in the ordinary manner, the animal was retained in that position for 6–7 days when the matter was ready for removal onto quills or into tubes; if using the latter, the liquid obtained had to be as clear as water or it was rejected. It was stated that the calves did not appear "to be at all inconvenienced by their confinement, but munch their food with zest and in fact get fat." During the summer months, animals "under process" were kept in the country, where they thrived to a greater extent than in town. Robbins and Lewis sent their vaccine to France, Egypt, China, Japan, and to all parts of South America.[23]

Dr. H.M. Alexander, of Marietta, Lancaster County, Pennsylvania, opened a vaccine farm in 1880. Bordering the Susquehanna River, it was considered by contemporaries the most complete virus farm in the world. The establishment began when a full-blooded Guernsey heifer became the victim of spontaneous inoculation. On being informed of this fact, Alexander had the animal watched. The usual symptoms of fever with the formation of a crust developed. On the eighth day, the crust was removed and a quantity of the purest bovine virus was extracted from the sore. The lymph was tested, found to be a preventive of great worth and the farm was established. In eight years, it grew from this start into a major vaccine-producing center, employing from 30–50 hands, including gatherers, packers, shavers, inoculators and shippers.

The stock used were Jersey, Devon and Holstein heifers ranging in age from 8 to 10 months, recruited by the gatherers from the surrounding farms, the farmers were paid for hiring out their animals. The heifers were transported to the vaccine farm in pairs, conveyed by a comfortable patent cart. Upon arrival, the animals were washed and fed a diet of oats and middlings (also known as "mill feed," an inexpensive, high-energy by-product from the milling of wheat) the first day and corn, oats and middlings the second day. This combination was known to cause fever, making the heifer more susceptible to the inoculation.

On the third day, the heifer was inoculated with a scarifier, similar to that used on humans, containing ivory points heavily coated with virus from former subjects, until the shaved flesh resembled raw beef. Once the serum dried, the animal was returned to the stable. By the third day, the pox appeared on the shaven portions of the skin; by day eight, the sores were ripe. The scabs, as large and thick as an oyster shell, were then removed and the sore sponged with tepid water, removing pus and foreign matter. Soon after, the sore discharged lymph, technically known by the expression "to weep." The operator then used fine brushes of camel hair to remove the lymphatic fluid and applied it to ivory points the thickness of writing paper, two inches long by one quarter wide. The points were then placed in racks of 50 each to dry. Each heifer yielded enough virus to supply from 600 to 1,200 points. In 8–10 days, the heifer recovered with no ill effects and was returned to its owner.

Alexander's Farm produced 30,000–40,000 points per day, all of which were packed in bunches of ten, placed in glass tubes and then put in wooden vials for shipment. The points preserved their virtue for 30 days, although shipments to China and Japan occupied six weeks to reach port, and a week or more before they reached their final destination. Statistics from this farm in 1888 indicated a 95 percent success rate for points sent to these countries.[24] An identical technique was later used in England at the Government Vaccine Institute, Lamb's Conduit-street.[25]

THE ANIMAL VACCINE STATION

The best-equipped and best-managed "farm" in England was this institution in Lamb's Conduit Street, known as the Animal Vaccine Station, under the care of Dr. Robert Cory and his assistant, Mr. Thomas S. Scott. It opened in April 1882, under the direction of the local government board. It used the same techniques as those of Robbins and Lewis, and the annual report for 1890–1891 stated that 280 calves were vaccinated, while 7,200 primary vaccinations (human) and 478 revaccinations (human) were performed. Human vaccinations at the station were done gratuitously.

Five calves were delivered each week to the quarantine station at Little St. James' Street, a spare animal always being kept on the premises in case of need. The calves were kept under observation for 8 days, fed principally on milk, with some hay, according to the age of the animal. The milk was boiled on the premises to prevent diarrhea.

The Building had two stories. The whole of the ground floor was made of cement to allow for free and frequent washing. Each room and stable was heated with hot water pipes, so arranged that the heat in any one could be maintained independently of the others. The rooms were lit with gas, including specially shaped gaseliers above the operating tables, necessitated by the London fogs.

The "Waiting Room" served to hold those who came for vaccination or revaccination. Besides a window on the south side, a skylight provided all the illumination necessary. The "Operation and Vaccination Room" was actually one large room extending across the building and divided by a centrally placed and incomplete partition about 7 feet high. In the half devoted to the operating room for calves, there were three large tables to accommodate the animals; at the sides were perforated India rubber mats ($4 \times 5'$) on which the operators stood. Beside the tables were three stands on castors, $17" \times 3"$, on which instruments rested. There was also a weighing machine, a fire extinguisher and a sink. A skylight as well as the gaseliers provided light.

The portion of the room devoted to vaccination was lit by two large windows; two washhand basins were supplied by nearby water taps. The room also contained three desks, a cupboard for books and 25 plain chairs. The instruments used in the operating and vaccination rooms were these:

Clamp forceps to clamp calf vessels;
Scalpels;
Lancets, ordinary bleeding, used in human vaccination;
"Points" made from ivory shavings, bought by the gross;
"Capillary glass tubes" bought by the gross;
Razors for shaving calves;
Plates, of the ordinary soup kind, to hold "charged points," etc.;
Wire gauze meat covers, 6 in number, to protect drying points from flies;
Cylindrical glasses for milk — used as "cremometers";
A pair of compasses used to measure percent of cream in milk supplied to calves;
Wooden boxes, small, to pack stores of lymph.

Besides the above, four separate registers were used to record vaccinations and revaccinations (human), registration of calves and calf vaccinations and special calf registrations. Printed forms and cards were also filled out here and given to patients.

The "Upper Story" of the building contained space reserved for the microscope room; the rest was occupied by the caretaker (first assistant) and his family. The "Microscope Room" (in actuality, a laboratory) was lit by two large windows. It contained two long, plain tables and a water tap over a sink. Shelves were arranged around the walls. Two stools and a chair completed the furnishings. The instruments included:

A Microscope;
A hot box for sterilization (wire trays);
An air pump used to dry "points" rapidly;
Filtering and boiling stands;
Flasks, pipettes and watch glass;
Glass measures and porcelain slabs;
Weighing machine;
Test tubes and test tube stand;
Bottles containing staining re-agents, carbolic acid and glycerine.

Employees included the following:

Title of Officer	Salary (£) 1892–93	1893–94
Director of Animal Station	400	400
Asst. Director	300	300
Clerk	7–8s/wk	30s
Attendant/Caretaker	100	100
2nd Attendant/ Caretaker	35	35

Stables for the calves had concrete floors and were well maintained, with openings into a well-trapped drain. Each calf had floor space of 36.7 feet. Partitions between the stalls were made of slate, capped with wood, sloping upwards from 3½ to 4½ feet. Troughs were made of iron. Maintenance of temperature was controlled by hot water pipes.

The "Yard" also contained the milk-boiling shed and an isolation stable.[26]

24

The Hoffman Block Outrage and Other Stories

A Doctor recently possessed a pet magpie, which constantly hearing his master's advice-gratis patients repeat, in answer to the solicitous inquiries of a valet, "Ah, Henry, I'm very ill!" learnt the phrase by heart, so as to speak it with surprising distinctness; it was, in fact, his distinct form of expression. The magpie escaped to the neighboring rural district, and was shot by a sporting peasant. The latter ran to pick up his prize. The dying bird opened his eyes, and said, looking up dolefully at his murderer, "Ah, Henry, I'm very ill!" The peasant's name was Henry. He dropped his victim and his gun, and took to his heels.[1]

A paragraph in the *Jones County Liberal* (IA), December 19, 1872, contained the following information: "A party of medical students at Cleveland, Ohio, a short time ago, in making a raid on a cemetery for "subjects," unfortunately exhumed the corpse of a smallpox victim. Result — Several students down with the disease, and a general panic in the college."

The incident became known as the "Hoffman Block Outrage," stemming from the fact the college dissecting room was in one of the upper stories of Hoffman's block and that was where the students took the disinterred body. According to reports, a student at the college witnessed the burial in the afternoon and that night "piloted a squad of medical students to a grave which they thought did not look like a fresh one but, as the guide declared he saw a body buried in it that day, the coffin was laid bare and robbed of its contents, the 'subject' being the putrid body of a man who died of small pox."

The students were apparently so enamored of their feat that they "indulged in a Bacchanalian orgy of the most hideous character," stripping the body of its clothing and tossing the garments, reeking with infection, about the room in drunken glee. The young men unknowingly spread the disease and eventually twelve cases were reported in Cleveland. Once the situation was uncovered, precautions, including widespread inoculation, were taken and an epidemic was averted. Had less care been taken, authorities believed a "pestilence would probably have resulted because the corpse of a small pox victim disseminates the disease more widely, more surely and in more malignant form than anything else."

The following month, however, three young men in Akron and Royalton became indirect victims of the incident. They caught the disease from exposure to others who attended a Thanksgiving Day party in Richfield that included one of the medical students from the Hoffman tragedy. The partygoers subsequently carried the infection to their boardinghouse, infecting others who eventually carried it home, exposing the three victims and perhaps others.[2]

Grave robbing was big business in the 1800s, and many medical students paid their way through college by turning "resurrectionist." The only tools required were a spade, keyhole saw and a piece of rope. After identifying an appropriate grave, half of the plot was marked off and dirt covering the upper part of the coffin was removed. When done by a professional this work was performed in eight minutes. After reaching the coffin, the saw was used at one side, cutting through the upper board and often through the shroud and flesh of the subject.

The manipulator of the saw then raised his own body with a hand on either side of the grave until a foot above the coffin's lid. He then loosened his hold on either side, precipitating his whole weight upon the lid, which gave way with a crash. The broken lid was then removed, and a rope with a slipknot lowered and arranged around the head of the corpse. Word was then given to "hoist away." Occasionally the head of the victim was pulled off in the process.

As soon as the body was above ground, the shroud was torn away and thrown back into the grave. This precaution was taken to avoid a technicality of the law that made it a felony to steal any article of apparel; stealing the corpse was only punishable as a misdemeanor. Once disinterred, the body was doubled up, dumped in a sack, placed in a wagon and taken to town, where it was deposited in a vat of considerable size. A vein in the neck was opened and arsenic run through to preserve it; there the "stiff" remained until called for.

Nearly all bodies were stolen from potter's fields and a team of grave robbers was capable of collecting 150 bodies during the summer season. The average corpse sold for $8, occasionally going as high as $12. Undertakers typically aided grave robbers by putting a "mark" on the plots of fit subjects. Catholic cemeteries were generally guarded and thus suffered fewer robberies; if the undertaker also happened to be a Catholic, he never marked the graves of one of his own class. According to one body snatcher, smallpox bodies were never marked, so professionals left them alone; those not of the trade and unfamiliar with the system took them by accident, as in the case of the medical students. Proving Americans had a sense of humor, an 1882 notice observed, "There is one good point about smallpox. If you are removed by it, body-snatchers will not search for you."[3]

Another aspect of death equally disturbing was the common practice of "working over" cemetery grounds numerous times. When cemeteries became overcrowded, workers dug anew into the ground, adding coffins atop decomposed remains; by the third time, bones of those underneath were simply scattered about before a new coffin was placed, usually no more than three feet deep. This practice often disturbed the resting places of those who had died of contagious diseases, posing a serious health hazard. Worse, after burial grounds had been worked over several times, corpses did not decompose as rapidly as they otherwise would in fresh soil, causing the development of miasmas tainting the atmosphere. In Davenport, Iowa, the noxious gasses produced were called "a mysterious visitation of Providence," which local citizens opted to blame on the poorer sections of the city, crying, "glucose works, glue factory, slaughter house, river slough, etc. when it is the graveyard in which the dark saturated earth and bones of corpses are daily being turned up to make room for new subjects."

In Paris, where the practice of working over cemeteries was common, grave diggers were affected by the gasses arising from opened graves, prompting a call for cremation. It was warned, however, that not only did fire fail to obliterate contagious germs, it also tended to spread them into the air. As proof, a brig arrived at the Philadelphia lazaretto carrying a cargo of wool and rags. The rags were burned on the quarantine wharf but the infected smoke carried contagion into the surrounding area, resulting in the loss of twenty lives from fever.

The problem of overcrowded cemeteries also plagued New Orleans, where major burial grounds were located near populous areas. Dr. G.H. Pratt, of the New Orleans Charity Hospital, warned of the danger, further stating that fluids and gasses from decomposing bodies were a frightful source of smallpox and yellow fever germs. Although, at the time (1878), the major disruption to health was considered the odor arising from the city ammonia works, Dr. Pratt argued that those from decaying bodies were ten times worse. Adding to the problem was the threat of opening a burial vault, thereby spreading disease that was believed to survive any length of time.[4]

"Malignant air" (miasma) was considered to be the carrier of many poisons during the 19th century and in 1853, when Hanover and northern Germany suffered from an especially virulent form of smallpox, the anatomist Langenback began a study to determine the "peculiarity of organic structure which disposes one man to catch a disease while his neighbors escape." He eventually confessed the mystery of smallpox eluded his search and the topic remained at the forefront of medical research.[5]

Such questions were naturally discussed among lay people as well, with varying degrees of wisdom. In 1871, editor Brigham of the *Commercial* (PA) accused the editor of the *Indiana Progress* of being a "dolt" for declaring that goods may be infected with virus. In his defense, the latter cited the case of a lady and child in Pittsburgh who died after being exposed to infection brought into the house on the clothing of an attending physician.[6]

Two similar cases of disease being reintroduced after a substantial period were discussed in the early 1870s. The first instance involved a house in Hoosick Falls, New York. In 1799, it had been used as a pesthouse, later serving as a private dwelling. Seventy years later, a workman hired to effect repairs contracted smallpox, to which he had not otherwise been exposed, raising the question of how long the smallpox virus could be retained in walls, floors and ceilings.[7]

The second case involved a former slave named Reuben Span, an artist in slack lime. He sued for $1,000, claiming that his employer had exposed him to smallpox by hiring him to fresco a dwelling in which a woman had died of the disease. He contracted smallpox and was confined to his couch for six weeks, cut off from his source of income and suffering terrible pitting of the face. Span lost the case on the grounds that he knew the condition of the house as well as his employer and therefore no negligence was demonstrated.[8]

Life — and Death — Go On

Although the numbers may seem ridiculously small today, the cost of maintaining smallpox victims took a heavy toll on state and local governments. For example, the Logansport, Indiana, board of health was presented the following bills covering care for smallpox victims:

Hebel & Hoover, for groceries:	$13.18
Fitch & Coleman, for medical attendance:	$44.00
G.W. Burrow, for lounge & mattress	$5.75
Mrs. McPherson, for board	$145.00

The board recommended payment of the first two but did not endorse the last, as the mayor complained that in smallpox cases, "everybody seemed to claim the privilege of bringing in a big bill against the city; that it would break the city up if allowed to go on." After discussion, it was decided the bill from the physicians was extravagant and the one for board the most reasonable. They finally agreed to pay her, less $13.18, the amount charged by Hebel & Hoover.[9] Nor was life easier for those who suffered from that loathsome disease. In another case, typical of the type found repeatedly in newspapers of the 1800s, a man was taken off a steamboat at Dubuque. When it was seen he suffered from smallpox, he was left on the levee exposed to the inclemency of the weather without any care for two days.[10]

Lacking a vaccination law established and enforced by the federal government (which would have been impossible to enforce in any case due to lack of consensus by legislators, the prohibitive cost and expanse of the nation), smallpox remained a constant of life and death in the United States. Without any major epidemics until the end of the century, pockets of infection continued to strike terror and inflict death. The average yearly mortality rate from smallpox in Wisconsin was somewhat over 100, with the average number of cases exceeding 400.[11]

On May 19, 1876, a case of smallpox was reported in San Francisco; by July, no part of the city was free of the disease, although nearly 16,000 persons were vaccinated. With supply of vaccine scarcely equal to demand, increased orders were sent east. The prevalence of disease did not stop people traveling to nearby Oakland and, according to local authorities, every case in that city was attributed to such intercourse.

Demonstrating the prevailing theory of transmission, leading physicians in Oakland believed smallpox was communicated by the patient's breath "and the miasma exhaled from the epidermis, as well as by exposure to infected clothing." Those whose system placed them in a favorable condition could also catch smallpox by merely passing close to a home in which the disease existed. The costs in Oakland for a three-month period were as follows:

August: $434 for professional services of 2 patients at the Pesthouse;
September: $679 for professional attendance of 6 smallpox patients, including two Chinamen
October: $132 for livery fees for physician plus $8 transportation.[12]

One of the greatest threats to the spread of smallpox actually came from inbound vessels. Most captains were ordered by their employers to smuggle infected passengers ashore in order to avoid quarantine; those who disobeyed were often threatened with discharge. By and large, however, the epidemic was blamed on the Chinese, and those found on the streets in the end-stages of disease were often ignored and left to die. By September, Dr. Meares, the health officer of San Francisco, organized a massive plan to fumigate Chinatown in a "determined crusade against the small-pox heathen."[13]

Statistics from May–September 1876 put the total number of known cases at 730; of those, 128 were white, 60 Chinese and 2 African. Considering most cases among the Chinese went unreported, the total number of victims was estimated at 1,000.[14] The situation was not improved by those immigrating to the City by the Bay: in April 1877, the *Alaska* brought in 950 Chinese, most of whom were suffering from smallpox. Significantly, the disease was epidemic in Hong Kong when the ship departed.[15]

The Chinese reliance on traditional medicines also confused the situation. Salted or dried and powdered scorpions and the skins of snakes and rhinoceros horn were considered efficient remedies.[16] The shell of a gourd was also suspended over the head of the bed occupied by children who had never had the disease, as it was believed the god of measles would empty the smallpox into the shell if it were placed convenient to his hand. More effective yet was to place an ugly mark on a child's face, for the god considered it useless to waste valuable smallpox on so homely a person.[17]

It is important to note here that superstition was widespread throughout the United States during the 19th century. In Pennsylvania, for example, where nearly every town had its witch or soothsayer, a sorceress named Granny Tribble was particularly famous. Her remedy for smallpox and the itch (diseases commonly associated) was to treat the disease with grease rendered from a black cat that died with its throat cut; for protection against smallpox, she advised carrying black fur from the left forefoot of a cat.[18]

With the disease always present somewhere, the virus was easily spread; by the summer of 1876, cases were reported in Virginia City, Emigrant Gap and Eureka, Nevada. Recognizing the danger, the C.P.R.R. ordered all its employees vaccinated.[19] In April 1877, smallpox reached Santa Fe, New Mexico, with the first death reported on May 27. Between that date and December, the death tolls were as shown below:

City of Santa Fe	93
Ranchos in the vicinity of Santa Fe	26
Aqua Fria	15
Cienega	8
Rio Tesuque	7
Tosuque pueblo	15

Out of the 164 fatalities, 83 were male and 81 female. Victims were of all nationalities commingled in the population, including Mexican, American, French and Indian. While Santa Fe suffered less than other parts of the territory — the ratio being less than 1 percent of the total population of 6,000 — in the Indian village of Tesuque, 15 out of 100 souls perished.

It was believed that smallpox entered New Mexico through El Paso del Norte and ascended the valley of the Rio Grande without deviation until reaching Albuquerque. The disease did not strike Albuquerque, the most important and central town of the Rio Abajo (and incidentally filled with puddles and swamps) but, "yielding to one of its familiar freaks," flew over the mountains as far as Manzano and then into Santa Fe. Because of the sporadic nature of the disease, long editorials were written disputing the fact smallpox was contagious, although authors grudgingly admitted the efficacy of vaccination and sanitary measures.[20]

By January 1878, smallpox had become rampant in Utah, where business in Ogden came to a standstill. In order to combat the disease, the quarantine physician of nearby Salt Lake City ordered that infected persons be isolated and that no individuals suspected of carrying smallpox be allowed to enter the city. He further demanded that railroad cars be disinfected and a "kettle of burning tar should be kept in each car sufficiently long to permeate every interstice and crevice with the fumes thereof, at least three times a week." Carbolic acid and water, in a ratio of 1:1, were also to be freely sprinkled over the floors and platforms of every car, every day.[21]

Rumors of outbreaks proved nearly as devastating as the actual disease and in the spring of 1879, accusations flew on whether smallpox prevailed at San Antonio. In response, authorities at Seguin advised that no Negroes or Mexicans from San Antonio be hired to pick cotton. By September, the mayor reported to the national board of health in Washington that the number of smallpox cases since January reached 850, of which 71 died: 49 Mexicans, 15 Negroes and 7 whites. In his opinion, the reason for the high death rate among the Mexican population was their opposition to vaccination.

Two weeks later, the *Galveston Daily News* reported that there was no way to secure immunity for San Antonio, as smallpox prevailed all along the Rio Grande, particularly in places where there were large Mexican populations. As the "Mexicans know nothing of vaccination," they suffered greatly from the disease, whereas there were only two whites out of 15,000–16,000 citizens down with the contagion.[22]

The Anti-Vaccination Movement— "The War of Bigotry and Ignorance"

The idea that vaccination was harmful to the human body began almost contiguously with the discovery of vaccination. Throughout the 1800s, lay people, physicians and associations registered numerous complaints on the dangers and ineffectiveness of the procedure, achieving an astonishing degree of success with their rhetoric and fear mongering. Advocates fought back with statistics on its efficacy. Two notices from the *Semi-Weekly Wisconsin* (October 3, 1869) present a common defense:

> The experience of last fall ought to teach a lesson, and we trust it will, despite the strong efforts being made by a certain class of Germans against vaccination.
>
> We commend the following statistics to those who are earnestly working against vaccination in our city — Previous to the introduction of vaccination the annual death rate from small pox was 3,000 to the 1,000,000, which has been gradually reduced in proportion to its being made compulsory; and last year the rate was only 202 to the 1,000,000.

Ten years later, with nothing settled, the *Galveston Daily News* (August 26, 1879) reported complaints that city officials failed to provide an "unflinching effort" to suppress an epidemic of smallpox, noting that "the anti-small-pox meeting, Saturday night, was largely attended by most respectable citizens, who passed resolutions, made suggestions, and partially relieved the mayor of responsibility."

In 1879, the as-yet-unorganized anti-vaccination movement in the United States gained traction when the *New York Evening Gazette* and the *New York Sun* began a crusade against vaccination. On August 16 the newspapers ran a series of highly selected statistics from Great Britain on the failure of the preventive, concluding that, "there are so many reasons why filth [vaccine], even in the form of disease, should not be put into the system at all." By September 13, one of the newspapers chided a proponent "for airing his belief in that popular madness known as vaccination." On September 27, the newspaper followed up with the argument that "there was absolutely no certainty of obtaining virus free from these diseases [scrofula and syphilis among others] even granted that the theory is all that its warmest admirers claim for it, but which we do not grant."

On October 7, 1879, the "First Anti-Vaccination League of America" was formed in the lecture room of the United States Medical College, 13th Street, New York. The movement was brought about by the efforts of William Tebb, a well-to-do Englishman. While living in the fashionable quarter of London, he took his second daughter to be vaccinated after the first attempt failed. The physician there advised him to take her home and let her alone. Since that incident, he had researched the preventive and determined that not only did vaccination fail to protect against smallpox, it also held the potential for harm. Resisting thirteen prosecutions for failing to vaccinate his children, Tebb came to the conclusion that compulsory vaccination was a tyranny "because it made people liable to take inoculable diseases, and did not insure them against taking small-pox." He encouraged his fellow citizens to resist the law, helped pay their fines and hired lawyers to defend them.

Tebb and his anti-vaccinationist tracts were present at the inauguration of the league. He lectured on the hardship poor families suffered paying fines after refusing to have their children vaccinated and related the experience of a physician who lost $2,500 a year by refusing to perform the operation. He further stated that in Montreal, where vaccine "was punctured into the people by law," public indignation was so strong that a mob of 10,000 threatened to tear down the building where authorities had assembled to pass a compulsory vaccination law.

The chair and president of the league was Alexander Wilder, M.D., who told converts that vaccinated persons were more susceptible to disease that the non-vaccinated and that bovine virus increased the chance of contracting smallpox. Other officers included J.W. Nickles, secretary; M.L. Hollbrook, treasurer; and doctors J.E. Briggs, Thomas A. Granger and R.A. Gunn serving as the executive committee. The object of their society was to "awaken the attention of the public to the evils of vaccination and to its inability, to put an end to its practice, and to prevent legislation for its enforcement."[23]

The headline for the November 29, 1879, issue of the *Evening Gazette* proclaimed "Killed by Vaccination," and recounted the history of a five-year-old child who had been vaccinated in August. The wound healed but he developed a rash diagnosed as chicken pox. Another physician considered the child's deteriorating condition to be the result of blood poisoning. After the child died on November 25, the attending physician determined the child did not have the strength "to throw off the poisonous matter in the blood." Despite what the bold-type headline proclaimed, the article avoided any direct link to vaccination, offering innuendo, instead: the undertaker "feared that the disease was small-pox"; the doctor signing the death certificate called the case "a very rare one," leading the reader to infer that death resulted from the vaccination three months earlier.

Reprinting an article from the *New York Sun,* the *Evening Gazette* (December 6, 1879) quoted Dr. Wilder as stating, "It is not the province of government, it is a crime against nature, to disease a human body on any pretext whatever. There is no fact more certain than that disease is always opposed to health; that corruption is opposed to soundness. Vac-

---

Correspondent Argues That Vaccination is an Evil to be Avoided by Intelligent Persons.

LETTER WHICH IS WRITTEN WITH THE INTENTION OF CLEARING UP THE MATTER FOR MANY HERE WHO DO NOT KNOW THE NAURE OF THIS PRACTICE.

The anti-vaccination movement was not limited to England or the United States. In this editorial from the *Daily Gleaner* (Jamaica, September 20, 1923), the author expressed a common "anti" theme that vaccination caused numerous diseases including tuberculosis and syphilis.

cination virus is corruption, loud, disgusting, and the source of constant disease. The crusade against it has the sanction of the highest motives of which man is capable — of religious veneration, paternal benevolence, and a pure conscientiousness."

Wilder went on to the argue that vaccine disease was "distinctly septicemic — a disease produced by actual corruption" and "an utter immorality," and finally quoting John Birch of St. Thomas Hospital, who stated that natural smallpox was a mild disease, only "rendered malignant by mistakes in nursing, in diet, and in medicine."

Using flashpoint issues, including personal freedom, religion, parental rights and immorality, anti-vaccinationists continued to gain converts through the rest of the century. Forced to fight back, proponents, including the influential publication *Scientific American,* conceded some statistics unfavorable to vaccination might be true, then countered with the fact that in New York City in 1879, the worst of human scourges had so thoroughly been brought into subjection that, with 1,100,000 inhabitants, only 14 cases were then reported. The publication concluded: "It is as manifestly unwise as it is absurd for our newspapers to lend themselves to the propagation of anti-vaccination nonsense."[24]

25

Smallpox in Canada and England Through the 1880s

> It is said that Confederate money is being circulated in Canada. So is small pox; but that does not make it good.[1]

The ebb and flow of smallpox in Canada was similar to that in the United States, England and Europe in that outbreaks, spread over vast areas, were often swift and deadly. Larger numbers of fatalities were reported in major cities such as Montreal, where over one hundred deaths were reported during a five-week period in December 1868–January 1869. In late December 1876, the disease appeared in Quebec, with authorities sounding the same tone of anger and desperation as those of their neighbors to the south and across the ocean.

By June, angry that smallpox had gone unchecked for six months, the newspapers noted "the city has submitted quietly to the disease and so far except in a few individual cases nothing has been done to get rid of it." The Marine Hospital was opened to smallpox patients but in the city of over 60,000 inhabitants, there was no semblance of an ambulance corps. Sick people were transported in public conveyances, providing a medium for the spread of the pestilence, while "the almost superstitious prejudice of the many people here have against vaccination and also the careless way in which the family linen is washed" presented an almost impenetrable barrier for disease control. Lacking compulsory vaccination and laws regarding the separation and washing of infected clothing, it was feared smallpox would spread all over Canada.[2]

The situation was not destined to get better, and, as dreaded, posed serious problems for the northwestern United States. In October 1876, the ship *Dakota,* lying in the port of Esquimalt, Victoria, BC, and bound for San Francisco, was found to contain numerous cases of smallpox. Fortunately, quarantine officers discovered the danger and sent the ship to anchor in the outer harbor, where it was fumigated and detained at least a fortnight. The *Dakota* had a heavy list of freight and about 150 passengers.[3] Spread of smallpox by land was equally to be feared, as its prevalence in Montreal and Sherbrooke, Quebec, quickly reached across the borders to Milwaukee and other points in direct communication with St. Paul.[4]

The fear of vaccination came to a head in 1876, when the largest city in the Dominion of Canada passed through its annual scourge of smallpox. "Through the blind fanaticism and vicious stupidity of a large portion" of Montreal's inhabitants, numerous citizens resorted to violent demonstrations against compulsory vaccination. They asserted that the vaccinated died from smallpox as surely as the unvaccinated, failing to distinguish the proportion of deaths from each group. In Quebec, for instance, out of the total number of cases reported, 27:100 unvaccinated persons died, while among the vaccinated the ratio was only 12:100.[5] Cold logic had little effect on public sentiment and a worse conflict would occur in 1885.

Smallpox Among Canadian Emigrants and Native Americans

In the fall of 1875, an Icelandic deputation visited Lake Manitoba with a view of colonization. Upon the deputation's approval, the first wave of colonists arrived in the spring of 1876, establishing a settlement named Gimli. When the summer proved unusually rainy, many of the new colonists moved farther north on the lakeshore. A further colonization occurred in the summer of 1876, when 1,156 Icelanders arrived on the west shore. Although they were in good health at the time, as winter approached, smallpox broke out, causing great suffering and loss of life. A very large number of men were thus prevented from continuing to obtain employment on the railway works, adding to further privation.[6]

Conditions continued to deteriorate: "The most terrible outbreak of small-pox ever known in the history of the northwest is desolating the Icelandic and Mennonite settlement of about 7000 souls on the east side of Winnipeg. The deaths average 180 daily" owing to want of ventilation and bad food. Compounding the tragedy, no medical men were among the colonists. The government quarantined the area, preventing anyone from communicating with the Province of Manitoba. Lieutenant-Governor Morris was vested with authority over the area and sent two physicians to the settlement. By late November, reports indicated that 18 Indians had also perished at Sandy Bar.

As the afflicted country was beyond the confines of the province, and the new seat of government known as the Council in Keewatin had not yet been appointed, Morris telegraphed to the Ottawa governor to pass an order establishing an official quarantine and to send another doctor. At Fort Garrie, Colonel Smith received orders to send a detachment of militia to assist the newcomers and enforce the law.

The scourge spread to the Fort Alexander Indians living on the west side of the lake, decimating their numbers. Hundreds died in settlements on the Qua Appalled River, forcing the inhabitants to flee south toward the boundary line. Lieutenant-Governor Morris sent a letter to the Indians at St. Peter's, warning them to have no contact with tribes to the north. The problem became so serious the United States secretary of the treasury ordered, "Refuse any entry of robes, pelts, and skins from districts infected with small-pox, unless accompanied with Consular certificate of noninfection."[7]

By December, while smallpox had not reached Peguis, Manitoba, smaller settlements reported isolated incidents. Unfortunately, the vaccine available to physicians proved ineffective, due to its being "very old stuff and also not properly cased to prevent it from losing its virtue." The health inspector ordered a new supply and proposed revaccinating those upon whom the former vaccine had no effect.

Complicating matters, the Indian Intoxicating Abstinence Act was to be subverted by government issuance of "skit-e-wah-boo," an alcohol-based concoction meant to mitigate the influence of smallpox encounters.[8]

The newly appointed board of health from the Council of Keewatin prevented the spread of smallpox throughout Keewatin, Manitoba and the Northwest Territories through vigorous efforts and the disease did not develop epidemic proportions.[9] Sporadic reports surfaced in Grand Forks, D.T. (southwest Canada), in 1878, but it was not until 1883, when

Above and opposite: Egyptian smallpox certificate, issued by the Ministere de L'Interieur, entitled, "Administration des Services Sanitaires et d'Hygiene publique." It is dated 1896 and bears the signature of the issuing officer and the official seal (from the authors' collection).

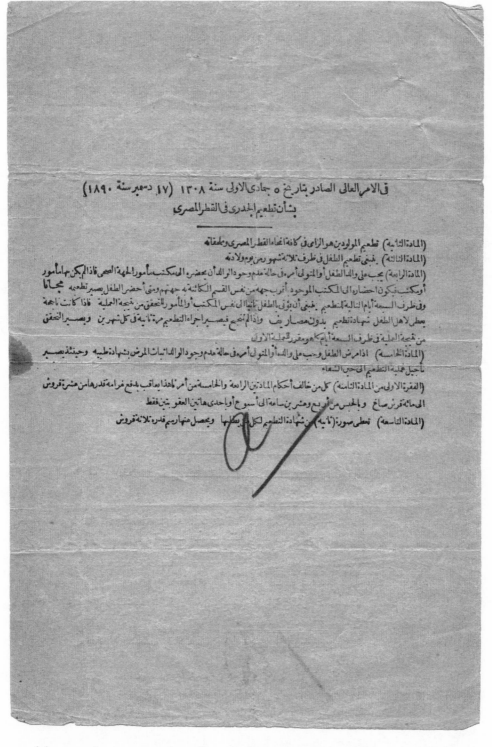

في الأمر العالي الصادر بتاريخ ٥ جمادى الأولى سنة ١٣٠٨ (١٧ ديسمبر سنة ١٨٩٠)
بشأن تطعيم الجدري في القطر المصري

(المادة الثانية) تطعيم المولودين هو الزامي في كافة أنحاء القطر المصري وطبقاته

(المادة الثالثة) ينبغي تطعيم الطفل في ظرف ثلاثة أشهر من يوم ولادته

(المادة الرابعة) يجب على والد الطفل أو المتولى أمره في حالة عدم وجود الوالد أن يحضره الى المكتب مأمور الجهة الصحي فاذا لم يكن به مأمور أو مكتب يكون احضاره الى المكتب الموجود أقرب جهة من نفس القسم الكائنة به جهتهم ومتى أحضر الطفل يصير تطعيمه مجانا وفي ظرف السبعة أيام التالية للتطعيم ينبغي أن يؤتى بالطفل ثانيا الى نفس المكتب والمأمور والتحقق من نتيجة العملية فاذا كانت ناجحة يعطى لأهل الطفل شهادة تطعيم بدون مصاريف واذا لم ينجح فيصير اجراء التطعيم مرة ثانية في كل شهرين ويصير التحقق من نتيجة العملية في ظرف السبعة أيام كما هو مقرر للعملة الأولى

(المادة الخامسة) اذا مرض الطفل وجب على والده أو المتولى أمره في حالة عدم وجود الوالد الاثبات المرض بشهادة طبيه وحينئذ يصير تأجيل عملية التطعيم الى حين الشفاء

(الفقرة الأولى من المادة الثامنة) كل من خالف أحكام المادتين الرابعة والخامسة من أمر ما لهذا يعاقب بدفع غرامة قدرها من عشرة قروش الى مائة قرش صاغ والحبس من أربعة وعشرين ساعة الى أسبوع أو بأحدى هاتين العقوبتين فقط

(المادة التاسعة) تعطى صورة (ثانية) من شهادة التطعيم لكل من يطلبها ويحصل منها رسم قدره ثلاثة قروش

a scandal concerning an escaped smallpox patient occurred, that the topic became headline news once again.

In May 1883, the Manitoba newspapers were abuzz with news of an escaped smallpox patient. The invalid's name was William Kittson (called Alexander in early reports), son of

Commodore Kittson. One night, while the attendant was away, he slipped through a window and escaped. A search party failed to find Kittson and early the next morning the search resumed. According to the *Pioneer Press* (St. Paul, MN), the body was finally discovered five miles distant, partially eaten by an eagle. A smallpox ambulance was sent out to recover the corpse although it was feared those who came in contact with the unfortunate were exposed to the disease.

An inquest held the following month detailed the wretched condition of the hospital, then without bedding or glass in the windows and smelling more like a dead-house than an infirmary. The staff was minimal, accused of sleeping on duty and drinking too much. Dr. Kerr, the health inspector, who testified at trial, later sued the *Times* (presumably the New York newspaper that ran several articles on the tragedy) for $20,000 for libel. On account of the smallpox outbreaks during the year 1883, the Province of Manitoba spent $8,065 for prevention measures, including $2,129.55 in the disputed (Keewatin) territory.[10]

A year later, in 1884, reports of smallpox outside Ottawa, Ontario, began surfacing in the township of Hungerford, Hastings County. The four villages in the county — George-town, Tweed, Stow and Thomasburg — were all connected with Peterborough by the Canadian Pacific Railway (C.P.R.). So great was the fright in Tweed that townsmen built fences around their houses and closed their doors against neighbors for fear that the scourge would be carried into their families. Those suffering from smallpox were neglected and left to die without assistance.[11]

By the spring of 1885, reports began surfacing that the disease had appeared in Montreal. The board of health denied the claim, stating that until recently there had not been a single case reported in the city limits since 1881. The report added there were isolated incidents but those were in an outlying municipality. The favorable picture did not last long. On August 16 and 17, there were 23 new cases reported with 13 deaths; on Tuesday, 24 cases and 6 deaths; Wednesday, 35 cases and 5 deaths; Thursday, 32 cases and 9 deaths; Friday, 34 cases, compelling authorities to order disinfectant used in watering the streets. The provincial government petitioned for the use of the Exhibition buildings for a smallpox hospital and asked for the construction of a new hospital. Economic reaction was swift: theatres closed, and fall orders of merchandise from the West were cancelled on account of the pending epidemic. Four public vaccinators were appointed to serve three months.

The same week, the disease spread through the west end, forcing residents to leave the county, carrying the disease with them. Floors were sprinkled morning and night with carbolic acid and physicians were besieged by hundreds of persons anxious to be vaccinated. Unfortunately, vaccine was scarce, compelling the board of health to send to the New England Vaccine Company for a fresh supply. When reports arrived from Halifax, Nova Scotia, that smallpox had made an appearance there, Montreal citizens crowded the religious services in Notre Dame Church to supplicate for aid. Contrary to expectations, smallpox numbers increased among the French residents, as the service drew the sick as well as the healthy, inadvertently spreading the contagion. The priests thereby promised dispensation to inmates of infected houses so they need not attend church.

Fifty-six patients crowded the smallpox hospital meant to accommodate 28 and while a new facility was hastily being constructed, a tent served to house the sick. To counter further spread, the village of St. Anne de Bellevue passed a resolution ordering the immediate vaccination of its residents. Nearby, in St. Jean Baptiste, 25 people died in one week, with many private homes simultaneously holding three or four cases of smallpox. Witnesses stated that nothing was done to stay the spread of the disease, with hardly a single house placarded.[12]

Travelers brought smallpox from Montreal to Toronto, and amid fears of a general epidemic measures were taken to prevent it from moving throughout Ontario, with the provincial health officer quarantining all towns on the boundary between the two provinces. In Quebec, a motion for the enforcement of compulsory vaccination under penalty was adopted.

Residents in upstate New York feared the disease would easily cross the border. Those in Cohoes were especially worried, as over one-third of the city's population comprised French Canadians, primarily from Montreal. In the era of inexpensive and relatively reliable transportation, the midnight trains were filled with people either coming from or returning to Canada, prompting locals to demand that extra precautions be taken.[13] Of like mind, many people in Oswego wondered why the health authorities did not institute a system of quarantine over the bargemen who arrived daily from Montreal, as it was reputed that the pestilence raged in the vicinity where the coal barges unloaded.[14]

In response to the epidemic, large-scale production of vaccine began on a commercial and government-sponsored basis in 1885 at the newly established Montreal Cow-Pox Institute. L'Institut Vaccinogene de Quebec began operation at Sainte-Foy, just outside Quebec City in 1886, operating with the support of the Quebec provincial government. By 1899, the L'Institut Vaccinol de Montreal was established as a privately funded company that received some financial support from the city.

The Ontario Vaccine Farm established at Palmerston became the first vaccine supply company in Ontario. Influenced by the 1884 outbreak at Hungerford and the 1885 epidemic in Montreal, it opened in 1885. Sponsored by the provincial board of health, the Palmerston Vaccine Farm was managed by Dr. Alexander Stewart. Later in the century Canada imported commercial vaccine, principally from the Pocono Laboratory near Swiftwater, Pennsylvania, founded in 1898 by Dr. Richard Slee.[15]

The Anti-Vaccination Movement in Canada

On March 20, 1882, the *Manitoba Daily Free Press* reprinted an article first published in the *New York Times,* detailing a speech given by the eminent Dr. Carpenter in defense of vaccination. Significantly, he delivered it to the monthly meeting of anti-vaccinationists. Carpenter argued that the state was "morally bound to intervene in such matters [of vaccination] between the parent and the child, for the good of both the child and the society at large." Among many statistics, he presented was the observation that within five years after the compulsory vaccination law was passed in Scotland, the death rate from smallpox fell to less than 12 deaths per year. In England, however, "thanks to the efforts of the society he was addressing, 'an unvaccinated residuum kept the disease alive.'" His words had little impact, as members decried "that hideous monstrosity vaccination," which was working "the physical deterioration of the human family."

Dr. Carpenter had previously written for the *London Times* on the subject of "Vaccination and Small-Pox." Considering facts supporting the procedure indisputable, he argued first that anti-vaccinationists of the present generation were ignorant of medical history of the last century when smallpox ravaged the world; second, they were reacting to the exaggerated claims of the pro-vaccinationists; and third, they were obsessed with the illogical idea that what is not complete protection is no protection at all. In this highly quoted article, he went on to stress the need for revaccination, concluding, "The experience of mankind is overwhelming in favor of vaccination."[16]

French Canadians in Montreal supported their brethrens' anger and on September 28, 1885, they took their anti-vaccination beliefs a giant step further. On the day compulsory vaccination was begun, between 900 and 1,000 French Canadians gathered by the branch health office for the east end of the city. They "broke in the windows, tore down the doors, smashed the counter and generally demoralized the place." After completing the ruin, the greatly augmented mob proceeded to a drugstore, which they mistook for the store of Alderman Gray, the medical officer. In 20 minutes they demolished the business, then marched on city hall, shouting, "Down with the Council! Kill the vaccinators! Burn the town!" and "Hang the English!"

At city hall the mob began an onslaught on the public buildings, including the central police station. There were few protectors, as most of the officers had been sent to the east end of town where the riot had been anticipated. Stones were thrown and shots fired by the fanatics, then numbering several thousand. When the police finally arrived a hard fight ensued before the agitators moved up the street, vowing vengeance on "the d — — d English paper [the *Daily Herald*] which favored vaccination."

Major damage was done to alderman Roy's house and that of a physician who belonged to the provincial board of health. By 1:00 A.M. the 2,000 remaining rioters declared they would rather die than be vaccinated and would not submit to "the English dogs." The English-speaking community considered the riot "the beginning of a war of races," adding that there was, at present, at least 4,000 cases of smallpox in the city.

The reading of a papal decree, which was considered as applying to the epidemic in Montreal, issued by His Holiness Pope Leo XIII on August 20, called on the faithful around the world, impressing upon Roman Catholics the efficacy of prayer in crushing "these regrettable calamities."[17] In response, the *Boston Post* observed, "We have not a word to say against the religious ceremonies in Montreal for the abatement of the small-pox, but faith without works is dead. Vaccination is one of the works."[18]

With a strong contingency of police on hand, quiet resumed the following day, but public feeling on both sides was aroused. The rioters vowed to remain quiet until there was a laxity in the present armed resistance, while the authorities stated their resolve to carry out the health laws, promising to take whatever steps were necessary for that purpose.[19]

Smallpox remained a threat and states near the Canadian border took precautions to prevent its spread into their jurisdictions. The board of health in Minnesota required lumberjacks working the Canadian forests to be vaccinated. Trains making the round-trip from St. Albans, Vermont, to Montreal were used only for that route and disinfected every day, while no through passengers going south were permitted to continue until they were vaccinated.[20]

On September 17, 1885, Washington issued an official statement authorizing inspectors to board trains in Canada before they crossed the Detroit and St. Claire Rivers to aid the state of Michigan. In regard to the introduction of smallpox by rail in Maine, New Hampshire, Vermont, Massachusetts and Northern New York, authorities advised that upon the request of individual governors, inspectors would be appointed.[21]

If the danger to citizens of the United States was great, the people of Canada were often in a worse way. Overwhelmed by the outbreaks, institutions were overcrowded and poorly staffed. One female patient told of how she was brought to a Montreal hospital suffering from a mild case of the disease and placed into a bed with dirty sheets. Aside from the horrific smells of the disease, body odors from patients too ill to care for themselves made the eight-bed ward unbearable. She stated there was no nursing care and food was delivered by children, themselves recovering from smallpox. No attendants were available during night hours, window glass was broken and bed linen often nonexistent. As soon as breath was extinguished, the dead were sewed in a sheet, and the corpse was dropped on the floor and dragged away.[22]

Reports from the Montreal Health Department showed 281 persons died from smallpox during the week ending October 9. Of those, 263 were French Canadians (who comprised about two-thirds of the population), revealing a significant disproportion of deaths between them and those of English descent.[23] Anti-vaccinationists continued to argue their points, however, and the disease persisted into 1886, causing Montreal a loss of six million dollars by slow business resulting from fear of smallpox contagion.[24] This forced the city council to raise one million dollars by means of bonds to help pay off the $13,000,000 debt incurred by the epidemic.[25]

Smallpox in Great Britain through the 1880s

In the year 1876, the death rate in England and Wales was lower than in any year since 1856. Fatal cases of smallpox and measles were more numerous in 1876 than 1875, but death from the other principal zymotic diseases declined.[26] In 1877, the death rate declined again to levels not seen during the prior 38 years, excluding 1850 and 1872. Considering the increase in population, the yearly report went so far as to proclaim London the healthiest of all cities. The claim was a stretch in that the death rate was 21.9 per thousand, while in Christiania it was 20.1 and in the major United States cities, the average was 21.2, with Philadelphia registering the lowest percentage of 18.8 per thousand. Other countries, however, were considerably in excess of London mortality rates. The three Indian cities of Calcutta, Bombay and Madras had a death rate three times that of London, due to the prevalence of cholera, smallpox and fever. London had its own problems with smallpox, where more than 2,500 deaths were attributable to the scourge, "sufficient to produce a marked effect on the death-rate."[27]

In early January, members of the Royal Household were revaccinated and as cases of smallpox in London "made the rounds," rapid converts were made of the "few followers of the Keighley Board of Guardians in revolt against Dr. Jenner." Hundreds of patients were turned away from smallpox hospitals.[28]

There may have been fewer anti-vaccinationists at Keighley, but the movement was growing in England. A paper on the "Increased Mortality from Small-Pox" read before the Manchester Literary and Philosophical Society by Joseph Baxendell in 1877, presented statistics asserting compulsory vaccination actually increased mortality by 132.5 percent. In commenting on Baxendell's data, the *British Medical Journal* countered the data by simple reanalysis and regretted that such a person was accepted as an authority on smallpox statistics by others as well as anti-vaccinationists.[29]

Politicians were not insensitive to the growing movement and discussion in the House of Lords centered around the "almost political character" of the societies. Great concern lay over the basic mistrust of lymph, either from contamination or loss of efficacy, as well as a resurgence of belief that it had become a vehicle for other maladies. Citing medical testimony from Dr. Simon, medical officer to the Privy Council, given 20 years past, as well as that of Dr. Marston, physician to the Small-pox Hospital in 1853, Earl Percy and others urged a consideration of animal vaccination. Obtaining lymph from cows had been successful in

Belgium and America, and he requested further inquiry. Others complained that the accumulation of fines for parents' refusal to vaccinate their children weighed more heavily on the poor, and made "martyrs" all over the country.[30]

In response, the following year, Mr. Pease, of the House of Commons, introduced a bill limiting the number of prosecutions to which parents were subject on the grounds of conscience. Opponents argued that if vaccination were to be compulsory, paying one fine of 20 shillings defeated the law and wished it were possible to remove children of objecting parents and submit them to the state for the "beneficent operation." Pease's Bill was defeated 271 to 82, although Earl Percy was in favor of referring it to a select committee.[31] Discussions such as these also had an effect in the United States, where editorials speculated that vaccination was a "mixed blessing," and questioned whether "its advantages compensate for its evils."[32] They also brought on a fresh outcropping of "cures," such as the one published in the *Liverpool Mercury,* where Edward Hine "staked his reputation as a public man" that cream of tarter (tartanic acid or potassium bitartrate) dissolved in a pint of water cured smallpox in three days.[33]

Parliament brought up the subject of vaccination again in 1879, when Dr. Cameron, MP, brought up a bill sponsoring the use of cow lymph. At a meeting of the British Medical Association, Cameron stated that fears of the present humanized arm-to-arm transfer "had practically proved fatal to the spread of vaccination" in England, and felt animal vaccination could be carried out at a moderate cost with a success equal to that of the present system. Dr. Warlamont, director of the Vaccination Bureaux at Brussels, then read a paper arguing that the use of animal lymph "was necessary to satisfy doubts, fears, imputations, and perhaps prejudices" in the public's mind. Results of bovine vaccination in his country had proven hugely successful. More than 10,000 children vaccinated with animal lymph between 1865 and 1870 survived the terrible epidemic of 1870–1871, not one of them contracting smallpox. Most attending the conference agreed with his position, supporting the transfer as a "nearly perfect system."[34]

The effort had little effect on those who refused to believe. In March 1881, a small pamphlet, entitled "The Fable of the Small-pox Hospital Nurses Saved from Small-pox by Re-vaccination" was published by the London Society for the Abolition of Compulsory Vaccination."[35] As an example of how far the debate had deteriorated, in May 1881, most schools in Dudley and the Black Country had to be closed, stemming from the belief that, as the population grew, Mr. Gladstone was "anxious to kill off little children" by the use of vaccination.[36]

Parliamentary Mortality Returns for England and Wales covering the years 1838–1877 indicated that between 1838 and 1853 (England), the average annual death rate per million of population was 22,386; Wales, from 1838 to 1853 (excluding the cholera years of 1846–1849), 21,840. From 1854 to 1877 (England), the average was 22,141; from 1868 to 1877 (Wales), 21,847. From 1847 to 1853 (England) inclusive, the proportion of deaths of all ages from smallpox was 305 per million; from 1868 to 1877 (Wales), 261. During the twelve year period 1838–42 and 1847–53, before compulsory vaccination (the only years prior to compulsory vaccination for which mortality statistics were available), the average death rate from smallpox was 420 per million; whereas, in the 25 years (1853–1878) of compulsory vaccination, smallpox deaths averaged not more than 216 per million, notwithstanding the exceptionally fatal epidemic of 1871–1872.[37]

Smallpox made a resurgence in 1880. During the 52 weeks ending May 29, deaths of vaccinated persons in London amounted to 90 per million, while the unvaccinated deaths totaled 3,350 per million. As further testimony to age differential, deaths of vaccinated persons under twenty years was 61 per million and unvaccinated 3,350 per million. Under five years of age, the vaccinated deaths were 40.5 against 5,950 in the unvaccinated.[38] By 1882, there were 88 deaths registered in London for the second week of May; 59 were reported in the second week of June and 82 in the third week. By the last week of September, a significant decrease showed only 7 smallpox deaths. Numbers continued to decline and by the first week of November, only 4 smallpox deaths were recorded.[39]

Reports from London in the year 1883 revealed very low numbers, averaging two per week, but 1884 provided far higher numbers. When an outbreak occurred in Chelsea in May, Dr. Graham was hired to provide vaccination in private homes, offering his "Vaporizer" for use.[40] Along with the "Vaporizer," various types of oral vaccination were tried (see a description of Dr. Landell's technique in chapter 17) as well as novel inventions. In 1875, for instance, the Reverend Henkle of Logan, Ohio, developed an instrument containing 30 odd, small, sharp needles that pierced the arm in a delicate manner. After administration, the skin was rubbed with oil-causing blisters, said to be an "infallible" preventive.[41] On the other hand, a man from Iowa who thought to save himself the price of a doctor, "cut a plug out of his arm, thrust in some virus from the arm of his sister, who had been vaccinated by a physician a few days before, tied up the wound with a piece of wet newspaper and awaited the result." A short time later, a surgeon was required to amputate the arm and the self-vaccinator found himself in the grave, "beyond the reach of small-pox and other contagious diseases."[42]

The year 1884 was another bad one for Londoners, with 1,000 cases reported at Hackney, a northern suburb. With so many deaths occurring, bodies were carted away during the night to make them less visible, but on May 29, a terrified mob gathered and threatened violence over the frequency of the dead wagon's visits. They had to be restrained by police escorting the vans. The district was black-flagged and isolated, but as there were no actual laws preventing infected persons from leaving smallpox hospitals (they could be prosecuted only for going about), the disease spread rapidly.[43]

To relieve overcrowding in local hospitals, the ship *Castalia* was purchased and fitted up as a hospital for 200 female patients, mooring at Long Reach with two converted man-of-war vessels, the *Atlas* and *Endymion*, holding 100 male smallpox victims. Interestingly, ads appeared in the newspapers seeking kitchenmaids, laundrymaids and cooks for the smallpox ships. Kitchenmaids could earn £18 per annum; laundrymaids £20 and cooks £40. All positions included board, lodging, washing and uniform but did not mention vaccination.[44] By mid–June 1884, the total number of cases in London reached 1,400. The greatest number under treatment during 1880–1881 was 1,650; in the mild epidemic of 1877–1878, the total reached 980, and in 1870–1871, the total was 2,027. The lower numbers for 1884 were attributed to prompt and proper removal of isolation cases as they arose.[45]

Despite that optimism, the number of new cases grew to 500 per week by the first week in December, with a mortality of 12 percent. Hospitals were overcrowded and were predicted to reach their limits within a fortnight. At Leicester, a serious outbreak occurred, believed by the authorities to have been caused or aggravated by the efforts of the Anti-Vaccination Society. The members continued to defy the compulsory vaccination laws and no fewer that 4,000 summons were issued, requiring them to appear before a court and show cause why their children should not be vaccinated. To counter their influence, the chairman of the Law Reference Committee said it ought to be publicly known that the chairman of the anti-vaccination committee of Fulham died of smallpox in early July. Anti-vaccinationists fought back by publishing a pamphlet intended to show that compulsory vaccination had cost Leicestershire $12,500,000 for doctor's fees and incidentals since 1840.[46]

Fatal Smallpox Cases in London, 1884–1885

1st week December	45
2nd week December	33
3rd week December	32
4th week December	33
1st week May	32
2nd week May	44
3rd week May	45
4th week May	28
1st week June	38
2nd week June	34
3rd week June	23
4th week June	21[47]

As there was no substantial evidence on the origin of smallpox, in 1884 the idea was proposed that the disease was carried on the air. Estimates on how far germs could travel ranged from 2–3 feet to 8,000 feet; some authorities even suggested the infection traveled like smoke and might strike a person 50 miles away. Dr. Day, the medical officer of Edmonton and Tottenham, suggested that germs might remain in the air for years until developed by atmospheric conditions.[48]

Killing germs in the air presented a problem, but germicides were one way to destroy topical contagion. People were advised that the best and most powerful of these, in order of their enumeration, were corrosive sublimate, chromic acid, acetic acid, alum and perhaps common alum, pyrogallic acid, tannin, sulphate of copper, permanganate of potash, boric, salicylic, benzoic and picric acids, nitrate of lead and chloride of zinc. The best volatile disinfectants were listed as turpentine, chlorine, iodine, bromine and sulphurous acid, made by burning sulphur. The most used and best fixed disinfectant and germicide was sulphate of iron, while carbolic acid was considered the best volatile one.[49]

In a very interesting study done by Dr. Ogle, superintendent of the Statistical Department of the registrar-general's office, England, he concluded that mortality among physicians was higher than that seen in seven other professions. Doctors died at a rate of 25.63 per 1,000; lawyers died at a rate of 20.23; while parsons showed a death rate of only 15.92.

Causes of Death Among Physicians and Nonmedical Men, Per Million

	Physicians	Nonmedical Men
Smallpox	13	73
Scarlet fever	59	16
Typhus	79	38
Diphtheria	59	14
Typhoid fever	311	238
Alcoholism	178	130
Suicide	283	238

In the matter of suicide, Dr. Ogle reported that poison was the preferred method. Liver disease was the primary killer of doctors, attributed to irregular dietary habits. One statistic from the list stands out: death from smallpox. The low percentage among doctors was attributed to the fact they took better care to have themselves properly vaccinated.[50]

Comparisons of Mortality from Smallpox
1877–1886 (British Medical Association)

Country	Compulsory Status	Average Death Rate
Vienna	Not compulsory	670 per million
London	Only compulsory vaccination for infants	250 per million
Berlin	Compulsory vaccination	10 per million

In England over the prior 62 years (1839–1901) there had been 19 smallpox epidemics. The highest number of deaths (7,912) came in 1871; the lowest, in epidemic years (206), occurred in 1893. In the epidemic of 1884, out of 1,000 mortalities, 86 were of vaccinated children under age 10, while 612 were unvaccinated children.[51]

While the number of smallpox cases in England remained low during the years 1886–1887, the smallpox war over vaccination continued to play out in the newspapers, with both sides arguing different interpretations of the same data. One major demand of the anti-vaccinationists was the repeal of the cumulative penalties clause of the Vaccination Acts. (Previously repealed in 1871 by the House of Commons, but defeated 8–7 in the House of Lords.) The contention that vaccine transmitted other diseases, the controversies over humanized lymph versus cow matter, deaths resulting from vaccination and the argument over personal freedom persisted. Pasteur's experimental "vaccination" or "inoculation" for hydrophobia and his studies for a vaccine to prevent cholera only complicated matters. The *Manitoba Daily Free Press,* July 12, 1880, regretfully noted, "A great many medical men and proportionately many more of the unlearned are at present strongly opposed to vaccination as a preventive of small-pox, and it is not supposable that inoculation for cholera will soon become popular."

The same paper suggested the vaccine be tried "upon the vile bodies of the people in India," and if successful that it be introduced to the people of the West. The idea of using "less desirable" human subjects was not a new one. In 1875, the prestigious *Scientific American* advocated using criminals "in the interest of science" in the study of diseases. The paper added, "We are disposed to think that the possibility of being made a subject for the study of small pox, cholera, typhoid fever, or even a bout of measles or the mumps, would restrain a pickpocket quite as effectively as the chance of a few weeks on the Island or a few months at Sing Sing. At least the knowledge gained by means of him, and others like him would go far to recompense society for all it might suffer from his depredations."[52]

26

"Providence does a great deal for us, the city fathers nothing"

Don't be afraid if small-pox be in your neighborhood. Get some Flour of Sulphur from any Drugstore, put a table spoon full on a tin plate, set it on fire with a lucifer match and fumigate your bedroom morning and night, and oftener, if you like. Perhaps you have been vaccinated; perhaps not; but don't rely on it, if you have been, for some persons have taken small-pox although vaccinated.[1]

The island being occupied in a war with invading Spanish armies, disease ran rampant through Cuba from the end of the 1860s into the 1870s. Reports out of Santiago stated there were so many cases of yellow fever and smallpox that it was impossible to properly bury the dead. Bodies were dumped into shallow graves and as a consequence, the stench from the cemetery became a pestilence in itself. Cuba was not alone: ships from its ports as well as those from Haiti (commonly spelled "Hayti") and many West India ports were quarantined upon arrival at the United States.[2]

The summer of 1878 saw another outbreak of smallpox in Havana but the primary cause of concern was yellow fever; American naval ships were primarily responsible for the inadvertent transport of disease-ridden mosquitoes to Key West, Florida. For the week ending July 20, Havana reported 122 deaths from yellow fever and 13 from smallpox; during the week ending September 7, death rates were 51 and 5 respectively. A year later, yellow fever still killed 28 per week but smallpox deaths had been reduced to one.[3]

Early in 1879, political corruption reared its ugly head. A Cuban girl arrived in Kingston, Jamaica, on January 15, from Santiago-de-Cuba. The steamer presented a clean bill of health, signed by health authorities at Santiago and countersigned by the British consul at that port. Nevertheless, the girl came from an infected district and developed a full-blown case of smallpox within a fortnight of her arrival. Jamaicans charged that if an epidemic developed from this exposure, it was directly attributable "through the indifference of the Cuban Health Authorities, and the culpable carelessness of the British Consul at Santiago-de-Cuba. It is not impossible, however, that the failure of the British Consul to perform his duty on the occasion in question was owing to something different from carelessness."

The writer, in a report dated February 24, charged the British consul of being a member of a Cuban commercial house and a long-time resident of Cuba. Refusal to endorse a clean bill of health already signed by Cuban authorities "would undoubtedly give offence to them and be highly prejudicial to his commercial interests. It is not long since an American Consul was compelled to leave Cuba, because he had sent to his Government an account of the wrong-doings of some Cuban officials." He warned that unless Jamaica had the pro-

VACCINATION IN CUBA.

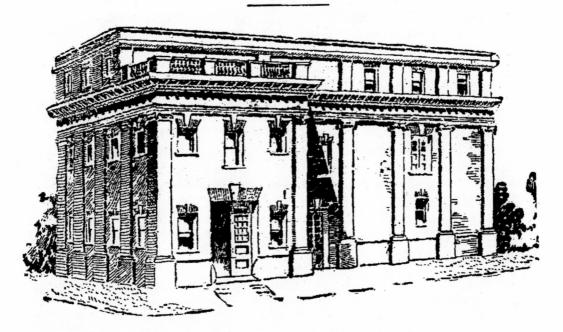

When the American method of vaccination was first introduced to Cuba it was met with a chorus of disapproval and citizens were dragged into the new Vaccination Hospital against their will. When the procedure proved unexpectedly successful, it soon became fashionable to undergo the procedure (from the *Daily Northwestern* [WI], December 7, 1898).

tective vigilance of a consul unhampered by business of his own, the people were subject to the importation of disease. The author proved correct, as subsequent events revealed.[4] In 1883, an epidemic of smallpox raged through Matansas, Cuba, prompting the United States consul to remark, "The only sanitary agents are the rains which clean the streets. There are no gutters, and no sewers. Providence does a great deal for us, the city fathers nothing."[5]

During the cooler months, yellow fever presented less of a problem, but smallpox remained. Reports from the United States National Board of Health dated March 5, 1881, gave statistics showing that at Havana, during the month of February, five patients died of yellow fever while 89 succumbed to smallpox. For the week ending March 4, no deaths were reported from yellow fever, while 31 died of smallpox.[6] During 1882, a brilliant comet was visible in the night sky on neighboring Haiti, striking the natives with awe. People believed the end of the world was approaching. They had reason to consider the comet a bad omen: after the appearance of a previous comet, 60,000 had died of smallpox.[7]

Smallpox in Jamaica

As feared by the February 24, 1879, report concerning the laxness of Cuban and British officials stated above, the girl who arrived in Kingston on January 15 did, indeed, introduce smallpox to the island. Officials quickly appointed public vaccinators. They also instituted a system of registration to keep track of those treated and gave thanks to the medical gentlemen who offered to serve for the inadequate compensation of £20 a month.[8]

The presence of smallpox invariably brought out anti-vaccinationists, who argued along established lines that the operation resulted in blood poisoning. They strayed from canon, however, by taking the position that pandemic diseases throughout history displayed a pattern of becoming weaker and less virulent over time. This being the case, the visitation of smallpox in a milder form across the world (variola) "cannot by any means be regarded as a consequence of vaccination, but as due to COSMO-TELLURIC INFLUENCES," or the Eternal Laws of Nature. Using religion to augment their case, they continued the justification by adding, "As the Creator of the eternal laws of Nature would not alter them on behalf of mankind, *these* epidemic pestilences [smallpox, cholera] arise under the influence of the Cosmo-telluric laws, which are gradually developed until they obtain a certain height, decreasing afterwards until finally disappearing, to give up their places for others of more or less virulent character."[9]

In spite of tremendous efforts to limit smallpox, cases continued to be reported throughout 1881. Discovering the 1879 importation to be far from isolated, citizens demanded that vessels from New York and other places where disease prevailed be quarantined upon entering national harbors.[10]

Vaccination was the only form of preventive immunization against infective diseases until 1880, when Louis Pasteur "developed the attenuation of virulence and protective inoculation of animals against anthrax and chicken cholera."[11] In discussing the recent medical congress in London where M. Pasteur and Professor Tyndall introduced the theory that artificial vaccines for use in humans and animals might be developed for other diseases, including cholera and "splenic fever," the *Gleaner* writer included a paragraph that would ring as true one hundred years later:

> With most of us, vaccination is a grim reminder of childhood, and to increase the number of inoculations and punctures to which a child must submit seems hardly desirable; but if the child can be secured from many of the ills to which in extreme youth it is heir to, then the temporary discomfort of the additional processes will be but a small price to pay for the blessings of health.[12]

In 1881, Pasteur recognized Jenner's contributions by proposing that his own procedures should be called "vaccination," and the substance used a "vaccine." This nomenclature remains common today, although the term "immunization" is often substituted.[13]

Smallpox in South America

In warm climates, smallpox went hand in hand with yellow fever, appearing with frightful prevalence in Central and South America. Reports out of Buenos Aires in October 1871 indicated 26,000 deaths during the summer; spreading across national boundaries, 30,000 more were recorded in the Province of Corrientes, Argentina. With little to prevent it, smallpox reached into Santa Rosa, Chile, particularly along the southern coastal towns. The following year, the combined diseases prevailed at Montevideo and "carried off" 8,000 of the 130,000 inhabitants of three Brazilian towns.[14]

News out of Ceara, in northern Brazil, in 1878, was horrendous. The town was filled with refugees from the interior who fled a famine so gripping rumors circulated that they were compelled to devour carrion and human flesh, and disease made swift inroads. Eyewitness accounts reported people dying with such rapidity and in such great numbers that it was impossible to supply enough coffins, compelling the living to tumble unshrouded corpses into ditches, 8–10 at a time. Open graves only led to more contagion, but by December, with death tolls reaching 500–600 daily and fear at a fever pitch, authorities were powerless to collect bodies for cremation.

The only positive note, and a grim one, was the effort of the Brazilian government to disperse the immigrants, scattering 30,000 of them over the country. Of this number, 1,000 were sent to Para and put to work by the Collins brothers on construction of the Mamora Railroad. This prompted Americans working on the railroad to flee, both from fear of contagion and an inability to become acclimatized. Some returned home, but most lacked the means and were forced to remain.[15]

The horrors in Brazil became the subject of many editorials in the United States, most of which blamed the tragedy on a total lack of communication with the outside world. Although the country suffered under the yoke of famine for two years, no word leaked out, leaving the people without international aid. The *Chicago Tribune* noted that vaccination had never been practiced there and thus epidemics spread throughout the country; singling out Fortaleza (also spelled "Fortalez"), the paper stated that disease was especially virulent there as no sanitary measures were taken to avoid or limit mortality, concluding disease was simply "allowed to wear itself out."[16]

H.H. Smith of *Scribner's Monthly* published a piece in the *New York Herald,* describing his trip into the infected districts and saying Fortaleza was the principal commercial town on the coast. Reiterating the theme of isolation, he concluded that since the city had no harbor and was thus cut off from world traffic, when famine struck in 1877 it required nearly a year for the government to make the outside world aware.

When smallpox struck in June 1878, no one, including the wealthier and aristocratic people, was immune. Panic ensued and by the latter part of November, over 500 people died per day. On the last day of the month, 574 deaths were recorded, bringing the total interment for that 30-day period to 12,000. On the single day of December 10, deaths from smallpox reached 1,000. With a city population of 300,000, that number constituted a greater percentage of mortality than that occasioned by the great London plague. After this black day, death rates declined and by December 20, they had dropped to 200 per day. The total for the year represented a staggering 21,000 fatalities. In all, it was stated that out of a population of 900,000, only 400,000 Brazilians remained.[17]

Reports of smallpox outbreaks continued into the next decade, but with better rates of survival. In September 1880, the disease reached Bogotá, the capital of the republic (Colombia). Fortunately, a strong board of health encouraged vaccination and, aided by newspapers that printed instances of its efficacy, losses were less than elsewhere in South America.[18]

Smallpox in Australia, New Zealand and Fiji

The January 20, 1877, edition of the *London Iron*, in speaking of New South Wales, remarked on the recurrence of smallpox, typhus and typhoid fever with the comment, "Perhaps this yearly visitation is beyond our control; at any rate it appears to be an accepted fact in the profession that all we can do is exercise caution." In regard to smallpox, it was noted the vaccinators were busy, then the question was asked, "Is not the spread of the infectious disorder more due to carelessness of sufferers, or those who have charge of them, than to the natural redundancy of the disease itself?" More vexing was the problem with public vaccinators who received free supplies of lymph but refused to share with private practitioners without a monetary reward.

With the appearance of smallpox in South Australian waters in July 1877, another familiar question arose: the necessity of establishing a permanent quarantine ground somewhere on the coast. Placing the quarantine on land would, it was hoped, eliminate the "folly and misery" of confining large numbers of immigrants on board a hulk and languishing, as was done during the late panic. Sanitary precautions were also debated, with special attention to the city of Adelaide, which suffered from unusually high mortality due to utter want of drainage.[19]

The fear of an epidemic led to increased vaccinations. In Sydney and suburbs, the number of children vaccinated was 5,236, and in the whole colony for 1877, a total of 16,881 underwent the procedure, upwards of 12,000 more than in 1876. No ill effects from vaccination were reported.

On June 15, 1881, an isolated case of smallpox was discovered in Sydney; the man was quarantined and laborers were employed to sprinkle water mixed with carbolic acid over the rooms he had occupied. Several new cases followed in quick succession, all of the victims being unvaccinated. An investigation revealed that the disease was introduced into the city by the steamer *Brisbane,* which arrived from China with a case on board. The report concluded, "Previous to this no epidemic of small-pox had ever occurred in the Australian Colonies."

This, of course, was untrue. An outbreak of what was probably smallpox occurred in 1789, at the recently established Botany Bay colony south of present day Sydney. Only the aboriginal population was affected and the disease spread through the interior. During the years 1829–1831, a second epidemic spread extensively through southeastern Australia. Two other notable outbreaks occurred from 1861 to 1866, along the southern coasts and from 1865 to 1869, along the northwest coast. The first outbreak among Europeans began in 1857, introduced by passengers on a ship from Liverpool.[20]

A hopeful report in August 1881, suggested the threatened epidemic had been averted, with patients in the quarantine station progressing favorably, but this proved overly optimistic. Later that month, cases were reported extending beyond the city limits, affecting unvaccinated children. By September, smallpox had assumed an epidemic character, with 16 fatalities. Great complaints were made of insufficient quarantine arrangements and a royal commission was appointed to investigate.

With the number of infected patients growing, a detached smallpox hospital was established and a vigorous cleaning of the city was undertaken. Houses containing sufferers were marked with yellow flags and guarded by police. A great deal of blame was placed upon the hapless Chinaman from the *Brisbane,* but the "diffusion of the disease is very largely due to the careless blundering of the Government." Calls for physicians went out, there being several medical men in Sydney who had considerable experience with smallpox epidemics in England. They refused to tend the sick, first, because they did not want to be quarantined and second, because they feared losing their practice if patients knew they treated smallpox victims.

Fear of seeing the disease travel from Sydney to Brisbane prompted health officers from the latter colony to unanimously pass new resolutions concerning the creation of new quarantine laws and the establishment of a fever hospital and ambulance wagon. Dr. Bancroft, who attended the meeting of the board of health, approved the proposals, adding that "if the whole of the population were thoroughly vaccinated the disease would soon be extirpated." As there was no lymph available in Brisbane, the government was urged to procure a supply from Sydney or Melbourne.

The health officer of Auckland, New Zealand, had other ideas. An anti-vaccinationist, he chaffed at the idea that quarantine and vaccination protected the citizens, stating that it was "a manifest absurdity and directly contrary to all experience" that such techniques provided protection. With his letter to the board of health, he "exonerated [himself] from all blame" in trusting a "delusion."

By October, the smallpox epidemic at Sydney was waning and there was hope it would soon be extinguished. Hearing that Dr. Benjafield of Hobart, Tasmania, had discovered a calf suffering from true spontaneous cowpox and was making good use by inoculating other animals to obtain a supply of lymph, the board of health sent for a supply that duly arrived. Unfortunately, by December 1, 1881, the outbreak had assumed a far more serious stage, with several deaths reported. It would not be until April that the cases finally abated to the point only one or two were being tracked; by July 1882, South Australia and Victoria were declared free from smallpox. On occasion, individuals still contracted the disease and in August 1884, an isolated case, traceable to Victoria, appeared at Napier, New Zealand, where the victim was quarantined at Auckland.[21]

The health of the Fiji Islands was of great concern to Great Britain, which had pecuniary interests there. The Colonial Office estimated the white population of the islands to be 2,000, about 1,700 being British subjects, mostly of Australian birth or of long residence there. The report stated that zymotic diseases such as smallpox and fever were "as yet nearly unknown in Fiji," as were remittent fever (malaria) and venereal disease. The three most common diseases were asthma, bronchitis and delirium tremens, caused by the popular "kava drinking." It advised that dysentery was the only disease Europeans had to fear.[22]

Although smallpox had not become endemic, in May 1879 the ship *Leonidas* arrived off Nasova with a cargo of 480 coolies, among whom there had been outbreaks of smallpox and cholera. Governor Des Voeux promptly quarantined the vessel until arrangements could be made to land passengers and crew on a small, uninhabited island, where they remained until the disease disappeared and they received "pratique" (a French nautical word meaning "freedom from quarantine"). In the meantime, the natives, fearing an epidemic similar to what they had suffered from measles, "were easily induced to submit to vaccination, and the islands have since completely preserved their immunity from small-pox."[23]

Smallpox in China

In early 1875, the *Peking Gazette* reported on the condition of the emperor, who was prematurely believed to be recovering from smallpox. In appreciation to those who attended him during his illness, numerous members of the royal family were given additional titles and an increase in salary, while the empress dowager granted a generous amnesty to all but the most serious offenders to mark their gratitude for the "safety from harm vouchsafed through the silent protection of the azure vault above."[24]

Vaccination had long been practiced by inhaling dried virus through a silver tube into the left nostril if the patient were a girl and into the right nostril in the case of a boy. Subsequently, virus was dissolved in water and taken into the nostril on a wad of cotton. Missionaries from Great Britain introduced the Jennerian method, and arm-to-arm transfer was practiced from the 1800s in the "Celestial Empire."[25]

Shortly before the emperor's death from the disease, rumors surfaced that the "Goddess of Smallpox "was paraded around the city of Pekin [*sic*] in solemn procession, and then taken into the very bedroom of the dying youth, where it was worshipped and honored with many propitiatory offerings. As, however, the goddess continued obdurate, she was subjected to a severe thrashing and other insults, and finally burned."[26]

Four years later, the European method of vaccination had become generally accepted in China. The sole objection to the technique was the belief that unless a Chinese girl had pockmarks on her face, giving evidence that she had passed through smallpox, she was considered as lacking one of the chief qualifications of a marriageable maiden.[27]

By 1880, acceptance of vaccination was increasing, although at the staff meeting of the Chinese Hospital, Shanghai, vaccinations were slightly decreased from 1879. Due to the success of the operation, however, smallpox was on the decline, not only in Shanghai, but also in the province generally. Vaccination was carried out at Soochow, Sungkiang, Kading and other places on the children of eager Chinese parents. By 1881, letters from Canton stated that an epidemic had broken out among the Chinese, especially at Tartar City, causing a rush for vaccination.

At Hangchow, smallpox ravished the city during the winter of 1881 and through the first quarter of 1882. In what likely referred to improper technique or ineffective vaccine, reports indicated, "those who have been inoculated after the native plan were able to withstand it, but many who had been vaccinated after the foreign method died with the smallpox."[28]

Smallpox in Japan

Although variolation had been used in China for thousands of years, it was not used in Japan until the mid–18th century. Introduction by the Chinese helped stem some of the worst outbreaks but it was not until 1849, when crusts used for vaccination were imported from the Netherlands East Indies, that control of the disease became possible. The World Health Organization noted, "Between 1850 and 1860, smallpox vaccination clinics were opened all over Japan, and their success helped to erode the Japanese inhibition about Western learning." After several severe outbreaks in 1870, a vaccine institute was established in Tokyo in 1874, and a comprehensive vaccination act created in 1876.[29]

Smallpox in India

Most reports of smallpox in the latter half of the 19th century included a discussion of the sanitary conditions of infected cities. The *Colonies and India* of London, July 14, 1877, described Bombay as suffering from defective drainage and an impure water supply, ascribing those deficiencies as the main cause of fevers and smallpox then prevalent. The health department gathered on the average 190 tons of night soil (human waste) per diem, carting it away from the city. However, owing to the want of a complicated drainage system and the presence of open, offensive side drains, the air remained polluted and deaths from cholera and smallpox remained ever-present.[30]

Weekly mortality rates from 1883 until the first quarter of the year 1884 at Madras, on the southeastern coast of India, revealed a staggeringly high death rate from smallpox and other causes, at about 85 per 1,000 per annum. Among the chief difficulties of coping with epidemics was the widespread superstition among Hindus that smallpox was carried by a goddess whose visits should not be interfered with in any way. In studying the history of smallpox, it should not be overlooked that this belief was not widely different than protests made throughout Great Britain, Europe and the Americas after the introduction of inoculation and vaccination. Various Christian groups argued the same point, that as God had visited the disease on mankind, the course of it ought to be accepted rather than fought.

Notwithstanding native opposition, the local council passed an act making vaccination compulsory and the viceroy's assent was obtained by telegraph. It was hoped by this means that mortality among children, the largest segment of the population to be destroyed by smallpox, would be significantly decreased.

The epidemic of 1884 caused great mortality in Rangoon and in cities in Upper India. It was described as "above the average" in Calcutta and appeared to a greater or lesser extent in almost every large city in the country. By early April, reports indicated the disease was raging in the Barolong territory, where many inhabitants perished; those surviving the plague often died from famine as the economy collapsed.[31]

Matters were destined to worsen. A letter written by Dr. Neve of the mission hospital in Cashmere and published in the *Civil and Military Gazette of Lahore,* indicated that English authorities had been able to carry out vaccination to some extent in the portion of India ruled by Great Britain, but Cashmere remained entirely unprotected. Neve was quoted as saying, "It would be nearer the truth to say that the population is annihilated than to say that it is decimated by the scourge of small-pox. Small-pox is epidemic in every village and town of Cashmere."

Dr. Neve's staff compiled a statement of mortality among 25 families, to which 190 children were born and of whom exactly 100 died of the disease. Two or three remained healthy, and the remaining 87 suffered but survived. He concluded, "There is not much room for hoping that these figures indicate any very unusual rate of mortality; and, of course, the evils inflicted by the disease are life-long in many who survive the attacks." The *London Standard,* which published the letter, added, "Here we have presented to us the state of things prevailing in a country where vaccination is unknown."[32]

One of the principal evils alluded to by Dr. Neve was blindness. Numbers from 1881 revealed that in England it was estimated fully one-fifth of sightlessness was the direct result of smallpox. According to the census returns in the United States, there was one blind person for every 1,900 of the population. This was considerably lower than other parts of the world, yet it left over 25,000 Americans "doomed to an existence that has not one ray of redeeming joy."

Germany had the next lowest ratio of blindness, 1:166; England, Scotland and Wales, 1:1,100; Ireland, 1:850; Austria, 1:1000; France, 1:950; Spain, Portugal, Turkey and Greece, 1:800; Russia, 1:900. Norway had the highest percentage of any country called civilized, at a ratio of 1:600. In Asia, statistics indicated a ratio of 1:500 and in Africa, 1:300, owing to the more general prevalence of smallpox. For the entire world, there was a blind population of close to 3,000,000 persons.[33]

In 1884, deaths in Calcutta for the week ending April 4 numbered 320, giving a death rate of 38.5 percent per thousand. In the previous week, there were 296 deaths. Of these,

11 were attributed to smallpox, 101 from cholera, 74 from fevers, 25 from tetanus and 5 causes unknown. The yearly mean for smallpox deaths stood at 11 percent.[34]

Smallpox in Africa

There is little certainty on the origin of smallpox in Africa, with the earliest records indicating one introduction of the disease possibly occurring in A.D. 568, when Ethiopian troops were exposed during the "Elephant War" at Mecca and carried it back to their homeland. During the 11th century, as Islam became a significant factor, pilgrims making the round-trip to Mecca likely contracted the disease and took it home. Arab traders colonizing the eastern coast may also have brought smallpox with them; by 1589, when the Portuguese had become a presence among the coastal towns, they reintroduced the disease, resulting in an epidemic along the coasts of Kilwa and Mombasa.

By the 17th century, the disease was widespread, brought into the interior by slave traders. The southern coast remained free of the disease when the Dutch settled Cape Town in 1652, but in 1713, a ship returning from India sent ashore infected laundry, starting an outbreak. The indigenous Hottentots and Bushmen immediately fell victim. A second importation from Ceylon in 1775 devastated several entire tribes and in 1767, a Danish ship instigated a third epidemic. European settlers, protected by variolation, were spared the worst of the disease, but the natives suffered terrible calamities. Interestingly, some form of variolation existed among Africans as evidenced by Cotton Mather's slave, who reported to him in 1706 that cutaneous inoculation was a common practice in some parts of western Africa.

Slave traders continued to spread the disease, not only to African ports free from smallpox, but also into the lands where they sold their human cargoes. Smallpox remained a severe endemic disease in northern Africa, while six epidemics were recorded in Ethiopia and the Sudan, in 1811–1813, 1838–1839, 1865–1866, 1878–1879, 1885–1887 and 1889–1890.[35]

With Africa assuming greater importance to the British, news of smallpox epidemics finally reached the newspapers. When the disease appeared across the globe in 1879, sanitary officers traced its entrance into South Africa by way of the Transvaal, where it spread rapidly. The news came as no surprise, as it was assumed to be imported through Delagoa Bay (which was still in the hands of the Portuguese), but near the coastline of newly acquired British possessions. The disease was predicted to travel through the diamond fields or the Orange Free State into Cape Colony, bringing into question antiquated quarantine laws and the need for a vigorous vaccination program.

Considering the epidemic that struck Cape Town several years previously did not compel the authorities into systematizing vaccination and relaxing quarantine laws "that are not only detrimental to commerce, but cruel and, in a sanitary sense, useless," it was suggested that the governments of Cape Colony, Natal, the Orange Free State, Griqualand West and the Transvaal create a confederation on sanitary measures with reference to zymotic diseases.[36]

The year 1882 brought an epidemic of smallpox at Cape Town, where 2,000 cases, primarily affecting natives, proved fatal to 600 people. The disease even reached into the military, and the city was declared "infected," meaning that all departing vessels would be quarantined upon reaching their destination. Great excitement prevailed in the diamond fields and all legal measures were taken to exclude infected persons. The streets were reported deserted and business was at a standstill.[37]

Several thousand victims at Cape Town had died by the end of the year when indications finally pointed to an end of the epidemic. The death toll was exacerbated by a disregard for sanitary measures, principal among them the transport of corpses in public hack-carriages and "the Malays hiring out small-pox ambulances for picnics and wedding parties." Quarantine regulations had not been lifted, however, and passengers on outbound ships were held over for six days before landing.[38]

Ships leaving Cape Town were still suspect in 1883, as word of the devastation became public. Advisors in the city notified the United States consul at St. Helena that during the prior two months, 9,000 people were affected with smallpox, of which 2,400 died. Epidemics continued and in 1884, advisors from Western Africa reported that smallpox raged at Coomassie, Ashantee.[39]

By the 19th century, inoculation appeared in many parts of Africa, although not significantly diffused to influence the general health of the population. Inoculation sites on the body varied from region to region — forehead, arm, leg and what was called "the anatomist's snuff-box," on the dorsum (back or posterior) of the hand at the base of the metacarpal of the thumb. The latter, along with the forearm, were also used as preferred sites in Afghanistan and Persia.[40]

Smallpox Gleanings from Around the World

As the world marched toward the 20th century, very little was settled pertaining to smallpox and vaccination, while "cures" continued to pop up with regularity. Norwegians, for example, were reported to wear a bag of sunflower seeds around their necks to keep smallpox away,[41] which may explain the high incidence of the disease in that country. In Prussia, after a smallpox victim escaped into the snow and remained uncovered all night, he was returned to the ward, where it was observed his fever had subsided and the pustules dried. Using this discovery, the temperature in the hospital was kept low and quantities of ice were applied to patients, resulting, it was said, in complete cures.[42]

A German physician stated his theory that smallpox originated from an excess of albuminous matter in the blood and suggested the disease might be cured by common salt, presumably to counter the over-sugared diets of modern society. Administration of organic acids like lemon juice was supposed to unclog the blood from too much albumen.[43]

The German doctor was far from alone; many who abandoned the name "anti-vaccinationist" began styling themselves "hygienists." The theme was the same, however, as they protested against the value of vaccination, saying instead that "smallpox is a disease of filth. It has never been known to make much headway among cleanly people. Those who live on meats, greese [sic], highly concentrated and stimulating food are not cleanly people, strictly speaking. Their systems are weakened by excessive stimulating and by gross food until the vessels are unable to carry off the necessary secretions of waste matter, and the result is corruption."

Using the American Civil War as an example, one of the new hygienists remarked that many Negroes in the South died of smallpox, while "Union forces were scarcely troubled by the disease." He based his theory on the strict rule among slaveholders to have their slaves vaccinated. Since vaccination did not save them, he inferred that Northern soldiers fared better from discipline and clean living.[44]

Along with modern diets and prejudicial pseudoscience, "aristocratic blood" proved a hindrance. Hygienists believed that due to luxury, pampered habits and overfeeding, children of this class suffering from the disease were not suited to provide vaccine matter; only "perfectly healthy children" were optimal, but such individuals were scarce. In Amsterdam, therefore, doctors went back to Jenner's first principle and "go to the calf direct to vaccinate babies." Mothers brought their infants to the Amsterdam General Hospital, where a calf was secured to a table ("the report says 'comfortably,' but of this the SPCA must judge") and the physician performed the operation by transferring lymph from the animal directly to the arm of each infant. Three-fourths of all vaccinations in Holland were performed in this manner and it was claimed that during epidemics, a "quite unlimited supply of calf lymph can be obtained in five days."[45]

The year 1882 witnessed a number of epidemics around the world. The disease was especially virulent in Panama, where both "confluent" and "black" smallpox claimed victims. Newspapers noted that health boards made recommendations, "but the local government are apathetic in carrying them out."[46] Death rates, from both smallpox and yellow fever, continued to climb as the neighboring city of Colon, Aspinwall, experienced mortalities, not only among laborers and strangers but also among officials of the Panama Canal Company. With an estimated population of 6,000 (including 2,500 canal workers), 100 died per month, leaving the city nearly void of people. The "ever increasing filth of the city" was ascribed as the cause.[47]

Not surprisingly, the United States surgeon general received a report from Brownsville, Texas, warning that black smallpox was causing great mortality in the towns of Tamailan and Periacon, Mexico, as well as in Guatemala, the victims being mostly foreigners.[48] A warning the following year indicated that visitors to the Mexican capital got vaccinated before they went, as the board of health made no attempt to isolate smallpox patients "and the people at large pay no attention to it."[49] With little to prevent smallpox, it continued to plague Mexico and in December 1885, Governor Ireland of Texas quarantined the Rio Grande border against its importation.[50] The order may have come too late, for in January 1886, Fort Stockton reported an epidemic there and had to be quarantined. Fort Davis, Murphyville, Marpa, Toyah Creek and many of the ranches stretching to the Rio Grande continued to be infected. The state health officer also quarantined Presidio del Norte, too late to prevent the counties of Pecos, Reeves and Presidio from suffering the scourge.[51]

The disease known as "black smallpox" raged through coastal towns and settlements in the southern interior of Mexico throughout the summer of 1887, and the threat of oncoming winter brought grim speculations on how many empty graves might be filled. It was believed to have spread through Nogales as far as Tucson, although in a milder form. "Carelessness along the coast" was blamed for the epidemic.[52]

Statistics from Prussia and the Compulsory Vaccination Law

Statistics indicate that up until 1870, mortality in Prussia had been fairly steady. But the great smallpox epidemic of 1870–1872 changed matters. In 1872 and 1873 respectively, mortality rose to 243 and 262 per 100,000 inhabitants. In order to control the disease, a law was passed enforcing vaccination in the first year of life and revaccination at age 12 years. The law went into effect in 1875. The following table compares mortality per 100,000 people between Prussia, where a vaccination law existed, and Austria, where no such compulsory law was in effect:

Statistics Comparing Prussia and Austria

Year	Prussian Mortality	Austrian Mortality
1875	3.6	57.7
1876	3.1	39.2
1877	0.3	53.7
1878	0.7	60.3
1878	0.7	50.8
1879	1.2	60.3
1880	2.6	82.6
1881	3.6	
1882	3.6	

On August 29, 1885, the *British Medical Journal* reported that not a single death had occurred in the German army since the year 1874. It was calculated that as the result of vaccination and revaccination in Berlin and other German cities, in the nine years from 1875 to 1883, smallpox mortality was 1.7 per 100,000 on average, against 25.83 in London and 89.29 in Vienna.[53]

Russia and the Russo-Turkish War

The Medical Bureau of Russia published its report on the health of the country for the year 1877, showing that in a population of 80 million, the mortality rate ranged from 30 to 50 per thousand, marking one of the highest death rates of any country that collected statistics. Diphtheria ranked as the number one disease, followed by typhoid fever and smallpox. Of the population, 14,000,000 sectarians did not allow vaccination, accounting for the large mortality from that disease.[54]

The seemingly never-ending conflicts of the century continued with the Russo-Turkish War (1877–1878). By April 1878, the Russian government estimated a loss of over 80,000 soldiers, but devastation to civilian populations was equally high due to maladies arising out of war. At Alexandropol, owing to the passage of 70,000 sick and wounded soldiers and the neglect of the sanitary authority to take requisite precautions, the death rate reached 55 out of 1,000 persons. At Titlis, doctors from the Red Cross were reported dead, while in the Caucasus plague was expected. As seen in all wars, prisoners carried disease with them; in this case, Turkish prisoners from Armenia spread epidemics in their wake. At Penza, smallpox and measles were so rife that schools and institutions were closed by order of the government.

Official reports stated contagious disease was present in every house, while near St. Petersburg, the black smallpox ("a form of the Persian plague") broke out among Turkish prisoners at Gatchina, causing great alarm in the capital.[55] Further reports from the office of the U.S. surgeon general dated July 12, 1878, gave information from Constantinople. It stated the bulk of the Russian army had removed to healthier campgrounds while most of the refugees had departed for Asia Minor and Syria, leaving 30,000 behind. Of this group, typhus, smallpox, measles and scarlet fever, which had prevailed extensively since the war, was slowly abating.[56]

Plagues persisted in Russia through 1879, with smallpox and typhus fever appearing to a large extent in Tiver, where out of 100 cases, 18 proved fatal. Great mortality from smallpox also occurred at Orsk, along with another "unknown" disease, followed by extensive reports of cattle plague.[57]

Always with an eye toward war, whether defensive or offensive, an 1885 report stated that owing to the constant vaccination and revaccination among European armies, smallpox deaths in Europe numbered 60,000 annually, but that mortality was confined almost entirely to civilians.[58]

27

Of Rags and Railroads

Small-pox is said to be equally as bad among the natives of Springfield, Mass. as among the immigrants in Minnesota. It is no respecter of persons or classes, and hence the importance of proper precautions everywhere. The disease is drifting southward from Cincinnati and Chicago, and the States east of the Mississippi are urging vaccination.[1]

The 1880s in the United States were characterized by a fear of spreading contagion. Nearly every newspaper carried stories of how smallpox was carried from one state to another, from city to city and by one individual to the next. The primary culprits were railroads and steamboats; however, while the finger of accusation pointed at specific vessels, immigrants came in for the worst of it.

From "sea to shining sea," foreigners were considered culprits, aided and abetted by the purveyors of mass transportation, who themselves were occasionally victimized by the disease. It was not infrequent to read reports such as the one out of Reno, where a "Chinawoman," recently arrived in that city from San Francisco, introduced the disease to Martin, the brakeman of the Virginia and Truckee Railroad, who died of it. This caused a scare in Virginia, where drugstores sold great quantities of disinfectants, the services of vaccinationists were sought and children wore bags of camphor around their necks.[2] The folk remedy failed, as the president of the Virginia Board of Health reported that for the first week of January 1882, there were 98 new cases being treated, of which "76 are colored and 22 whites." The city experienced five new cases a day. The following year, smallpox was introduced into Wheeling, West Virginia, by a tramp who had taken sick while en route through the country. The disease spread with alarming rapidity and within two weeks, 40 cases were reported, with 15 deaths.[3] Not surprisingly, the *Burlington Hawkeye* reported that steamboats from St. Louis were distributing smallpox along the river towns.[4]

As much as states feared contagion from San Francisco, the city remained a magnet for foreign and domestic émigrés, and with them came disease. Prior to the smallpox epidemic of 1876–1877, vaccination was by no means general, even among the American population. But during this crisis, the board of health made vaccination compulsory for every child attending public schools. No fewer than 34,020 children were vaccinated between 1877 and 1881, with an additional 60,000 vaccinated with heifer lymph. Vaccination was not enforced on the Chinese, however, and consequently, the disease remained prevalent. The danger of contamination was obvious, as artists and laundrymen frequented the city but nothing was done to allay the danger.

After a steady importation of smallpox from eastern cities threatened the general welfare, the disease became epidemic in November 1880, rising from 65 the first week to 147 by the end of the month. Thereafter, cases declined everywhere but in the Chinese quarter. With a population of 233,700 in 1881, nearly one-tenth of that number were Chinese. The death rate of all nationalities stood at 18.27 per 1,000; for whites alone, it was 17.2, and for the Chinese, the rate climbed to 21.2 per 1,000.

On November 9, 1881, the board of health requested that the governor issue orders for inspection and quarantine of all trains approaching the boundary of the state. This was immediately complied with, special emphasis being placed on the Central Pacific Railroad that ran from Chicago. There was also fear of having the disease spread from New Tacoma, Washington Territory, where 69 cases were found; already, physicians reported smallpox had spread to the Puyuhys Indian Reservation by two Indians who had recently visited New Tacoma. Across the ocean in Honolulu, Hawaii, deaths from smallpox persisted among the natives, although few cases were reported among the whites. Infected locals were taken to a reef and isolated, although little could be learned from them as to the ravages of the disease.[5]

As the disease penetrated into the better sections of San Francisco, a rush for vaccination occurred (there being no anti-vaccination league in the city) and the supply was soon exhausted. As soon as new supplies arrived, fresh cases became rare, with only 10 or 12 reported out of 94,000 children vaccinated in the five preceding years. The conclusions drawn by the city fathers were these:

1. The dire effects of what may be called a smoldering fire of smallpox in keeping up a source of infection in the Chinese quarter that might break out into renewed conflagration;
2. The non-limitation of smallpox infection to any class of society;
3. The protective power of efficient vaccination.

Railroads continued to take blame for spreading smallpox and in 1887, officials of the Northern Pacific Railroad requested the state board of health to investigate their culpability, or lack thereof, in Los Angeles, where 30,000 "points" had recently been requested to aid in vaccinating the public.[6]

The Spread of Smallpox "in mysterious ways"

As the self-styled "Queen of the West" and an important railroad hub, Chicago stood out as both an — unintended — importer and an exporter of smallpox. Additionally, in January 1881, citizens complained that no one shoveled the 723 miles of sidewalks and the local government was in the process of licensing 2,000 "low, disreputable places, where vice and immorality abound." Ten years after the legend of Mrs. O'Leary's cow setting fire to the city, thousands of defective flues, seldom inspected by authorities, presented the omnipresent danger of repetition. Though $2,000,000 lay in the city treasury, it was concerned citizens who donated 25 cents into a fund that helped the poor pay for coal.

Life, in the general sense, was good, but death from smallpox still averaged 10 percent per week, with diphtheria, scarlet fever and croup remaining prevalent in certain districts.[7] At a meeting of the Illinois State Board of Health, the cause of smallpox was attributed to foreign immigrants. As Chinese labor in Chicago was being used in a new paper brick factory, members urged Congress to pass a law requiring all immigrants to be vaccinated immediately upon arrival in the United States. Significantly, the request fell short of demanding compulsory vaccination for residents.[8] The national board of health recognized the need, and sent to the president regulations requiring all immigrants arriving in the United States from any port where smallpox existed to undergo vaccination (unless protected by previously having had the disease) and kept in quarantine for 16–17 days. The request was approved, with authorization given November 14, 1881. In like manner, acting postmaster-general Hatton issued an order allowing local postmasters to refuse mail from cities under quarantine.

Smallpox continued throughout the year, with 118 Chicago deaths in December. On December 9, word circulated that San Francisco had established quarantine against Chicago. The chief medical officer remarked that if this were true, the only thing Chicago could do would be to quarantine against New York.[9] Vaccinations offered a second solution and during the month, 30,000 free vaccinations were issued and arrangements for 50,000 more were planned for January. This seems to have been effective, as the number of new cases dropped from 15 to 4 per day.[10]

Local quarantine was also put into effect but efforts at control were ineffective. In January 1882, a case drawing national attention concerned a smallpox carrier who escaped Chicago authorities and took the Pullman on the Baltimore and Ohio to Wilmington. The national board of health attributed to him the spread of the disease in that city, as well as in Baltimore. The report further indicated that smallpox prevailed in 18 states and territories, and was considered epidemic in Philadelphia, Pittsburgh, Allegheny, Cincinnati, Chicago, some parts of Indiana, Illinois, Missouri, Michigan, Minnesota, California, Oregon and the Montana and Indian territories.[11]

Steamship companies proved capable of screening passengers, but railroads required a more formal arrangement. Out of $50,000 appointed by Congress for its use, the national board of health paid for train inspections that were at least somewhat effective in curbing the spread of smallpox. The question of how long federal subsidies would continue to support such inspections was never far from the minds of state authorities, who would have to assume responsibility in the event funds dried up.

Along with states, counties and municipalities worried about the financial costs of smallpox. In Bellevue, Iowa, for example, during the winter of 1881–1882, smallpox bills aggregated to about $3,800, of which the county paid $2,600, leaving the city to pay $1,200. The cost, directly and indirectly to the town, including loss of business, amounted to $50,000. During 1882, Baltimore had 480 deaths from smallpox out of a reported 2,825 cases. During the year, 90,000 vaccinations and revaccinations were performed. The expense to the public was $100,000.

Perhaps the most apt observation of cost came from the *Newport Mercury* (RI), April 14, 1888: "The bill for taking care of the late small pox patient which has just been presented amounts to $377. Of which sum one dollar and forty cents is for medicine. At the above rate it will not pay to have many cases of small pox in town."

In an innovative collaboration between government and business, the New Orleans Sanitary Commission and delegates from the Cotton Exposition devised a plan to permanently eradicate smallpox from that city. It called for the employment of 15 physician sanitary inspectors, to be paid at $100/month; 10 sanitary police at $50/month and the appropriation of $500 for the purchase of vaccine. The Cotton Exchange and chamber of commerce approved the plan, with $5,000 appropriated to carry it into effect.[12]

Cooperation of a more insidious nature occurred in Indianapolis. After newspapers reported new cases of smallpox, businessmen demanded that the information be suppressed, "since it would deter persons from visiting this place and do business here." One editor observed, "The idea is a wrong one, but such is human nature. The Indianapolis papers are being soundly berated" for publishing the statistics.[13]

In relation to the above, a more guileful practice was to lie to the public concerning the presence of smallpox. At Bloomburg, British Columbia, in 1881, for example, railroad workers contracted the disease and the death of one was covered up in order to prevent stoppage of work. On a larger scale, health officer Bramble of the New York Sanitary Department withheld the real facts regarding the ravages of smallpox, issuing false numbers on August 24, 1882, to make it appear the disease was far less widespread. Although he refused to offer any explanation, it was supposed his purpose was to create the illusion he was ridding the city of smallpox, and to protect trade from being injured.[14]

Mr. Bramble was not alone. "Cheap doctors" could often be found who would conceal the fact of smallpox in private homes in consideration of an extra fee, while "old" physicians who had been practicing before the establishment of health boards often declared such public institutions held no authority over them. These instances went along with the "war on quack doctors" that the *Newport Daily News* (March 6, 1882) declared was being lost. Many erstwhile physicians were exposed for having no diploma, but they went right on with their business. "After exposure they generally get up some sort of partnership with regulars of the shyster order, and as these have diplomas they cannot be interfered with while they keep within the law. The 'whack-up' principle is carried out of course, and the quack can laugh at authority."

New York City recorded 300 vaccinations per day in January 1882, the largest number since the vaccinations bureaus were established in 1875, but reports of contagion continued to spread, with immigrants being the easy target. Canadian French were blamed for the isolation of Sioux City, Dakota, resulting in loss of United States mail delivery and the refusal of railroads to enter its depots; cities in Pennsylvania and the city of Troy, New York, likewise blamed outbreaks on French Canadians; the first smallpox epidemic in Boston since 1874, when 1,040 persons died, appeared in early 1871, and was blamed on the importation of smallpox from Europe. The *Scientific American* blamed a shipload of Italians for bringing smallpox into the country and even cats were blamed for spreading smallpox: owners were urged not to let their pets roam about.[15]

On January 20, 1882, the national board of health in Washington, DC, declared, "There is no doubt that the disease [smallpox] was originally imported. Countries from which persons emigrate to America are almost without exception infected with the disease. There were between 1,200 and 1,400 deaths in Philadelphia from small-pox during 1881, and about 700 fatal cases in New York." The executive committee then declared smallpox to be epidemic in the United States and appropriated $2,000 to prevent smallpox in the District of Columbia.[16] Yet everything was not smooth sailing in Congress, as Mr. Cox of the House of Representatives offered an amendment to abolish the national board of health after September 1, 1882, on the grounds it encroached on state boards "and had no right to investigate small-pox any more than measles." He was ultimately forced to withdraw the amendment.[17]

Danger from Rags

When immigrants were not directly accused of introducing smallpox, the culprit most often blamed in the 1880s was the humble rag. The United States health officer in London, Dr. Hill, sent a report to Washington, asserting that the exportation of rags into America from England (primarily used in the manufacture of paper) was fraught with great danger. Quantities of rags were collected in London and the Continent, where disease was prevalent. Without undergoing any type of disinfectant, they were packaged into bales and shipped, often with countries of origin obscured. In one case, 23 bales were shipped to New York on the *Lydian Monarch* upon representation they had not been collected from infected districts. Investigation showed they actually came from Dunkirk, France, where epidemic cholera was present.

Lacking national regulations and effective inspections, death rates from exposure to smallpox by infected rags continued to inflict small but significant numbers. In 1882, the town of Pepperell, Massachusetts, was infected through rags used in the paper mill. Taking matters into their own hands, the state board of health recommended that paper mill owners make evidence of successful vaccination a prerequisite for employment. Little, if any, national improvement was made, and as late as 1889, imported rags from Egypt spread smallpox to women employed in the rag-room in Windsor Locks, Connecticut.[18]

Rags, of course, were not the only medium through which smallpox was spread and isolated incidents were the rule rather than the exception. An outbreak on a small island in the Mississippi River near Harrisonville, Illinois, started after an infected mattress, thrown into the river, lodged upon its coast. A tenant, tearing down wallpaper in his room that had been on the walls during a previous scourge, contracted the disease from it and died in the pesthouse.[19]

This post–World War I advertisement from the *Dunkirk Evening Observer* (NY), April 3, 1919, extols the benefits of cleaned and sterilized clothes similar to those supplied by the U.S. Army for the boys in the trenches. Considering that rags imported from Europe for paper manufacture were a secondary cause of transmitting the smallpox virus, the point was well taken.

Potentially more dangerous were two instances of infected mail occurring within several days of one another. On January 18, 1882, Cincinnati newspapers reported the "latest form of vengeance," which took the form of enclosing several smallpox scabs in a letter with the announcement, "I have sent you the small-pox d — n you, now go home and die!" On January 20, an undated and unsigned letter was received at Richmond, Indiana, containing two smallpox scabs and a similar letter, merely omitting the profanity. The *Columbus Times* believed the scare was perpetrated by someone hoping to force the postmasters to resign.[20]

If rags and mail did not kill the American of the 1880s, that person stood a fair chance of dying from believing what they read in the newspapers. There were also incidents like that of the East Atchison, Kansas, inventor who sold barrels of his concoction, "Small Pox Bitters," as a preventive but actually filled the bottles with cheap whisky.[21]

Smallpox in Daily Life

Doctors wore rubber suits when treating smallpox patients, yellow patches flew above houses to warn away visitors (red flags were also used for the same purpose), wagons scattered chloride of lime throughout the streets and burning tar barrels were used to ward off germs; yet smallpox continued to be epidemic in some states and as isolated cases in others. In Kansas City, flooding of the Missouri River not only carried away the island on which a pesthouse had been established, but the waters also bore coffins toward St. Louis. By 1888, Wisconsin was surrounded by infected states contiguous to its borders. In order to promote prevention and restrict occurrences, circulars promoting free vaccination were printed in English, German and Norwegian.[22]

In an appealing human-interest story, a drug clerk in San Antonio relayed that men undergoing vaccination tended to "squirm and flinch like they were having a leg taken off. It is not affectation but mere fright.... The idea is prevalent that ladies are timid and easily frightened. My experience has proven the contrary. After the flesh is bared for the operation they undergo it with the greatest fortitude, and with

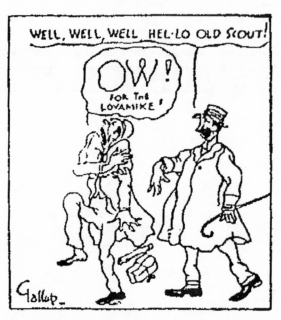

When slapped on the arm by a cordial friend a sense of deep annoyance sets in.

This cartoon from 1916 uses humor to depict a common scenario. The caption reads, "When slapped on the arm by a cordial friend a deep annoyance sets in." The victim cries, "OW! For the Lovamike" and drops his parcels. Interestingly, vaccinators often observed that women were braver than men when receiving the smallpox vaccine (from the Waterloo *Evening Courier* [IA], March 22, 1916).

none of that flinching that one would expect from a lady." He added that ladies not wishing to have visible scars often asked to have the procedure performed on their legs; when they did have the vaccination on the arm, they invariably preferred to have the sleeve ripped than remove their waist or jersey and disclose their corsets. The clerk noted that Negroes and Mexicans were ignorant of the value of vaccination, although they would bring in their children while denying it for themselves. Mexicans, especially, shunned doctors, erroneously believing they would be arrested if a case of smallpox were found in their house.[23]

Tragic errors in misdiagnosis were not uncommon, although the case of Miss Angeline M. Brown differed from the typical newspaper report. Miss Brown, a successful New York City florist, brought suit against Alfred S. Purdy and his son, Alfred E.M. Purdy, both physicians who had treated the plaintiff in 1879. She alleged that upon being called to treat her, the Purdys determined she suffered from smallpox and notified state authorities. Despite strenuous protestations that her face had become marked from scratching and her bilious condition was brought on by a druggist prescribing some compound pills that made her vomit, she was sent to the reception hospital on 16th Street and in the morning was transferred by boat to Blackwell's Island during a pouring rain.

Physicians at the smallpox hospital as well as Dr. Janeway of the health department all declared she actually suffered from eczema and should never have been brought there. Because her name was published as a smallpox patient, her customers refused to patronize her business. She testified that she made a yearly profit of $2,000–$8,000 and sued for $10,000. The ante was higher in a California case, where Mrs. Hattie McLand brought suit against the Los Angeles municipality for removing her daughter to a smallpox hospital, where she died. The plaintiff sought $100,000 damages.[24]

A case of a different sort occurred in Steubenville, Ohio, where a youth named Benton Coulter, formerly an actor in Sells Brothers Circus, came down with smallpox. He was mistakenly identified as a man named Wise, who was wanted for the attempted murder of a boy. Coulter was on his way to recovery when the warrant was served on him; immediately after hearing the charge, he suffered a relapse and died. Adding disgrace to the fatal mistake, Coulter's remains were kept in an outhouse for four days before they were interred.

A case actually brought to trial had an unanticipated ending when the sequestered jury believed one of its members had come down with smallpox. Although it was later determined to be no more than a case of nettle rash, the jurors bolted, forcing the judge to declare a mistrial. On the other hand, Governor Blackburn of Kentucky came under criticism for refusing to grant a reprieve to a condemned murderer on account of his dying from smallpox. The date for his hanging was set a week in advance and there were doubts the criminal would survive long enough to be executed.[25]

Deaths from smallpox of individuals belonging to a more noted class included David Navarro, the Fat Boy of circus fame, who died at a pesthouse on March 7, 1882, while Mrs. Caroline Richings Bernard, the famed English opera singer who was born in London but came to America at the age of one year, died at Richmond, Virginia, in January 1882, of the "worst type" of smallpox. Members of the Mozart Musical Association attended her funeral and she was buried in Hollywood Cemetery, not far from the tomb of President James Monroe and the grave of Confederate general J.E.B. Stuart. (Later in the decade, Dr. Erasmus Garrett, chief medical inspector of Chicago's health department and one of the most eminent authorities on smallpox in the world, died of heart failure.)[26]

Ancient and Modern Theories Concerning Germs and Scars

Dutch businessman and amateur lens grinder Anton van Leeuwenhoek (1632–1723) refined the single-lens microscope in the 17th century, giving rise to a new science that expanded theories that had actually began nearly two thousand years earlier. Classical Greek physicians such as Hippocrates held the premise that disease arose from imbalances in the four basic humors: red blood, yellow bile, black bile and mucus. If any of the humors became out of balance, they were believed to erupt through the skin in the form of sores or blisters.

The Persian-born physician Abu Bakr Muhammad Ibn Zakariya, better known as al-Razi, or "Rhazes" (circa A.D. 865–925), expanded the humoral idea of disease, posing an "innate seed theory," which suggested within each human there existed the germs of smallpox and other maladies. Changes in atmospheric conditions could germinate these seeds in the form of sores on the skin.[27] Fear of contracting disease in such a manner likely mutated into the idea of miasma or "unhealthy air," widely believed throughout the 19th century to cause contagious diseases such as smallpox, yellow fever and cholera. Throughout the 1800s, numerous references from physicians, lay people and sanitary commissions warned of draining swamps and cesspools. The idea of liming outhouses and drying standing water certainly had a positive effect on eliminating mosquitoes (and thus yellow fever), but not for the reasons supposed at that time.

A brilliant theory developed by an Italian from Verona named Girolamo Fracastoro (1487–1553) took Rhazes' ideas further by stating that "seminaria" (small seeds of disease) could be transmitted from person to person through a variety of means. In his paper, "De Contagione et Contagiosis Morbis et Eorum Curatione," he suggested smallpox and measles possessed unique seminaria.[28] Contemporary scientists had the added benefit of receiving the translated works of Rhazes, published at Basil in 1543.

On the return of Christians from the Crusades, the writings of Rhazes and Avicenna became better known. Significantly, Rhazes, who entertained a profound reverence for Galen, pointed out that ancient authority left no description of what could be positively diagnosed as smallpox. It is a fact that neither the Greeks nor the Roman physicians described any disease that is unquestionably identified as smallpox.[29]

With van Leeuwenhoek's improvement of lenses, the presence of microscopic organisms was demonstrated, giving new appreciation to Fracastoro's theories; ideas postulating that the spread of smallpox was due to "animalcules" (miniscule animals) became widely discussed. In 1772, Thomas Fuller further developed the idea that disease was spread through unique "seeds" or animalcules in his "Pharmacopoeia Extemporinea": "The Pestilence can never breed the Small-Pox the Measles ... any more than a Hen can a Duck, a Wolf a Sheep, or a thistle Figs."[30] Unfortunately, the smallpox virus was too minute to be detected by early microscopes and the concept of miasma continued to dominate medical thinking.

During the late 1800s a plethora of medical discoveries were made, among the more significant of which concerned germ theory. Already, Louis Pasteur had put forth his proposals on curing hydrophobia by inoculation; further research by other scientists developed the relationship between germs and disinfectants. In 1884, the *Gesundheit* published the theory that it was extremely probable that the germs producing smallpox were "present in the form of living bacilli in the fluid which is the principal bearer of the infection — the lymph removed from the pustule. The degree of vitality of the bacilli varies in the different kinds of lymph, that from the cow-pox losing vitality much more readily than the so-called human lymph."[31]

A year later, Professor S.A. Forbes, of the Illinois State College at Champaign, identified a spherical germ causing remarkable mortality among the perch in Lake Mendota, Wisconsin. Described as "about one-twenty-five-thousandth of an inch in diameter," it attacked the liver and kidneys of the fish, forming abscesses and destroying the cells of the organ. The professor classified the germ as belonging to a group that produces smallpox, chicken pox and hog cholera.[32]

Although seldom a topic of discussion in the United States, the German Medical Convention at Berlin determined that several pustules (as opposed to a single pustule) should be used to ensure protection. In supporting the theory, Dr. Robert Koch's research of 703 patients at the Stockwell Hospital revealed that of those who died, 47 percent had no scars; 25 percent had poor scars; 5.3 percent had one scar; 4.1 percent had two scars; 2.3 percent had three good scars and mortality among those with four or more scars resulted in a death rate of only 1.1 percent. Koch therefore took the position that the protective power of vaccination was in direct relation to the number of vaccine pustules. In this, the authorities Grosshelm, Siegel and Arnsperger supported him.[33]

Although the relationship between tuberculosis and smallpox was not fully understood, the Congress on Tuberculosis, 1889, announced the fact that persons who had smallpox were peculiarly liable to tuberculosis and concluded that those pitted with smallpox should never work around tuberculosis wards.[34] And for those interested in conclusions drawn from observation, Southey's *Commonplace Book* reported that a physician who had seen over 40,000 cases of smallpox stated he had never met with the disease in a person with red or light flaxen hair.[35]

Moving into the last decade of the century, perhaps nothing better summed up the American entrepreneur's "take" on smallpox than the following:

The Chicago Sanitary News says that during the prevalence of small pox in Paterson, New Jersey, Dr. David Robinson, a physician and preacher circulated a tract setting forth his views on the subject of contagious diseases. He has now filed a bill amounting to $5,000 against the city for lowering the death rate of the city by means of his circulars. He charges $1,500 for showing by means of his publications that the ravages of small pox can be stopped by the use of hot tea.[36]

28

School Boards Win Some
and Lose Some

Let us abide in the hope that the Jenner centennial celebration, provided by this association and to be a part of its exercises at the annual meeting in 1896, may bring out the boundless blessing of the discovery of that immortal Jenner in such wise that all men shall see and acknowledge its protective powers, and even the wayfaring man, though a fool, may not err by further causeless cavil.[1]

The 1890s in the United States were characterized by outbreaks of smallpox across the country, the debate over compulsory vaccination, the waxing and waning of the anti-vaccinationists and a Supreme Court decision. Aside from the latter, the decade differed little from its predecessors.

After 8 years of almost complete freedom from smallpox, the disease appeared in Ohio, Pennsylvania and Illinois in January 1892. These states were situated at the crossroads of the east-west railroad trunk lines, and authorities in Indiana urged all local boards of health to enforce measures for prevention and suppression. By July, when it became obvious that smallpox was also being transmitted along the Great Lakes, Ohio and Mississippi rivers, the United States Marine Service was called upon to quarantine and supervise vaccinations of passengers on contaminated vessels. Continuing into the next year, local physicians at Logansport, Indiana, called for massive vaccinations as the city was vulnerable because of its location as a railroad center.[2]

It did not take long for epidemics to occur in major cities: New York, Pittsburg, Cincinnati, Detroit, Boston and Chicago all reported smallpox by the end of the year. As a safeguard, the War Department ordered every army post in the country to apply good sanitary conditions, so that if disease did appear it would not spread on account of unhygienic conditions.[3]

Reports from Chicago indicated that immigration continued to be a problem. In April 1893, Chinese actors coming to the city to perform at the fair were found to be infected. Unfortunately, all had been allowed to depart on the steamer *Mogul.* On further investigation, it was discovered that none of the Chinese merchants visited had certificates of health inspection. At New York, where contagious arrivals were crowded on Hoffman and Swinburne islands, mass vaccinations were begun to try to contain the disease. The year 1893 proved to be a record-breaking one for vaccinations in New York City. In a twist on physicians visiting private dwellings to perform the service, vaccinating corps visited large department stores, providing protection to customers and employees alike. It was estimated that by the end of the year, 175,000 vaccinations would be performed, 65,000 more than in 1892.[4]

Across the nation, governors and mayors began issuing orders for compulsory vaccination. In Waterloo, Iowa, for instance, where there had been no general vaccination for the past ten years, the mayor felt it was the "proper time" to begin vaccinating children. In Reading, Pennsylvania, fines of $100 per violation were issued to parents who sent their children to school without being vaccinated within the previous seven years.[5] Difficulties of a different nature came from the Amish of Holmes County, Ohio, who believed every person had an appointed time to die and if God wanted to remove them by smallpox, it was not their right to question.[6]

Representatives from Wisconsin, Minnesota, Indiana, Michigan and Illinois held a secret meeting on April 19, 1884, to determine whether they should collectively quarantine Chicago. According to the *Chicago Tribune,* there were at that time 200 cases in the city and that precautions against the disease were insufficient. The newspaper blamed commissioner of health Reynolds for being unable to cope with the disease, which had been mildly epidemic for several months. In pure Chicago-style, the editorialist added, "If Mayor Hopkins can spare a little time from the running of his political machine, laughing at the side-splitting humor of coquetting with the Garfield gamblers' association, and puzzling over Rubens' veto messages," he might spur Reynolds to action.

Including quarantine to keep out Chicagoans, authorities from surrounding states suggested compulsory vaccination in their own districts. They also considered warning officials at Winnipeg, as that city was only two days removed from Chicago. If there were to be an exodus from the plague-ridden city, refugees were as likely to go there as anywhere.[7]

Matters grew worse: smallpox results for Chicago from January 1 through April 21, 1894, were: January, 128; February, 233; March, 305; April 1–21, 296, for an average of 14 per day. Vaccination was vigorously promoted, with 300,000 persons receiving protection during that time. Washington, DC, had its own smallpox scare on October 25, with over 5,000 people rushing for vaccination. The Interior Department had three cases of the disease among its employees and granted leaves of absence for those engaged in rooms contaminated by victims. Five days later, as a precaution, Dr. O'Reilly vaccinated everyone at the White House.[8]

As outbreaks crept into 1895, suggestions on how to control smallpox in private households filled the newspapers. Along with his recommendation of home treatments of cream of tartar, a local "electro-therapeutist" from Chicago stated that Roentgen rays (X-rays, invented by Wilhelm Konrad Roentgen, 1845–1923) were proven to kill the bacteria of cholera, diphtheria, typhoid, tuberculosis and like diseases. Ideas such as washing the pet dog and shooting the pet cat (which was said to carry disease in its fur) were offered. Caregivers were ordered quarantined inside infected houses and free vaccinations were supplied around the country.[9]

Smallpox and African Americans

It was seldom easy being an African American in post–Civil War America, as attitudes of mistrust abounded. Not surprisingly, this carried over into how the black population was educated about smallpox and how they responded to vaccination. Often, small groups were left to their own devices, while those in major cities were treated with contempt and often misplaced humor.

In Lynch's Prairie, Grand River, Oklahoma, 1882, after reports that the population was "dying off right and left" from smallpox, a concerned citizen took the trouble to write the newspaper and correct the misconception. It was not the white citizens who were dying but only the African Americans. The outbreak spread rapidly because "the [N]egroes, at first, did not believe it to be the small-pox, and by mischief and neglect, let the disease take good hold of them." Outside Negro neighborhoods, he added, "health was never better."[10] A typical event was reported along the Georgia coast in a small community called Harris Neck in Liberty County, populated mainly by African Americans, where a total of 85 cases of smallpox were reported in 1891. Lacking a board of health, surgeon White of the marine hospital service was sent to take charge. Besides the fresh cases, he reported 18 deaths, 32 convalescent and 42 older but active cases. He expected more to follow.[11]

Two years later in Lynchburg, Virginia, the outcome was less encouraging. During an epidemic there, orders were given for every inhabitant to be vaccinated. The program went smoothly enough until the authorities attempted to vaccinate the African Americans, who refused on the grounds it was "some scheme of white people to kill them off." They were not alone in their fears; blacks in Atchison, Kansas, complained they had not been treated fairly by city officials in the matter of quarantine.[12]

Smallpox in Maryland during the early part of 1895 was confined to "colored people." Education, or lack thereof, would seem to be the problem here, as "many of them have unreasonable prejudice to vaccination and but few have taken any precautions to protect themselves by the ordinary means." Any person believed to have the disease was removed to the "suspect camp," from which, if disease were confirmed, they were "hurried off to the hospital."[13]

When smallpox became epidemic in Atlanta, Georgia, in 1897, local authorities carried out "wholesale vaccinations." Escorted by police, physicians went down Decatur Street, where a large number of citizens were treated. "Not a few [of the Negroes] objected to the process, but these were soon brought into humble submission by the iron grasp of the officer and in less time than it takes to tell they were gazing with eyes of wonder at a small wound of their left arm." The article continued:

> Much fun is had [as] Negroes of all sizes and shades were vaccinated yesterday and about half of them objected most strenuously to having their arm "skint".... Many Negroes of the old type were anxious to know why they should be vaccinated and wanted to know all the details of the cause for the sudden move on the part of the board of health.... The Negroes talk of nothing else on the street but the smallpox and the mention of it among them starts a panic to get out of the way or much discussion. They are aroused to the highest pitch of excitement over it, and while all of them fear it, they do not think they will be visited.[14]

The state of affairs in Virginia does not appear much improved by 1898, when smallpox was alarmingly prevalent "among the colored population." On October 4, a Negro with the disease appeared in front of the city dispensary in City Hall Square in search of medical assistance. He was left in the street for 1½ hours with no more done than a police squad's being summoned to keep people away. He was finally taken to the pesthouse and the board of health ordered all persons who had not been successfully vaccinated to undergo the procedure.[15]

Two Sides of the Native American Equation: Slaughter and Vaccination

In the immediate post–Civil War era, Union generals who remained in the service were inevitably assigned to confront the "Indian Problem." Although the United States should have been celebrating the end to a disastrous conflict, there was little charity for those emancipated or those whose ancestors had roamed the landscape before the Pilgrims. In 1865, what passed for an amusing anecdote read, "The Digger Indians have a splendid remedy for the small pox. When one has it, he closes the door of his hut, kills his dog and then shoots himself, which effectually removes the disease."[16]

Squibs of the time reflected more of the same. From the *Virginia Tresspass* (Nevada), September 15, 1868, came this note: "The small pox has made its appearance in this place to the great terror of the Piute Indians. The noble red devils are awfully frightened at the appearance of small pox in the land, and now, for the first time, have asked for vaccination."

Less humorously, the semiannual payment made by Dr. M.M. Davis to the Wisconsin Indians in August 1865 consisted of $5 for every brave, squaw and papoose. From a total of $10,000, that left $1,600, which first went to pay funeral expenses for those who had died during the year, and second to provide for the needy. Those two items were unusually large that year owing to the prevalence of smallpox. The total number of Indians paid was 1,600, the number steadily decreasing at the rate of about 150 per year.[17]

Reports from 1869 and 1870, usually no more than a few sentences, continued to pour in. Smallpox broke out among the Crow Indians in Montana; General Sully, Indian superintendent, reported 500 deaths (half the entire tribe) among the Gros-Ventre Indians from smallpox. He added, "They are committing suicide by blowing their brains out with revolvers." While whites suffered a mild form of varioloid, dead Indians "strew the road from the Forks to Mill River. They demand the Indian agent to act as mediator with the Great Spirit to stop the disease." From Benton, Montana, Indians at camps on the Moras were dying at the rate of 25 per day from smallpox. A follow-up added, "It seems that the most friendly tribe of Indians in Montana, are to be killed off by the old Puritan mode of letting them die with small pox. By this kind process they have been reduced to 1,200. Those that will not commit 'outrages' so as to be killed and scalped by civilized soldiers, must be killed off by contagion. Our Indian policy has many suspicious circumstances."[18]

The latter referenced one of the largest and most savage attacks by United States soldiers on American soil. The massacre had its beginnings several years before, as the Piegan and Blood Indians were known to have raided small settlements in northern Montana. The point of no return was reached in the winter of 1869–1870, when a brave named Owl Child stole several horses belonging to Malcolm Clarke. Clarke eventually captured Owl Child and beat him in front of members of his tribe. Humiliated, the brave and a band of warriors retaliated by killing Clarke and several other whites.

Application was made by General Sully to arrange a retaliatory attack. Brevet-Colonel (Major) Eugene Baker was designated to lead an attack from Fort Shaw north toward the Marias River, where the target Indians under Mountain Chief were believed to camp. Departing January 15, 1870, the cavalry suffered from extreme cold but reached the bluffs at the bend of the Marias River on January 23. Although apparently warned by army scout Joe Kipp that they had actually arrived at the camp of Heavy Runner, where most of the inhabitants had been suffering from smallpox for two months, "half a dozen dying daily," the chief was shot dead, initiating a slaughter that savagely took the lives of 173 Piegan Indians, of which only 15 were fighting men. More than 90 of the dead were women, many elderly; 50 were children.

After 140 captives were turned loose in freezing weather to walk 90 miles to Fort Benton, Major Baker headed downstream to find his actual target. One company was left behind to dispose of the corpses on a pyre; Lieutenant William Pease, the Piegan Indian agent, calculated the body count. The following day, Baker's troops found Mountain Chief's camp abandoned. After burning what remained, they left for the Northwest Fur Company's fort. Only one soldier died in the two-day massacre.

A message from General Sully, dated February 26, stated that the Gros-Ventres and Assinaboines, after hearing that the Piegans had declared war on the whites, sent a large party toward the latter's camps to retaliate on them for stealing their horses the previous fall when their warriors had been smitten with smallpox. As the Piegans, including Big Jake's band, were also afflicted with the disease, Sully predicted they were completely susceptible, with no means of sustaining life and faced starvation unless fed by the government.

Expressing no remorse, Union Civil War hero William T. Sherman wrote to another well-known officer, General Philip Sheridan, on March 7, remarking that permission for the attack was sought by General Sully and those in the Interior Department, so they had no right to be "shocked" at the outcome. General De Trobriand, commanding the district in Montana, issued a report, expressing "gratification" in the "complete success" of the endeavor. Sent by Sheridan, Inspector-General Hardie reported the Piegans were guilty of many murders and robberies of whites, concluding the "chastisement was necessary."

A letter to the editor published in the *New York Times,* March 14, aptly observed, "Whole tribes must not be responsible for the outrages of those of the tribe who break away and steal, kill and destroy on their own account." The author continued, "Shall our gratitude to our military men for their noble efforts during our late struggle [Civil War] cause us to attempt to extenuate their crime, while as a nation we cover our faces with shame before the world." What little outcry there was in Congress quickly faded away.

By April 17, the *New York Times* ran an editorial advising foreign critics of the debacle to reconsider, considering that "notwithstanding late bitter collisions [the federal government] is now taking the most active steps, through its agents, to stop the ravages of smallpox among the Indians." Large quantities of vaccine were sent for distribution, despite the fact the "poor savages" feared the prophylactic would make them "ox-faced" or "like onto beasts." With hypocritical piousness, the author added that this, certainly, should be "set down by Christendom to the permanent credit of the authorities at Washington."[19]

Smallpox did not go away. In April, Superintendent Sully to the Montana Indians reported the ravages of disease among the Gros-Ventres and Assiniboines were "frightful," although "through the efforts of the citizens," the disease was being checked. By June, the River Crow Indians, scattered all over Montana, were suffering greatly but refused to be vaccinated. The following month, 750 out of 1,900 Gros-Ventres had died, reportedly infected by discarded Piegan clothing. Perpetuating the cycle, buffalo robes worn by the dead, the bodies of which were left on the open ground covered with brush, were stolen by traders. Sold to local merchants, the robes were crated and sent back East by railroad, thereby spreading smallpox to entirely new locales.

In October, in order to prevent the spread of disease in Minnesota, the commissioner of customs at Pembina was instructed to refuse all buffalo robes and skins arriving at that port from infected sites along the Red River. Little seemed to help. A month later, smallpox was reported at the Nez Perce reservation in Washington, introduced by other Indians who had been across the mountains to hunt buffalo. By December 1, smallpox was blamed for the deaths of thousands of Plains Indians: "The decaying corpses are lying all over the country, filling the air with a terrible stench."[20]

The year 1871 saw no relief. Smallpox broke out among the Blackfeet on the Upper Missouri. From one camp of 900 Indians, 600 had the disease and 310 died. In consequence, when the fur trade on the Red River ended in August, only 1,340 robes, valued at $24,000, were sold in the market, down from 8,500 robes ($65,000) and $33,000 worth of mink and furs the year before. By November, the spread of smallpox in Philadelphia reached 576 in one week, attributed to robes taken from the Piegan and Blackfeet camps. Although traders had been prohibited from selling the robes (speculated to have been gathered by army incursions), they merely moved into new districts and shipped from there.

After a particularly disastrous outbreak in Canada during 1869–1870, the disease persisted through the 1880s in Upper Gatmeau, where over 100 deaths were reported, as tribes divided and moved north, leaving their dead unburied. Smallpox also persisted in Northern Wisconsin, with infected Indians "allowed to roam and care for themselves as best they can." In 1882, the commissioner of Indian Affairs reported the prevalence of smallpox along the Missouri River and ordered vaccine virus forwarded to agency physicians. A year later, smallpox raged among the Creek Indians at Okmulgee, Indian Territory. Whether or not they were also beneficiaries of receiving vaccine virus, attempts at education were futile, as the medicine men were "adopting very unwise treatment, which kills many patients." Settlers at Muskogee, however, were spared the scourge by taking precautions. Toward the end of the year, smallpox was so prevalent in the Cherokee Nation, Oklahoma, it was feared the schools would not be allowed to open and Santa Claus might be prevented from visiting the orphan asylum.[21]

In lieu of vaccination, ancient remedies for curing the fever of smallpox by use of cold water became more popular with Indians in the 1880s. The treatment was also taken up by non-vaccinationists, "not always with success." Clearly, vaccination was the only way to stem the tide of this disease, but reports of scattered and occasionally large-scale outbreaks were depressingly frequent, indicating an overall failure of education and effort to prevent smallpox among the Native Americans. In 1883, the half-breed settlement near Neche, Dakota Territory, suffered from the disease "to an alarming extent," the number of cases being very large. The same year, smallpox was reported to be making terrible inroads among those from Itasca County, Minnesota. The death toll from two small towns, entirely without medical aid, reached eighty-five.

In 1885, smallpox was reported among the Piute of Mason Valley, Nevada, while an epidemic in 1888 struck the Blackfoot reservation 60 miles east of Calgary. The Canadian government sent vaccine matter sufficient to vaccinate 1,500 persons, but it was feared native superstition would delay widespread acceptance. Concurrently, at Green Bay, smallpox raged among the Menomonees, losses totaling between 40 and 50 within a month. They were considered "miserable in the extreme," but no mention was made of preventive measures.

Across the compass, Indians at the Allegany Reservation, Pennsylvania, suffered from smallpox and a strict quarantine was placed against them. It was believed the disease was imported from Buffalo, New York, where smallpox was prevalent on the Cattaraugus Reservation. Here, Neely & Company druggists imported fresh vaccine virus daily and offered special rates to physicians. It was stressed that quills not used within three days would be exchanged for fresh ones. Dr. Beal, the state health officer at Allegany, indicated that the Indians were "submitting willingly to vaccination," and that cases rapidly decreased. Not all health care providers were willing to cooperate, as a blurb from a Pennsylvania newspaper indicates:

Randolph has a new trust. Physicians have formed a vaccination combine and will charge $1 per stab. Is this an M.D. or a D — M trust?

Lack of education on the benefits of vaccination, an inability to reach scattered tribes, superstition, ineffective quarantine, medical costs and a combination of disregard and prejudice all marked national and state policies on the treatment of Native Americans. To that list, graft should certainly be included. One typical example came from the Dakotas, where the distribution of rations and medical supplies was based on population. In 1890, it was discovered that instead of the reported 7,500 individuals served by the Rosebud Agency, there were actually only 5,166. A query was placed to Indian agent Wright, who blamed the discrepancy on an epidemic of smallpox. Unfortunately for agent Wright, only 19 deaths from smallpox and measles had been reported for the year ending June 30, 1890, and an investigation was ordered.

In one ray of sunshine, the prognosis for members residing in the Indian Territory commonly referred to as "the five tribes" (or "the five civilized tribes") was significantly more favorable than their brethren. Composed of the Cherokee, Chickasaw, Choctaw, Creeks and Seminoles, numbering 65,000, a systematic form of government greatly aided the distribution of medicine and medical supplies. Expenses for the nation in 1883 amounted to $183,000, of which $21,508 went to the health office for use in suppressing smallpox.[22]

The year 1892 brought a smallpox epidemic to Canada, affecting Indians in the Thunder Bay district. Orders were immediately given for all children and others on the reserve who had not been recently vaccinated to undergo the procedure. Fresh supplies, amounting to some 1,000 points, were sent, and the Indians were ordered to keep to their own areas. North Dakota immediately established quarantine along the Manitoba frontier and in consequence of the general scare, citizens from Victoria made a great exodus, giving the city a "rather desolated appearance."[23]

Compulsory Vaccination and the Courts—A "Signal for War"

Cases across the country challenged the legality of state boards of health and education to mandate compulsory vaccination, either for the general population, or, more specifically, in reference to children who were entering the public educational system. Decisions varied widely, sending conflicting and contradictory signals.

Two prominent cases were brought in Wisconsin in 1894: the first involved Reverend J.H. Schlerf versus the board of education. Schlerf filed a writ of mandamus to permit his son, Carl, to attend public school without undergoing vaccination. In his affidavit, Schlerf offered his opinion that the operation afforded no protection and that it endangered the health and life of the person vaccinated. Under questioning, he stated that "the vaccination lymph is like Koch's lymph — a humbug," and argued the only reason it was pressed on parents stemmed from the fact physicians made money on it. The school board countered that smallpox was a very contagious disease and that vaccination afforded protection and served as a preventive. A similar case was held at Beloit under Judge Bennett and was titled *The State of Wisconsin ex rel T.J. Adams, of Beloit, against ex-Assemblyman R.J. Burdge and the School Board.* The circuit court ultimately invalidated the idea of compulsory vaccination and it was taken to the state supreme court (see below).[24]

In 1895, the courts sustained the Shelby, Iowa, board of health in excluding children from school who had not been vaccinated. An irate editorialist for the *Cedar Rapids Evening Gazette,* February 2, 1895, sneered, "The boards of health, on behalf of the doctors, have power to compel vaccination. The boards of education (possibly in behalf of the undertakers), have power to lock the doors and needlessly expose children to bad weather and possibly to disease and death." He added, "Schemers should be compelled to keep hands off." In 1896, a different tack was taken by the *Burlington Hawk-Eye,* March 15, when the newspaper warned that the law of the state mandated that boards of health could be held responsible for neglecting the public health, and pleaded, "Above all, don't let the insane ravings of a few loud-mouthed anti-vaccination cranks deprive the public of the goodly heritage they have in vaccination."

The same year, a question—"Is the requirement of the Board of Health and the Board of Trustees, that pupils, before attending the public school, shall be vaccinated, a reasonable one?"—came before the Supreme Court of Pennsylvania. Rather than address the issue concerning the validity of vaccination, the case was decided on the grounds the school board had the right to "preserve the public health." In 1896, Judge Cheney quoted from this decision in a case brought before him in Reno, Nevada. His decision was based upon the premise that there were conditions when individual rights had to be made subject to the greater public welfare: "To leave it to each individual to determine for himself, would destroy all order and government." Thus, he concluded that arguments in the case did not warrant issuing of the peremptory writ and dismissed the proceedings.[25]

In 1897, the Wisconsin supreme court reviewed the Beloit case. Despite a vocal outcry from local boards of health and education arguing that their work had been considerably hampered by the Rock County Circuit Court decision, the high court affirmed the decision on February 23. Considering there had been no epidemic of smallpox when the first decision had been reached and the supreme court did not address that issue, it was hoped this

VACCINATION IS UPHELD

Medical Society Unanimously Favors It.

IT PREVENTS SMALLPOX

Members of the Society Very Emphatic in their Advocacy of Vaccination—Would Have it Made Compulsory if Possible—Approve of the Board of Education Preventing Unvaccinated Children from Attending School—Mr. Critchlow Says Such Action is Legal.

The debate over whether or not to admit unvaccinated students into the classroom was a hot-button issue throughout the 18th, 19th and 20th centuries. Those in favor declared that personal freedom did not give any individual the right to potentially harm others, while those against mandatory vaccination argued that the pursuit of liberty and religious freedom granted them the right to refuse any treatment they considered unsafe or unsound. In this case, the local medical society supported the board of education's stance on requiring vaccination in the classroom, but did not go so far as to make vaccination mandatory. Such halfway measures only complicated the situation and left the debate open for future lawsuits (from the Salt Lake *Tribune,* January 11, 1900).

left open the question of whether the issue would be revisited if smallpox became epidemic. Educators promptly called for legislators to "pass some law that is constitutional regulating the powers and duties of the state board," while the board of health declared, "If some law is not enacted in the near future to provide for vaccination, the state will be liable to an outbreak of smallpox within the next decade that will be disastrous."[26]

The situation in Illinois mirrored that of Wisconsin, where the state supreme court had struck down compulsory vaccination for school children in 1897. In Berkley, California, attempts to enforce the vaccination law brought the city to the verge of "war." After the pros and cons were discussed, "in a manner that a condemned criminal would consider the advisability of submitting to be hung," many suggested that enforcement was not only injudicious, but criminal. Although defended by the health officer, those gathered considered past efficacy "stretching the point too far in order to give an excuse for the enforcement of an obnoxious measure."[27]

"Moving On" to the 20th Century

The last decade of the 1800s represented both the good and the bad in the fight against smallpox. Although women's suffrage was a long way off, Dr. Amelia Fendler Abrams became a member of the New York Vaccinating Corps in the fall of 1892. At 18 years of age, this distinguished person graduated from the New York College of Pharmacy and earned the position of druggist at the Northeastern dispensary. At 21, she completed the courses at Women's Medical College, Baltimore, and returned to New York. Besides working on the vaccination corps, she joined the board of health and was instrumental in vaccinating children.[28]

While yellow flags still floated above private dwellings and surgeons donned their rubber suits to treat the infected, more states fell in line behind the effort for vaccination. Maryland (1898) enforced compulsory vaccination of schoolchildren; compulsory vaccination was declared to have been "completely successful" in eradicating the speckled disease in Georgia (1898) and Governor Bushnell of Ohio ordered the vaccination of all 2,200 state prisoners (1898). The senate and house in Arkansas appropriated $5,000 to help eradicate smallpox (1899), while the Maryland Board of Health required employees of small fruit farms and canning houses to be vaccinated (1899). Iowa passed a compulsory vaccination law for all citizens (1899), while Vermont eliminated language requiring vaccination of schoolchildren from school board resolutions (1899). Mississippi was moving ahead with a law on compulsory vaccination (1899), and the Choctaw authorities in the Indian Territories began a vaccination crusade (1899). Further proof of vaccination protection came from Los Angeles. During the year 1899, of 119 cases reported, 59 had been protected at some point in their lives and 60 were unvaccinated. None of the vaccinated died, while 22 of the unvaccinated perished.[29]

In 1895, the New York legislature approved $75,000 for a Pasteur institute over objections that it was throwing away money "in vain and foolish experiments." The same year, the world mourned the passing of Professor Louis Pasteur, who gave to humanity, among other revelations, the cure for rabies.

Tracing the route of transmission in two varied cases illustrates the power of the disease. In the first instance, smallpox traversed the water from Cuba ("where it always runs riot") into Florida. The following table illustrates the path it was believed to have taken:

Transmission of Smallpox from Cuba Throughout the U.S.

State	Date of Epidemic	Number of Cases
Florida	January 19–February 20, 1897	62
Alabama	March 1897–ongoing	1161
Tennessee	April 1897–January 1898	152
Georgia	October 1897–April 1898	374
South Carolina	January 1898–ongoing	33
North Carolina	January 1898–ongoing	—

State	Date of Epidemic	Number of Cases
Florida (reappeared)	January 1898	12
Kentucky	February 3–March 14, 1898	177
Virginia	February 1898–ongoing	2
West Virginia	February 1898–ongoing	5
Washington, DC	February 1898–ongoing	2
Ohio	April 1898	7
Pennsylvania	May 1898–ongoing	Just begun

In Georgia and Alabama, it was stated the disease was almost wholly confined "to the colored race, among whom vaccination is extremely difficult to accomplish, as they evade the law in every possible manner."[30]

A more localized path of transmission that might be called a comedy of errors were it not so serious began on April 29, 1898, when the Joshua Simpkins One-Horse Company opened at Dunkirk in upstate New York. A man named Pickett from Fredonia (about 3 miles away) traveled by trolley line to see the show. Two weeks after returning home, he was taken ill and diagnosed with chicken pox. His children quickly sickened and soon the outbreak became general. Not until a traveling salesman visited the Pickett home and correctly identified the disease was it recognized as smallpox. Quarantine was established but proved difficult to maintain as smallpox had been absent from the town for more than a dozen years. In light of the fact "cranks and certain doctors" believed vaccination worse than the disease, few adults were protected or acknowledged the danger.

From Fredonia, the disease traveled to Dunkirk, where many cases were reported. The show company played at Norwich on May 9, then moved westward through Cortland, Groton and Moravia. A spectator at Groton became ill two weeks later and spread the disease through his community. At Moravia, one of the male members of the company fell sick; instead of quarantining the company, local physicians ordered it out of the vicinity. The order came too late, however, as laundry left behind with a washerwoman infected her; she, in turn infected other members of the house. The physician who attended them called another doctor for consultation, but the telephone connection was so poor the message was not clearly understood. By the time he arrived, the sick had grown considerably worse.

A schoolteacher who attended a performance at Groton later went to a Spiritualism meeting at Freeville, then returned to the house of a doctor with whom she boarded. When she became sick, he diagnosed her problem as "some contagious skin disease" and no quarantine was established. The teacher returned to work and infected children in her class. Eventually, she was properly diagnosed, but health officials disputed it. Finally, at Geneva, the Joshua Simpkins Company was corralled and sent to a boat anchored on Seneca Lake. Two members escaped, one going to Rochester and the other to Buffalo, carrying contagion with them. The latter, passing through North Tonawanda, began an outbreak there before moving on.

A victim of the disease spread by the company visited Syracuse and was taken sick at the home of a physician. The doctor failed to make a proper diagnosis and other members of the house fell ill. One of them left, buying a ticket to Union Springs, where she spread smallpox. In all, 180 cases were directly attributable to the One-Horse Show, although conservative estimates place the number at twice that.[31]

In summing up the American state of affairs regarding smallpox at the turn of the century, Dr. Hibbard of the American Medical Association noted:

While a century of experience has convinced the great body of intelligent people that vaccination is the true and only prophylactic for small pox, it has not carried conviction to the extent its merits deserve, and the welfare of the people demands. The cause of this is not difficult to discern; vaccination and other forms of sanitation have prevented a visitation of the epidemic smallpox in this country for a generation, and the people have lost the fear of its contagion, through ignorance of its nature while progressing, and its sequels, if its victims survive. Add to this the disorders that sometimes follow the insertion of pure vaccine in a system, and the greatest evils arising from the use of spurious or imperfect vaccine, and careless vaccination, all open to the observation of the public, and subject to amplification by cranks and the maliciously ignorant, and we cannot marvel that there is a positive distaste for vaccination among a considerable portion of our population, and a carelessness about securing it on the part of a much larger number....

Under these circumstances it seems to me the reasonable duty of the association, at this time, to declare and proclaim its unabated faith in the virtue of vaccination to protect from smallpox; to render persons as immune against variola, as an attack of variola itself, and that it is innocent of all mischief when vaccination is done by a vaccinator who is a competent judge of both the purity of the vaccine and the fitness of the vacinee.[32]

Brilliant words, eloquently expressed. To counter them, two small articles follow, the first an advertisement:

A Case of Smallpox is not the worst thing a city like Fort Wayne could have; five cases would be five times as bad. Of course, a small-pox patient is to be pitted [*sic*, the word should be "pitied"), and so in one sense of the word are the men and women who make themselves miserable ... by worrying for fear they will have it.... Take the money you spend for things you should not eat and buy good, clean, well-made suits, overcoats and furnishings. We have overcoats from $4.00 to $30.00. Suits from $4.00 to $25.00.[33]

The second, equally distasteful article, warns people that the sanitary authority in Ohio planned on taking away "one of the luxuries of life" by putting a stop to the practice of unscientific kissing, or "kissing which is not carefully restrained by sanitary laws." Citizens were also warned of the dangers of using the same cup during communion and urged not to allow the kissing of babies "by every chance comer." The report continued: "The most ardent manifestation of masculine devotion may be the means of planting the seeds of disease, which will bring forth a fruitful crop of maladies sent down through generations. So says science."[34]

So says science. Dr. Hibbard and his colleagues had a long road to travel.

Anti-Vaccination Hysteria
in Great Britain

A curious incident of the vaccination muddle in England is that Lord Aldenham
and Lord Feversham voted for the compulsory vaccination in the House of Lords,
while their equally conservative associates, Mr. Gibbs and Mr. Duncumbe, voted
against it in the Commons. The older generation in England can remember when
smallpox was a common and menacing plague.[1]

During the 1890s, England took center stage in what can be described in no lesser
words than anti-vaccination hysteria. If newspapers and letters are any judge, the abolition
of cumulative penalties on parents for refusal to have their children vaccinated, the with-
drawal of any and all laws requiring state mandated vaccination, and ultimately the discon-
tinuation of vaccination altogether raged throughout Britain with unparalleled force and
vitriolic rhetoric.

Nearly everyone had something to say, from physicians to politicians, senior fellows
of King's College, Cambridge, to the man on the street. Editorials in bold type and capital
letters proclaimed, "the evil effects of vaccination"; "repressive effect of vaccination"; "the
anti-vaccination campaign"; "conservatives and anti-vaccination." On the other side came,
"vaccination vindicated"; "defenders of vaccination"; "preserving vaccination from reproach."
The *London Echo* ran a column titled "Hear All Sides," but no one was listening. Minds
were made up and logic vanished amidst clenched fists and poisoned pens.

Statistics were quoted to support each writer's viewpoint: when the vaccinationists
asserted that 450 physicians of the "Blue-Book" supported the preventive, anti-vaccinationists countered by asserting that number paled by comparison to the 3,000 physicians
in London who opposed it. The claim that genuine vaccine taken from the cow was pure
was argued against by calling it a "bastard poison." When statistics giving numbers saved
by vaccination were published, these were offset by warnings that hospitals and drug shops
had seen an 80 percent increase in smallpox-related business. Testimonies proving the safety
of vaccination were challenged by other medical authorities, who claimed it transferred
syphilis, "ophthalmia [severe irritation of the eye], storrhoea [obscure; probably similar to
pyaemia, a type of septicemia], fluor albus [*Leucorrhoea;* a white, secretion from the vagina,
similar to gonorrhoea], prurigo [chronic skin disease marked by itchy papules]."[2]

A typical statement from the executive committee of the London Society for the Abolition of Compulsory Vaccination, 1893, reads, "That this Committee protests against Sir
Walter Foster's assertion that small-pox killed annually 3,000 per million before the discovery
of vaccination. Without denying the existence of such a small-pox death-rate in particular
years of severe epidemics, the committee deny indignantly that this was ever a small-pox

mortality.... That the committee desire to criticise the statement that only one death from primary vaccination occurs in 14,159 operations, and to express their disgust at the indifference thus shown to the legal murder of children, which amounts, according to the Registrar-General's admission, to about one a week for England and Wales." They went on to add:

> The committee desire to point out that the actual number of deaths from vaccination must be far greater than this, for that many deaths, really due to vaccination, are not so recorded, either because (1) the evidence connecting the cause and effect is not regarded as conclusive; or (2) that the doctor, who certifies the death, is anxious to preserve vaccination from reproach, and that, independently of the deaths caused by vaccination, there are cases of life-long injury, which do not find their way into any official record.[3]

One portion under consideration of the so-called "Mr. Asquith's Vaccination Bill" of 1893 was used to clarify sections 29 and 31 of the Vaccination Act of 1867. In that bill, section 29 required only one fine for conviction of refusing compulsory vaccination of a child, while section 31 stated that if the same child were not vaccinated after the first fine, repeated convictions up to the age of 14 years were possible. Rather than have the ambiguous language clarified, anti-vaccinationists demanded its total repeal.[4]

Further debate in the House of Commons pitted Mr. Hopwood — who said "the law compelling parents to vaccinate infants and young persons is unjustifiable and ought to be repealed" — against those of the Royal College of Surgeons, who regarded "as a national calamity any alteration in the law which now makes vaccination compulsory."[5]

Playing out in a smaller venue, at the Greenwich police-court in April 1893, a parent stated he wished to "place his faith in the living God, and to adhere to the Bible, which said the laying-on of hands and the prayer of faith would save the sick." When asked by the magistrate, "Don't you think we ought to do what we can ourselves," the defendant replied, "When God has laid down rules we ought to abide by them." A second defendant stated that he "would rather lose his child to small-pox than from vaccination." Fines of 10 shillings and costs of 2 shillings were inflicted in most cases.[6]

Situations such as that at Lewisham were not unique. The Union Guardians, "affected with the anti-vaccination craze," excused all parents "who, from obstinacy or mere whim, or any other inadequate reason, state they do not wish to have their children vaccinated." The original notice, published in the *London Blackheath Gazette* November 15, 1895, brought numerous letters in defense of and against the Guardians (published November 29, December 13 and 20; February 7 and March 20, 1896). The opponents typically remarked that public officials ought to be required to follow the letter of the law, while the supporters praised them for their courage.

The *Blackheath Gazette* continued the thread with a similar story from Gloucester (March 13, 1896), where several years before, the board of guardians had taken it upon themselves to suspend the Vaccination Act. This "prepared the soil, as it were, for an epidemic of small-pox, and at last the epidemic has come, and brought with it, not only panic and death, but disasters to trade and reputation from which Gloucester will not recover for some time to come." (Less than two weeks later, in consequence of smallpox still raging, the show of the Glocestershire Agricultural Society was abandoned.) Espousing the vaccinationist perspective, the article continued: "It is hardly necessary to say that the result of this state of things is panic — utter panic. The people are rushing in thousands to be vaccinated and revaccinated, and among them, it is reported, are some who have been leaders of the anti-vaccination movement. This is just what might be expected of people whose 'convictions' or 'conscientious objections' are based upon ignorance." Proponents of anti-vaccination used the sanitation argument, stating the outbreaks were "mild" and confined to those who lived in overcrowded dwellings or where drainage was defective.[7]

While the dean of Gloucester, Mr. Spence, appealed for help with the epidemic, he stated it would be well "if the serious object-lesson which Gloucester now presents is laid to heart by other cities of England which neglect vaccination." Sanitationists repeated that "small-pox fears neither the vaccinated nor the unvaccinated unless they are clean. If they are clean, and their environment be in accordance with sanitary laws," smallpox would not come near them. The lessons to be learned, which the "antis" argued, actually lay in the impurity of the water system, the disposal of sewage and overcrowding.[8]

The Gloucester Sanitary Committee's returns with reference to the smallpox epidemic for the week ending April 24, 1896, were: Fresh cases: 168, against 201 and 211 in the two preceding weeks; total number of cases from the beginning of the outbreak: 1,470; discharged from hospital, 18; died in hospital, 18. Death rates between unvaccinated and vaccinated were "more than 14½ times greater among the former than the latter." The grand jury at the Gloucester Quarter Sessions heard from a number of town councils that the vaccination authority, rather than the board of guardians, should be responsible for overseeing vaccinations.[9]

The Jennerian Centenary

On May 13, 1896, the *Guardian* reported only 81 fresh cases of smallpox at Gloucester, down 51 from the previous week; that brought the total number of smallpox cases to 1,682. The report noted that the guardians "have decided to enforce the Vaccination Acts, which have been in abeyance in the city for ten years." The following day was celebrated as the centenary of the first vaccination in England, May 14 being the day Dr. Jenner performed the operation on James Phipps. The *Church Weekly* pointed out that the "best memorial to Dr. Jenner is the grand result that has followed his discovery to the almost total blotting out from modern Bills of Mortality of the very name of smallpox."

Before the celebrations were over, the Royal Commission on Vaccination (appointed May 29, 1889) finally presented their report to the Queen on August 13, 1896. Lord Herschell (chairman), Sir James Paget, Sir Charles Dalrymple, MP, Sir Guyer Hunter, Sir Edwin Galsworthy, Mr. Dugdale, QC, Professor Michael Foster, Mr. Jonathan Hutchinson, Mr. Samuel Whitbread, Judge Meadows White and Mr. J.A. Bright signed the document. Two commissioners, Mr. J.A. Picton and Dr. Collins, were unable to subscribe to the majority's recommendations and drew up a report of their own. Three of the original commissioners died while the report was in progress; two places were left open and Mr. Bright filled the third. Their findings caused ripples that would affect smallpox vaccination around the world.

FINDINGS OF THE ROYAL COMMISSION ON VACCINATION, ISSUED IN 1896

1. The commissioners reported that "vaccination has a marked effect in reducing both the prevalence of, and mortality from, smallpox, and that revaccination had prevailed to an exceptional degree.

2. Immediate hospital isolation for 16 days could be of high value in diminishing the prevalence of smallpox, but no considerable number of smallpox patients should be kept together situate in a populous neighborhood and ambulance arrangements should be organized with scrupulous care. They added that isolation could not be regarded "as a sufficient substitute for vaccination."

3. In effect, that though some dangers attended vaccination, yet "when considered in relation to the extent of the vaccination work done, they are insignificant."

4. They recommended only calf-lymph prepared with glycerine be used. The age when vaccination was obligatory should be six months instead of three.

5. Noncompliance with the law should no longer be enforced.

The commissioners suggested that only duly qualified medical men be permitted to vaccinate and said these men were entitled to a fee then paid only to the public vaccinator.

In their separate report, Dr. Collins and Mr. Picton maintained that "more effective and less objectionable modes of stamping out smallpox were available" (improved sanitation, i.e., antisepsis), while Sir Guyer Hunter and Mr. Hutchinson expressed the view that not only should vaccination remain compulsory, but also that revaccination should become compulsory by 12 years of age.[10]

In a scathingly satirical summary, the *East Ham Express*, August 15, 1896 (referencing an advanced copy), summed up the seven-year project: "Vaccination will be approved as a safeguard against small-pox, but compulsion will be thrown overboard."

In speaking of vaccination at the annual meeting of the British Association at Liverpool, Sir Joseph Lister (1827–1912), the brilliant surgeon who pioneered antiseptic surgery, noted: "While we cannot be astonished that the centenary of Jenner's immortal discovery should have failed to receive general recognition in this country, it is melancholy to think that this year should, in his native country, have been distinguished by a terrible illustration of the results which would sooner or later inevitably follow the general neglect of his prescriptions." He added that with revaccination, "we have the means of making Jenner's work complete." In commenting about the Guardians of Gloucester, he stated that through their "misguided, though well-meaning" beliefs, epidemic raged and while their "praiseworthy exertions" in later enforcing the vaccination law so that "their city is said to be now the best vaccinated in Her Majesty's dominions ... they cannot recall the dead to life, or restore beauty to marred facial features, or sight to blinded eyes."

On the seven-year Vaccine report, he stated, "I understand that the majority of the Commissioners who have recently issued their report upon this subject while recognising the value and importance of revaccination, are so impressed with the difficulties that would attend making it compulsory by legislation that they do not recommend that course, although it is advocated by two of their number, who are of peculiarly high authority on such a question." He quickly dismissed the legislative difficulties by citing Germany, a country that experienced no difficulty in carrying out compulsory laws. Smallpox was "a matter of extreme rarity in that country, while it is absolutely unknown in the huge German army, in consequence of the rule that every soldier is re-vaccinated on entering the service." He concluded:

> Whatever view our Legislature may take on this question, one thing seems to me clear — that it will be the duty of the Government to encourage by every available means the use of the calf lymph, so as to exclude the possibility of the communication of any human disease to the child, and to institute such efficient inspection of vaccination institutes as shall ensure careful antiseptic

arrangements, and so prevent contamination by extraneous microbes. If this were done, "conscientious objections" would cease to have any rational basis. At the same time, the administration of the regulations on vaccination should be transferred (as advised by the Commissioners) to competent sanitary authorities.[11]

Perhaps in anticipation of calamity once compulsory vaccination was eliminated, the General Accident Assurance Corporation issued a "Combined Policy" covering *a weekly allowance for disablement caused by Small Pox.*[12]

Incidence of Smallpox
Worldwide Up to the
20th Century

As Dr. MacVail writes, "Never believe anything that an anti-vaccinationist, as such, says, without obtaining independent evidence as to its truth." And whenever I read an anti-vaccinationist effusion, Shakespeare speaks to me of the author of the same, "Now what a thing it is to be an ass."[1]

Unlike consumption, where mortality rates showed little fluctuation, smallpox statistics tended to reveal wide variance, at times giving the false impression of unsanitary conditions in a city ordinarily well maintained. In the *Revue d'Hygiene,* June 1887, Dr. Jacques Bertillon, chief of the Bureau of Statistics, Paris, provided a comparative sanitary report of mortality for various diseases:

Smallpox Mortality 1886
(Number of deaths per 100,000 of population)

City	Number of deaths
Marseilles	573
Rheims	110
Buda Pest	358
Saragossa	221
Rome	128
Milan	64
Zurich	106[2]

Outbreaks in Canada during the late 1880s and throughout the 1890s did not reach epidemic proportions and most cities managed to control the disease. During this period, most outbreaks came from immigrants: in 1888, the steamer *Parthia* of the China and Japan Line discharged passengers who infected eight persons in Vancouver as well as the local Indians, who contracted smallpox from clothing thrown overboard. In January 1890, the steamer *Premiere* brought in new cases and in December the *Empress of China* introduced several infected passengers; in April, and again in the end of June, the *Empress of Japan* discharged a number of contagious Chinese to the city.

Forty cases of smallpox appeared in the province of Montreal in October 1891, in consequence of an infected passenger from the steamboat *Brazilian* that had departed at Quebec. In order to stem a spread into the city proper, authorities threatened to prosecute all doctors or others hiding cases of smallpox or varioloid. By February 1892, the threat ended as the

Quebec provincial board of health declared the city free from disease, the outbreak having causes 151 cases and 32 fatalities.[3]

On July 11, 1892, Washington issued a report from Assistant Surgeon Maginder, notifying the public that smallpox was epidemic at Victoria, BC, with 25 known cases. The disease apparently came from immigrants traveling the new Canadian steamship line from China and the East to British Columbia. Toronto's medical health officer, Dr. Allen, noted the absence of proper quarantine on the Canadian Pacific coast and the lack of enforcement for quarantine, as none of the passengers from the steamer were isolated. He warned that as smallpox, cholera and leprosy were common in countries along shipping routes, quarantine arrangements should mirror those at Atlantic ports.

In order to limit person-to-person contact, health authorities requested that clergy hold but one Sunday service and discontinue Sunday-schools. The subject of vaccination also became an important issue along the Pacific coast and newspapers published advice from English physicians urging the protection. By July 29, the disease was reported in Manitoba and the situation was considered serious enough that Governor Andrew H. Burke of North Dakota declared quarantine against the province. Premiere Greenway expressed dismay at the order, declaring there was no epidemic.

Either Premiere Greenway was correct or the physicians of British Columbia and Manitoba were particularly effective. By the second week in August, the disease was "under control" and Canadians poked fun at the "celebrated Dakota quarantine." This did not lessen the fear of contagion from a "stream of immigration from Russia into Manitoba," which was described as "almost constant at present, and it has been so throughout the present season." Citing the approved construction of a quarantine wharf to be built at Grosse Isle, Montreal, at a cost of $100,000, and a new wharf for large vessels approved for Albert Head, B.C., home sanitation was still argued as the best way to prevent infection.

The city council of Winnipeg took matters into their own hands in April 1893, when they made vaccination mandatory, while in Montreal, the large French Canadian population continued to resist the procedure. By 1897, few inroads had been made. When smallpox threatened the city, Archbishop Bruchesi, chairman of the Catholic school board, refused to enforce vaccination in Catholic schools. The situation had worsened by 1898, when 300 were reported dead from smallpox. Mass vaccinations among the Canadian English proceeded well, but resistance among factory workers compelled the government to demand they receive vaccination or submit to dismissal. The poor were also supplied with disinfectants free of charge, health authorities making the rounds to ascertain if they were used.[4]

Smallpox in Jamaica

The year 1886 brought renewed outbreaks of smallpox in Kingston, beginning in March. By July, health officer Ogilvie reported 241 cases, of which 196 were in hospitals. Arguments over where to construct a new smallpox hospital became acrimonious, with the leading newspaper expressing disgust over the "dilly-dallying" of the city council, charging that the members cried out "against hospital expenses! Do they realize how much the city suffers from the reputation which has gone abroad that it is a pest hole?" With the island quarantined by outside interests, the economy suffered and demands were made to sanction the Preservation of Health Bill, taking smallpox matters out of the hands of municipal boards and putting them under the central board of health.

In response to the epidemic, His Excellency Sir Henry Wylie Norman, governor of Jamaica, issued the following proclamation in the local *The Daily Gleaner*, August 5, 1886:

1. All parishes must provide temporary hospital accommodations for smallpox patients.
2. Suitable vehicles for transport must be provided; no public conveyances shall be used.
3. Officers shall be appointed to inspect private residences to ascertain whether smallpox is present.
4. Smallpox patients are to be kept isolated so long as danger of infection exists.
5. Placards must be placed (black printing on yellow background), outside places of contagion.
6. All places where smallpox existed must be thoroughly disinfected once the contagion is passed.
7. If bedding or other articles must be destroyed to prevent infection, the Board of Health shall replace them.
8. No children from infected houses may attend school until 14 days after the house is disinfected.
9. Bodies of persons dying from smallpox shall be buried underground at a depth not less than 4 feet, if possible within 6 hours after death.
10. Head of families or lodging-houses must notify the Commissioner of Health as soon as the presence of smallpox is made known.
11. All persons living in a house or lodging where smallpox is present must be vaccinated/revaccinated if not done within the past 10 years.
12. Copies of these regulations to be posted at police stations, churches, markets and other public places.

The same year, the steamer *Atlas* departed from Kingston, destination Panama, likely bringing workers for the Panama Canal. Some of them carried smallpox and introduced it into Colon. Thereafter, Mr. Ward, doing double duty as superintendent of the Panama Railroad and harbor master, ordered "quarantine observation" against Jamaica, meaning that, whenever grounds justified, vessels must anchor in the stream for 48 hours before going into the wharf. Ward also ordered tents erected for the isolation of contagious individuals.

By November 1887, ships departing Jamaica reported smallpox on the increase, with 482 cases, of which half were fresh, adversely affecting work on the Panama Canal, as most of the laborers came from the island. This forced contractors to hire laborers from Africa and China, who signed contracts for a year to work on the canal for bread, lodging and nominal wages. Few of the laborers "ever survive[d] the deadly diseases of the swamps and jungles." Neighboring Martinique suffered a smallpox outbreak during 1888; reports in June indicated that out of 250 victims, 56 died. As the island was under French control, the Chamber of Deputies voted 1,000,000 francs (£4,000) for relief of the sufferers.

Nor was Jamaica immune from anti-vaccinationists. In 1884, Mr. W.B. Hannan, member of the city council, proposed repeal of the vaccination laws (believing vaccination spread serious disease and diminished the vitality of children), substituting "cleanliness and proper sanitation." Over the next several years, this launched a series of defenders and critics of vaccination, greatly exacerbated by the report of the Royal Commission in England. By 1898, Jamaican anti-vaccinationists rejoiced at the introduction of the "Conscience Clause," and even vaccinationists urged that when the reforms were passed in England, Jamaica should immediately follow suit.[5]

Cuba and the Spanish-American War

The so-called Ten Years War for Cuban Independence (1868–1878) ended in failure for the nationals, leaving Spanish colonial authorities in charge of the island. Although great concern existed in the United States for the people of Cuba, the Monroe Doctrine (1823) specifically omitted the island, and the U.S. government did not intervene in the Spanish conquest.

Considering the close proximity of the United States and Cuba, the two countries shared blood ties and commerce. Both factors played heavily in the potential for the spread of smallpox. Santiago de Cuba had a large and direct steamship trade with the United States; vessels connected with it directly from Havana and between that port and New Orleans, Key West and the southern states. The smallpox epidemic of 1886–1887 in Jamaica also affected Cuba and great fears were entertained of a general epidemic. In May 1887, newspaper articles began appearing, blaming the Cuban government for neglect in enforcing the vaccination laws: in Santiago de Cuba alone, out of a population of 40,000, nearly 30,000 were unvaccinated. As the residents were without protection, 500 cases were reported, and as the disease spread across the island, a death rate estimated as high as 60 percent caused widespread panic. Without quarantine enforcement, by July, 1,000 fresh cases were reported in Havana, with deaths averaging 14 per day. The disease did not lessen until the fall; returns dated October 25 indicated that for the first fortnight of the month, Santiago de Cuba registered 10 cases of smallpox resulting in 6 deaths.

In 1895, revolutionaries made a second attempt for independence. A surprise attack failed and the guerrilla forces settled in for a long struggle. General Arsenio Martinez de Campos, followed by General Valeriano Weyler y Nicolau, commanded the Spanish troops who were ordered to quell the rebellion. United States consul Hyatt reported on May 6, 1896: "Small pox is epidemic in many parts of Eastern Cuba, and between the lack of sanitary discipline and moving troops bids fair to continue until between the disease and vaccination, the culture field is exhausted." Reports of June 26 were worse. Dr. Caminero, the official at Santiago, reported that smallpox was raging epidemically and cases by the hundreds were occurring daily. The American consul at Cienfuegos reported 49 deaths from smallpox.

The following year, widespread starvation set in, with an estimated 175,000–220,000 persons suffering from the lack of necessities of life. The poor were driven into towns by the military authorities and were at the mercy of the soldiers, "who are careless of their fate. Indeed, it is tacitly understood that the widespread misery resulting from the awful system of concentration is part of the captain-general's [Weyler] plan of campaign, and that just what has happened was duly expected."

Due to forced vaccination in January, February and March at Matanzas, 46,000 underwent the operation and thus numbers suffering from the disease were low. Such was apparently not the case elsewhere, as large outbreaks were reported at Guines. Later statistics indicated "little of the smallpox vaccination is effective. With foresight thousands of pacificos might easily have been saved by vaccination." Smallpox increased dramatically by November, with people at Sagua La Grande, a town of 12,000 in the province of Santa Clara, being stricken, while 35 cases presented in the "Lazaretto." The former took on special significance as the port of Sagua Le Grande was used by vessels departing for the United States.

As tensions between the United States and Spain increased, a former Havana resident gave an interview in May 1898, describing the deplorable conditions in Cuba. He averred "smallpox has killed more than any other disease. The people are unable to keep clean, unable to be vaccinated, even if willing, and they died by tens of thousands." He added that after a death from smallpox, victims were "hurried away to the graveyard and buried as soon as possible. During certain rainy seasons I have known hundreds of deaths per day to occur from contagious diseases, and with the present conditions the daily death list may run into thousands before the middle of the summer."[6]

President William McKinley sent the USS *Maine* to Havana and on February 15, 1898, it was destroyed by a massive explosion. On April 19, Senator Henry Teller of Colorado proposed the "Teller Amendment," promising that the United States would not annex or assume control over Cuba and entitling the president to use force to gain Cuban independence. Spain broke off diplomatic relations with the United States on April 21, and the United States Navy initiated a blockade of Cuba. War became inevitable, lasting a brief period of months before the official end came on December 10, 1898, with the Treaty of Paris.

Smallpox from Mexico to Africa

As oil became more and more important to the United States, capitalists looked to Mexico for untapped sources. Searching in the vicinity of Tabasco in the late 1880s, explorers found abundant pitch or bitumen, but smallpox was an annual threat, appearing as soon as winter weather set in. Along small coastal villages such as Tuxpan, natives died at a rate of 25 per day, causing authorities to quarantine seaside areas. During periods of high mortality from smallpox, yellow fever and cholera, a wagon was sent around nightly to collect bodies. They were taken to the "dead lot," a high-fenced area where bodies were sorted the following day and buried. It was not uncommon for persons to be collected prematurely; waking to find themselves in the corpse wagon or in the dead pile, they disengaged themselves and ran away.

Throughout the 1880s and 1890s, outbreaks of smallpox were common and counted in the mortality rates of Mexico City along with typhus, tuberculosis, dysentery and yellow fever as a matter of course. Contamination necessarily spread across the border, and notices such as the one provided by the *San Antonio Daily Light,* January 13, 1887, stated that epidemic smallpox in Paso del Norte quickly spread to El Paso. The extent of the disease was not known, "as the authorities are keeping the matter a dark secret." Since no quarantine existed between the two cities, disease had easy access across Texas via the Southern Pacific railway running between San Antonio and El Paso. Reports of railroad workers dying from smallpox appeared with some regularity.

Plague struck Campeche, Mexico, in 1891, where 1,200 cases were reported. Unfortunately, many of the sufferers throughout the country felt smallpox was a "visitation of God's displeasure," and little was done to prevent further outbreaks or to cure the sick. Many people held the tenet that "God has cursed them and there was no use to try to cure the disease." There was little vaccination, and the only preventive measure practiced by Mexicans was to expose children to the disease at an early age in the hope they would become immune in later life. Those living on the Texas side of the Rio Grande often brought their own children into Mexico, where the disease was prevalent, for the same purpose.[7]

Although Chile was being modernized by the introduction of the electric light in 1886, smallpox "made sad ravages in the Chilean Republic, particularly in Santiago, the capital, and it is expected that vaccination will be made compulsory." Reports did not get any better: in July, the smallpox epidemic proved fatal to 60–70 percent of victims, and on two days alone in July, 27 sufferers were sent to the hospital.

The headline "Guatemala's Sad Condition," from December 1890, accurately represented the state of affairs. Journalists arriving in San Francisco reported that the country was "besieged by smallpox." In the prior seven weeks, 1,200 deaths were registered throughout the country, with new cases on the increase. Because few sanitation precautions were taken at the start of the outbreak, the people "were mowed down by hundreds." In the city of Guatemala, dozens of deaths occurred daily.

The epidemic in Brazil in 1889 covered not only "Rio Janlero," but ran through all the states within a 2,000 mile radius of the city. The death rate for three days at Santos was 70 percent, "and the people who could do so were leaving in droves." Pernambuco, called the "Ven[i]ce of South America," suffered an epidemic of smallpox in 1890 and 1891; in August of the first year, there were already 4,000 cases, with an average of 20 deaths daily. By the following April, hospitals held 400 cases, with 15 deaths per day. Ladies going outside used handkerchiefs saturated with camphor to protect them, while gentlemen "carried umbrellas." A description by United States consul Charles Negley said, "The countenance of about every other [N]egro we meet is frightfully pitted, for chiefly among the colored people was the small pox raging."[8]

Following the geographic line, it was inevitable that Africa would continue to suffer from smallpox outbreaks, exacerbated by British importation of indentured servants from India to work the rich agricultural fields of their colonial possessions. The Indians kept in contact with their native country, causing repeated outbreaks of "Asiatic smallpox" (variola major; see below) in Natal (South Africa), Kenya, Uganda and Tanganyika (German East Africa). After a major outbreak in 1881, vaccination was made compulsory in Cape Colony, a law that remained in effect throughout the Union of South Africa in 1919.[9]

The year 1898 witnessed outbreaks at "Johannesberg," Natal, where eyewitnesses described the disease as "seething." In September, 300 cases were reported. The local sanitation board had limited power, and despite frequent visits from deputations requesting the government take action, that body remained "indifferent." It was feared the remainder of South Africa would quarantine the town.[10] A severe drought in Kenya between 1897 and 1900 drove people from outlying areas toward cities, resulting in fertile ground for smallpox and by 1899 the country suffered a severe outbreak.

Significantly, toward the end of the 1800s, an endemic disease, locally referred to as "amaas," a mild form of smallpox (later identified as variola minor; see below) affected the black population. From the 1900s onward, it became endemic, causing numerous outbreaks.[11]

A striking insight into smallpox came from the firsthand account of Henry Morton Stanley, the famous African explorer. In 1897, at the beginning of his expedition, Stanley had the foresight to order surgeon T.H. Parke to vaccinate the entire community aboard the expedition ship, having previously "procured a large supply of lymph for this purpose, because of the harsh experience of the past."

On September 4, 1888, after camping at Batundu, Stanley wrote, "Here we halted two days, during which we became aware of certain serious disadvantages resulting from contact with the Manyuema. For these people had contracted the small-pox, and had communicated it to the Madi carriers. Our Zanzibaris were proof against this frightful disease, for we had taken the precautions to vaccinate every member of the expedition on board the *Madura,* in March, 1887. But on the Madis it began to develop with alarming rapidity."

By September 24, the situation had worsened. "We had the small-pox raging among the Manyeuma and Madis, and daily creating havoc among their numbers...." The entry for September 21 included, "But early in the morning, Tam, a native of Johanna, raving from small-pox, threw himself into the rapids and was drowned." By September 30 Stanley wrote, "We also had fifteen cases of small-pox, who mingled in the freest manner possible with our Zanzibaris, and the only suicide, Tam, had thus far been attacked." By October 4, his observations were particularly poignant:

> As the men were being transported across the river opposite the landing-place of the Bavikai on the 4th, I saw a dozen Madis in a terrible condition from the ravages of the small-pox, and crowding them, until they jostled them in admirable unconcern, were some two dozen of the tribe as yet unaffected by the disease.... Never did ignorance appear to me so foolish. Its utter unsuspectingness was pitiful. Over these human animals I saw the shadow of Death, in the act to strike.

Finally, on October 18, as the party approached the Amiri Rapids, a second Zanzibari showed symptoms of smallpox.

> So far we had been remarkably free of the disease, despite the fact that there were from ten to twenty sufferers daily in the camp since arriving at the settlement of the Batundu. Out of 620 Zanzibaris who were ordered to be vaccinated, some few constitutions might possibly have resisted the vaccine; but no more decided proof of the benefits resulting to humanity could be obtained from Jenner's discovery than were furnished by our Expedition. Among the Manyuema, Madis, and native followers, the epidemic had taken deadly hold, and many a victim had already been tossed into the river weighed with rocks.[12]

Vaccination progressed slowly through Africa. In 1890, when outbreaks of smallpox appeared in small villages in Egypt, the government granted £2,000 to defray the cost of vaccination; seven years later, in a report from the "Soudan" (Sudan), the Emir Zain arrived in Wady Halfa from the South, requesting to have his two children vaccinated: "His knowledge and appreciation of European practice in connexion with the disease caused some surprise among the officials at Wady Halfa."[13]

The islands of Hawaii were especially susceptible to the importation of smallpox from China and Japan. In a report dated April 14, 1896, statistics from the quarantine station were:

CHINESE

New vaccinations, 261 good (including 12 women); old vaccinations, 11; not vaccinated, 3; had smallpox, 71. Total, 346.

JAPANESE

Old vaccinations, 412 (80 women); not vaccinated, 86 (10 women); had smallpox, 82 (13 women). Smallpox, 1.

Total, 581.

From this number, 14 Chinamen and 498 Japanese required vaccination. At the same time, all the guards and policemen (excepting the two Chinese interpreters who had previously contracted smallpox) were vaccinated. A steamer was sent to Kauai for virus and returned with 20 tubes.

The law in Hawaii required all school children to be vaccinated, but adults were exempt on the grounds they were supposed to know enough to look after themselves. In the face of probable epidemics introduced from abroad, it was suggested the law be expanded to include everyone, thus safeguarding the community and serving as a "protection to commerce, both interisland and international."

The same year, in discussing smallpox before the board of health, Dr. Russell argued that the adult population had "little or no immunity against smallpox," and argued for a general vaccination, stating, "If the real advantages of vaccination were better known, very few people would fail to profit by the great discovery." In 1898, however, during debate in the Hawaiian senate, the efficacy of vaccination in Japan, Hong Kong, China and Formosa was questioned. Rather than credit or increase vaccinations, physicians argued for continued quarantine within those countries, as the "enforcement of those regulations has been of immense value to this country."[14]

Smallpox in India, China and Japan

Smallpox was endemic in India and Asia at the end of the 19th century. In the "Report on Sanitary Measures in India," 1890–1891 (volume 24, p. 181), the Army Sanitary Commission concluded that as to the North-Western Provinces of Oudh, "the mortality from small-pox was somewhat higher than it was in 1889, but records of the past few years seem to the Sanitary Commissioner to indicate that vaccination is exerting a decidedly repressive effect."[15] Anti-vaccinationists immediately touted the first part of the quote and used the report's statistics to prove the point.

Statistics from India 1885–1890

Year	Number of Vaccinations
1885	697,610
1886	713,916
1887	751,875
1888	764,190
1889	800,757
1890	989,169

Year	Number of Smallpox Deaths
1885	14,593
1886	10,486
1887	8,492
1888	25,000
1899	48,243
1890	55,394[16]

The author of the report quickly clarified his comment by stating the statistics were "not intended to call into question the utility of vaccination." Rather, due to high birth rates, the numbers could not be interpreted at face value.

Anti-vaccinationists were not through. By 1893, they attributed leprosy in India to vaccination, apparently based on numbers published in the *British Medical Journal*, indicating that lepers in India increased from 1851 to 1881 at a rate of about 30,000 every ten years. Anticipating pro-vaccinationist arguments, "antis" continued: "One of the most pernicious assumptions of the vaccination-monger is that strong suspicion is to go for nothing. We know that leprosy in Hawaii has been spread mainly by vaccination ... and [also] in New Caledonia. Why should we not expect the same results in India?"

Among the various medical authorities practicing in India who gave credence to the above was Dr. A. Mitra, chief medical officer of Kashmir, who stated, "I have on three occasions searched for [smallpox] bacilli. In one instance I found them in lymph from a vaccinated leper." Even the English in India expressed concern over advances in science, a number of them writing to the British government calling for subscriptions to create a "Pasteur Institute" such as the one "to be got up in England under the patronage of the Prince of Wales" to be rescinded. In the same letter (dated August 3, 1891), the pro-vaccinationist writer addressed this new threat by stating, "With regard to the spread of leprosy in Hawaii and the West Indies, Dr. Arning has shown it to have been brought about by the culpable carelessness of non-medical vaccinators."[17]

Fortunately, during 1894–1895, a total of 6,869,271 persons were successfully vaccinated in India, an increase of 153,137 from the previous year. Results were best in Punjab and Bombay, where 57.4 percent and 57.3 percent respectively of the children born during the year (estimated at 40 per 1,000 of the population) were protected against smallpox. In the central provinces and Berar, the percent was over 50; in the northwestern provinces and Oude, the percent was 29.8; 14.2 percent in Bengal and 9.3 in Coorg.

In lieu of a compulsory vaccination law, "which, for obvious reasons — in a country where the cow is sacred to the Hindus, and the medicine of the English is liable to racial distrust," present significant obstacles, the government was still able to impose the necessity of vaccination upon large sections of the populace by insisting on it as a qualification for government employment. In 1896, the North-Western Railway of India instituted this type of requirement (with the approval of the government) and it was hoped that the thousands of vaccinated natives working the line "must gradually permeate the country with knowledge of the safeguard against smallpox."

Results in Burma were promising. By 1894, a total of 1,737 deaths were attributed to smallpox, a noticeable decrease from 1893, when the total reached 3,081. The chief commissioner expressed regret that due to the decrease, "a certain casualness on the benefits of vaccination" had occurred in some districts and he urged the district civil surgeons to make the efficacy of vaccination clear to the people. There ought to be less difficulty in persuading them to come to the stations, seeing that the operation can be performed more cheaply now than it could a year ago."[18]

The *Japan Mail* of August 31, 1885, published a report concerning infanticide in China. While generally disputing the idea, evidence was given that in Newchwang incurable infants and smallpox children were literally "thrown out to the dogs." This was done on the supposition that if the child were allowed to die under the parental roof, its spirit took possession of the next child born there.

"Sure cures" such as utilizing drum banging to ward off smallpox went hand in hand with the old method of inoculation. A description of this from 1893 is taken from health officer Dr. Edward Henderson's report, published April 7, in the *North-China Herald*.

1. In the absence of vaccination, inoculation was universal.
2. In Shanghai and surrounding districts, the 11th, 12th, 1st and 2nd moons — December, January, February and March were invariably selected, the object being to secure cold weather during the subsequent development of the disease.

3. Children only were inoculated; the age varied from 3 months to 1 year.
4. The full constitutional manifestation of smallpox was considered essential.
5. Inoculation was considered a branch of the medical profession and those practicing it devoted themselves to it exclusively.
6. In Shanghai there were 30–40 native doctors performing the operation.
7. Fees were typically $2 for a boy and $1 for a girl

Dr. Henderson noted that until the people were prepared to accept vaccination, it was probably better for the government to allow inoculation, as long as those individuals stayed outside municipal limits. That said, he believed that soon the edict granted by the Taotai in 1870 that peremptorily forbad inoculation should be enforced and vaccination substituted. To ease the transition, he suggested the accumulation of large amounts of lymph, first by importation and then by local cultivation of calf lymph, on "farms" similar to what had been created in Japan. Afterward, revaccination, almost totally unknown, had to be instituted. As in India, where a Pasteur Institute was proposed, Dr. Henderson's desire for the establishment of one at Shanghai was deemed impracticable on account of the large expenditure of public money.

On the subject of safe removal and disposal of persons having died from smallpox, he stated that however careless the Chinese might be from exposure to the living, they disliked contact with the dead and promptly buried bodies. Chinese coffins, excepting the very poorest, were of great strength and thickness and, as nearly as may be, hermetically sealed. In the case of smallpox deaths, a layer of quicklime, often mixed with charcoal, was placed several inches thick in the bottom of the coffin. Henderson did, however, urge the establishment of formal cemeteries outside municipal limits.

In a report to the Municipal Council, Dr. Henderson gave details of imported lymph:

1. Calf lymph emulsified; imported by Messrs. Llewellyn & Co. from Yokohama. Result: almost uniformly *nil*.
2. Calf lymph pure; imported by Messrs. Voekel and Schroeder from Japan and certified as pure calf lymph by the Director of the Lymph Institute at Tokio [*sic*]. Result on use: good.
3. Calf lymph, pure; imported by Messrs. Mactavish & Lehmann from London through Maw, Son and Thompson, London. Results on use: good.
4. Calf lymph prepared by triturating the scrapings of the pustules with glycerine, and termed, "glycerine pulp"; imported by Llewellyn & Co. from the Pasteur Institute, Saigon. Results on use: good.

Dr. Henderson noted that the latter method was a significant breakthrough in that it preserved the lymph in hot weather (see chapter 31). He advised that with the problem of revaccination it was difficult to get a significant number of people together at the same time; thus, one tube of Saigon lymph that provided enough to vaccinate 12–16 persons was wasted if only two or three presented themselves. He noted that if a "vaccine farm" were to be started in Shanghai like the one in England (see chapter 23), the start-up cost, not including a microscope, would not be less than £150.

Two stations offering gratuitous vaccination were opened at Shanghai in 1894, the official notification ending with the words "and do not be suspicious." By 1898, the governor of Hong Kong announced that while the Chinese scornfully reject most Western medical science, it was practiced with great frequency under his watch. This primarily stemmed from the fear that steamers coming from all parts of the world frequently introduced smallpox and once it gained a foothold, it was often fatal.[19]

The Japanese held a firmer belief in vaccination and in 1886, they enacted a law expanding vaccination in the first year of infancy to include at least two subsequent revaccinations at intervals from 5 to 7 years; so by age of 15, the child would have been vaccinated three times. Additionally, during epidemics, authorities were granted the power to require vaccination of all inhabitants in their districts, irrespective of the vaccination required by law.

This was put into practice in 1893, when the governor ordered compulsory vaccination during a particularly severe epidemic. There was no opposition shown and a steady diminution in fresh cases resulted. In 1896, during yet another outbreak in the towns of Hiogo and Kobe, the United States consul listed the port of Kobe as "infected."[20]

Institutes for the production of calf vaccine began operating in Japan in 1874. By the year 1896, the famous bacteriologist Kitasato made an important contribution to the preparation of bacteriologically sterile vaccine and helped promote its use.[21]

Smallpox in Germany, Prussia and Russia

In speaking on the benefits of vaccination, Dr. Koch of Berlin offered statistics from Prussia during the years 1800–1870, when there was no compulsory law. He showed that from 20 to 60 out of every 100,000 inhabitants died annually from smallpox. After the great epidemic of 1870–1872, where mortality rose to 262 per 100,000, a law was passed enforcing vaccination. But since the mandatory vaccination law in 1874 (that began to be enforced in 1875), mortality from smallpox decreased from 3.6 percent to .07 percent out of every 100,000. He noted that as the mortality had remained unchanged in Austria, England and France, its decrease in Prussia could be ascribed only to compulsory vaccination.

When anti-vaccinationists attempted to cite statistics from the Royal Commission on Vaccination regarding failure of the operation in Bavaria, Arthur F. Hopkirk, one author of the above report wrote to correct the misconception. He stated that of 29,429 cases of smallpox among vaccinated persons, 25,435 (86.4 percent) recovered and 3,994 (13.6 percent) died. Of the 1,313 cases among the unvaccinated, 523 (39.8 percent) recovered and 790 (60.1 percent) died. Of 776 cases among the revaccinated, 712 (91.8 percent) recovered and 64 (8.2 percent) died.

Deaths in Germany After
the Compulsory Vaccination Law

Year	Deaths
1886	198
1887	169
1888	110

Of the 110 deaths in 1888, most occurred in parts of the empire immediately bordering countries not protected by vaccination. Comparing the death rate to other countries, smallpox was 136 times greater in Austria, 30 times greater in Hungary, 16 times greater in England, 24 times greater in Belgium and twice as great in Switzerland.

Comparison of Mortality Rates, 1899

Country	Population	Fatal Cases	Percentage of Mortality
Germany	54,000,000	28	0.52
58 Austrian towns	4,000,000	77	20
72 Belgian towns	2,414,000	126	52.2
33 English towns	11,404,400	145	12.7
116 French towns	8,668,000	600	69.2[22]

By 1888, the majority of vaccinations in Prussia were carried out using calf lymph, and in Berlin and Saxony calf lymph was obligatory. An "Animal Farm" was established at the Central Cattle Market to ensure proper technique and supply. Importantly, a report issued by the Bundesrath stated that there was "no existing active agitation in Germany against the use of vaccination." Although in Magdeburg, some resistance was reported, "gradually all opposition to compulsory vaccination is wearing away." The use of calf vaccine had much to do with the improved regard of the populace, especially in Berlin, while the authorities printed instructions for parents in regard to post-vaccination care, saving much suffering to the children. Dr. Bouardel presented these statistics to the French Academy of Medicine in 1891, hoping to convince physicians to take greater care and encourage vaccination, as the mortality in France at the time was 43 per 100,000. In a further step forward, the Royal Scientifical Medical Commission, Berlin, issued its findings on the question of whether smallpox vaccination produced a disposition to tubercular diseases by stating there was no proof of such a link.[23]

Data from Russia was difficult to obtain due to government suppression, but information out of St. Petersburg in December 1891 indicated that famine and smallpox were wreaking havoc on the population. The villages of Voatka, Samara, Validimre, Kursk, Orenburg, Peterhoff and Sartoff were hit especially hard by the "loathsome disease," nearly destroying the will to live as many were said to prefer death from disease over the slow torture of death from starvation.[24]

Ironically, Russians celebrated Edward Jenner's centenary with portraits and articles in the newspapers. Smallpox, however, as described in the *Moscow Daily News,* "spares neither rich nor poor, peasant nor king" and continued to run rampant five years later. Although Alexander I had been a great believer in vaccination, and it had been the law since 1805, the law was poorly enforced. That and the national custom of kissing the dead and distributing the victim's clothes among friends accounted for the unchecked spread of infection.[25]

Depressing news of a different sort was presented to the Academie de Medecine de Belgique in 1894. In arguing that a compulsory law was required, one author said:

> While it is to be hoped that in case of another war we should not again see, as in 1870, 25,000 of our own people succumb to smallpox, as against 600 on the German side, still there is in the scheme for mobilization an important category of soldiers placed in the auxiliary services who, having never served before, may not have been vaccinated, and run in this way the risk of becoming a danger of contagion.[26]

The Changing Face of Variola Major

Until the 1890s, smallpox (variola major) was a deadly disease: unvaccinated persons contracting the disease suffered horrible, debilitating skin eruptions that resulted in prolonged illness. If the individual was fortunate enough to survive, he was left with deep pitting on the face and, occasionally, blindness. In 1896, however, a mutant strain struck Pensacola, Florida. Later called "alastrim," or "variola minor," it quickly took hold in the state. Variola major prevailed during the summer of 1897, but thereafter disappeared except for small outbreaks. In its place, alastrim assumed predominance. This disease resembled smallpox but consisted of a mild form, rarely resulting in death. Symptoms were similar to chicken pox and the two were frequently confused.

In 1898, Florida reported 3,638 cases of alastrim with 51 associated deaths. Alastrim spread quickly and within four years it had extended over the whole continent north of the Mexican border. Before the century ended, variola minor had become endemic in the United States and South America, eventually replacing variola major as the predominant form of smallpox. Moving into the 20th century, this mutant strain would eventually replace the more deadly form of smallpox around the world and change the perceptions of the disease, not always for the better.[27]

In one hundred years, huge strides toward control, if not eradication of smallpox, had been achieved. Depressingly, however, even with so many advances to be thankful for, the minds of many were fixated on armed combat. They, at least, would not be disappointed.

New Century, Old Problems

Less than a century ago smallpox was as common as scarlet fever is today, and it was as unusual for one to escape its attack as it is now for a person to grow to adult life without having suffered from this pest of childhood. So almost inevitable was it that it became a common practice to inoculate people in early life, as the disease so produced was found to be milder than that arising from contagion. Then vaccination was discovered, and as it became general smallpox ceased to be the scourge it had been.

The above paragraph, taken from the January 6, 1900, edition of the *Ironwood Times* (MI), began a summary of how one writer viewed smallpox at the turn of the century. He noted "there is no remedy that will cut short an attack of smallpox," but added that skillful medical treatment and careful nursing could "do wonders in the saving of life and in warding off the evils which may follow the disease." Isolation of the patient was mandatory; items such as curtains and upholstered furniture were to be removed from the room to prevent contamination and the sick area was to be kept wet with disinfectants such as chloride of lime or carbolic acid. The author concluded by reminding his readers that the only "sure preventive of smallpox is vaccination," and that, as this effect weakened over time, revaccination was required.

Unfortunately, his enlightened message did not reflect a universal attitude. Simply stated, the year 1900 began as 1899 had ended: variola major was endemic in most countries except Australia, and outbreaks persisted throughout the world. There was no abatement over the argument of compulsory vaccination, and anti-vaccinationists continued to promote their platform of eliminating the procedure altogether.

Science attempted to convert the skeptical by explaining how the process worked:

Bacteriology has demonstrated not only the germ theory of many diseases, but the study has also shown that during the existence of the disease these bacteria cause the production of certain substances known as toxine and anti-toxine.... Now when a person has smallpox there is produced in his blood an anti-toxine which prevents him from having the disease again for several years. My belief is that vaccinia is a modified smallpox. Smallpox is inoculated on the cow and the disease after passing through several members of the bovine species is greatly modified in virulence so that its reinoculation on the human animal produces only a slight sore, but it has not lost its power to produce the anti-toxine which gives immunity from another attack for quite a number of years. The result is the same as if a person had had smallpox.... This is vaccination.[1]

That reason did not win the day was exemplified by the fact that in the United States, increasing reports of smallpox exacerbated rather than eliminated the debate over whether vaccination should be required of all children attending public schools. Boards of health were divided over the issue and depending on how strong anti-vaccinationists were, laws supporting the preventive were either defended or stricken from the records. In Vermont, medical societies "universally favored vaccination," but not uncommonly they were forced to defend themselves against the assertion that they supported the practice "by motives of pecuniary benefit." When those against vaccination charged that England had modified its compulsory laws to allow for "conscientious scruples," pro factions countered by stating that since the new act had been passed two years earlier, evasions of vaccination were down 40 percent, and "vaccination was more general in England now than it had ever been before."[2]

VACCINATION

THE FOLLOWING, written by an eminent physician, Secretary of the Massachusetts State Board of Health, is interesting in connection with the general alarm caused by the outbreak of small-pox in several cities:

At the turn of the century, people were eager to learn more about smallpox. The advertisement under this heading promoted the *World Almanac and Encyclopedia for 1901*, from the *New York World*, January 10, 1901. It offered a preview of the book, describing the discovery of vaccination, Dr. Waterhouse's introduction of vaccination to New England and statistics of how the procedure nearly eliminated smallpox from Germany.

The board of health of Lowell, Massachusetts, reported that primary causes of death in their jurisdiction stemmed from cholera infantum and other diarrhea diseases, tuberculosis and marasmus. Deaths from smallpox did not reach alarming levels but authorities warned that vulnerability to the disease was "thoroughly cosmopolitan," and persons were liable to exposure anywhere at any time. Medical men added their concern that with decreasing numbers, citizens were neglectful of vaccination.

Record of Deaths in
Lowell, Massachusetts, from Smallpox

Year	Deaths
1848	17
1849	41
1854	18
1855	20
1866	18
1870	178

Record of Expenses in
Lowell, Massachusetts, from Smallpox

Year	Cost of Smallpox
1871	$22,794.37
1877	$9,246.58
1886	$1,603.54
1894	$7,850.86
1899	$1,039.52[3]

They had reason to be concerned, as outbreaks around the country mounted. In January 1900 reports from the Indian Territory indicated that a very contagious form of smallpox prevailed in patches throughout the territory as well as in Oklahoma. Dr. V. Berry, national physician to the Seminole Nation, reported that a very malignant form of smallpox had struck the Chickasaw Nation. He also took pains to distinguish the epidemic from chicken pox, noting it struck adults as well as children and that those vaccinated showed no symptoms of the disease.[4] Also in January, the *Iowa Health Bulletin* stated that outbreaks of smallpox were more numerous than for any month in the history of the state.[5]

By February, reports from the midwestern and southern states indicated that smallpox was epidemic. The generally accepted theory suggested that in 1898, during the Spanish-American War, a mild form of smallpox first made an appearance at Key West, Florida, before being carried to military camps further north. Unsanitary conditions fostered the disease and after peace was declared, soldiers returning from Cuba, Puerto Rico and the Philippines further spread the contamination. Commercial travelers had great difficulty getting through some rural communities due to quarantine restrictions; schools closed, and at points along the Canadian border, mails were delayed by disagreements over which side was to undertake fumigation.

Thirty-five counties in Kentucky were affected and members of a dozen boards of health resigned became they did not have money to fight the plague. The Indiana State Board of Health reported 1,500–2,000 cases; Mississippi reported 4,000 cases since September, and the legislature argued for compulsory vaccination; Alabama, Tennessee, Washington and Colorado reported increasing cases; while Kansas established quarantine against Oklahoma. Smallpox was reported in nearly every town of the Cherokee Nation, leaving only Michigan, Minnesota and South Dakota relatively free of the disease.[6]

The Misdiagnosis of Smallpox

The problem with the misdiagnosis of smallpox was not a new one, frequently contributing to events of major significance. An epidemic of wide proportions occurred in 1885, when an infected individual left Chicago for Montreal. Because the traveler's ailment was diagnosed as chicken pox, he was never isolated. The disease spread and eventually over 3,000 people were affected. In 1893, in Muncie, Indiana, the diagnosis of smallpox was received with incredulity and ignored. In consequence, no quarantine was established and it was not until several deaths had occurred that people woke up and took notice.

The exceedingly mild form of smallpox in the early years of the 20th century vastly contributed to the problem. With fewer fatalities recorded, the disease failed to frighten as it had in previous centuries. (One individual in 1909 was quoted as saying that if the disease were the genuine smallpox, "someone would be dying from it," and that a funeral was the only thing that would convince him there was smallpox in the city.)[7] This led to a decrease in vaccination rates but, more specifically, the lack of severe epidemics left many physicians totally unaware of the early manifestations of smallpox, leading, in turn, to misdiagnosis, either from ignorance or intent. Headlines such as, "No Truth in the Rumor" were frequently accompanied by statements from select authorities, typically avowing outbreaks to be chicken pox or a new disease called "yaws." ("Yaws" was the name used in the British West Indies and on the coast of Africa for a "peculiar disease of the skin among [N]egroes." The medical name, first applied in 1761, was "framboesia," from the likeness of the eruptions to a raspberry. Yaws was actually caused by a spirochaete, *Treponema pertenus,* transmitted from person to person by direct contact, producing chronic, deforming and incapacitating lesions.)[8]

Denying the presence of smallpox, authorities in Iowa attributed the prevailing disease among "the white and colored people" to the Negroes, noting that for many years, it was thought yaws peculiar to the African Negro, spread by them to the East Indies, affecting the Malays. Because of recent contact with the Malay nations, this suggested a link in the spread of this disease to the United States.[9] Arguments became heated when a patient in Toledo contracted a disease physicians could not diagnose, one side considering it smallpox and the other yaws. The distinction was believed to be significant, as yaws was "simply a skin disease and is not serious," while smallpox was often fatal.[10] Actually, although rarely fatal, yaws caused marked fever, joint pain and eruptions, often leaving the sufferer disfigured and disabled.[11] In fact, the mild form of smallpox prevailing in the United States was variola minor, a close relative to variola major (true smallpox).

Complicating matters, doctors and laymen alike used misleading names to describe what they could not diagnoses. Expressions such as "yaws," "Cuban itch," "Spanish itch," impetigo, "Georgia bumps," "Bold chicken pox" or simply chicken pox led to confusion. Others simply described symptoms as "the disease," refusing to give it a name, but persistently refusing to call it smallpox. When closely questioned, many doctors, claiming to be authorities on the subject, acknowledged they had never seen a case of smallpox. Unfortunately, "they were still able to affirm that the cases were not smallpox even when pronounced smallpox by the city authorities and state inspectors." This inability to distinguish between diseases often led to serious consequences both for the victims and the community, preventing quarantine and vaccination measures to be instituted.

Even if "the disease" attacked only the unvaccinated, or was seen in adults (chicken pox being primarily a disease of the young), few wished to hang the onerous diagnosis of smallpox on a patient, and by association the community. By 1901, when epidemics of "mild variola" (variola minor) had spread from Florida as far north as Canada and across the country from Philadelphia to San Francisco, the failure of family physicians to correctly diagnosis the illness was believed to be responsible for the rapid and unusual extension of the infection.

The nonfatal American strain of variola minor (alastrim) soon became the predominant form of smallpox in North America (excluding Mexico), leading to greatly reduced numbers of primary and revaccination and augmenting the unenlightened view that people "would rather have smallpox than be vaccinated, for everybody has it and everybody gets well." A case highlighting the problem of variola major and minor concurrently infecting a community occurred in Washington in 1905, when a carpenter had an eruption on the skin but continued to work and visit relatives. It was not until his brother was diagnosed with smallpox that the infection was traced back to its source.[12] Whether the brother died of true smallpox or was a rare victim of a fatal case of variola minor, it underscored the danger of neglecting vaccination that would likely have saved his life. As serious as the situation was, Americans found a way to make light of it.

Unsuccessful Diagnosis
(What the Doctors Agreed on in Regard to That Cough)

The man's cough got worse, so he resorted to the physicians.

"From the stomach, I think," said Dr. Simtom.

"Pardon me, there is no such thing as a cough from the stomach," answered Dr. Modern.

"From the effects of vaccination, I should say," announced Dr. Nature. "Indeed," replied his colleague, Dr. Serum. "Let me remind you that (except tetanus, blood-poisoning and graft), there are no evil effects of vaccination."

"Well," said Dr. Experiment, "it is not expected that we should all [be] agreed —"

"On one thing we are agreed," cried Dr. Getrox, "that is to charge five dollars apiece."
But the widow refused to pay.[13]

Not everybody was laughing, however. In a bold editorial from the *New York Times,* April
30, 1900, the author opined:

> Smallpox had practically disappeared from this country when the war with Spain began, but since
> then our soldiers returning from foreign service have established centres of infection in many
> States. In most instances, of course, prompt and thorough vaccination has conquered the disease
> at once, but in the remaining cases, ignorance, carelessness, or criminal fanaticism has prevented
> the utilization of this invaluable safeguard, and as a result the Marine Hospital officials are obliged
> to make the humiliating report that in the past three and a half months there have been in the
> United States 7,267 cases and 402 deaths of a malady which no civilized human being has a right
> to contract. We seriously incline to the opinion that the time has come to hold the so-called
> victim of smallpox legally responsible for the danger he creates for others.... Years and years ago
> it was absolutely demonstrated that vaccination and safety from smallpox are synonymous. The
> continued existence of the disease among us is therefore a crime, and on recognized crimes penalties
> should certainly be imposed.

A similar stance on the subject of vaccination was taken by the *Salt Lake City Tribune*
(UT), February 3, 1900, when it categorically stated, "Whenever the church and the State
come into conflict, one must give way, and that one must not be the State, it must be the
church." Clearly this was easier said than done. In 1901, at Sioux City, Iowa, the teachings
of Christian Science were held responsible for the widespread exposure of pupils to a well-
defined case of smallpox. While schoolrooms were being fumigated, the afflicted child
(whose mother was a strong believer in Christian Science theory) stated the pustules on his
face were the result of "eating pancakes and pork gravy." An investigation revealed an
advanced case of smallpox "and much indignation was caused by those interested."[14] Abetting
anti-vaccinationists were practitioners of osteopathy who often allied themselves with Christian Scientists "and other mental and psychic systems." Defending their position, they cited
the "distrust of the laity to drugs." They added, "Suggestion is a prominent factor in medicine
and is the one underlying principle in all methods of mental healing."[15]

Fear was not limited to health concerns. Businessmen often protested against a diagnosis
of smallpox in their communities to preserve commerce. One typical letter to the editor
reminded fellow businessmen, "In the first place what is going to suffer most — the business
of the city and then the people? Is there a member of the Merchants' association who does not
realize what it will mean to him if this epidemic increases? Small-pox is the most loathsome
of diseases and no one from outside is coming to a city to do business which is filled with it."[16]

As New York City began a compulsory vaccination campaign in December 1901, authorities traced the recurrence of disease path through the upper part of the state. According to
the state board of health in Albany, in 1898 a traveling theatrical troupe introduced contagion
in every town in which it performed. By November 1900, another colored minstrel company
from the South, in whose personnel smallpox had been discovered, infected people in the
capital, Schenectady and Gloversville, and may have ignited the epidemic in New York
City, as well.[17]

As reports dribbled in that outbreaks were diminishing, others announced more dire
news. Michigan and Minnesota were "affected with it worse," while other notices warned,
"Pestilence Breeds in Country: Rural School Districts of the State [NY] become a Hotbed
for Smallpox." Although the percentage of fatal cases remained low, at 2–3 percent, experts
were concerned that "within the next two years the probabilities are that smallpox will

become much more widely epidemic than it has been among civilized people at any time during the nineteenth century."[18]

List of Cases of Smallpox, Health Report, March 22, 1901

State	1901	1900
California	20	3
Colorado	1,190	33
Idaho	205	10
Indian Territory	16	75
Iowa	40	30
Kansas	2,236	690
Louisiana	142	2,146
Minnesota	1,981	223
Missouri	134	80
Montana	218	100
Nebraska	1	—
New Mexico	4	—
North Dakota	60	—
Oklahoma Territory	690	55
Oregon	8	5
Texas	432	517
Utah	556	22
Washington	25	350
Wyoming	4	4[19]

Dr. Victor C. Vaughan, of the University of Michigan, spoke in plain terms, outlining cause for fear:

1. The time is ripe for a widely spread epidemic of smallpox.
2. The agitation of anti-vaccination fanatics has led thousands to refuse the only safeguard against the disease.
3. Criminal commercialism of some manufacturers of vaccine points in putting out worthless vaccine has resulted in thousands more being susceptible, although they believe they are immune.
4. Already there are now prevailing epidemics, which, fortunately, are light.
5. The remedy: vaccination and repeated vaccination after a lapse of a few years. To insure effective vaccination there should be state laws, regulating the output of the virus.[20]

The January 1, 1901, report of the Marine Hospital Service revealed that smallpox was present in 45 of the 51 states and territories, with a total of 9,229 cases, of which Ohio had 1,732; Tennessee 1,405; Minnesota 1,199; Texas 674; North Carolina 587; Nebraska 467; Wisconsin 412. The disease had spread quickly: from the beginning in 1898, it was confined to four localities in three states (New York, Tennessee and Alabama). At the close of the year, it was reported in 151 localities in 24 states.[21]

With the facts before them, the Utah State Legislature passed a bill making illegal the exclusion of unvaccinated children from public schools. Governor Wells promptly vetoed it, but anti-vaccinationists threatened to override the veto. In presenting this news item, the editors of the *Post-Standard* (NY), February 15, 1901, added, "The people of Utah who object to smallpox have our sincere sympathy."

Along with the bad news, there were occasional glimpses of grim humor. One physician in New York had a slight scratch on his thumb and inadvertently touched the virus he was using to vaccinate patients. Within 48 hours, the virus "took," and he was out of practice for a week. Another physician scratched a pimple on his nose while vaccinating and within a few days found himself in seclusion, nursing a huge red, purple and blue proboscis.[22]

American Indians and African Americans

A report from Washington dated October 30, 1900, indicated that it was feared cold weather would greatly increase smallpox epidemics on the western Indian reservations. According to Lieutenant-Colonel Randall, in charge of the Kiowa Indian Agency, Oklahoma, smallpox was already epidemic on the Wichita reservation, at Cache Creek Mission and St. Patrick Mission on the Apache, Kiowa and Comanche reservations. From the Colville agency at Miles, Washington, agent Anderson reported that smallpox was prevalent among the Indians on the Coeur D'Alene Reservation. From the Fort Hall agency in Idaho, agent Caldwell reported smallpox increasing. Complaint was also made on the quality of vaccine supplied, as only 3 of 50 primary vaccinations of small children proved successful. United States senator Shoup of Idaho reported that smallpox was prevalent at Black Foot and Pocatello and feared the disease would spread to the Indians. Smallpox was also reported from Valentine, Nebraska, the shipping point for the Rosebud agency.[23]

Nearly one year later, reports of a more alarming nature surfaced. At Black River Falls, Wisconsin, Indian agent Alex Jaconson discovered 30 cases of smallpox, including a number of deaths among the Winnebago, coupled with 50 cases in the towns of Brockway and Manchester. With "no end in sight," the state "practically refused to come to the aid of the town, and the Indians come and go at pleasure," spreading infection.[24] Warnings in Grand Rapids immediately went out that, as many Indians came to that section of the country to pick cranberries, growers ought to be careful whom they hired.[25] Simultaneously, the 3,000 residents of Sturgeon Bay were exposed to smallpox after the local physician misdiagnosed the condition as chicken pox.[26]

In September 1901, the Department of Indian Affairs ordered agent Caldwell of the Fort Hall Indian Agency to have all Indians on the reservation vaccinated, as they had suffered very severely from the disease in the past, and "to some extent, understand the value of vaccination." The work was promised to begin as soon as "points" could be secured.[27]

During the late summer of 1901, the *Cedar Rapids Gazette* (IA) was given official information by agent Malin concerning the lack of smallpox on the Indian reservation, Tama County, Iowa. When this proved incorrect, editors noted, "The Gazette [did] not wish to create the impression that the towns of Tama, Toledo and Montour [were] endangered, and guided by this idea, sought to minimize the rumors, that [now] appear to be founded on facts of the gravest kind, so far as the reservation is concerned. There is additional proof of the incompetence of the men in charge, and the government should make a rigid investigation."

Benjamin Thompson, M.D., sent a corrected report to the newspaper, stating that on September 23, an Indian from the Winnebago agency, Nebraska, visited the Tama Reservation, occupied by 600 Sac and Fox. Shortly thereafter, he became sick with an eruptive disease. Nothing was done to diagnose the disease and friends visited him at will. About two weeks later, others became stricken and it spread rapidly. Again, no effort was made by the government to ascertain the true nature of the illness and whites visited the camp daily.

On October 22, a local from the city of Tama reported the smallpox outbreak to Dr. Thompson, who visited the reservation with Dr. Carpenter. They found nine well-marked cases of smallpox, three convalescents and four who had already died. On their way out, they encountered a hack carrying 16 tourists, who informed them Indian agent Malin indicated there were no contagious diseases in camp.

That night, the physicians held a joint meeting with the boards of health of Monitor, Toledo and Tama. Agent Malin did not accept their findings and demanded another inspection. On Wednesday, Doctors Thompson, Carpenter and Linn returned to the reservation and reconfirmed the presence of smallpox. The three townships immediately ordered quarantine, "as the white people in the vicinity are much alarmed at the prospective spread of the disease."

Malin refused to accept the findings and did nothing more than supply the Indians with provisions. Cases increased rapidly, with the chief reporting 70 cases. After deploring the fact nothing was done for "a people who could not care for themselves," Dr. Thompson concluded, "If it was some scheme to send a missionary to some far distant land to corrupt [convert] the heathen, money would be found to send them. Here we are, in one of the wealthiest portions of the great state of Iowa, and yet 400 poor, forlorn people are left to die like dogs and the government reports no funds for quarantine work; no effort made by a Christian people to assist them in their dire extremity."

In defense, agent Malin stated that he "made daily inquiries of the Indians as to the existence of small pox in the camp and invariably elicited a negative reply." Early in September, he received orders from the Indian Department to vaccinate the Indians and nearly 200 received the operation. He added that many of the older Indians insist there was no smallpox in camp and that the health of the camp was normal.[28] Coincidentally, local papers reported that Indians at Tama refused vaccination, "and there is no state law compelling it." The Indians also objected to quarantine and for the purpose of avoiding legal complications (see below), the board of health recommended police be stationed on land adjacent to the reservation. Ten days later, a report from Grinnell, Iowa, reported smallpox in the vicinity, reputed to have been introduced by Indians from Tama.[29]

Among the Indian deaths from smallpox at Tama was Lillie Puck-a-Chee, a young woman who had earlier attracted much attention from a court case in which the government attempted to appoint a guardian for her as a means of compelling her to attend school at Toledo. Judge Shiras ruled the state courts were without jurisdiction over the Indians.[30]

In a rapidly degenerating standoff between unnamed parties (principally Dr. Thompson and agent Malin), the physician declared that the state board had done nothing to relieve the condition of the Indians and had not even communicated with the health officer of Tama. He stated the death toll had risen to 35, with new cases appearing daily, while Malin reported there were but 4 cases. Thompson urged the construction of a warm house and "at least as good care as we give our animals," but feared nothing would be done, as another physician who inspected the reservation (at Malin's request) confirmed "they decided to do nothing and let the disease die out of its own volition." Malin's response was that "someone had been poisoning the minds of the Indians until they believed that the whites had them quarantined for the purpose of poisoning and wiping the whole tribe off the face of the earth." He suggested this had been done by personal enemies who desired to "make him as much trouble as possible in caring for the Indians."[31]

Governor Shaw telegraphed Secretary Hitchcock of the Interior Department, stating that doubts existed over the authority of the state board of health to quarantine. Hitchcock replied, "Government will be glad to co-operate with state authorities in protecting the people of Tama against smallpox among the Indians and will also instruct the Indian agent in charge. Under the exigency shown in your telegram your state board of health and government authorities may take any necessary action."[32]

Similar situations were occurring in other communities. In September 1901, when smallpox struck, remnants of the Cocopah tribe crossed the Mexican side below Yuma. While "scores" were dying, an armed guard kept them away from Yuma, their sole source of supplies. As a result, they suffered from a lack of food, with no medicine but their own "concoctions." In October 1901, Sheriff Cloggett of Mille Lacs County, Minnesota, reported smallpox among the 500 Chippewas "squatting on the shores of Mille Lacs lake." When the village authorities of Robins tried to keep the Indians from circulating by setting a guard, armed braves turned out in force, chasing the whites away. It was believed "a clash between the settlers and Indians is probable at any time."

Also in October, 90 cases of smallpox were discovered on the Bad River (Odanah village) Reservation, Wisconsin. The Northwestern Railway Company was ordered not to stop trains at the reservation, but the Indians left by boat and through the timber, causing alarm that the disease would spread to Red Cliff Reservation, Bayfield, Ashland and nearby Michigan. A "shotgun quarantine" was maintained. By November, the disease had become epidemic among the Indians near Spooner, and Senator William O'Neill of Washburn, Wisconsin, ordered all logging camps on the Bad River Reservation closed, putting nearly 1,000 men out of employment.

Including the above, the Indian Bureau (October 10) reported smallpox cases among reservations at Leech Lake, Mille Lac and Fond du Lac, MN; Devil's Lake, ND, Yankton and Crow Creek, SD, Seger Colony, OK, Pima, AZ, and Bloomfield, Nebraska. By October 15, the bureau added the Southern Ute Reservation, Colorado, the Kickapoo Indian boarding school in Kansas and outbreaks among Mexicans at Phoenix, "in uncomfortable proximity to the Indians."[33]

For one editorialist, at least, the situation was summed up thusly:

> The difficulty of taming and civilizing wild things is well illustrated in the case of 1,500 Indians upon one of the western reservations. Smallpox is decimating their ranks, and they will neither submit to vaccination nor quarantine. The state has no control over them, and the general government humors their whims. The reservation is surrounded by a thickly settled community of white farmers, who fully realize what a nuisance the red man can become.[34]

The situation was little improved by 1923, when a journalist wrote of the Yaqui, living outside Tucson: "Nobody pays much attention to them until the smallpox gets so bad the health authorities have to take notice. That is about the only time a white physician is ever seen among these Indians." Left to their own devices, the tribe depended upon their medicine man, who would "sprinkle something over one, puff smoke into the ear of another and perform some sort of mummery over the head of another," before retiring to his shack to commune "with the good spirits."[35]

Even though the century had turned the figurative page on America's "domestic problem," African Americans garnered little respect, with the invisible line of "them" and "us" affecting everything from education to health care. The same edition of the *Des Moines Daily News,* July 27, 1900, that carried a scientific discussion on modern germ theory resorted to word of mouth by printing, "It has been found that the darker the skin of the person the greater the susceptibility of that individual to small pox. The [N]egro is far more attacked by the disease than the white individual." The *Moberly Weekly Monitor* (MO), January 3, 1901, went further, dismissing the contagion as "the itch," while noting the observation of a political attaché: "It's the [N]egroes who have it, don't think it's smallpox. It's that disease the soldiers imported from Cuba."

Life for African Americans did not get any easier when reports from Charleston, South Carolina, indicated that when the appearance of smallpox prompted health authorities to impose mandatory vaccination, those chosen to perform the operation on the black population were undergraduate medical students rather than certified doctors. All "semblance of a scandal" was averted by the discharge of the young men.[36] When smallpox was discovered in Petersburg, Virginia, $1,000 was set aside for the establishment of a detention camp to be used for [N]egroes, who were reportedly the only section of the population affected.[37]

In 1920 in North Carolina it was reported that 20 cases of smallpox had occurred, "nearly all of them among colored people." Health authorities warned everyone to be vaccinated, as an epidemic of preventable smallpox "reflects on the intelligence of the people, whether white or colored." The warning worked in the latter's case, as within 10 days over 95 percent of schoolchildren in the colored schools were vaccinated, with success due to the cooperative effort of the teachers and the "non interference of their parents."[38] There was less success at St. Louis in 1923, when municipal health authorities proposed a plan to vaccinate all Negroes coming from the South. Members of the powerful anti-vaccinationist group American Medical Liberty League out of Chicago thwarted the idea by circulating through the southern states, advising the Negroes to resist the action.[39]

The American Medical Liberty League, Incorporated, persisted in its anti-vaccination campaigns, charging in 1927 that the procedure "frequently caused the death of the patients, the loss of an arm or in the pollution of the blood stream by the introduction of organisms which produce foul diseases." (Surgeon general M.W. Ireland countered by stating that in the United States Army there had been no deaths, no lost arms and no cases of syphilis among the 7,000,000 soldiers vaccinated during the previous 25 years.) The League also challenged the historical success of vaccination, questioned vaccine purity and maintained the right of citizens to refuse vaccination on the grounds of personal liberty. Arguing against the League, Dr. William Brady of Wisconsin, wrote, "The so-called 'medical liberty' corporation is not medical at all, but is rather a league of cultists, pathists, mail order tradesmen, quacks, and nostrum makers, interests that demand, not liberty, but license, special privilege, impunity from the law or exceptional relaxation of the rigor of the law to favor their extraordinary methods." Unfortunately, the League and other anti-vaccination groups had the support of George Bernard Shaw, who declared in 1926, "Vaccination kills more persons than smallpox. America is a hundred years behind the times." Shaw's anti-vaccination views were not lost on the American public. In 1933, under the notice, "Smallpox is spreading in India," a writer observed, "Those five words will interest George Bernard Shaw and change objection to vaccination, if he is still in India on his journey around the world."[40]

Glycerinated Lymph

The question of whether Americans could trust vaccine lymph to be "pure," or free from contaminants, continued to be a major issue. Statements made by Dr. Walter Reed, surgeon, United States Army, given before the DC Medical Society in June 1895, warned that he had examined samples from six of the leading makers of vaccine and found "colonies of bacteria" in every one. To this was appended the fact that the manager of the Mutual Life Company did "not care whether applicants for insurance are vaccinated or not. Here is vaccination pushed aside as though it were just common Hood's Sarsaparilla."[41] Events were about to change.

The greatest advance in vaccination since the discovery for the need of revaccination came from Sydney Arthur Monckton Copeman (1862–1947), an English physician. The son of Reverend Canon Arthur Charles Copeman, LL.D, Monckton Copeman was educated at King Edward VI School, Norwich, and at Corpus Christi College, Cambridge. He graduated with a bachelor of arts in the Natural Sciences Tripos in 1882, and took his clinical studies at St. Thomas' Hospital. He married Ethel Margaret, youngest daughter of Sir William Boord, Bt., MP, in 1899, and together they had one son.

Well aware of the inherent dangers of vaccination as it was then practiced (attenuation of the virus by repeated human transmission; the danger of transmitting other diseases, including sepsis from contamination or the use of unsterile equipment) and the repeated failures of the procedure to "take," Copeman began his research. He started by demonstrating that the lack of efficacy of calf lymph resulted from a loss of potency "when kept in the fluid state dried on ivory points," therefore becoming less reliable than humanized lymph. He also addressed the growing concern regarding germs found in "pure lymph" (frequently cited by anti-vaccinationists as a reason to abandon vaccination) by subjecting lymph to temperatures that should kill the bacteria. This did not prove effective, as Copeman observed in 1898: "Some method of readier application and requiring less delicate manipulation was therefore obviously desirable. This I at length found in the addition to the lymph or rather to the vesicular pulp obtained from a vaccinated calf, of a selected 50 per cent solution of glycerine in distilled water."[42]

The significance of glycerin (alternately spelled with an "e" at the end of the word and used alternately with "glycerol") was that it provided "the selective germicidal action on the extraneous bacteria of calf vaccine lymph." By destroying these germs, Dr. Copeman thus achieved as "pure" a vaccine as possible, making vaccination considerably safer. He was not the first to use glycerin, which he readily acknowledged. In 1850, Dr. R.R. Cheyne promoted the idea in an article published in the *Medical Times*. Vaccine centers in France, Belgium, Holland and Germany had also experimented with the technique, while Müller reported that vaccine lymph could be diluted with three times its bulk of glycerin and remain effective.

Like Edward Jenner, Copeman achieved what the others did not: he caused the scientific community to stand up and take notice. Glycerin not only acted as an effective antibacterial, it also helped make the vaccine stick to the skin and permitted the maintenance of the vaccine in liquid form, ensuring long survival of the active vaccinia virus when distributed in capillary tubes.[43] Once these facts were established, physicians around the world quickly adopted the technique. During 1896 and 1897, Copeman traveled with Sir Richard Thorne, medical officer of the Local Government Board, to Paris, Brussels, Berlin, Cologne, Dresden and Geneva to study preparation, storage and distribution of vaccine lymph. Discovering that glycerinated calf lymph "had become almost universal," Dr. Thorne recommended the following:

1. Vaccination carried out by the British Government should be performed exclusively with vaccine derived from calf lymph.

2. Distribution of calf vaccine by the National Vaccine Establishment should be limited to glycerinated, or similar preparations, in airtight tubes or other glass receptacles.
3. The board's Animal Vaccine Station should include a properly equipped bacteriological laboratory.

The Vaccination Act of 1898 and the Vaccination Order of 1898 of the Local Government Board incorporated these suggestions and a new laboratory was established at Chelsea under Dr. F.R. Blaxall, with distribution of glycerinated calf lymph begun on January 1, 1899. The Government Lymph Establishment was created in 1907, under Dr. Blaxall, incorporating the entire process of lymph manufacture and distribution.[44]

By March 1900, when defending the virtues of vaccination, the Illinois State Board of Health included this in its report: "No danger can result from vaccination properly performed under aseptic conditions with pure virus. This Board advises the exclusive use of glycerinated lymph."[45] Two years later, the *Waterloo Daily Courier* (citing the *Saturday Review*) remarked on the subject of the theoretical danger of vaccination by concluding "the modern method of glycerinated calf lymph has now destroyed even the remote possibility of such intrinsic danger." In fact, during the latter part of the 19th century, glycerolated calf-derived vaccine greatly contributed to a decrease in smallpox in countries where it became available.[46]

Anti-vaccinationists were hardly convinced, however, continuing the trend of discounting scientific evidence. One Canadian objector wrote the following:

> The use of government glycerinated calf lymph in vaccination is a grave source of danger. Glycerine is a nutritive medium for the growth of putrefactive and other germs, and, being fluid, the germs soon pervade it throughout. As a matter of fact, in India glycerinated lymph soon becomes putrid and septically dangerous. This precious concoction of vaccine lymph, thymol solution, and glycerine caused the infection of 320 persons with a loathsome contagious disease at Rugen, in Germany, through vaccination.... Sir George Buchanan, M.D., F.R.S., chief medical officer to the local government board, alluded to glycerinated calf-lymph as a "preposterous adulteration of vaccine."[47]

A 1905 objector used more inflammatory language by writing, "I am told, referring to 'tubes and points' that calf-lymph-glycerinated vaccine, 'the pure' will be used. Pure Poison! Think of it parents! Pure pus-rottenness — think of it! Pure calf-lymph from calves 'filthy sores' put into the arms of innocent babes and school children. 'Pure!' Why it is virtually beastly calf-brutality thrust into our children's budding humanity!"[48]

The argument did not go away. In 1913, two opposing sides were presented on the question of vaccination. The supporter claimed there was no danger associated with vaccination because the glycerin "destroys all disease germs such as tetanus, erysipelas, tuberculosis, etc." citing Ricketts' work on Immunity and Serum Therapy (published by the American Medical Association Press) by quoting, "Glycerinated lymph has many advantages, the most important of which relates to the bacteriological action of the glycerine by which the lymph is freed from the pathogenic bacteria which in former times caused serious complications in vaccination."

Countering this, Dr. J. Deason of the American School of Osteopathy, was cited as having "found that all the samples of glycerinated lymph, coming as they did from different houses, contained disease germs. As many as twenty varieties were found in a single sample." The anti-side then noted that between 1900 and 1908, there were 82 deaths caused by vaccination; 47 of the patients had lockjaw.[49]

Not surprisingly, a physician named Fraser took exception to the above article written by Dr. Andrews, choosing to answer him in the April 11, 1913, edition of the *Algona Courier* (IA). Dr. Fraser informed his colleague, "The glycerine should kill all disease germs that are likely to be present in the lymph. It will not kill spore-forming bacilli. The lockjaw bacillus is a spore-forming bacillus, but had it been present when the lymph was collected it should have been discovered. If it was not present when the lymph was collected it could only gain admission through carelessness."

Dr. Andrews replied in the April 25 edition of the *Courier,* noting rather sarcastically that Dr. Fraser did not believe the 47 lockjaw deaths stemmed from vaccination. "Such argument," he wrote, "is parallel with the saying ... 'The operation was a success, but the patient died.'" Andrews went on to question the use of glycerin as a germicide by stating, "Sternberg in the Reference Handbook gives a list of 65 with glycerine occupying 63rd place with the antiseptic (not germicidal) strength two-thirds that of table salt. The lymph in the vaccine virus tubes is 50 per cent glycerine, giving it an antiseptic strength one-third that of table salt.... Referring again to the Reference Handbook we read, 'Of the various micro-organisms that have been discovered in lymph by different observers, the most common are Staphylococcus albus, S[taph] pyogenes aureus, and S[taph] cerreus flavus.... According to Copeman one or another of these is to be found almost universally in every specimen of lymph examined.'" Quoting from Ricketts again, Andrews added, "The bacteriological power of glycerine has been overestimated, and while it kills pyogenic (pus) cocci within two weeks when kept at body temperature, such organisms may live for months in glycerine when kept in the ice-chest; and of course our glycerinated virus is kept in the ice-chest.'"

The Progression of Vaccine Procurement and Technique

When giving a history of vaccination, in the *Oelwein Daily Register* (IA), March 28, 1914, the author opined that the danger of vaccination had been "entirely removed by the discontinuance of the use of humanized lymph and the universal employment of pure glyc-erinated bovine virus." Gone were the days when wounds were expected to suppurate (create pus): the modern vaccinator was "as scrupulously particular about the purity of his virus, the asepsis of his instruments and the site of the vaccination, as the surgeon who is about to undertake a major operation."

The 1914 description of vaccination noted it was a "trifling operation," where a slight scratching of the skin did not cause blood to flow. A moment's application of the aseptic vaccine, then several seconds to allow it to dry, and the operation was concluded. In 10 or 12 days, a little blister or vesicle formed, the size of which depended on the surface denuded by the operator. The vesicle dried, a small crust or scab formed and several days later dropped off, leaving a scarcely perceptible scar.

During the manufacture of aseptic vaccine, every precaution was used to exclude con-tamination. Only healthy young heifers were selected and these underwent a test for tuber-culosis by a veterinary surgeon before the process continued. Inoculation rooms were airy and well lit, with walls and floors constructed of an impervious material capable of being easily flushed and disinfected. After the heifer was manipulated onto a table and firmly secured, the surface of the abdomen was surgically cleaned and shaved to provide a sterile field. The scarification was then performed, and the virus applied and allowed to dry. After-ward, a sterile dressing was applied to prevent germs from contaminating the skin.

After the usual waiting period of five days, the animal was returned to the operating theatre, the vesicated region sterilized with water and disinfectant and the external crust removed. Serum exuded from the pulpy portion (or base) of the vesicle and was gathered and placed in sterile receptacles containing pure glycerin. This mixture was then taken to the laboratory, where it was placed in a machine and mixed into a perfectly smooth, homogeneous state, at which time a dilutent was added and the mixture again emulsified.

Before being certified as pure vaccine lymph, it was tested by a bacteriologist to insure freedom from pernicious germs and physiologically tested to determine activity. After passing examination, the vaccine was put in sterilized glass tubes, hermetically sealed and placed in a refrigerator. In order to preserve vaccine from deteriorating, it was recommended that exposure to temperatures above 60°F be avoided. When vaccination was correctly applied, the resultant vesicle resembled an ordinary blister; as the fluid contents were absorbed, the vesicle depressed in the center and eventually dried into a pearly white crust. This differed significantly from the technique of the early and mid–1800s, when red, swollen and painful arms, accompanied by constitutional disturbances, were looked upon as proof of success.

By contrast, when an anti-vaccinationist described the above process, it sounded completely different:

> A calf is tired to an operating table, the belly shaved for about a square foot, on which exposed surface about one hundred incisions are made. Into these incisions, vaccine seed or glycerinated lymph (the pus of smallpox, and perhaps cancer, syphilis, and tuberculosis, taken from persons having these diseases) is thoroughly rubbed to ripen into vesicles filled with pus that produces the matter which is later injected into perfectly healthy human beings.[50]

Time did not significantly modify the language of anti-vaccinationists. In 1950, the process described above was followed by this:

> To this mass of rotten matter glycerine is added and the "stew" is stirred and mixed. It is then placed in another crucible and passed through a sieve to remove pieces of decayed flesh, hair, etc. The mixture is again beaten and mixed, placed in tubes and distributed throughout the country as pure calf lymph — how "pure" it is you can imagine.[51]

32

Vaccination Creeds,
Homeopathic Pills and Lettuce

Dr. James Nevins Hyde says, "If a modern traveler could find himself transported to the streets of London as they appeared one hundred years ago, it is probable that no peculiarities of architecture, dress or behavior would be to him so strikingly conspicuous as the enormous number of pock marked visages he would encounter among the people at every turn." In the village of Ware, it may be stated, where accurate records were kept, after the epidemic of 1722, 2,443 persons survived, 2,141 of whom, or 88 per cent, had the indelible marks of smallpox upon their countenances.[1]

In many respects, the battle over compulsory vaccination in schools was encapsulated by the struggle in Pennsylvania. The Act of June 18, 1895, section 12, provided that "all principals or other persons in charge of any public, private, parochial, Sunday or other school are required to refuse the admission of any child to the schools under their charge except upon a certificate, signed by a physician, setting forth that such a child has been successfully vaccinated, or that it has previously had small pox." Section 21 of the same Act provided that any principal who violated the above requirements be fined not less than $5 and no more than $100. If in default of payment, the said person was to undergo imprisonment for a period not exceeding 60 days.[2]

Protests of the new act began immediately; ten years after its enactment, Dr. Nathan C. Schaeffer, superintendent of public instruction, submitted a report stating the unsatisfactory results of the Act:

1. It failed to make vaccination universal.
2. It disorganized schools in communities where there was no smallpox danger.
3. It punished the innocent instead of the guilty.
4. It did not exclude unvaccinated children from other public places.
5. It did not impose vaccination upon teachers.
6. It subjected teachers to enforce a duty for which parents, physicians and health officers should be held responsible.[3]

In addition to the above, one of the major issues to come out of compulsory vaccination was the contrivance to usurp the law by the issuance of false certificates.[4] In 1906, Dr. Samuel G. Dixon, state health commissioner, responded to the growing trend against vaccination by stating, "The wildest literature is circulated depicting alleged horrors of vaccination. In some districts you will find that the death of nearly every child in the community is being laid to vaccination." He warned parents, "Unchain the horrible monster—smallpox — by taking away vaccination, and inside of two generations our prosperous state would have her industries paralyzed and her cemeteries overcrowded with the victims of that dread disease."[5]

Dr. Dixon's words had little effect, compelling him to take more drastic action. He determined to make a test case against the public school authorities of Waynesboro, Franklin County, who had thrown open their institutions to unvaccinated children. Of the 1,200 students in Waynesboro, only 300 had been inoculated. After "very acrimonious correspondence between the state health department and leading anti-vaccinationists of that community," Dixon ordered schools closed a week before Christmas (1905). "The opening of the schools Tuesday [January 2, 1906] was the result of a council of war between the directors and teachers."[6]

Commissioner Dixon had the support of the state's attorney general and a number of legislators, including Assemblyman Walter S. Reynolds. Speaking at the Lawrence County School Directors' Association in defense of compulsory vaccination and the difficulty of convincing "people of the present day" to accept science, he noted, "Vaccination was introduced in an age of superstition, witchcraft and necromancy. Nothing is harder to eradicate than superstition, and the opposition to vaccination is largely handed down, robbed of its grosser features, from generation to generation, but it still retains its hold."[7]

If you read it in the newspaper...

Part of the problem in the acceptance of vaccination was the influence of the printed word under what might be considered "if you read it in the newspaper it must be true." Anti-vaccinationists used the press as a tool, making sure that letters to the editor filled columns, while leading spokesmen skillfully garnered headlines. Under the heading "Vaccination Fight On," a typical story ran in the *Washington Post,* August 16, 1909: "Having read Sunday magazine[s] and newspaper articles on the subject of vaccination and convinced himself that the generally accepted method of prevention is more to be dreaded than a case of smallpox," a local proprietor determined to make a legal fight over a compulsory order.

If that were all, the case for vaccination might have convinced the majority of people by presenting case histories and statistics, but frightening headlines sold newspapers. Exchanges picking up the stories often found it to their advantage to pursue the topic. On that subject, the March 29, 1900, issue of the *Iowa Postal Card* ran a paragraph from the *Sumner Signal,* commenting on the propensity of reworking sensational (in this case, smallpox) stories: "The reason why so many papers pick up such matters is because there are too many human phonographs pushing pencils on country papers. Some one agitates a matter and the others pick it up, twist a couple of words around and an original (?) editorial. They give no credit, and in many cases the originator should be thankful for it."

Worse, newspapers and physicians often suppressed the true epidemic nature of smallpox "from a false sense of duty." On December 26, 1900, the *Cedar Rapids Gazette* published an article out of New York, indicating that a reputable physician had reported 4,000 cases of smallpox in greater New York; the writer further stated that between the Atlantic Ocean and Mississippi River, there were probably 25,000 suffering from the disease, adding, "It is no secret that many cases have been concealed, and to this fact is attributed the spread of small pox wherever it has appeared." In his opinion, the first 16 cases in the state were identified around March 1900. The victims were employees of the largest department store in the city; they were quickly removed to the pest hospital on North Brother Island in the East River. The doctor concluded: "The newspapers of the city were requested by the proprietors of the store to omit any mention of these cases, and their request was granted. For similar reasons — the fear that the commercial prestige of the city might be injured — subsequent outbreaks of the disease have passed unnoticed or have been so minimized that the average reader would never suspect the real danger."

Going one step further, the city council of San Antonio, Texas, passed an ordinance providing for the punishment of any person who was found guilty of circulating false, willful or wanton reports of the existence of yellow fever, cholera or smallpox.[8] It is not a stretch to envision this law being used to suppress legitimate reports of contagious or infectious diseases.

Tragically, headlines such as "Parents Object to Vaccination" and "School Board Negligent in Enforcing Vaccination Law," "On Vaccination: Doctors Disagree as to Its Usefulness,"[9] "Compulsory Scratching of Arms Opposed,"[10] and "A Sacrifice to Liberty"[11] persisted.

Of wider-scale importance and ramifications was an article in the *Evening Record* (PA), March 16, 1906, entitled, "Defiance to Law Is Bred by Utterances of Some Papers with Demoralizing Editorials." In reference to the *Mercer County Herald*, which "continues its [ill] advised tirade against the efficiency of vaccination as a protection against smallpox," the newspaper astutely pronounced:

> It is such papers as these which are the comforters of the violators of law and which really incite to a resistance to law, as no publication is so violent or so radical but what it will have some adherents who accept its doctrines as the truth and who blindly follow them without reasoning whether or not they are justified, these poor deluded followers being all the more easily led because of the fact that such papers generally make a blatant declaration in their editorials as to how they are law-abiding and respectable members of the journalistic fraternity and that they ever stand for a full enforcement of the laws enacted by the state and nation. On one hand it is an obedience to law; on the other an open defiance and an invitation to resistance. It is the utterances of such inconsistent statements which breed anarchy and which result in the assassination of rulers and the overthrow of good government by the misled rabble, who rely upon the newspapers for their information and to mould their opinions as to the right and wrong.

In debunking the arguments made by the *Herald* (that vaccination was a disease and had no virtue against smallpox; that it was unscientific and that health was the best preventive against smallpox), the *Evening Record* sarcastically concluded:

> The last argument is one worthy of a master mind and doubtless physicians and scientists all over the country will be much elated over this wonderful discovery. And its truth is not to be denied, as all will admit that so long as a person is in good health he cannot be diseased. Therefore, if you would live long and never be sick, always keep well. We concede this truth.

The above complements a brief paragraph published by the *Mansfield News* (OH), December 14, 1903: "Bulk of scientific authority still holds that universal and compulsory vaccination of every child at its birth is the one effective remedy for smallpox and, that, strange as it may seem, the United States is the one civilized country which still has to make a fight against this preventable disease."

In commenting upon newspaper reports regarding unsanitary conditions in Cuba, the 20th Annual Conference of the States and Provincial Boards of Health of North America, meeting in 1905 at Washington, DC, declared, "Whereas, sensational and misleading articles have recently appeared in American newspapers, based upon the report of alleged sanitary experts ... in part untrue, in part exaggerated and in toto misleading," they resolved "that these publications are condemned by this conference as unwarranted by the facts as injurious to international amity...."[12]

Occasionally, a newspaper article would inadvertently promote the cause of vaccination. Returning to the United States from Florence, Italy, after the death of his wife, Samuel L. Clemens and his two daughters were caught in a smallpox scare aboard the *Prinz Oscar*. On July 13, 1904, after a baby was diagnosed with the disease (later claimed to be chicken pox or flea bites), the family, along with 40 other first class cabin and 300 steerage passengers, were required to undergo vaccination.[13] It is not unreasonable to suppose that if someone as famous as Mark Twain underwent the procedure without protest, his followers would feel more compelled to protect themselves and their families.

Conversely, there were instances when a well-meaning reporter without proper background in his subject misinterpreted his data, leading to great potential harm. Grant Wallace, a distinguished newspaperman and war correspondent of the *Sunday Bulletin* (CA) specialized in pithy comments on current events. On January 1, 1905, he widened his repertoire by offering an expose on vaccination. Wallace began by announcing that within the past few months, 3 or 4 children in the Bay Cities had died of lockjaw or blood poisoning due to vaccination. He added, "The statute books are still marred by this law forcing us to engraft matterated [*sic*] cow virus upon our children at say $1 a head." After saying "quinine is known to be good as a preventive of malaria," he asked, "Do we have to make laws to force our neighbors to take quinine"? He also offered the common belief that "small-pox is no more of a dread disease than measles or whooping cough."

In a spirited reply, Dr. J.F. Rinehart expressed consternation that "a great many people who have not taken the pains to inform themselves of the subject" would believe the "wild statements" and "garbled statistics" of a writer known for his veracity. The physician offered statistics of his own.

Comparison of Mortality Between Vaccinated and Unvaccinated Persons Around the World (Death Rate per 100 cases)

Place/Years	% Unvaccinated	% Vaccinated
France, 1816–1841	16.1	1.0
Quebec, 1819–1820	27.0	1.1
Verona, 1825–1829	46.6	5.6
Milan, 1830–1851	38.5	7.6
Breslau, 1831–1833	53.8	2.1
Wirtemburg, 1831–1835	27.3	7.1
Vienna Hosp., 1831	51.2	12.5
Lower Austria, 1835	25.8	11.5
Bohemia, 1835–1855	29.8	5.2
Galicia, 1836	23.5	3.1
London Smallpox Hosp., 1836–1856	35.0	7.0
Vienna Hosp., 1837–1856	30.0	5.0
Epidemiological Soc. Returns	23.0	2.9
Illinois	48.6	6.1

After refuting Wallace's charges (lockjaw resulted from contamination of the site, not vaccine virus; it was illegal to engraft; it required extensive efforts to drain swamps and educate the public on exterminating mosquitoes, which was far more effective than quinine; smallpox was potentially a fatal disease and minimizing measles and whooping cough to triviality revealed "blatant ignorance"), Rinehart sadly concluded, "A profound brain may sometimes fail to grasp a very simple proposition, especially if there has been no pains taken by the said brain to become informed upon the subject."[14]

On the political side, the opening paragraph of an article entitled, "Somerset Recrudescence," read: "Some of our Somerset county contemporaries injected the vaccination question into the late Republican primaries possibly in the belief that there wasn't enough virus in the campaign."[15]

Finally, but certainly not last, there was the following from the *Titusville Morning Herald* (PA), September 10, 1906:

> From the rousing protest that is going up all over Pennsylvania it looks as if State Health Commissioner Dixon may find it difficult to enforce his compulsory vaccination law, in spite of court decisions. In Erie the anti-vaccinationists have found three crippled persons whose condition came about from vaccination. They are being held up to the eyes of the public and there is a genuine stampede away from the school house.

By the end of the year, the school board of Altoona gave notice to principals and teachers that if any felt disposed to violate the vaccination law, they would have protection from the directors. The question then arose, "But what will the taxpayers say about spending their money to defend persons guilty of violating a state law?" Commissioner Dixon responded to the action by exercising the prerogative of his office to visit the schools to guard against violators. "Heretofore, it has been the custom to take the word of those in authority. It is hardly likely this course will be continued."[16]

Despite the notice on February 1, 1907, that Edward Gulden, living within a few miles of Franklin County where people were protesting, died of smallpox,[17] Porter F. Cope, one of the leading anti-vaccinationists, continued his efforts to pass a state anti-vaccination law. In the state legislature, representatives sought to place such a bill on the calendar with the comment "vaccination has been a curse in this state for the last twelve years and the people are not going to stand it any longer," but failed to succeed on the larger issue. The house did, however, pass a bill requiring compulsory vaccination "only in the event of an epidemic of smallpox." Known as the "Watson bill," it was vetoed by Governor Stuart.[18]

The Vaccination "Creed"

Smallpox spread throughout the United States during 1902 and 1903, although in a milder form than usual. Long immunity from the disease made people careless, with few adults bothering to be revaccinated. In the central western part of the country, Des Moines, Iowa, was considered "the blackest plague [smallpox] spot" that had "brought more or less scandal on the entire state." Matters became so bad the national post office considered the question of fumigating all mail from Iowa. The city of Chicago passed quarantine against Des Moines and the traveling public was "shunning it whenever possible." Indiana, Wisconsin and Illinois were similarly affected. In 1902, to the delight of anti-vaccinationists, Cleveland abandoned vaccination for a total reliance on disinfection. Within one year, there were 1,248 cases of smallpox and 224 deaths. One hundred and seventy physicians were appointed public vaccinators and 195,000 persons were vaccinated at public expense. "The result was that in three months the disease was practically stamped out."[19]

Of the major cities, Chicago stood as one of the few with low smallpox rates, "owing to the vigorous measures" of the board of health. There, vaccination was "made compulsory, no excuse, subterfuge, or alleged religious scruples" permitted.[20] In fact, the Chicago department of health circulated a "Vaccination Creed" that gained wide circulation:

Vaccination Creed

1. True vaccine, repeated until it "takes," always prevented smallpox.
2. Properly conducted vaccination never did and never will make a serious sore.
3. Vaccination left a distinctive scar and was the only conclusive evidence of a successful vaccination.
4. No untoward events ever followed vaccination; on the other hand, thousands of lives were sacrificed annually through neglect.[21]

In contrast to beliefs of the 19th century, those of the early 20th held that there were more cases of smallpox in winter than summer. As the disease lingered through the beginning of 1902, hope for warm weather turned into concern when the disease failed to abate. With little improvement in conditions, the dawn of a new year saw Indiana claim the dubious honor of leading all states in the number of smallpox cases and deaths resulting from the disease. The marine hospital report indicated 500 fatalities, but local newspapers claimed a more accurate count would place the number at over one thousand. As in other cities in other times, the case was laid at the feet of anti-vaccinationists and a general apathy among the public.

The *Fort Wayne News,* February 4, 1903, called for enforcement of existing laws, but more specifically, it urged employers to demand general vaccination of all employees. The idea was not a new one but would grow in prominence. In 1901, for example, John S. Fulton, secretary, state board of health for Maryland, issued a notice, warning truck farmers and small fruit growers to engage only those pickers recently vaccinated.[22] The same year, the Maine Central Railroad Company issued orders that all its employees, station agents and trainmen be vaccinated within the next two weeks.[23] In 1904, after a case of smallpox was found in a "Slavonian" settlement where thousands of stockyard workers resided, orders were issued for the vaccination of 3,000 workers.[24] All was not smooth sailing, however, as Miss Grace Vorhees, an employee of Truax, Green & Company, sued for $50,000, claiming she was required to be vaccinated or lose her job. She averred the procedure was not done properly and in consequence she would never be able to return to her job that paid $100 a month.[25]

In lieu of vaccination, there continued to be any number of "cures" or preventives for those who did not want the traditional method. Primary among them was the homeopathic idea of an internal application of "variolinum" administered in pill form. In 1902 homeopathic physicians in Des Moines went to court, charging that school boards failed to recognize the certificates they issued. They were denied on the grounds no form of vaccination through the stomach would be recognized. Authorities based their decision on the resolution adopted at the conference of State and Provincial Boards of Health of North America, 1902. Their definition read: "An inoculation by scarification puncture or injection beneath the epidermis of a vaccine which produces with some constitutional disturbance, the typical vaccine vesicle, which leaves, after the pock has healed, its characteristic scar."

The argument continued into 1906, but the board of health refused to legalize the homeopathic method, as it would then be forced to "recognize the new osteopathic method of guarding against smallpox." They ultimately referred the matter to the legislature. In Iowa, Senator Young introduced a bill in 1906, reviving "the old fight between homeopathic physicians and those of the old school." Young's intent was to clarify state law into acknowledging only vaccination as a preventive.[26]

After winning the battle in Iowa when internal (oral) vaccination (variolinum) was accepted as a substitute for bovine vaccine virus by school and state authorities, the annual convention of the International Homeopathic Physicians at Pittsburg, Pennsylvania, affirmed that "the now established practice of vaccination by internal variolation [is] a sufficient method of prophylaxis, and that it is the only method consistent with hygiene and the modern conception of asepsis." By 1911, however, an outbreak of smallpox in an Iowa school for the deaf made headlines, as vaccination of students was done

Small-Pox

And Vaccination, Like all Serious Diseases, Greatly Reduce the Vital Powers, Causing Nervousness, Headache, Backache, Depression, Nervous Exhaustion and General Debility.

Dr. Miles' Nervine

Speedily Restores the System and Strengthens the Vital Powers.

It was commonly believed that every organ in the body was under the control of the nervous system. In order to prevent "great debility," concoctions such as Nervine (a liquid likely containing burnt sugar and alcohol or cocaine) were the answer. Such nostrums earned substantial sums for the promoters (from the *Des Moines Daily Leader,* February 28, 1902).

entirely on the homeopathic plan of internal vaccination. Although "anti-internal vaccination adherents" had been "routed" in 1908, the present outbreak "has renewed, in a slight measure, discussion of the merits of the two plans."[27]

If relief were not to be found in pills, the idea of eating lettuce as a preventive received wide exposure through the newspapers. The theory stated that as smallpox was a scorbutic disease similar to scurvy, eating fresh lettuce (an anti-scorbutic) would act "a thousand times better than vaccination." Celery and onions were also good for this purpose, but as the time between harvest and consumption was often prolonged they tended to lose their anti-scorbutic properties.[28]

For those with dogs, news that vaccination had become popular for household pets may have caused them to make a trip to the veterinarian. A Philadelphia practitioner advocated the new idea, stating that as many valuable dogs died of smallpox (a false assertion), inoculation was necessary. He performed the operation by shaving a spot the size of a silver dollar on the animal's back (where it could not reach to scratch) and injected the vaccine. He advocated every pup's vaccination.[29]

A Sensational Case — Boston Anti-Vaccinationist Versus Smallpox

Few cases drew such attention as that of Dr. Emmanuel Pfeiffer of Boston. Pfeiffer became a regularly registered physician of Massachusetts, "although making vigorous and even violent war against the system and laws which supported it." An ardent anti-vaccinationist, he held that proper diet, cleanliness and hygienic conditions were the only means required to ward off disease. Frequently indulging in verbal tirades against the authorities and physicians who enforced and advocated vaccination, Pfeiffer believed the mind was supreme in its power over the physical system and "because of his peculiar opinions" was made president of the American Psychic Society. He practiced hypnotism and earned notoriety by fasting for 31 days, surviving because he took "command of his digestive organs."

Dr. Pfeiffer was in interesting company. Other leading anti-vaccinationists in Boston included Alfred Russell Wallace, the codiscoverer with Darwin of the theory of natural selection in 1858. Since that time, however, he had paid little attention to biology, concentrating on phrenology, anti-vaccination, spiritualism and table-tipping. Professor Cruikshank was a bacteriologist, one of the few ever known to reject vaccination. The third was Herbert Spencer, a philosopher without a medical background.

In January 1902, Pfeiffer spoke before the committee on public health, then considering a bill to repeal compulsory vaccination. His argument in support was based on the fact the legislature was not a medical body and therefore unfit to judge medical questions; he further stated that compulsory vaccination was a violation of constitutional rights. Around this time he became aware of Dr. Samuel H. Durgin's offer to permit leaders of the "anti movement" access to Gallups Island, where smallpox patients were held, in order that they might see and more fully understand the disease and its treatment.

Pfeiffer approached Durgin, chairman of the Boston board of health, seeking permission to visit Gallups Island. This was granted and the doctor went to the hospital on January 23, where he was required to wear a white robe and cap as protection. During his stay, he examined no patients, displaying "no interest in the cases whatever." After observing that he smelled no bad odors, it was suggested he draw closer and smell the breath of a sufferer. This he did. Upon leaving the wards, he was required, as were all visitors, to wash his hands, face, beard and hair with a disinfecting liquid.

After his visit, Pfeiffer publicly boasted that he had exposed himself as much as possible, smelled the breath of a patient and freely used a handkerchief in his examination of patients, subsequently shaking this cloth in the faces of his friends at a public meeting immediately after his return. Physicians accompanying Pfeiffer at Gallups roundly denied he ever used a handkerchief, then widely believed to be a source of contamination, or closely inspected any inmates.

Fearing he might be contagious (being unvaccinated), authorities closely followed Pfeiffer until Monday, February 3, when he disappeared from sight. He was not located until late on February 6, when he and a woman named Mrs. Broadman took a public hack to the residence of Dr. John T. Simpson. The pair was not seen again until Saturday, February 8, when they were found at Pfeiffer's home in Bedford. The doctor was dangerously ill from confluent smallpox, compelling his son to notify authorities (the law required all cases of smallpox to be reported) and call for a doctor. Dr. Shea confirmed the diagnosis and issued quarantine on the house and its occupants.

The board of health and Dr. Durgin were criticized for permitting Pfeiffer to break the rules and visit the smallpox hospital without benefit of vaccination. Durgin defended himself by the simple explanation that as a physician, Pfeiffer expressed the wish to familiarize himself with the disease so he might be enabled to make a ready diagnosis. He had permitted doctors and advanced medical students to examine patients at Gallups for over 20 years and never had a single person contract smallpox before Pfeiffer.

To allay public fears of contamination, the board issued a statement that the hack drivers who transported Pfeiffer and Broadman had come forward. They had their carriages thoroughly disinfected and underwent revaccination.

In a telephone interview on March 9, Pfeiffer's son (who underwent vaccination) declared his father to be "as strongly opposed as ever to vaccination." He stated his father was "not much marked or pitted," and expected to return to his office within a fort-night.[30]

The case of another anti-vaccinationist roused extreme ire in New Brunswick, New Jersey, in 1902. Dr. Samuel Long permitted a fellow physician suffering from smallpox to enter the city and visit him in his office. When the fact became known, indignant citizens hanged him in effigy. On the effigy the placard read: "This doctor does not believe in vaccination — Long."[31]

33

Vaccination Is Un-American

Resolved, That the Allen County Medical Society [Indiana] deems it unnecessary to treat the proposed legislation against vaccination seriously, inasmuch as the immunity against smallpox granted by vaccination, like the rotundity of the earth, is too well established to be overthrown.[1]

If that were only the case, smallpox might have been eradicated decades, perhaps a century, earlier. But it was not and costs, in human life and suffering as well as treasure, continued to mount.

As far as money was concerned, one point agreed upon by everyone was that treating and preventing the disease was expensive. In Rochester, New York, for example, for the smallpox season of 1902, the sum of $50,000 was appropriated for stamping out epidemics. The same year, fearful that the arrival of cold weather would usher in a return of the disease, Dr. Lederle, president of the New York City Department of Health, requested $20,000 for immediate vaccination. It was observed that last year "nothing was done at this time, which the Health Department officials now consider to have been a great mistake in view of the prevalence of the scourge during last Winter." During the year 1902, smallpox cost the state of Michigan over $1,500,000 and Bay City alone spent $30,000 on the disease.

In 1904, Pennsylvania experienced a mild outbreak of smallpox. Despite only 18 serious cases and 4 deaths, the cost for treatment of these alone reached $5,400. This paid for vaccination, maintenance, formaldehyde fumigation (the current standard), destruction of infected materials, clothing, bedding and guards. One year later at Williamsport, the city expended $284 for each of its 18 cases of smallpox, while spending only 20 cents each to vaccinate healthy individuals.

Under the heading, "Smallpox Is Expensive," commissioner of health Dixon reported, "At the lowest estimate it costs the state $350 for each person outside of cities quarantined to prevent the spread of smallpox. This means that during 1905 more than $2,000,000 of state money was expended, or, as well put by Dr. Dixon, was wasted simply to gratify a whim of those who opposed vaccination." Dr. Dixon's remedy for controlling costs was to impose a tax on those who refused vaccination. Not for the first time it was noted, "Veritably, smallpox is a 'luxury and not a necessity.'"

Broken down into specifics, for the period June 15, 1906–June 15, 1907, Washington County, Maryland, spent $417.50 on vaccinators; $63.17 for physician services; $300 for the health office; $610.49 on drugs; $93 for fumigation and $172.90 for antitoxine. In contrasting cases, the value and economy of vaccination in the control of smallpox was aptly demonstrated in two Michigan cities during 1910. Saginaw, which suffered a severe outbreak in which 48 people died, spent approximately $75,000 in combating the disease. Grand

Rapids spent $2,693.86 for vaccination and not a single case occurred in the city. Making the same point in 1915, doctors in Davenport and Scott counties, Iowa, stated that the cost of $3,000 per month spent fighting an outbreak of smallpox would have been unnecessary had citizens taken the necessary precaution of having themselves vaccinated.[2]

Following the expense of vaccination came the money drain from quarantine. The 1905 conference of national boards of health declared that restraining the spread of smallpox among the unvaccinated by means of quarantine alone was doomed to fail. Dr. Simmons of South Carolina spoke for the majority when he said, "Vaccination is the only way to prevent the contamination."[3] Across the country, states and counties began questioning the value of quarantine: in Iowa, for example, law required a "smallpox sign" be placed on a smallpox house as a warning; inmates were restricted from leaving the premises. The theory against a widespread quarantine was expressed as this: "Why should you expect the municipality and the quarantined individuals to spend large sums of money in an attempt (often fruitless) to protect you from smallpox by means of a rigid quarantine when you can protect yourself by so simple and inexpensive a procedure as that of vaccination?" In other words, if you do not care to protect yourself, "take your own chances."[4]

North Carolina spent $170,000 in 1910, trying to quarantine against smallpox as a means of protecting the unvaccinated. Using the same theory that vaccination was in the reach of everyone, the 1911 general assembly enacted a new health law, leaving out quarantine entirely.[5]

No One Dares Pass a Vaccination Law

The Marine Hospital and Public Health Service's report for January–June 1908 indicated 23,544 cases of smallpox, of which 55 proved fatal; the total for the year was 35,174, although John W. Trask of the Marine Hospital estimated a more accurate count would have been 70,000. For the same six-month period in 1909 (encompassing 42 states at 651 different localities), 13,851 cases were reported, with 59 deaths. Even considering that the incidence of disease was grossly underreported, facts indicated that the mild form of smallpox prevailed.[6] Even these statistics were too high for Henry S. Mathewson, former assistant surgeon, Marine Hospital and Public Health Service. In a bulletin entitled, "The Prophylactic Value of Vaccination," he noted that in Germany, where compulsory vaccination had been in force for 30 years, smallpox was virtually eliminated. Avowing that the presence of smallpox in the United States was entirely unnecessary, he called for vaccination and revaccination as the only means of "removing this pest."[7]

While smallpox was only one killer, advances in the medical sciences achieved significant results:

Records from Geneva

Century	Life Span/Years
16th	21.1
17th	25.7
18th	33.6
1801–1883	39.7

The average life span of women was greater than that of men in almost every country, and was increasing at a more rapid rate. It was speculated that if the present rate of improvement could be continued for a century, the average life span could reach 70 years![8]

Even with those statistics, anti-vaccinationists persisted. The April 9, 1910 issue of the *Indianapolis Sunday Star* warned, "There is today no state in the Union that can pass or dares to attempt to pass a vaccination law, such is the natural antipathy of the people to such an invasion of personal rights, due to their instinctive dread of the dangerous operation." Doubtless, the writer would have stood by a notice in the *Racine Daily Journal* (WI), November 15, 1910, stating, "There were twelve deaths due to small-pox in England and Wales in 1908, and twenty-nine deaths due to the effects of improper vaccination." Quite damning by itself, but when put in context of the vast numbers vaccinated, hardly worthy of a stand-alone notice. Possibly both would fall under the heading "Disease Causes False Reports," beginning, "Whenever smallpox makes its appearance all sorts of rumors concerning the disease and vaccination begin to be spread around. Just why this should be so with reference to small-pox we don't know unless there is some connection between smallpox and mendacity."[9] On the lighter side, all three articles pale in comparison to an event in Brooklyn never before accomplished in medical history: the vaccination of a large part of the city directory, tombstones and hundreds of door plates. Apparently, physicians were assigned the task of vaccinating 100 persons per day in specified districts. Finding it impossible, they copied names at random. "It made a fine record, and the fraud was only discovered by accident. About the only satisfaction that Brooklynites get out of the whole matter is that they ought to be able to visit graveyards, read the directory and ring door bells with no risk of smallpox."[10]

Smallpox Struggles in Upstate New York

Newspapers, letters and public meetings across the country questioned the value of vaccination and the sundry laws concerning the right of unvaccinated children to attend school. A representative case study from upstate New York gives an overview of the situation mirrored around the United States.

In July 1911, several mild cases of smallpox were discovered among the citizens of Olean. In August, the school board followed state law and excluded all unvaccinated children from the public schools. This immediately caused outrage among anti-vaccinationists, eventually resulting in half of the 2,800 children staying out of the classroom. Faced with irate parents and the threat of citywide agitation, Allan J. Hastings, president of the Olean Board of Education, wrote a letter December 8 to Frank B. Gilbert, chief of Law Division, New York State Education Department at Albany, asking for advice. Hastings stated that only one-fifth of schoolchildren were vaccinated and that 18 cases of smallpox then existed in the city. In defense of the school board's order to enforce the vaccination law and refuse admittance to non-vaccinated students, he referenced the constitutionality of the law as sustained by the New York Court of Appeals, Vlemieseter case, 179, N.Y. 235.

Hastings then touched upon the compulsory education law, questioning whether the board might be in violation, as only 15 of 200 children refused admission subsequently received any form of study during their expulsion from the public system. Gilbert replied on December 11, supporting the Olean school board and directing that action be brought against parents who refused to have their children vaccinated and who subsequently neglected to provide equivalent instruction, citing the case decided before the Appellate Division of the Third Department, *Shappee v. Curtis*, 142 App. Div. 155. On the same day these letters were published, 22 local physicians signed a letter expressing sympathy for the efforts of

The Anti-Vaccination

the school board, noting that the most common way the scourge spread was from direct contact between pupil and pupil.

On December 15, the renowned smallpox expert, Dr. Edward Clark of Buffalo, appeared in Olean, speaking in favor of vaccination. The prime emphasis of his speech, however, was to seek support for the health officer, Dr. W.E. McDuffie. Remarking that the position was always an unpleasant one, Clark said that in times of smallpox outbreaks it was made doubly so "by the ill-advised opposition of certain, perhaps well meaning

forces are standing firm and the Cursed VACCINE Dogma must be crushed forever in Olean, and this infamous law repealed.

FIGHT FOR YOUR FREEDOM. Don't be a slave to a graft scheme. Relief from Albany is expected hourly.

The Anti-Vaccination League met last night and appointed a committee to go to Albany and bring about, if possible, a satisfactory adjustment of the school question and to insist upon the rights of the taxpayers of Olean to enjoy school privileges without the vaccine dogma being imposed on the school children.

Anti-Vaccination League

In a significant and complex case involving the right of local boards of health and education to enact laws requiring students to be vaccinated before attending public schools, the Anti-Vaccination League took issue with authorities in Olean, New York. Warning its followers not to be "a slave to a graft scheme," both members of the league and the health authorities went to Albany, seeking a definitive decision from the state (from the Olean *Evening Times* [NY], January 23, 1912).

people, who do not understand and who are not conversant with the difficulties under which he labors."

Four days later, Dr. McDuffie issued a statement confirming the existence of 26 cases of mild smallpox, but assured the people things were well in hand: the schools were closed for Christmas, the sick were under quarantine and it was perfectly safe to do business in the city. Toward that end, he included statements by the presidents of the chamber of commerce and merchants exchange, reiterating the above.

The same could not be said for central and western New York. While Syracuse was free from contagion, Courtland, Tompkins, Chenango, Broome, Cattaragus, Wyoming, Allegany and Erie counties were infected. State commissioner Porter reaffirmed his belief that vaccination was the only dependable measure, both for prevention and suppression of the disease, and urged the cooperation of officers and physicians to stay the spread of smallpox.

Three days after Christmas, a pro-vaccinationist meeting was held in Olean. Health officer D.M. Totman, one of the department's experts, reminded everyone that in 1875, Syracuse was swept by a smallpox outbreak numbering in the hundreds, causing a business loss that ran into the millions. The desperate businessmen of the city banded together and compelled everyone to be vaccinated or to leave town "at once." That, he declared, was "what you people of Olean should do in a similar case." The meeting was sparsely attended.

Evidence that his message was not heeded came in a petition to the board of education, January 15, 1912. Signed by 84 local businessmen, they demanded that the 1,574 unvaccinated children be allowed to attend school "at once," in order to alleviate the controversy over vaccination that had been "very injurious to the business and reputation of the City." Allen Hastings responded, "The Attorney-General has in a written opinion ... held that the law is mandatory and the Board has no discretion in the matter.... The members of the Board understands the foregoing petition as asking the Board to ignore and violate the law, and their plain duty." The meeting ended when the board ordered the chief of police to preserve order. Anti-vaccinationists countered with the following published notice:

THE ANTI-VACCINATION

forces are standing firm and the Cursed VACCINE Dogma must be extinguished forever at Olean, and this infamous law repealed.

FIGHT FOR YOUR FREEDOM. Don't be a slave to a graft scheme. Relief from Albany is expected hourly. The Anti-Vaccination League met last night and appointed a committee to go to Albany and bring about, if possible, a satisfactory adjustment of the school question and to insist upon the rights of the taxpayers of Olean to enjoy school privileges without the vaccine dogma being imposed on the school children.

The school board convened on the same day (January 22) and decided to send a delegation to Albany along with anti-vaccinationists to confer with commissioner A.S. Draper of the state education department. On January 25, word came that in light of the outbreak having passed, Commissioner Draper had announced the matter had been put on the health board of Olean and that "in all probability the pupils will be permitted to attend school without much further delay."

The commissioner's decision brought to the fore one of the most seething questions regarding compulsory vaccination of schoolchildren: while the health law declared that all children admitted to schools be vaccinated, thereby excluding children who were not, the education law required that all children of school age be required to attend school. "In other words," Draper wrote, "there is an inconsistency between the provisions of the health law and those of the education law bearing upon this subject. Both of these statutes can not be strictly enforced." Reversing his previous position, Draper decided that while the board of education took the correct stance in excluding unvaccinated pupils, he was "of the opinion that some discretion is intended to be reposed both in the board of education and in the board of health laws, and that, pending the consideration of the conflict between these laws which it is proposed to ask of the Legislature, your board will be justified in rescinding its action excluding unvaccinated children from the schools, unless such action is insisted upon by the board of health."

The news spread quickly. One day later (January 26, 1912), the *Titusville Morning Herald,* Pennsylvania, ran the headline, "New York Vaccination Law Must Be Amended; Provisions Found to be Conflicting; Pending Action at Albany, Law Can be Disregarded by the Cities." On March 1, Assemblyman Cheney introduced a bill into the New York legislature, striking out the compulsory vaccination clause unless the local board of health (as opposed to the school board), announced an emergency. A similar bill introduced by Assemblyman Baumes was killed in committee.

In reaction to the above, the *Buffalo Times* (reprinted in the *Olean Evening Times,* August 6, 1912) noted that there was "a marked lack of uniformity and that legal requirements for general vaccination exist only in Kentucky, the Philippine Islands and Porto Rico. Arizona, Hawaii, Maryland, New Mexico and North Dakota have laws requiring the vaccination of children which, if enforced, would in time produce a population of which a large portion would have been vaccinated at least once." The editorial concluded, "A survey of the whole situation, shows that the need is not for abolition, or mitigation of vaccination requirements, but for an extended system of legislation on the subject. Aside from local regulations and State laws in a few States, very little preventive law exists."

Three years later, the subject in New York had not been settled. Medical men from all parts of the state opposed the passage of the Jones-Tallett Bill, which provided for compulsory vaccination of schoolchildren only if a smallpox epidemic existed. As an indication of how far matters had deteriorated, favoring the bill were state health commissioner Hermann M. Biggs, deputy commissioner Linsly Williams, assistant commissioner of education Thomas F. Finegan, Senator J.A. Jones (introducer of the bill), and J.A. Loyster of Madison County. The same year, Assemblyman James B. Montgomery introduced a bill repealing sections 310 and 311 of the public health law to the same effect. Little had improved by 1917 when authorities at Albany promoted the "desirability of vaccination" for those persons traveling about the state, as smallpox was prevalent there and in Connecticut, where the disease had been epidemic since June 1916.

In 1918, Hermann M. Biggs, state commissioner of health, dispatched a bulletin, advising that since January 1, there had been 375 cases of smallpox and new reports were daily received. The New York State Chamber of Commerce, "realizing the threat to the business interests," inaugurated a campaign with the department of health for an active effort on behalf of general vaccination. Biggs also reported that a recent outbreak of smallpox on one of the Indian reservations cost taxpayers more than $8,000, *"expended for the quarantine measures for the protection of the inhabitants of the surrounding towns"* (italics added).[11]

Fortunately, resisters did not go to the lengths demonstrated by fanatics in Chicago. After smallpox was discovered in Zion City, Dr. C.E. Crawford, state health inspector, attempted to use persuasion to convert the Dowieites, whose beliefs forbad such practices. Wilbur Glen Voliva, who had succeeded the late John Alexander Dowie as overseer of the city, ordered his followers to refuse, warning, "If the state authorities come up here and try to vaccinate us, we'll take shotguns and blow 'em to hell." (Other newspapers cleansed the quote by substituting, "blow them where they belong.")[12]

The following year, a St. Louis newspaper became the champion of anti-vaccinationists when it editorialized on an unfortunate incident in West Hammond, Indiana, where two boys died of lockjaw after being vaccinated. Reprinted as an advertisement throughout the country, the gist of the message was this: "Compulsion in medicine is un–American. It violates every principle of liberty and justice."[13] The argument was debated pro and con, missing the larger issue that had been looming for decades: did the injection of vaccine cause tetanus? State health authorities across the country were virtually universal in their condemnation of the idea, reporting that if tetanus developed, it was caused by the introduction of foreign matter into the wound. Yet the idea (also including malignant edema and anthrax) persisted, remaining one of the most effective weapons in the anti-vaccinationists' arsenal.[14]

Somewhat tongue-in-cheek, a 1916 editorial remarked that for those uninterested in vaccination, they might take note that when traveling to the Orient a legal certificate of vaccination was required, "lest you cause an unnecessary funeral in a foreign land."[15]

President Wilson Confounds Fanatics and Chicago Cubs Fumigated

Being infected at the workplace was a common and frequent danger for early 20th century employees. Standing side by side on an assembly line, crisscrossing paths with thousands of travelers on railroad lines, digging coal deep within the earth or even using a common roller towel presented numerous opportunities to contract smallpox germs. Without compulsory vaccination and adult revaccination, no one could reasonably feel themselves safe from contagion. Employers had three options: to move proactively and order vaccination for all their employees before an outbreak struck, to respond retroactively and order vaccination after contagion was discovered, or to do nothing and let the disease take its course.

During the second decade of the 1900s, most employers opted for the second choice, ordering vaccination after the fact. In December 1911, a case of smallpox was discovered in a young child attending public school in Chester, Pennsylvania. Dr. H.M. Hiller, the state health officer, inspected all pupils and teachers at the school and recommended revaccination in some cases. The child's older sister, who worked at the American Viscose Company in Marcus Hook, was also discovered to be afflicted. Having already been closed once by the state board of health after a previous case of smallpox was discovered, company authorities responded more quickly this time, ordering everyone to be vaccinated.

In what might have been used as an argument for compulsory vaccination of school-children by demonstrating how one unprotected child easily infected another, forcing an enormous retroactive response, a child exposed to the first victim also came down with smallpox, contaminating everyone in the household. That compelled the ownership of the Thurlow plant of the American Steel Foundries, where the child's father was employed, to order vaccination for its workforce of 450 persons.[16]

The next year, in light of the prevalence of smallpox about Cadosla, orders were issued to employees of the O & W Railroad working between Cadosla, Norwich and Scranton to report to one of the company's doctors and be vaccinated at company expense. The order also included all members of the workers' families because of the risk they might have been contaminated.[17] Smallpox persisted in Scranton and in 1915, authorities closed a dance hall, forcing 147 young men and women to be vaccinated; a nearby hotel was also raided, and 50 men found crowded there were refused exit until they underwent vaccination. After all other places of public entertainment were shuttered, officials at the coal mining company in nearby Jessup announced that none of its 2,000 miners could work until they presented a certificate that the miner and all family members had been vaccinated.[18]

The gravity of the smallpox situation in Alton, Illinois, during 1918 brought together 17 representatives of manufacturing plants, who agreed to demand vaccination of their employees. Among the companies were Alton Boxboard and Paper, Western Cartridge, Illinois Glass, Federal Lead, Alton Steel, Stanard Milling, Sparks Milling, Roxana Oil Works, Luer Brothers, Alton Brick, Brokaw-Eden, Beall Foundry, Duncan Foundry, Ginter-Wardein, A.B.C. Bakery, Nolls Bakery and Standard Oil. While the representatives felt this would "prove a burden," it was better than a complete shutdown of business and manufacturing interests. Schools, churches and places of entertainment were expected to follow suit by demanding certificates of vaccination. The process did not go smoothly but apparently the state board of health was satisfied that some progress had been made.[19]

Even the federal government was not immune to reacting to smallpox scares. In 1913, after several employees were discovered to have smallpox, Mr. Garrison, the secretary of war under President Woodrow Wilson, ordered a general vaccination of employees in the health department. Those included medical inspectors, food and sanitary inspectors, clerks, and members of the disinfecting service, as well as chiefs of the various departments. Press correspondents soon found that they, too, fell under the order. The information was conveyed by a messenger, who informed them, "The Secretary of War desires that the gentlemen of the press at their convenience, to submit themselves to the medical corps for vaccination." As Garrison had also submitted to vaccination, they could hardly do otherwise.

On a more far-reaching and unprecedented level, after massive flooding in Ohio and Indiana, the new president ordered three steps taken. First, crews and equipment of the federal government were sent to the afflicted areas to prevent a repetition of the calamity. Second, President Wilson ordered the secretaries of treasury and war to send all available medical officers of the public health and army to establish quarantine and stamp out existing epidemics. This was the first time federal officers had been ordered into a region to prevent the occurrence of epidemics and disease. Lastly, astutely comprehending that smallpox and typhoid often broke out after such natural disasters, the president ordered 10,000 vaccine points and 1,000 ampules of anti-typhoid serum sent to Ohio and Indiana for use in preventing epidemics. The American Medical Association praised the president, writing that the nation was fortunate to have "as its chief executive a man who does not fear official red tape, moss-grown precedents or the opposition of the ignorant and fanatical followers of fantastic cults, but who will calmly, fearlessly and sensibly place at the disposal of any stricken or afflicted community all the available resources of the government and of modern science for the prevention of disease and the saving of life."[20]

On a less serious note (unless you happened to be a Chicago Cubs fan), a sampling of headlines in the United States and Canada on April 1913, read, "Whole Minneapolis Team in Danger of Smallpox; Cubs are Scared," and "Ralph Comstock, Miller Pitcher Has Smallpox; Consternation in Chicago." There was reason for concern, despite the fact the baseball season had not yet begun. During an exhibition game between the Cubs and the Minneapolis Millers of the American Association on April 8, the Minneapolis players used the visitors' dressing rooms at the local clubhouse. It was subsequently discovered that a young Miller pitcher named Ralph Comstock had smallpox and he was immediately taken to the city pesthouse. Infielder Wade H. Killifer also had eruptions on his face and was diagnosed with smallpox. Minnesota officials failed to alert club Cub president Murphy, who discovered news of the outbreak by reading it in the papers. He declared "the clubhouses will be fumigated under the direction of the health department," and all Cub players, except those who had recently been vaccinated, were to undergo the procedure. President M. Cantillion of the Millers ordered the same for his players, even though it "will likely cause many sore arms."[21]

No More Sore Arms—The Three-Insertion Triangle

While the Cubs and the Millers were rubbing their sore arms, that sad fact of life was already changing. In August 1911, Dr. John Nivison Force of the University of California, Berkley, vaccinated the entering class with a new method he had devised. It entailed the use of a dental scaling chisel held perpendicularly to the skin, denuding the epiderm by rotation of the chisel. Three circles of epidermis, 2mm in diameter, were removed, glycerinized vaccine was applied and gently rubbed in. The resultant vesicles were remarkably uniform. The set-up required:

Rotary chisel, 2½ mm
Sealed capillary vaccine just out of the refrigerator
Rubber bulbs for same

Sterile gauze square for dressing
Absorbent cotton
Acetone for washing arm
Burning alcohol
Alcohol lamp
Zinc oxid rubber tape
Scissors
Sterile gown.

After sterilizing the rotary blade in 98 percent alcohol, then passing it through a flame, the instrument was set aside to cool. The deltoid muscle of the upper arm (traditionally the left arm was selected because most people were right handed) was tensed by pressure and the chisel was used to remove the epiderm only to the point were reddish dots appeared, representing the loops of the capillary blood vessels. The drawing of blood was to be avoided as it might float away the lymph and prevent absorption, and deep scarification was more likely to be followed by excessive inflammatory reaction.

After aseptically breaking off the ends of the sealed capillary glass tube, the vaccine was deposited on the three denuded surfaces and gently rubbed into the surface by the flat side of the chisel. The wound was then covered with a sterile small square gauze pad and held in place by zinc oxide adhesive tape.

Some authorities, including Dr. Hall of Canada, felt the best method of vaccination was to inject a drop of vaccine into but not under the skin by use of a hypodermic or a sterile needle (intramural puncture) as it left little or no scar. Force and his associates considered the lack of an easily identifiable scar a drawback rather than an advantage, as its character constituted visible evidence of protection.[22]

Advantages of the Three-Point Chisel Denudatation (Triangle Form)

1. Chances of a "take" were increased threefold.
2. Local reactions were less severe.
3. Rotundity of vesicle and scar tissue were insured; the vesicle did not break as easily.
4. The pitted scar area conformed to recommendations of the Local Government Board of England.
5. Reactions of immunity were easily read.
6. If all 3 insertions took, they were only ⅓ as great as a 1-point insertion.
7. There was no sloughing, no caustic.
8. The danger of secondary infection was greatly reduced.
9. Scabs came off on an average of 3 weeks as opposed to 6 weeks.
10. Dressings and after-care were reduced by one half.
11. A reduction of at least ⅔s occurred where axillary glands became involved.
12. The method was particularly adapted to health department work on account of its simplicity, rapidity of operation, ease of aseptic technique and characteristic scars that were able to be read for at least 7 years.[23]

John Force (1877–1938) received his degree of doctor of medicine an 1901, and earned a master of science degree for work carried out in the newly established Department of Hygiene in 1910. He interned in the United States Marine Hospital Service and at the outbreak of World War I he was appointed captain in the Medical Corps and served in the Canal Zone. As a result of his research on smallpox, he was appointed special expert in the U.S. Public Health Service and spent some time in 1921 in Washington studying the potency of smallpox vaccine. He did much to awaken the attention of the public in methods of preventing communicable diseases.[24]

The Los Angeles City Health Department used the three-insertion triangle method almost exclusively from 1924, covering 75,000 vaccinations by 1933. As early as 1914, the Oakland Board of Health utilized the technique, where nurses performed the procedure. Noting how the operation had advanced, Miss Schmits, a nurse responsible for vaccinating schoolchildren in Oakland, remarked that the operation had become practically painless. Abrading the skin with cotton-soaked antiseptic, she used a small steel instrument to prick the skin in three places close together, then rubbed vaccine-soaked cotton across two of the punctures, leaving the center one untouched. She explained the purpose of leaving one untouched was to allow her to compare the color of the three spots. If the pupil were immune, the two outer punctures were slightly pinker than the other, proving that the vaccine would have taken, had not the condition of immunity existed. By the old method, she explained, there was no telling what had gone wrong. The nurse was capable of vaccinating as many as 100 students in an hour and had never had one "pay a tragic price for his little scars."[25]

"Paying the price" had another meaning, as exemplified by the city of Cincinnati. Since the beginning of the smallpox epidemic, which lasted from October 1917 to March 1918, the cost of smallpox was placed at $13,000. During that period, there were 192 cases in the city, while Ohio at large reported a total of 7,547. The breakdown of Cincinnati's 6-month expenses were:

Hospital costs	$6,397.41
Quarantine	$200
Fumigation	$140
Vaccination of exposed persons	$600

Loss of wages covering 145 working adults, figured at $2 a day for the average quarantine period of 17 days, was $5,930. If this ratio were applied to the entire state, the cost would reach $1,000,000, a low estimate considering that the city had required vaccination of schoolchildren for years and had a comparatively low rate of infection.[26] It was much worse for the city of Chicago Heights, Illinois, where the population of 30,000 was threatened with complete quarantine. Mayor Hood attributed the disease to "the importation of (N)egro labor from the south."[27]

As the World Turns —
The Continuing Scourge

Nothing is easier than to emphasise the negative. "Thou shall not" is the beginning
of morality, but only the beginning, and is always promulgated with thunder. It
is what we do that makes us, not what we avoid doing.[1]

The opening of the 20th century in England continued what the 19th had left behind —
anti-vaccinationists and the controversy over "conscientious objection." Working a new tactic, boards of health not inclined to support vaccination cited cost as an overwhelming
burden. The guardians of the Wandsworth and Clapham Union complained that in 1895,
the total number of vaccinations had been 2,420, at an expense of £361 1s. 7d, while in
1899, the number had increased to 3,164, at a cost of £1,037 9s. 6d. This meant an expenditure of nearly £1,000/year "for something the people did not want, and which was forced
upon them." Hackney Union had, for the previous 20 years, been conspicuous for a decreasing disregard for vaccination. Exemption certificates were difficult to obtain but the number
of "escapees through untraceable removals" more than trebled.[2]

At Hull, expenditures on the smallpox outbreak for the fiscal year were £20,000. Up
to the end of December, £28,000 had been spent, with estimates reaching as high as £41,000
for the fiscal year. This did not take into account £12,000 spent by the public for vaccination
and revaccination.[3] Anti-vaccinationists in Glasgow used numbers provided by the health
committee to state that from the present outbreak of smallpox until May 19, 1901, there had
been 341,108 revaccinations. Vaccination cost 2s. 6d. and revaccinations 1s. 6d., making a
tidy sum for the medical profession, who "clung to false, fraudulent and mischievous superstitions."[4] London as a whole, during the half-year July–December 1901, spent £75,000 on
public vaccination, while the Metropolitan Asylums Board was committed to an expenditure
of £600,000 for maintenance of patients.[5]

The last major epidemic in London came in 1901–1902, with 3,723 reported cases
between May 1, 1901, and January 10, 1902, with 807 under treatment at the latter date.
The death rate was given as 11 percent for those vaccinated, 65 percent for those with
doubtful vaccination and 50.5 percent among the unvaccinated. Overcrowded plague ships
were anchored 15 miles down the Thames, forcing authorities to erect temporary barracks
along the shoreline to accommodate 800 patients. An outbreak in Liverpool followed in
1902–1903, with 2,280 cases and 161 deaths.

Medical authorities traced the outbreak of smallpox in London to travelers. In January,
a person recently arrived from Paris, where the disease was prevalent, carried smallpox; in
February, an officer on a ship was attacked because he had the disease; in May, a woman
recently arrived from Egypt was infected; in June, a case was discovered among Russian

Jews in Bethnal Green. The same month, another gentleman from Paris fatally infected the nurse who attended him; cases traced to laundries spread smallpox throughout other districts. By August 24, a total of 16 smallpox patients had been reported; from this date, the outbreak was considered general and by September, only six boroughs were left disease free.

Clearly, others introduced smallpox to London, but by 1903, as numbers rose, tramps were accused of spreading it. These homeless men, who shunned pest- and workhouses, wandered the city and along country roads. Infected persons could not be detained if the diagnosis were doubtful and as London authorities had no power to act against them, their wanderings brought them into contact with the unsuspecting. By 1910, a new, albeit familiar, threat was recognized: the common housefly, noted to be "very much more dangerous in carrying the disease [smallpox] than many people supposed."[6]

One method for containing disease came from clause 6 of the Factory and Workshop Act. This law called for any employer knowing the presence of smallpox or scarlet fever among his workers to report it. Failure to do so would result in a fine not exceeding £10. Because of this stringent measure, infectious diseases were discovered in 301 establishments, including those of 11 butchers, 8 bakers, 4 blouse makers, 13 confectioners, 20 dressmakers, 8 greengrocers, 9 hairdressers, 11 milkshops, 8 mangling houses, 8 eating houses, 10 grocers and 8 oilmen.[7]

Three principal factors weighed in the spread of smallpox. Similar to those in the United States, British physicians failed to recognize its symptoms, causing delayed or erroneous diagnoses. Laxity and conscientious objectors accounted for the fact 33 percent of London schoolchildren were unvaccinated. Third, nonexistent or incomplete protection in some sections of the country stemmed from the acceptance of "one-mark vaccination," whereas most physicians required two or three "points" (in this case meaning "areas") showing proof the operation "took."[8]

Compounding the situation, none of the vaccination acts adequately and legally defined vaccination. The only definition was found in "The Local Government Board's Order of 1898": "[T]he Public Vaccinator should aim at producing four separate vesicles or groups of vesicles, not less than half-an-inch from one another." However, this order applied only to public vaccinators, and the phrase, "aim at producing" proved too vague to be effective. Therefore, persons bearing between 1 and 3 marks were, by law, counted as vaccinated. The following table demonstrates cases of smallpox, classified according to the vaccination marks borne by each patient. The study was conducted over a period of 25 years and included nearly 6,000 cases.

Classification According to Vaccination Marks

Number of scars	*Number of deaths by percent*
1. Stated to have been vaccinated but no cicatrix	21.75
2. Having 1 vaccination cicatrix	7.50
3. Having 2 vaccination cicatrix	4.12
4. Having 3 vaccination cicatrix	1.75
5. Having 4 or more vaccination cicatrix	0.75
6. Unvaccinated	35–50[9]

A firm believer in vaccination, King Edward VII not only demanded those in the castle be vaccinated, he required all merchants delivering goods to show certificates. In October, in a display of royal support, the King's physician ordered all officials and men-servants at the royal mews, Buckingham Palace, to be revaccinated. Their wives and children aged 10 and up also underwent the operation. The total came to about 150 persons. Revaccination was also carried out in all military garrisons.[10] The king also yielded to popular custom by wearing a red armband signifying he had been vaccinated, demonstrating that "not only his arm but his temper is thus preserved." This custom originated during a period of nation-wide vaccination, when a number of women conceived the idea of wearing a red ribbon on the sleeves of their left arm to prevent vaccination sores from being jostled in crowds. The idea was elaborated on, and the "badge of suffering became a thing of beauty."[11]

The same month, a vaccination league, sponsored by surgeon Jonathan Hutchinson, F.R.S. (member of the Royal Commission on Vaccination), Sir Alfred Baring Garrod, F.R.S. (who held the post of Physician Extraordinary to Queen Victoria) and Professor Charles Stewart, F.R.S. of the Royal College of Surgeons, was established. The object of the league was to further vaccination, preventive medicine and practical sanitation among the public.[12]

By January 1902, smallpox cases reached 900 in London, fueling concern that London would be in quarantine when King Edward was officially crowned in May. Taking preemptory action, transatlantic lines ordered crews working the London-New York ships to undergo vaccination, in an effort to fend off an American embargo. Once this preliminary step was complete, orders were to be issued that all passengers be vaccinated to avoid financial losses due to detention. In this respect, England was ahead of America, as the United States consulate had taken no steps to protect home ports.[13]

The United States government's report, issued in February 1902, indicated that smallpox was present in 23 countries and every quarter of the world. Even in Germany, the best-vaccinated country in the world (where medical students had to be sent to England to study smallpox),[14] 3 cases were reported in Berlin.

Endemic smallpox was eliminated in Ireland in 1907 and subsequent importations were rare and quickly contained. Variola major was prevalent in Scotland from 1900 to 1905, with 6,628 cases and 641 deaths, over half in Glasgow. Thereafter, only one outbreak exceeded 80 cases but importations continued from Spain and the United States. Cases of variola minor occurred between 1927 and 1930, reaching a maximum of 154 in 1927 and a minimum of 146 in 1928.[15]

While life insurance companies in the United States showed little regard for whether a person was vaccinated, in England, there was a rush for "half-crown smallpox policies." Rates were graduated according to vaccination. At Lloyd's, the cost was 2s. 6d. per £100 if the applicant had been recently vaccinated and 3s. 4d. if some years had elapsed since the applicant's vaccination. Policies ran for a year and money was paid if the insured contracted smallpox. No medical certificate was required at the time of purchase, but in the event they took the disease, medical evidence of prior vaccination was required. During the week January 27–February 2, 1902, Lloyd's sold between £50,000 and £60,000 worth of smallpox insurance, some opting for £500 or even £1,000 policies.[16]

Anti-Vaccinationists Win the Day

As they had in America and around the world, anti-vaccinationists became more and more powerful in England. One major victory was the Vaccination Act of 1907, whereby a parent was granted the right to make a statutory declaration that he believed vaccination to be detrimental to the health of his child. Eliminating the step of applying in person and claiming conscientious objector status that might not be granted according to the dictate of the sitting magistrate, the act required no more than a written avowal made within the first four months of a child's birth. Considered a retrograde step by many medical officers, contemporary data from 1907 and 1908 indicated an uneven distribution of exemptions. Generally, the more populated an area, the slower parents were to give up vaccination, while those in rural districts were more prone to abandon the protection.

Exemptions between July 1 and December 31, 1908

Births	Exemptions	Percent
942,611	162,800	17.2[17]

A Ministry of Health report indicated that since the Act of 1907 had taken effect January 1, 1908, the number of exemptions doubled. In 1908 alone there were 910,640 births and 160,350 exemptions, or 17 percent, while the number of primary vaccinations fell to 594,792, or 62.3 percent. From that time, the number of vaccinations to births continued to decline, so that by 1922, between 50 and 60 percent of children born within that time frame remained unvaccinated.[18]

The *British Medical Journal* noted that the number of children left unvaccinated "must sooner or later be a matter of grave anxiety to the health authorities in this country. A considerable number of parents are merely indifferent and careless, and an effort should be made at least to bring before the notice of such as these the serious importance of the subject."[19] The homeopathic method of "internal vaccination" was also extant in England, with hundreds of practitioners offering smallpox protection.[20]

John H. Bonner, leader and organizer of the National Anti-Vaccination League, promoted the idea in a populist manner, by avowing, "Always assuming that people were not crowded together like sardines by rack-renting landlords, that they had fair wages and lived under fair conditions, the risk of smallpox was infinitesimal."[21] Brought to New England in 1909 by those interested in a crusade against compulsory vaccination, Bonner advocated "the true observance of nature's laws, which is immunity from disease." Noting "vaccination begins at the wrong end of the stick," he predicted a time when "cow-poxing will be obsolete," warning physicians that their true mission was to stamp out disease, not "impregnate contagion."[22]

Spreading disease was the last thing of which any physician wished to be accused. Although the unvaccinated segment of the population apparently did not fear infection by commingling with smallpox patients, there was surprising backlash against physicians who treated them. "Do doctors carry disease?" was a pressing question with no easy solution. A medical correspondent gave his opinion that physicians carrying germs from one patient to another "are almost unheard of." To make doubly certain, however, the writer informed

DANGER—VACCINATION SPREADS SMALLPOX
Do not be deceived; join the Ohio League for Medical Freedom and demand your rights under the Constitution. FREE "Horrors of Vaccinations" and Creed. 14897 Detroit Avenue, Cleveland, Ohio.

The League for Medical Freedom and the National Anti-Vaccination League were two of the most outspoken opponents of vaccination. Members pressed for the repeal of all vaccination laws, demanding that the choice of vaccination (which it did not support in any form) be left to the individual. In this small advertisement, the league promised a free copy of its publication, "Horrors of Vaccinations and Creed" (from the Steubenville *Herald-Star* [OH], December 20, 1924).

the public that doctors wore long dustcoats over their civilian clothes before treating a patient with an infectious disease. After leaving, precautions dictated that he bathe his face and hands in disinfectant. This explanation did not satisfy the Grantham Board of Guardians, who, in 1908, demanded a new vaccination officer after learning the usual doctor had attended a fatal smallpox case.[23]

Scotland suffered its own epidemic in 1920, as smallpox raged in Glasgow, creating a fiscal crisis. Apart from £30,000 set aside for smallpox precautions not including treatment and maintenance of patients, the 1920–1921 health budget included £20,000 for payment to physicians providing free vaccination. By September 1920, more than £11,000 had already been paid, indicating that unless the epidemic rapidly abated, fees would far exceed estimates. Other costs included £600 for medical students to provide house-to-house vaccinations; £2,154 for inspectors on smallpox duty; £750 for temporary epidemic inspectors; £4,140 for the maintenance of contacts in reception houses; £500 for calf lymph and £150 for vaccination sundries. The year before, Glasgow had only spent £2,596 on calf lymph and £1,418 on the maintenance of contacts in reception houses.[24]

In October 1922, an outbreak began at the Poplar E. Poor Law Institution (workhouse) and quickly spread to London, being of a particularly virulent nature. By November, 39 cases were reported. The government lymph establishment at Hendon worked overtime to provide adequate supplies of vaccine, sending out 5,000 tubes (one tube vaccinated one person) daily. The East End of London was considered particularly vulnerable, as the populace was exposed to ships in the Thames arriving from abroad. This led some to the conclusion that the epidemic was introduced by "alien settlers, overcrowding, lack of houses, neglect of vaccine, and the liberty of so-called conscience objectors, and 'peculiar people,'" with a warning that the "radical striking distance of smallpox atmosphere was 4,000 feet."

All over London the idea of wearing the red badge of vaccination became popular again, perhaps because the fatality rate reached a staggering 18 percent and people wished to inform strangers they were not contagious. This encouraged doctors to warn women to get vaccinated because as a group, they were far less protected than men, who had been revaccinated in the army. Others more liable to infection were undertakers and those who worked in laundries and lodging houses. Major employers promoted "in bulk" vaccinations, while the Westminster guardians moved to call upon the government to repeal the clause in the Vaccination Act permitting conscientious objection by parents. In December, as the epidemic abated, new cases were reported in South Wales, prompting the minister of health to warn local guardians that their stance in neglecting to have nonexempt children vaccinated would not be tolerated.[25]

Of importance was the fact that while civilian cases of variola major persisted, reaching 2,486 in England and Wales for 1923, reports from the War Office, 1924–1925, indicated no cases of smallpox among the troops. This was attributed to the King's Regulations specifically requiring vaccination or revaccination upon enlistment; refusal to comply was cause for discharge.[26]

By Any Other Name

As early as 1902, and again in 1919, variola minor was imported to England from the United States. Described in the United Kingdom as a disease similar to, but not precisely resembling, smallpox, authorities called it "alastrim" or "Kaffir pox" and debates raged over whether it was actually related to smallpox, or chicken pox or was some entirely unknown disease. It went by many names (Cuban itch, milkpox, pseudovariola, variola minor, West Indian smallpox and whitepox),[27] and Sir James Cantlie, writing in the *Journal of Tropical Medicine and Hygiene* (1923), described it as a mild form of smallpox that responded to vaccination. It was originally thought to be of Brazilian origin, spreading throughout South America, the West Indies and South Africa before making its way to Europe.[28]

In the early 1920s, alastrim appeared in Gloucester (already infamous for its refusal to endorse vaccination at the turn of the century). The "extraordinary obsession" of its citizens to proclaim the disease a mild form of chicken pox finally reached Parliament, where the health minister was forced to confirm the disease was truly smallpox and that vaccination was a protection against it. Dr. Walter Hadwen, Britain's most prominent anti-vaccinator and antivivisectionist, denied smallpox existed in Gloucester, writing an article, "The City of Dreadful Lies," protesting any other view. He was countered by the Bishop of Gloucester, Dr. A.C. Headlam, who preached "to refuse to be vaccinated was wrong from a Christian point of view," and took the medical profession to task for their "lack of propaganda in support of vaccination." As few of Hadwen's followers were church people, this presumably had little effect. The city was boycotted, but medical men were torn as to the nature of the disease. In 1930, Reverend Headlam opened a national campaign for vaccination to combat smallpox.[29]

Not surprisingly, Gloucester again proved the case for vaccination in 1923, when 319 out of 350 admissions to the hospital for smallpox were unvaccinated. Each case represented a cost of £200 to the community, with the loss of trade and commerce far greater.[30] Altogether, alastrim was rare in England during the early 20th century, one outbreak being in Nottingham, attributed to fomites sent from Salt Lake City to a Mormon convention. It spread to several other cities and then died out.[31]

Lax vaccination enforcement led to continuing outbreaks in England during the 1920s. In 1926, one article proclaimed "a number of English villages are swept with a pox epidemic such as has not been seen in nearly half a century." In 1927, new cases of smallpox were reported in Sheffield, resulting in a rush for vaccination. As supplies of lymph ran low, urgent telegrams were sent to the Ministry of Health, which rushed 3,000 additional tubes to the stricken.

The same year in July at the Royal Sanitary Institute at Hastings, research showed that smallpox was becoming more prevalent every year, beginning with 51 cases in 1918, and reaching 10,205 cases in 1926. Up to June 1927, over 10,000 cases had been reported. Poor revaccination rates were discussed as a factor, while one member suggested that the virulent and nonvirulent varieties of smallpox should have distinctive names to allow for a distinction in case reports.[32]

As testimony to the fright smallpox continued to elicit, when two liners from India arrived in England with passengers suffering from virulent smallpox, the French cabinet met to discuss the possibility of the disease spreading. Without conferring with British authorities, they issued an order on April 16, 1929, to take effect the following day, declaring that anyone entering France from England either through the channel ports or French airports, must show a valid vaccination certificate dated within the past two months. Reaction in England was swift and negative, especially in light of the fact tourist season was just beginning and many Americans already in England were also to be affected. Efforts were made through diplomatic channels to have the order modified, as a dozen cases could not be called "epidemic" and the incubation period for those aboard the liners was about to expire.

The French order was temporarily suspended and French and British health authorities met at Calais to mitigate the crisis. Failure to do so prompted Louis Loucheur, minister of labor and health, to reissue the order on April 22. Amid growing anger in England, it was officially announced that there were only 202 cases of smallpox in London and "that France's death rate from smallpox from 1919 to 1927 was 29 per million persons whereas England's was only 0.46."[33]

Finally, in July 1940, the British Parliament made vaccination compulsory in the United Kingdom.

Smallpox in Canada

Authorities believed smallpox crossed the border into Canada from Dakota in 1900, where a number of cases were reported. The following year, outbreaks were believed to have been spread by persons entering the dominion from the Northwest Territories. Dr. A.H. Simpson, provincial health officer, Manitoba, urged railroad authorities to detach cars carrying infected persons, fumigate the facilities and leave the victim where he was to be treated. He also advocated quarantine of foreigners from countries where the disease was present.[34] Quarantine had already been imposed against the city of Sault Ste. Marie, Michigan, in 1901, by placing an inspector at the dock on the Canadian side; this inspector demanded to see certificates of vaccination or show scars before passengers were permitted to land.[35]

Dr. Montizambert, director general of public health in the Dominion, called for a general vaccination throughout Canada to protect citizens from smallpox "directly traceable to the United States." He stated the disease had been prevalent there for the past five years, working its way northward from the infected Southern States. Although characterized as mild, his faith in the efficacy of vaccination would prevent a general epidemic. By November, upward of 50,000 vaccine points had been sold.

Authorities in Montreal heeded the call. In view of the prevalence of smallpox, the city council passed a compulsory vaccination by-law, requiring everyone to be vaccinated or show a satisfactory certificate or face a fine of $40 or 60 days imprisonment. It did not take long for Winnipeg citizens to form an anti-vaccination league, citing the report of the English Royal Commission as proof that civilized countries no longer accepted compulsory vaccination.[36]

By 1905, Dr. Simpson announced that vaccination continued to be reported satisfactorily, with few cases coming across the border, and in 1911, in order to see vaccination laws carried out in Montreal, 18 public vaccinators were hired to visit factories and shops. The same year, prosecutions against 34 municipalities were undertaken after authorities failed to comply with compulsory vaccination legislation.[37]

Once variola minor became established in Canada early in the 20th century, it became the predominant type of smallpox. Although less serious than variola major, vaccination remained the only preventive. After 100 cases were reported in Hamilton, Ontario, in 1912, Dr. Roberts, M.H.O., and William Farrar, chairman of the board of health, warned that if people would not protect themselves, vaccination would be made compulsory. In regard to those doctors who avowed the disease to be chicken pox, Roberts pithily declared, "The man who makes statements of this kind makes a particular ass of himself and does not deserve the safeguard the medical act gives him."

When the smallpox hospital in Manitoba opened February 17, 1914, the number of patients was 54, all but one being unvaccinated. Many were exposed to cases of reputed chicken pox and had circulated freely until full-blown symptoms of smallpox developed. All too often, children were the victims; fathers escaped by being well vaccinated, but neglected to provide the same protection to their offspring.[38]

The first smallpox vaccine farm in Canada was established in Ontario in 1885. Sponsored by the provincial board of health, the Palmerston Vaccine Farm was managed by Dr. Alexander Stewart until his death in 1911. Dr. Herbert Coleman then assumed responsibility for the Ontario farm and produced "points" until 1916, despite increasing imports of higher quality glycerinated vaccine. Thereafter, the Palmerston facility was transferred and upgraded by the Antitoxin Laboratories, University of Toronto. The name was changed in 1917 to "Connaught Antitoxin Laboratories and University Farm." Eighty years later, the Pocono Laboratory in Pennsylvania would become Connaught Laboratories, Incorporated, eventually becoming the United States division of Aventis Pasteur.

At the antitoxin labs, vaccinia virus was introduced into the belly of calves and the infected vesicles were harvested and processed into glycerinated points. With the assistance of Dr. William H. Park, director of the New York City Department of Health, Dr. Robert D. Defries of the Connaught lab was able to obtain a "New York vaccinia strain" (see below) descended from a strain originally used by Dr. Jenner. The strain having first been brought to the United States in the 1850s, Park's laboratory had begun large-scale production of it in 1876. "Since 1916 and then refreshed every two years since 1927, the New York strain served as the primary seed virus [that which was inoculated into an animal for the purpose of obtaining vaccine lymph] of all smallpox vaccine produced by Connaught." This vaccine was sold at cost to provincial Canadian governments for free distribution.[39]

In Alaska, where vaccination was promulgated solely for preventive measures, the federal government dictated that entrants first receive vaccination. However, if ship passengers could prove they had not been exposed to smallpox within the past two weeks, they were exempt from the rule. Although sources declared no smallpox in Alaska in May 1911, by June an outbreak had occurred at Dawson. Canadian authorities in all parts of the Yukon rigidly enforced compulsory vaccination, fining those attempting to evade the order $400. Dr. Foster, of the U.S. Marine Hospital Service at Eagle, released those who escaped Dawson in boats, provided they had been vaccinated any time during the past year. On July 16, with no new cases reported, quarantine was lifted, although compulsory vaccination was still enforced in all towns and along the creeks. As health officials toured the country with vaccine points, they encountered no resistance.[40]

Outbreaks of smallpox across Canada occurred with some regularity into the 1920s. In 1919, the United States government ordered all travelers passing into the country from Toronto to show proof of vaccination or undergo the procedure (compulsory vaccination had been abolished in this province); Canadian authorities adopted similar regulations in Manitoba to prevent the epidemic in Ontario from spreading. In the fall and winter of 1920–1921, there were 600 cases of smallpox reported in Ottawa; at Hull, despite the threat of an epidemic, the city council voted against compulsory vaccination.

When compulsory vaccination for schoolchildren was repealed in Edmonton, Alberta, in 1916, the number of smallpox cases rose from 101 cases in 1919, to 386 in 1920, with no decrease in cases in 1921. In 1923, the province of Manitoba reported 445 instances of smallpox, brought under control by a "vigorous vaccination campaign." Matters were more volatile in Toronto during 1924, where citizens blamed Mayor Montgomery and the police department for the Toronto epidemic. They, in turn, blamed the board of health, while smallpox outbreaks across the border in Lansing, Michigan (400 cases in January and 505 February), were attributed to the widespread prevalence of black smallpox in Canada.[41]

With an outbreak of smallpox in Ottawa striking 101 persons between October 1 and October 27, 1927, compulsory vaccination for all children was ordered for the first time. Free clinics were opened and no student was permitted to attend class without a certificate. Smallpox was identified in Camrose, Alberta, in 1929 and in 1930. Forty lumbermen exposed to the disease walked freely about Saskatoon, prompting the health authorities to complain that for years past, when the lumbering camps broke up in the spring, infected workers had often put citizens in danger.[42]

Vaccinia Virus and Smallpox Production

It is important to note that sometime in the 19th century the nature of the virus used for vaccination became altered from the standard cowpox virus originally used by Jenner to another *Orthopoxvirus* that came to be known as "vaccinia virus." The origins of vaccinia are unknown: It may have transformed into a hybrid between cowpox and variola virus, or it may have been derived from cowpox or some other *Orthopoxvirus* by serial passage under artificial laboratory conditions. Vaccinia virus is a distinct species of *Orthopoxvirus*, and DNA strains are different from those of all other *Orthopoxviruses*, including cowpox and variola. It did, however, offer a high degree of protection to individuals vaccinated against smallpox.

During the 1920s, scientists agreed that biological products prepared for use in human beings should be "bacteriologically sterile." Legislation in some countries was introduced to enforce this mandate, but the process of obtaining lymph from animals carried with it the inherent risk of contamination. As the World Health Organization observed, "Smallpox vaccine was the only vaccine for which both the public and the health authorities accepted the fact of contamination by exogenous microorganisms."[43] Confusion over the type of vaccine employed became an issue with anti-vaccinationists in Massachusetts in 1923. Their argument was twofold: that the form of vaccine prevailing in 1855, when the child vaccination law was passed, had been entirely, almost "surreptitiously" changed, and that the law did not define vaccination. "Anything which the public health authorities may choose to call 'vaccination' will pass for vaccination as the law stands. Having changed from cowpox as the basis of the manufacture of vaccine virus to smallpox, the state laboratory may at any time again change to something else, such as sheeppox, horsepox or chicken pox. Even if peculiar virtue is conceded to reside in cowpox virus, it does not follow that any kind of virus which our health officials may agree to call 'cowpox' has the same virtue."[44] Clearly, it was a point well taken.

Smallpox in Asia

For the first three decades of the 20th century, smallpox was endemic throughout the mainland countries of eastern and southeastern Asia, in Japan and the larger islands. Tibet remained the worst, as vaccination did not reach there until 1940. Variola major was highly endemic in China through 1940, occurring primarily as a seasonal disease, from December to the end of May, with epidemics in 1902, 1904, 1907, 1910 and 1913.[45] The Municipal

Council, Shanghai, meeting on November 13, 1902, proposed new "bye-laws" pertaining to infectious diseases. The first four regulations dictated that medical practitioners were required to report in writing any persons under their care suffering from smallpox or other infectious diseases; if infected persons were not properly quarantined, they were to be removed to an Isolation Hospital; no person suffering from an infectious disease should appear in public; every person above the age of 6 months was to be vaccinated or a $5 fine would be imposed for each conviction.[46]

Public health reports continued to show extremely low numbers of smallpox cases, but Governor Truppel noted, "I understand that the local magistrate assured the German visitors that there is no small-pox in this vicinity, a remarkable statement in view of the thousands of known cases and the tens of thousands of probable cases within a short distance of his yamen. Of course it is notorious that the Chinese pay no attention to such an infantile ailment as small-pox, and poke fun at foreigners for their stringent measures against the disease. This year the epidemic is rife among adults as well as children. Any sort of quarantine regulations are simply useless. We depend on vaccination and all reasonable precautions for immunity." An excerpt from Stewart Lockhait's "Report on Wiehaiwei" further observed that "the Chinese did not take to vaccination so far as was practiced by Europeans and attempts made to induce the natives to present themselves voluntarily were not successful." A grim observation from the health officer's report for 1903 added that, by hard work, 500 Chinese babies had received free vaccination, but after the rumor started that their eyes were being taken out, no more babies were brought.

The municipal report also urged cremation as being more economical, referencing the price of Japanese cremation as under 10 yen. Authorities hoped to purchase a Japanese furnace in order to put the procedure in the reach of Chinese of ordinary means. In respect to outsiders, the report added, "Small-pox, the most obviously preventable of all diseases, still kills in that section of the foreign community which neglects vaccination," not failing to underscore that "alcohol, that comfortable poison," was another means by which foreigners died.[47]

The health officer's monthly statistics continued to report favorably on vaccination, reporting in April 1904, that the laboratory issued over 3,000 tubes of vaccine, or the equivalent of 15,000 vaccinations. The May report noted that 2,865 tubes of Aseptic Glycerinated Vaccine prepared in the laboratory were issued. By December, however, rising numbers of smallpox cases "of the severe type" were cause for concern. By January 1905, a total of 315 Chinese had died from smallpox; thereafter cases decreased, with only 189 deaths in February.

Efforts were made to increase vaccination and 233 vaccinators were employed during 1904 and 1905, urging residents in Shanghai to be vaccinated every three years until it no longer took. Despite such work, the number submitting to the operation was only 1,166,588 against 1,254,324 in 1903. Part of the problem stemmed from local prejudice, indicating that vaccination performed in the autumn and winter was "no good." Another concern, more successfully addressed, was the idea that people visiting the health office needed "best clothes" before presenting themselves.

Official statistics remained relatively low until the winter of 1908 and the spring of 1909, when smallpox "raged," killing large numbers of children. The situation was complicated by outbreaks of measles and pneumonia. During the same period, Kobe, Japan, also suffered a serious epidemic of smallpox; between January 1 and 11, 1908, there were 801 cases reported. Prior to 1909, when a new law requiring vaccination of every infant within three months of birth and two subsequent revaccinations during childhood was made compulsory, vaccination in Japan suffered from inefficient administration. In the 12 years before the new law went into effect, the yearly average of cases had been over 28,000, with an average mortality of 7,700. Within 6 years of enforcement of the new law, the average yearly number dropped to 91, with an average mortality of 20.[48]

Health authorities in China continued to indicate smallpox was very common throughout the country in 1911, but less frequent in Shanghai as vaccination was more generally practiced among the Chinese there. After the establishment of the First Republic in 1913, some attempt was made to promote vaccination but it was too little to be effective. In the winter of 1916–1917, a virulent outbreak of smallpox in Hong Kong caused great concern. During this period, 471 cases were reported, of which 380 proved fatal. Not surprisingly, local newspapers reported that since the victims were of the poorer class of Chinese, there was no "cause for alarm" until the disease spread to local Europeans. Thereafter, authorities were "at their wits' end" to know how to cope. Complicating matters, the Chinese dumped contagious bodies into the streets, "to be collected by anyone who cared to do so."[49]

Edwin R. Embree, secretary of the Rockefeller Foundation, returned to New York after organizing the Peking Medical College in 1921. He stated that lack of scientific attention to public health in China caused numerous fatalities, particularly among smallpox patients who went about the streets in an active state of the disease. It was hoped the new college and hospital would bring some relief to the sick while offering fellowships to Chinese doctors and nurses. During a 1922 conference of medical professionals in Shanghai, discussions on the benefits of wide scale vaccination in the Philippines were lauded, contrasted with California, where "faddists" had upset all the good work by introducing "conscientious" regulations, leading to the spread of smallpox "in the state after it had been completely eradicated."

In conjunction with the Chinese YMCA, health commissioners pursued a campaign of vaccination, reporting a total of 6,766 free vaccinations given during the latter part of December 1922, but reported the disease was still "smouldering." For the year, nearly 30,000 vaccinations were performed at the Shanghai branch health office, but authorities still feared the coming winter would usher in an epidemic greater than normal. They advised that the best time for vaccination was in October or early November, before winter set in. While there was some scientific basis for the belief, attitudes such as that expressed by an Illinois physician that he "wasn't doing much" about vaccination at present "because I do not believe that this is the time of year for vaccination" was contrary to common sense. As the newspaper dryly observed, "If he saw a rattlesnake approaching a child would he say this is not the season for killing rattlesnakes?" The reporter added, "When there is infection anywhere in the neighborhood the best policy by all means is safety first." By 1939, the Tientsin Railway Bureau (under Japanese control) required a vaccination certificate of anyone traveling by train through North China.[50]

Between the two World Wars, Southwestern Asia (the Ottoman Empire and Persia) suffered from endemic smallpox. When the territories were divided, numbers of new cases varied, falling to low levels by the late 1930s. In Afghanistan, recognized as an independent state in 1921, variolation was extensively practiced and it was not until the 1930s that modern vaccination service was established, with 3 million people receiving the protection between 1936 and 1939.[51]

The Netherlands East Indies suffered severe outbreaks of smallpox early in the 20th century; an outbreak in Borneo claimed 3,000 lives in 1905. In 1913, Java suffered 18,000 cases, with 5,000 deaths; severe outbreaks in 1918–1919, 1922 and 1924 spread to the outer islands. Primary vaccination was begun around 1926; by 1933, about 10 percent of the population had been vaccinated or revaccinated and by 1937, endemic smallpox had disappeared.[52]

Smallpox in the Caribbean Islands

A mild form of smallpox struck the Caribbean Islands in early 1902, rapidly expanding into epidemic proportions. Not unlike nations elsewhere, a general disregard there for vaccination and the overwhelming misdiagnosis of the disease greatly contributed to its spread. Contemporary authorities placed the origin of the outbreak in Trinidad, but during 1902, the majority of cases were reported in Barbados. By September, when the total number reached 473, Governor Hodgson called for universal vaccination. The plea was disregarded, in part due to the parochial treasurer of the Metropolitan Parish, who incidentally happened to be the proprietor of the newspaper, "run chiefly to defend his interests, and who is an anti-vaccinationist." Riots occurred on September 25 at Tweedside, and as the number of infected continued to climb, reaching 500 in October, the "lower orders [who] were at first violently opposed," changed their minds, "with hordes of labourers clamouring to be vaccinated." This proved insufficient, as October's returns showed 784 cases, of which 29 died, 107 were cured and 648 remained under treatment.

Nathaniel Nicolai, of the firm of Messrs. Parke, Davis and Company, visited Barbados at the outbreak of the epidemic and secured exclusive rights for his firm to supply vaccine. Promoting the value of vaccination, he claimed that with the advent of "Asceptic Vaccine" in the form of glycerinated virus, instances of septicemia could only be brought on by personal uncleanliness of the patient or neglect of the vaccinator to sterilize his scarifier. His experience indicated that among the West Indians of Barbados, natives were harder to vaccinate due to the thickness of their skin, often requiring revaccination.

Nearly as significant to the local population was the injury to trade, described as "incalculable." Bridgetown, the distributing port for the Windward and Leeward Islands, was completely blockaded and the introduction of any article from Barbados was prohibited. In British Guiana, all ships from Barbados were required to be fumigated with sulphur, all clothing and bedding thoroughly aired and the vessels inspected. No passengers were allowed to depart until quarantine had expired. The governor of Granada issued similar orders, increasing the quarantine period to 21 days. Citing the Quarantine Ordinance of 1895, authorities at St. Vincent followed suit.[53]

Frederick M. Martinez, a representative of English commerce in the West Indies, reported in October that smallpox was rife, with natives disliking the proposed compulsory vaccination law passed by the House of Assembly. Because the island was so densely populated and Negroes crowded together, disease quickly spread from one to another. Pelican Island was used as a quarantine area, but the natives hated to be sent there, and even medical men had to be obtained from Antigua. Referencing the riots, Martinez thought there were enough soldiers to contain the violence but strongly disagreed with Chamberlain's policy of loaning £200,000 to improve conditions. He felt most of the money went to planters at 6 percent, and might as well have been "thrown into the sea." His outlook on the sugar crop was dismal and in consequence unemployment was high. Martinez concluded, "It is a pessimistic view of the situation, but it is the true one."[54]

The above conclusions were echoed in the *London Times*, which reported that until 1901, Barbados had been the first port of call for Royal Mail boats from England. From there, a fleet of intercolonial steamers conveyed goods and passengers to Demerara, Trinidad, St. Lucia, St. Thomas, Tobago and other British islands. Quarantine gave a "knockdown blow" to trade already grievously suffering from depression in its one substantial industry, the growth and export of sugar. Somewhat prejudicially, the article added that many natives would rather be taken care of in a hospital than "get up in the morning and work till sundown." Taking a different approach, the governor of the Windward Islands, who had 9 years experience in Gambia, remarked that natives in that colony proudly accepted vaccination "as placing them on a footing of equality with the white man, and go about proudly showing on their arm what they call 'The Queen's mark.'" Less sentimentally, Barbadians were induced to submit to vaccination "in the form of the head of the Sovereign stamped on half-a-crown, children going to the doctor for a shilling." (In contrast, chocolate was used as an inducement in some regions of England.)[55]

The story was slightly different in Trinidad, where government medical men categorically denied the existence of smallpox or any contagious disease on the island. In order to protect their own territory, authorities in Barbados sent Dr. J.F.E. Bridger to assess the situation. His report, published in early March 1903 and widely distributed among the Caribbean Islands, declared that smallpox not only existed in Trinidad, but also was "spreading furiously." Newspapers in Trinidad berated Dr. Bridger's qualifications, as he had "only graduated in his profession five or six years ago," and called their own council. At that meeting (March 10), the Medical Board of Trinidad declared there was "no such disease as mild small pox" and that the eruptive fever then prevailing was not small pox, but "something new." Quarantine measures were promptly taken against Trinidad, finally prompting the medical officer to issue a leaflet in May (omitting the word "smallpox"), detailing recommendations to the public on how to deal with and prevent the spread of "the prevailing epidemic."

The following month, the *Port of Spain Gazette* published an account of affairs in Trinidad, reporting over 5,000 "cases of pox" since February, equaling 4 percent of the population. The epidemic was classified as being of "a varioloid type, chiefly chicken pox of a serious type, with a very few sporadic cases of smallpox."[56]

The situation in Jamaica was exacerbated by the fact so many coolies were imported from Calcutta for work on the sugar and banana plantations or on a stopover to the Panama Canal. Many were not vaccinated when they arrived, or had gone through the arm-to-arm transfer (inoculation), leading the former to be susceptible to smallpox and the latter capable of spreading infection to the unvaccinated.

Maintaining an adequate supply of vaccination was aided by importation from the Jenner Institution, with the lymph proving more reliable after being stored in an ice box (refrigeration unit) registering between 65° and 68° until required. When samples were tested for purity, results were variable, the best obtained from Pretoria, where a "Vaccine Establishment" was in operation.

Reports from September 20, 1904, indicated 18,530 successful vaccinations, down 8,066 from the previous year. (Unfortunately, most of these were arm-to-arm transfers due to a lack of vaccine.) The superintending medical officer, Colonel Kenny, attributed the decrease to the large number performed the previous year and the prevalence of yaws, which put vaccination "in abeyance." He also noted that no amount of persuasion could induce the adult population to undergo the operation and that, while children were typically well vaccinated, they frequently rubbed off the lymph, negating effectiveness.

A One-Day Sample of the Prevalence of
Vaccination, Kingston Public Hospital, 1905

Vaccination marks	93
No vaccination marks	41
Doubtful marks	38
Those with smallpox	12

Due to a £200 grant, the importation of lymph was expected to rise from 40–50 tubes of lymph delivered every fortnight to 180–220 tubes.

The West Indian Quarantine Conference was held in Barbados in April 1904 and required every colony to notify every other colony of the presence of contagious diseases in their territory. The conference described proper methods of sanitary inspection, isolation and disinfection, and required, "in the case of smallpox," vaccination and revaccination to be secured. Not inconsequentially, noting that the quarantine system of the islands was a "complete failure," the conference instituted regulations that sought to remove and relax restrictions on trade and communication within the colonies. (In this regard, delegates were aware that, as Jamaica was on the direct line between Europe and the future Canal, the island could not afford to be quarantined.) The regulations were to be in effect for 5 years.

Jamaica passed a quarantine law in 1905, but it was never brought into force. At the other extreme, because of poor salaries and stringent medical laws requiring foreign doctors to take an examination upon entering the country (excluding men with British qualifications), they were critically short of physicians. The solution for this problem was either to import doctors from Canada (where many young Jamaicans went for a "cheap and first class education") or establish a local medical college.

Anti-vaccinationists in the Caribbean tended to question why local laws were not adapted to reflect those in England, where conscientious objectors were permitted to refuse vaccination, as well as echoed doubts expressed in America over its benefits. Lending aid to the cause was the governor, who made arguments against vaccination in opposition to his own medical authorities, among whom the most prominent was George C. Henderson, M.D.[57]

During the year 1911, medical reports from Montego Bay indicated several hundred cases of yaws, most responding to treatment. Children were fairly well protected from smallpox but protection among adults was "practically nil," with greater than 90 percent having never been revaccinated. The same statistics were reported for Buff Bay, Black River and Stony Hill. Authorities observed that if the regulations of Germany, where children were revaccinated during their last school year, were carried out in Jamaica, the rising generation would have satisfactory protection against smallpox.[58]

As demonstrated in England, "Kaffir Pox" (alastrim) made an appearance in Jamaica during August 1920, first reported at the village of Hampstead, and quickly spreading to Kingston, Port Maria, Bailey's Vale and Oracabessa. Reports for the week ending September 18, 1920, revealed 496 cases of this mild smallpox. Because the disease was not attended by mortality, the tendency on the island was to ignore it, prompting some health authorities to remark the people were living in a "fool's paradise," as there was no assurance the virus would not turn lethal. Since no one knew exactly what alastrim was, however, Jamaican physicians considered vaccination optional.

The eminent authority Dr. J.C. McVial considered the outbreaks in England and Jamaica as the same type as was seen in Trinidad (1901–1903) and New South Wales (1913–1914). In a 1919, lecture he described two types of the disease: the severe, or African, type and the mild, or American, type, seen in Trinidad and New South Wales. Without having positive proof whether the severe and mild types were related, he concluded both infections were variolous (as opposed to bearing a relationship to chicken pox) as both responded to vaccination.

The appearance of smallpox in Port-au-Prince during 1921 (which had been under American administration the preceding five years) and the endemic smallpox in Haiti brought fresh concerns to Jamaicans. To stem the disease, they placed new regulations on passengers from Colon, Panama, Carthagena, Porto Colombia, Santa Marta, Haiti, San Domingo, Mexico and the islands of St. Andrew and Old Providence, requiring them to be 14 days out to sea or to possess a recent certification of vaccination before landing.

By September 1923, sections of Jamaica adopted compulsory vaccination against the spread of alastrim, "fairly well" protecting children so that by October, the disease had decreased. Figures published by the Island Medical Department in 1923 revealed that in 1920, when alastrim first made an appearance, 70,000 persons received vaccination, but as the scare died away, only 35,000 received the prophylactic treatment in 1922. With a population of 900,000, large numbers remained unprotected. Reflecting on the significance (or lack thereof) of vaccination, directly above an article describing the mindset of those who derived satisfaction from being in a minority (in this case, decrying the protection offered by vaccination), editors placed an ad reading: "Protect Your Piano, Let A.A. Russell take care of your Piano. You will appreciate the difference of tone and touch."[59]

In 1926, the question of vaccination for alastrim was broached again, this time for fear that tourists might believe the authorities were not handling the ongoing crisis and therefore would avoid the island. It was particularly noted that Jamaica was losing "an enormous sum of money annually, and will cost still more if the Government will not act, and act quickly." To press home the point, it was noted the Prince of Wales was to have visited six years ago, when the disease first found its way to the island, but he did not come in consequence of it. Although immigration authorities required vaccination in imitation of "America, Cuba and elsewhere," frequent letters to the editor of the *Daily Gleaner* demanded vaccination be made compulsory. A like number of "anti" letters appeared to argue the contrary. By the 1930s, vaccination certificates were required for Jamaicans desiring to enter any other country.[60]

Smallpox in Panama, Cuba, Central and South America

On July 20, 1906, the Royal Mail Company's steamer *Orinoco* arrived at Kingston, having previously touched in at Barbados, Trinidad and Colon,

Placed directly above an article (dealing with persons who took pleasure in finding themselves in a minority, in this case, anti-vaccinationists) with the title, "On Cranks and the Workings of Their Minds," the editor chose to run an ad warning people to "Protect Your Piano." It leads to the speculation that it was done on purpose to underscore how people took more care of possessions than their own, or the lives of loved ones. The article was written for the *London Daily Mail*, reprinted in the *Daily Gleaner* (Jamaica), October 23, 1923.

Panama. It was found to be carrying smallpox and the yellow flag was hoisted, initiating quarantine regulations. An earlier ship, the Colon *Starlet,* for July 12 reported that smallpox (endemic in South America, Panama and Bocas del Toro) had broken out in Colon (47 miles from the city of Panama), introduced from Cartagena, Colombia, in May. Natives there kept the extent of the epidemic from medical authorities, but fortunately the disease was of a mild form. Worse, smallpox was to be found almost constantly along the San Blas coast, making it a "standing menace" to the Isthmus and work on the canal. One commercial traveler noted "the Indians know nothing whatever of vaccination and the disease causes much suffering among them." Not surprisingly, the newspaper observed that, with the prospect of increased canal work and a large influx of Americans and others, it would be in the interest of public health to send a commission to the San Blas Coast to report on the matter.

Dr. W.C. Gorgas, superintending medical officer on the Canal Zone, "made his name famous for the admirable work of scavenging and cleansing," as well as enforcing the law that all emigrants to Panama were compelled to be vaccinated or submit proof of recent vaccination. Every ship entering the port was required to fly the yellow flag (indicating the presence of smallpox) and crews were strictly quarantined until proven safe. Poor lymph and vaccination techniques hampered his efforts but perhaps more damaging was the work of Joseph Collinson, author of the pamphlet "What It Costs to Be Vaccinated," directed against pro-vaccinators. His arguments were powerful enough that even the *Daily Gleaner,* typically very positive on vaccination, questioned whether vaccination was no more than a "fetish."[61]

Fortunately, the incidence of smallpox in Panama and the Isthmus remained low, with few reported cases. Contagious individuals typically arrived from incoming vessels, resulting in fumigation of the ship and vaccination for the crew. Regulations required that passengers in transit who had not been on the Isthmus for 14 days, and passengers from Mexico and Guatemala who desired to land, had to be 14 days out, or show the surgeon of the vessel marks of recent vaccination, submit to vaccination on the voyage or complete the remainder of the two-week period at the quarantine station. All travelers continuing to Jamaica were also required to follow the above restrictions.[62]

After a mild epidemic on the Isthmus in 1929, it was discovered that about 20 percent of the inhabitants of tenement houses in Panama had never been vaccinated. From that date until 1932, it was believed most received protection. With the population shifting from outlying districts into the city, a new vaccination campaign was begun as a preventive measure on the grounds that epidemic smallpox tended to recur every 5–8 years. During the month of August 1932, chief health officer Colonel J.F. Siler announced that 1,200 persons had been vaccinated in Panama and 1,500 in La Boca. In stressing the value of vaccination, Siler noted that between 1881 and 1904, during the French occupancy, there were 761 deaths among the French and Panamanians. From 1904 to 1929, when the United States assumed control for building the canal and inaugurated a vaccination campaign, there were only 6 deaths, 1 in the Zone, 2 in Panama City and 3 in Colon.[63]

Few in Puerto Rico would have described vaccination as a "fetish" in 1901. Instead, newspapers contained reports of the tremendous success the operation had on the island. The turnaround came quickly: in 1896, surgeon general Hoff reported no fewer than 3,000 cases of smallpox.

Early in 1899, after American occupation, General Henry, the governor, issued an order for universal vaccination that was strictly enforced. Aiding the cause was the establishment of a government vaccine farm. It was claimed 800,000 natives were vaccinated at a cost of about 4 cents each. Dr. Azel Ames, director of General Henry's vaccinating department, held the island up as an example of amazing success, contrasting sharply with the United States and Great Britain, where anti-vaccination forces enabled the rapid and general spread of the disease. Of the success in Puerto Rico, he concluded, "Vaccination alone did it, and will do it effectively wherever compulsory legislation, properly enforced, secures its benefits to all."

In the intervening years, vaccination was less strictly enforced, so that by 1907, cases of varioloid were diagnosed. On the recommendation of Governor Post, the executive council reissued a compulsory vaccination order. Six hundred points were ordered, with work to start in the Guayama district where the disease was most prevalent.[64] A severe outbreak occurred in May 1916, with 85 cases reported in one week, 47 being from San Juan. A vaccination crusade was begun, with preparation for a million and a quarter inhabitants. By July, the 6-week epidemic was considered under control, with a total of 159 cases placed in quarantine. The vaccination of 100,000 individuals was credited with preventing a worse outbreak, but authorities vowed to put in force a compulsory order if more citizens did not present themselves for the procedure. Prisoners from the penitentiary were used to clean up San Juan as a secondary means of ending the spread of disease.[65]

In Guatemala smallpox was described as the disease "which has been the scourge of the nation since the white man first settled there," and epidemics ran rampant into the 1900s. Finding the epidemic beyond his control, Dr. Juan A. Padilla, surgeon-general of the Marine Hospital and Quarantine Service, made strong representations to President Estrada Cabrera on the necessity of immunizing the Indians, who were spreading the disease. The president issued the appropriate orders and for three months, vaccination was performed. Thereafter, incidence of smallpox was reduced to extremely low levels and restrictions on travel were lifted.[66] Fresh cases in Kingston, however, presented a new concern, as vessels from the coast were constantly arriving. Contagious diseases easily passed from one country to another via water trade routes; one major epidemic in Panama was believed to have originated from Ecuador.

Considerable alarm was caused in Cuba during November 1914, when an outbreak was reported in an outlying district of Havana. While the sanitary authorities were considering the advisability of compulsory vaccination, those in the customs service or connected with the port of Havana were ordered to undergo vaccination at once.[67] In 1919, a passenger off the French steamship *Venzia* introduced an outbreak in Havana. More than 25,000 persons were vaccinated within 5 days, but a shortage of vaccine limited the procedure to those living in the infected zones.[68]

An epidemic of smallpox broke out in Nicaragua in January 1929, causing President Moncada to call for help in securing vaccine. Admiral David F. Sellers, USN, collected 3,500 tubes from Panama and forwarded them to Managua. On April 18, Moncada issued orders for a general vaccination; reports indicated people were standing in line to receive protection.[69]

Immediately south of Nicaragua, Costa Rica suffered an outbreak of smallpox in April the following year. With 12 cases isolated in a camp outside the capital and new victims "appearing daily," the government ordered that every person show a certificate of vaccination or be vaccinated. On June 7, sanitary authorities issued a despatch, stating the last 14 cases in San Jose had been cured and there was no further danger of smallpox in Costa Rica. The outbreak caused "few deaths."[70] Smallpox also appeared in Honduras in 1930, believed to have come in through the Atlantic route. As Costa Rica did, Honduran sanitary authorities ordered vaccination throughout the leading cities.[71]

Variola major was endemic in all the larger countries of South America during the opening years of the 20th century, with Brazil and Chile having the highest rates of infection. In 1921, the worst epidemic in the history of Chile reached 10,000 cases (out of a population of half a million) in the city of Santiago alone. Between September and October, estimates placed the number of dead between 500 and 1,000. Thousands were isolated in smallpox hospitals and "rigid enforcement of the vaccination requirements" was put in place. Vaccination certificates were required of those attempting to enter or leave by train, or to attend racetracks and other public places.[72]

Brazil suffered severe epidemics of smallpox in 1903 and 1904, with 3,800 deaths in Recife and 3,600 deaths in Rio de Janeiro. In consequence, the government issued compulsory vaccination orders but they led to riots by anti-vaccinationists, delaying the implementation of mass vaccinations. In consequence, large epidemics with high numbers of fatalities occurred in 1907–1910; in 1926, an episode of variola major in Rio de Janeiro caused 2,000 deaths. Variola minor first appeared in Brazil in 1910, spreading throughout the country and producing an estimated 250,000 cases in 1910 and 1911; by the late 1920s until the early 1930s, variola minor became established as an endemic disease. In 1910 at Parana, 6,000 persons became infected, with a fatality rate of 2.3 percent. Over the next 20 years, variola minor displaced variola major, but the more deadly form persisted in Chile and Argentina throughout the 1920s.[73]

Smallpox in Mexico

Unlike the United States and Canada, where variola minor slowly replaced variola major, Mexico continued to suffer the fatal strain of smallpox.

In an interesting letter to the editor responding to an anti-vaccinationist who happened to be president of a local chiropractic board (newspapers often cited chiropractors for refusing to vaccinate their patients), Charles Tarver, M.D., described his experiences during a long residence in Mexico. With smallpox being endemic, he witnessed several very bad outbreaks. Of the nonimmune (those who had not previously suffered from smallpox), he indicated fully 90 percent of the population was attacked, with 30 percent mortality. At the time, vaccination was reserved for "the better class," and as no precautions were taken, the disease eventually died out "for want of material."

While working in Santa Rosalia, a city of some 12,000 inhabitants, Tarver convinced Mayor Salcido to order compulsory vaccination. As chief executives were "never hampered by court interference," the request was approved and carried out. That season, when a severe epidemic struck La Cruz, a town only 6 miles away, no cases were found in Santa Rosalia, despite the fact no quarantine or sanitary precautions were taken, and many residents of La Cruz came to Dr. Tarver for treatment. He further added that as the health officer for Maverick County, he oversaw vaccination there and in spite of the fact many Mexicans carrying smallpox crossed the border, none of his patients suffered from the disease.[74]

After the Tampico Affair of April 9, 1914, where 9 American sailors were arrested by Mexican authorities for entering an off-limits area in Tampico, Tamaulipas, rumors of an arms delivery to the Mexicans prompted President Wilson to order the port of Veracruz seized. A show of force by the navy and Marines on April 21 prompted the defenders to retreat and the Americans occupied the port city under U.S. Army general Frederick Funston. Responsibility for public health and sanitation passed from Mexican to American physicians and when the navy left on April 30, the army assumed the job.

Chief surgeon Colonel H.P. Birmingham promptly reorganized public health into three departments: civilian, military and quarantine. Tuberculosis, measles and particularly smallpox were the primary contagious diseases and the task faced was enormous. Veracruz had a contagious disease reputation equaling that of Havana and Panama, and world ports were constantly enforcing quarantine against it. To counter contagion, medical men began a thorough sanitation by literally scrubbing the town: stagnant pools were drained or oiled, and a general smallpox vaccination was begun on May 18, 1914, with virus obtained from the States. Through June 30, there were 41,404 out of 60,000 persons who had undergone the procedure, with the expectation that just as the army contained smallpox in the Philippines, it would have equal success in Mexico. Fifty percent of adult vaccinations and 80–90 percent of children's vaccinations proved successful. Unfortunately, success was short lived. Once the army departed, standards of sanitation were relaxed, resulting in an outbreak of black (confluent) smallpox that led to high mortality rates. By 1917, however, the department of public health, Mexico City, reported that smallpox had been successfully combated by widespread vaccination, including the entire army, schoolchildren and occupants of prisons.[75]

With a population in the range of 14 million in 1920, Mexico reported between 5,000 and 13,000 smallpox deaths annually during this decade, making it the highest incidence of smallpox in the world.[76] In order to combat these horrendous numbers, 117,000 persons in the federal district were vaccinated over a seven-month period during 1923. Statistics from the health department of the City of Mexico showed that between May and December 1923, as many as 58,745 residents also received vaccination; 1,897 were vaccinated for the first time.[77] Variola minor was first reported around 1932, probably imported from the United States, but unlike other countries, it did not supplant variola major. Desperate to combat the disease, Rotary Club members and their wives vaccinated 20,000 persons in Veracruz in 1926, while in 1930, several dozen senior medical students in Mexico City were forcibly vaccinated by companions after they refused to submit willingly.[78] Between 1932 and 1943, major epidemics of smallpox caused over 8,000 deaths.[79]

Smallpox in Africa

By 1900, smallpox had become established throughout Africa and remained so for the first 25 years of the new century. Egypt suffered smallpox epidemics in 1904–1905, 1909, 1914–1915 and 1919–1920. In response, vaccination programs were instituted in 1919 and 1926. With assistance from the colonial powers of France, Spain and the United Kingdom, vaccination campaigns reduced smallpox to low levels, with only one major outbreak in Egypt in 1932–1934, which did not spread to other North African countries. By the end of the 1930s, endemic smallpox in Northern Africa had been virtually eliminated except for Morocco.

The Sudan, long a central road along which pilgrims passed going to and returning from Mecca, suffered heavily from endemic smallpox and by 1925, variola minor had become epidemic in the south and east, coexisting with importations of variola major from the west. In Uganda, Arab and other traders were primarily responsible for importing smallpox, creating endemic conditions that resulted in over 20,000 deaths between 1914 and 1920, a fatality rate of 23 percent.[80]

A published account of Captain J.F.J. Fitzpatrick's experiences in Nigeria from 1907–1922 included information on smallpox in this African nation. While exploring an "unsettled" area he received word that the disease raged in one high-altitude community. Taking an interpreter and a tube of vaccine lymph, he went into the village of the Out-and-Out, where the elders told him that 60 persons had already died and every hut contained at least one afflicted individual. He vaccinated all he could until his supply ran out; after seven days, when the vaccinations had "taken," he inoculated the rest with virus from the sores. During the 15 years he spent in Africa, Fitzpatrick noted he had vaccinated thousands of people and never knew one to contract smallpox or experience any ill result from the procedure.[81]

Importation of variola major from India into Eastern Africa during 1920s and the 1930s remained a constant danger. But seed vaccination from India was supplied to Nairobi in the 1930s, to supply most of the British colonies in that region, and endemic smallpox was eliminated from Kenya in 1930.

During 1927–1931, a severe epidemic of variola major in the Sudan was apparently introduced by Ethiopian immigrants, while an extensive outbreak was seen in the south between 1932 and 1934.[82] During the first 6 months of 1937, medical authorities vaccinated 116,534 citizens of Addis Ababa and the surrounding country. Although rumors circulated that the effort was made by Italians "to insert deadly poison into the Ethiopian blood stream," the Italian press stated that this obstacle was overcome by "persuasive action followed by the government," resulting, for a time, in low rates of the disease.[83]

As an island separated from the epidemics of the continent, Madagascar had endemic smallpox for a time in the 19th century, but authorities were able to control it and the disease eventually died out. Afterward, the major cause of smallpox came from periodic importations from Africa and India, with a severe outbreak in 1901, causing 98 deaths from 262 reported cases. Vaccine production began in Antananarivo in 1899, and compulsory vaccination and revaccination was instituted in 1909. During World War I, Madagascar became the first country in Africa to eliminate smallpox. After this time, only sporadic cases were reported each year between 1925 and 1931.[84]

Smallpox in Oceania

Australia, New Zealand and the islands of the Pacific Ocean were spared major epidemics of smallpox because of their isolation. By the time a passenger from Europe arrived by boat, whatever symptoms he suffered had usually dissipated; as methods of travel improved with the development of the airplane, the introduction of smallpox became more problematic.

What outbreaks of variola major did occur in the 1800s and early 1900s caused considerable panic and discussion among health care providers and anti-vaccinationists. But with vigilant vaccination control, the disease never became endemic. Low case reports and opposition to vaccination led to dangerously low infant vaccination in the early 20th century, but the requirement of current vaccination certificates for incoming travelers and monitoring of incoming ships and, later, aircraft, prevented major outbreaks.

Because smallpox outbreaks were rare, when the second city and port in Launceston, Tasmania, was exposed to an importation of smallpox, agitators in the capital of Hobart called for effective quarantine and isolation in the affected city. This led to a generalized antipathy against Hobart and an uprising around the country, rendering the system of vaccination and quarantine "farcical."[85]

The last significant outbreak in Australia came in 1913, with the importation of alastrim.[86]

Smallpox Visitations Around the World

At the turn of the century, 40,000 annual deaths from smallpox were reported in the Philippines, smallpox accounted for one-third of all cases of blindness. One of the most important contributions Americans made in the Philippines was the administration of vaccine. By 1908, more than 5,000,000 operations had been performed. In the six provinces around Manila (Cavite, Batangas, Celia, Bataan, La Union, Rizal and Laguana), where an annual death rate averaged 6,000, mortality decreased to the point where no deaths were officially reported. In 1907, the board of health completed systematic compulsory vaccination throughout the islands, with the result that "the disease, once so prevalent, is almost eradicated." The only American deaths from smallpox were those who neglected vaccination; the contagion was thought to have been imported from Kobe and other Japanese cities, where the disease was more common. By 1914, only 700 cases were reported.

Success did not mitigate anti-vaccination fervor, "antis" claiming the drop in mortality to be "mere coincidence."[87] In 1916, after the transfer of power to local authority, vaccination efforts were relaxed; in 1918 and 1919, a very severe epidemic caused over 64,000 deaths.[88] Without considering the circumstances, by 1922, anti-vaccination publications were filled with editorials, such as that demanding, "Why Is Smallpox Increasing in the Philippines?" published by the Medical Liberty League. Dr. A.C. Young, an authority on smallpox, responded to the question by bluntly stating the epidemics were "due to the want of a continued and systematic vaccination of the people." Dr. Heiser, former director of health for the islands, agreed with that conclusion. (Curiously, one of the arguments put forth by the Medical Liberty League stated that "for a century and a quarter vaccination has been largely required in the Philippines." That set the timeline back to 1797, the year before Jenner's vaccination thesis was published.)[89] Vaccination efforts were strengthened, and by 1931, smallpox ceased to be endemic.

With smallpox raging in the United States at the turn of the 20th century, the Hawaiian board of health opted to take a proactive stance to prevent the disease from spreading to the islands. The two principal means of contamination were believed to be through the mail and directly from incoming ships, primarily those from eastern Asia and San Francisco. Regarding the mails, discussion centered around payment for fumigation: it was believed the United States quarantine service and the postal authorities would cover the cost; the board accepted responsibility for incoming ships. Of the latter, doubt was expressed over whether a strict quarantine could be enforced when no epidemic was officially announced at the last port of departure.

At the end of the 19th century, regulations required persons landing in Hawaii to report to the boarding physician of the board of health, but it was felt stronger measures were required, especially toward steerage passengers, "who were more exposed to conditions which would bring on the disease." By 1903, a bill was entered repealing all vaccination laws; but it was later substituted with one requiring children to present a certificate of vaccination before entering school. It also allowed the board of health to compel vaccination, while prohibiting any physician from using any but bovine virus for vaccination or be liable to a $500 fine.[90] The only significant outbreak in the 20th century occurred in 1911, when 52 cases of variola major were reported in a detention camp for illegal immigrants from the Philippines.[91]

In Russia, health authorities were confounded by the religious practices of the peasantry. It was commonly believed that any child dying of smallpox (especially the "black smallpox," called "God's sickness") immediately became an angel. Instead of isolating the child, the family assembled around the sickbed in order to rejoice in the fact that the patient was under the protection of Providence, smallpox being regarded as a mark of divine favor. Consequently, attempts to prevent the terrible prevalence of the disease and more particularly, to enforce vaccination, was met with stiff resistance by the lower clergy, who regarded preventive measures as a "most damnable sacrilege."[92]

In 1907, eighty cases of smallpox in Vienna in 10 days led crowds to besiege the free vaccination stations. Lymph gave out and physicians were required to order fresh supplies by telegraph.[93]

A smallpox outbreak in Stockholm in 1913 resulted in 35 cases being hospitalized, causing a rush for vaccination. This resulted in a new social fad called "vaccination parties," where Swedish residents invited a physician into their homes to vaccinate guests, completing the ceremony with a dinner party. The demand for vaccination was so great, supplies were quickly exhausted, requiring enough vaccine for 100,000 persons to be ordered from abroad.[94]

In Hungary, compulsory vaccination of children in their early years and revaccination before entering school was reported to have virtually eliminated smallpox by 1925. Employing an extensive plan of health services, physicians visited villages every year and an innovative plan of "sickness insurance" was adopted, whereby workers and employers shared equally in the expense of the policy. All hospital bills and medicine were paid by the insurance company and the worker received a percentage of his wages until recovered. Four universities trained doctors and the government paid for doctors to serve one-year fellowships in the United States or England.[95]

Soldiers, the Law and Old-Fashioned Smallpox

Appropriations for the control of epidemics has not kept pace with the growth in population.... We hereby appeal to the people of Oklahoma to take every precaution against contracting and spreading all infectious and contagious diseases. A repetition of the present epidemic would render us helpless to furnish state aid for want of funds. Moral: Prevention is safer, better and cheaper than cure.[1]

With the atmosphere if not the actuality of war tainting the air at the dawn of a new century, more attention was paid to an army that might be called upon to serve at any given moment. Military cohesiveness and camaraderie did not unite America's fighting forces, however, when it came to vaccination.

With 2,300 recruits from Boston camped on the banks of the Assawamsett in July 1902, feelings were "anything but pleasant" after the soldiers were informed vaccination would be strictly enforced. Many, including the captain of Company K, claimed they would rather be court-martialed than be vaccinated. Aside from personal prejudice, the claim was that the camp at Lakeview was "neither the time nor place to perform the operation," as they could not be properly treated if the weather proved unfavorable.[2]

That smallpox proved to be a viable threat was aptly demonstrated in January 1904, when the presence of the disease at Jefferson Barracks, outside St. Louis, caused compulsory vaccination of all the men in the 4th and 8th cavalries. Affected men were moved to quarantine.[3] While the health of the army was reported to Secretary Taft in October 1905 as "improved," enlisted strength of the army as shown upon the monthly sick reports was 60,139, with 79,586 "admissions to the sick report" during the year, 406 deaths from all causes and 1,377 discharges for disability. Advancing from third to first place on the list of diseases was "immoral habits," causing 16 percent of admissions to the sick report. Pneumonia was the leading cause of death, followed by tuberculosis; 21 men were killed in action and 42 wounded, with 27 soldiers committing suicide; 10 were victims of homicide and 45 drowned. As proof that vaccination served as a preventive, alcoholism, dysentery, typhoid fever, malaria, measles and mumps placed American forces highest on the list of hospital admissions, with soldiers in Russia ranking last. The Prussian, Bavarian and Dutch armies reported a total absence of smallpox. Surgeon R.M. O'Reilly's report to Taft noted, "More care in vaccination would give like results in other services."[4]

By 1911, as more troops amassed, the plan for massive revaccinations for smallpox was changed to include only those whose first attempt failed to take. It was understood that this number was comparatively small. Antityphoid serum was also required of soldiers, but little resistance was reported over this series of injections. Underscoring the importance of protection, Sir William Osler, surgeon, British Army, declared in 1914, that "the army today marches on its brains not on its belly. The bacillus is more deadly than the bullet." Preaching that typhoid, dysentery, smallpox and other contagious diseases slay more men than enemy fire, he advocated health along scientific lines for those about to embark for the continent. Americans, both military and civilian, were reminded of these words as statistics continued to prove that no great epidemics of smallpox or typhoid fever struck the armies.[5] Once mobilization began, those soldiers assigned to patrol the Mexican border were vaccinated. As one recruit noted, "The Mexicans have smallpox with them always.... The government is bound that we shall not die a natural death at any rate." Not all efforts came soon enough, as smallpox broke out in the mobilization camp in Kentucky, forcing immediate vaccination.[6]

Typical of most states, Virginia's educational law stated that every child was required to be vaccinated upon entering the school system, but it also granted local authorities latitude to set the law aside. As many counties availed themselves of the privilege, it was estimated that not less than 35 percent of Virginians entering the service lacked vaccination, while 80 percent had no protection against typhoid.[7]

With the prospect of vaccinating many thousands of soldiers and citizens who had slipped through the loopholes of law, some by choice, home-front editorials took a hard stance on personal responsibility, looking beyond government for the answer:

> Modern hygiene and preventive medicine have recognized long ago that the individual can no longer claim liberty in his actions, independent of his neighbor. Our provisions for quarantine, vaccination against small-pox, and diverse other regulations in the interest of public health have, in the past, been enforced only with the annoyance that comes from lack of cooperation and from personal resentment together with the indifference for restrictive rules that is bred in a community of "free" people. Yet now you see, in the combined enterprise and altruism of modern employers, protective devices put into operation to secure, without friction or resentment, the same sort of welfare results that the federal government or state or municipality would find difficulty in getting under way.

The editorial added that under the unexpected conditions created by war, no device or agency that contributed to the health of soldiers was to be omitted; it urged the cooperation of everyone in this endeavor.[8]

Cooperation was still a dream of the future and loopholes persisted, occasionally arising from carelessness rather than intent. When 29 cases of smallpox appeared on the warship *Ohio,* resulting in 5 deaths, anti-vaccinationists were out in force, demanding to know how, with vaccination the policy of the navy, an outbreak could have occurred. Subsequent investigation revealed that no vaccinations had been performed on the crew of the *Ohio* for a period of 2 years preceding the epidemic. Of the 100 recruits joining the vessel before departure, all had been vaccinated and none suffered smallpox.[9]

Problems of a different sort occurred in October 1917, when it was reported that 2 out of 5 deaths reported in Memphis stemmed from lockjaw contracted through vaccination. The Washington Bureau of Public Health and the Secret Service began an investigation, considering the situation so serious that physicians in Memphis and Shelby counties were ordered to cease all vaccinations and druggists were told not to sell vaccine until the investigations were completed. War paranoia suggested "enemies of the country might be responsible."

Authorities in Washington responded on November 1, stating that of the ten deaths from tetanus following smallpox vaccination dating from July, several of the fatalities were traced to one of the country's largest vaccine manufacturers, largely patronized by army and navy purchasing agents. The deaths occurred in Ludington, Michigan, Cincinnati, Washington, DC, and Jacksonville, Florida, half coming from Jacksonville. None of the acknowledged deaths came from Tennessee and none occurred at military camps. Although an analysis of the manufacturer's product failed to disclose tetanus, the entire output on the market was recalled. Surgeon general Rupert Blue, chief of the public health service, pleaded with people not to panic, assuring them that all manufacturers were carefully monitored before putting their product on the market. It was further stated that the manufacturer whose vaccine may have caused lockjaw was "not a German" and was "not under suspicion." He was a veteran chemist, close to the government, who had always borne an excellent scientific reputation.[10]

Three years later, the United States public health service issued a warning to physicians not to use denatured ethyl alcohol containing phenol (carbolic acid) when prepping the skin before vaccination. It was believed such cleansing would materially decrease the likelihood of successful "takes," as phenol caused a rapid corrosive action on tissues. Soap and water or ether was preferred.[11] Vaccinators continued to favor alcohol in skin preparation despite the fact further research indicated that if it did not completely evaporate, the vaccine might become partially inactive. Ultimately, scientists determined no skin prep was necessary.

A different use for phenol was discovered while scientists worked on the problem of slowly decreasing bacteria in glycerolated pulp. Several months were required before counts were low enough for use but Gins (1924) and Lehmann (1937) developed the technique of adding phenol to a final concentration of 0.5 percent that greatly accelerated the process. D. McClean popularized the use of phenol in 1949. Liquid vaccine was dispensed in glass and later capillary tubes in single dose lots or in amounts sufficient for 20 vaccinations.[12]

On the subject of post-vaccination care, surgeon general H.S. Cumming warned in 1928 against the use of any shield or dressing on the wound site. Studies over several years showed that bandages caused severe "takes," and that dressings promoted the development of complications such as lockjaw, as tetanus germs found in soil, dirt and dust could easily contaminate bandages. Cumming advised that with proper vaccination the natural covering of the skin would suffice. Should an open sore develop, he suggested an antiseptic dressing, such as several layers of gauze pinned to the inside of a loose-fitting sleeve. If attached to the arm, the dressing should be large, with adhesive strips applied loosely and as far away from the site as possible.[13]

World War I and Its Aftermath

Although smallpox did not have the major impact on countries involved in the First World War as it had in previous armed conflicts (typhus and influenza being the major disease concerns), outbreaks caused considerable problems.

By 1900, variola major ceased to be endemic in Germany due to high levels of vaccination, but such was not the case in Russia during the period of 1900–1919, when low vaccination rates precipitated the prevalence of smallpox, making Russian travelers a threat to neighboring countries. More significantly, the importation of large numbers of agricultural workers and skilled craftsmen from that country into Germany reintroduced the disease, causing numerous outbreaks. After the creation of the USSR in 1917, V.I. Lenin ordered mandatory vaccination, but epidemics continued.[14]

On the active war front, smallpox presented a major obstacle to German forces occupying Poland. Encountering epidemic cases of smallpox, typhoid and rabies, medical officers not only had to contend with a lack of medical supplies, but also a distrust of the natives, who offered a distinct opposition to vaccination "that was overcome only with difficulty." Tracing the path of smallpox in a northeasterly direction, between 400,000 and 500,000 persons along the route were vaccinated. This curbed the epidemic but was unable to end it, as a lack of personnel and vaccine prevented covering the entire population.[15]

News out of Berlin indicated that the great number of prisoners taken early in the war presented a growing problem for the country, as many suffered from contagious diseases, including smallpox. Those prisoners put to work on the roads underwent compulsory vaccination and, when absolutely necessary, typhoid immunization. In all instances, however, care had to be taken, as great concern was expressed in the press and public meetinghouses concerning favored treatment of prisoners.[16]

In light of the above, it is odd to note that the German Reichstag made a motion to appoint a commission to study widespread opposition to vaccination with an eye toward amending the present law allowing for compulsory vaccination during outbreaks. The motion failed only by a tie vote, but the power of the anti-vaccinationists continued to grow. They claimed that 32 deaths were caused by the procedure in Prussia in 1912 and asserted that obtaining pure calf lymph was almost impossible. They further cited Great Britain, with its liberal conscience clause, as a model for Germany.[17] As war dragged on, conscience played less of a role, as cold, hard reality set in. Outbreaks of smallpox in the civilian quarter grew worse. One such outbreak, attributed to underfeeding and unsanitary conditions, occurred at the Krupp gun factory at Essen, where "black smallpox" raged among the workmen, resulting in 4 to 5 daily fatalities.[18] Shifting populations also led to outbreaks as those carrying the disease passed through populous railroad centers.

Smallpox increased in postwar Russia and Poland, spreading to Germany, Austria, and Sweden. By the end of the 19th century, variola major had been eliminated as an endemic disease in Sweden due to vaccination control, but outbreaks became more numerous in the postwar era due to importation of infected individuals. This was especially true in 1917, when soldiers returning to Russia from Germany caused large outbreaks in their wake. After 1920, Sweden suffered only isolated cases. Denmark and Norway also remained free of endemic smallpox throughout the 20th century, witnessing only isolated cases. Despite the persuasive anti-vaccination movement in Great Britain, the country escaped without major epidemics due to the relatively few travelers coming from Russia. The last outbreak of variola major in the United Kingdom came in 1902–1903.[19]

During the war, smallpox remained endemic in Italy, Romania and Yugoslavia (in the region that later became Czechoslovakia). Postwar conditions were worse. Between 1919 and 1920, severe epidemics killed 28,000 in Italy. Smallpox control in Portugal was almost nonexistent, causing 14,000 variola major fatalities at levels rivaling Africa and Asia. Spain was little better off. Germany reported 1,500 deaths, while in the USSR 186,000 cases of smallpox were reported. In grim comparison, Switzerland survived without a single epidemic due to its closed borders.

Smallpox was prevalent in Vienna in 1915, where 1,566 cases were reported, of which only 34 had been vaccinated. Of the 350 fatalities, only 2 had previously undergone the procedure. In contrast to the Polish population, which was largely unvaccinated, the Jewish people, who had their children vaccinated in infancy, were little affected by the disease.[20]

In France, smallpox continued to be a health concern, as compulsory laws were not enforced. The principal centers of infection were Paris and Marseilles, particularly the latter, as it served as the main port of entry for passengers and goods from endemic countries of North America and western Asia. The one bright spot was the French army, where vaccination was mandatory; from 1914 to 1917, no cases were reported among soldiers.[21]

Because vaccination was not well established in Africa during the war years due to poor vaccine and inadequate funding, over 100 separate epidemics were started in 1916 when survivors of the Carrier Corps (Kenyans who served as porters during the British invasion of German East Africa) returned from Nairobi to the home districts. Immediately after World War I, outbreaks of variola major occurred in South Africa; during 1920–1921, over 1,000 cases were seen but with low mortality.[22]

During 1916 in Greece, a major epidemic affecting both adults and children struck Athens with particular virulence, rapidly spreading into Piraeus, the port of Athens. Complicating matters, bubonic plague in Egypt and cholera among refugees from Asia Minor prompted quarantine.

Authorities in Athens ordered compulsory vaccination, but, lacking sufficient vaccine and hampered by the movement of demoralized troops into the interior, people reverted to the old ways, placing reliance on sacred icons or images of Christ. The icon of St. Barbara of Nicomedia, in Asia Minor, was brought out with "every pomp and ceremony from the ancient church of the convent of Daphine near Athens," and set out in the quarter where smallpox took the heaviest toll. Each morning, during the transport of the holy icon, bells rang in every church as black-robed priests carried it along the "sacred way." Belief was strongest among the "simpler Greeks," especially the artillerymen and firemen, who held her as their patron saint. In Greece and other countries, her day was celebrated on December 4, in honor of her martyrdom in 235.[23]

With the restoration of public health measures in the period between the First and Second World Wars, variola major fell into decline. In the early 1920s, however, the importation of alastrim from the United States caused it to become established as an endemic disease, producing over 10,000 cases each year between 1926 and 1930. By 1922 this typically nonfatal strain of smallpox became the primary form of smallpox in Finland, Germany, Switzerland, Egypt, Cuba, Jamaica, South Africa and sections of the United States, Great Britain and Canada. Alastrim occurred concurrently with variola major in Spain and Portugal in 1936. The only other sustained outbreak of alastrim in Europe occurred in Switzerland, where over 5,000 cases were reported in 1921 and 1926.

Failure to enforce vaccination laws as rigidly after as before World War I caused the minister of public welfare to reprimanded officials of the Prussian board of health. In an edict of 1927, the minister criticized "the extraordinary number of cases of evasion of the law ... and the disproportionate number of cases of vaccination on record compared to the total number of inhabitants." He enjoined all officials to enforce compulsory vaccination to the letter of the law.[24]

Despite mandatory laws enacted in 1917, smallpox continued to plague Russia, and in 1924 the law was altered to require vaccination in infancy and revaccination during teenage years. Epidemics in 1931, 1932 and 1933 led to intensified vaccination campaigns that finally succeeded in eliminating smallpox as an endemic disease in 1936.[25]

In a different aftermath of war, the Kingdom of Saudi Arabia was established from the country that since 1927 had been known as "The Kingdoms of Hejaz and Nejd." Arguing that there was nothing in the religion or laws of Islam justifying an attitude against science, King Ibn Saud established a number of hospitals and encouraged vaccination against smallpox.[26]

Smallpox remained endemic in large sections of China, especially Shanghai, where tourists were warned to undergo vaccination before sightseeing and shopping. For permanent residents, revaccination was recommended every three years. Widespread outbreaks in 1929 prompted the government to declare March 1 National Vaccination Day. Unfortunately, by 1932, a very virulent form of smallpox spread through Shanghai, proving fatal in half the cases. Dr. Wu Lien-Teh, director of the Chinese maritime quarantine service, reported the heaviest tolls were in the vicinity of overcrowded camps of warfare's refugees. At Hong Kong, Saigon and other refugee centers, 142 cases were reported in the second week of March. Foreigners were particularly susceptible and E. Koechlin, French consul-general, contracted the disease and died from it.

Steamers entering or leaving Shanghai were required to take precautions against smallpox, while Hong Kong ordered that all persons arriving there from Shanghai be vaccinated before entering the port.[27]

The Effects of Alastrim

The American strain of alastrim affected North America as far south as the Mexican border, South America, Europe, Australia and New Zealand. The African strain differed in several biological properties, being endemic in southern Africa until 1973. A similar disease was reported in eastern and central Africa, usually coexisting with variola major.

The dichotomy of the two strains was most apparent by how they were received by the public: variola major was regarded as a serious threat, while variola minor tended to be overlooked because of its mild symptoms. In contrasting the two, three factors were of epidemiological importance:

1. The infectiousness of the individual;
2. The number of contacts the infected individual had with other susceptible persons;
3. The degree of protection afforded those whose vaccination was of long standing.

As described in *Smallpox and Its Eradication*, published by the World Health Organization (chapter 8, pages 316–317), "The Incidence and Control of Smallpox Between 1900 and 1958," there were four patterns of endemicity:

1. In well-vaccinated communities, variola minor could not be established and the variola major that did occur originated from disease imported into the country.
2. In countries with highly organized health services (the U.S. and the UK) but lacking properly enforced compulsory vaccination, outbreaks of variola major tended to be selective and were brought under control by isolation and vaccination. Variola minor elicited no serious concerns.
3. In highly populated countries (India and Mexico), variola major dominated because of its greater capacity to infect and spread.
4. In countries where there was virtually no vaccination (Ethiopia), endemic variola minor replaced variola major, probably because the former could persist in small nomadic groups, whereas the latter would have been spontaneously interrupted.

By the late 1930s, as vaccination improved, endemic smallpox had been eliminated from most European countries except Turkey, Portugal and Spain, which suffered a major epidemic after the Spanish Civil War, killing 1,500 individuals between 1939 and 1940.[28]

United States civilians were spared occupation in World War I, but the country's soldiers were exposed to smallpox overseas. Statistics from the United States Army during the war years of 1917–1918 showed that during this two-year period, the number of men under arms reached its maximum of 3,551,447 in October 1918, the mean annual for the year being 2,518,499. Over this 24-month period, a total of 728 cases of smallpox were reported, or a ratio per 1,000 of 24 percent. Compared to the single state of Wisconsin, which had nearly one million fewer persons than were present in the army in 1918, there were 3,760 reported cases of smallpox.[29] Wisconsin continued to be a trouble spot six years later when smallpox was discovered at Camp Douglas, where state national guardsmen were assembled. One thousand vaccine points were ordered and rushed to the camp, where vaccination was considered imperative.[30]

A Tougher Stance on Vaccination

The winter of 1917–1918 was predicted to be a bad smallpox year. Although 1,000,000 men enrolled in the United States armed forces had been vaccinated, vaccination among civilians was shockingly low. Using the same tried and true words in the same old ways, medical men warned that neglect, carelessness, indifference and ignorance would lead to epidemics across the country. And so it did, not only confirming the dire forecast but also extending its reach.

American newspapers were filled with reports of smallpox outbreaks from east to west, but this time, there was an edge to the reaction. People had seen for themselves the positive results of compulsory military vaccination: soldiers still died of bullets and they died from TB and dysentery, but for the most part they did not die from smallpox. In 1918, the Texas Supreme Court overturned the court of civil appeals, finding that compulsory vaccination of schoolchildren was valid. Justice Greenwood's opinion held that it was not the purpose of the law to impose compulsory vaccination on minors (in this case, Christian Scientists), but to deny them "the privileges of the school" until they complied with the ordinance passed for their own and others' protection.

In Ohio, after suffering two disastrous years (the winter and spring of 1917, where more than 10,000 cases were reported, and the same period of 1918, where 434 cases were reported in November alone), the Department of Health lamented that the expense of the more recent epidemic of 8 months reached $600,000, "all of which could have been saved by general vaccination." In Ohio, the board of education declared, "The fact that it is the policy of the state to encourage education, and to enforce attendance at school does not render invalid a rule which required vaccination for

HEALTH ORDINANCES DECLARED VALID

[BY ASSOCIATED PRESS.]

Washington.—Municipal ordinances authorizing boards of health to enforce vaccination against small pox and take other precautions to prevent epidemics are valid, the supreme court held.

The *Janesville Gazette* (WI, November 13, 1922) ran this headline declaring that the United States Supreme Court had just ruled local boards of health had the authority to enforce vaccination. Despite the ruling, the controversial subject remained open to question.

small-pox as a condition of admission to the public schools" (*State ex, rel. v Board of Education* 7 0. C.C. (N.S.) 608). Judge Gillan of Chambersburg, Pennsylvania, echoed a similar sentiment:

> The law is well settled beyond pre-adventure of doubt that the school authorities of every school district are required to exclude from schools all children who do not produce a certificate signed by a physician, setting forth that said child has been successfully vaccinated or that it has formerly had small-pox.

The Texas State Board of Health, observing that smallpox had been practically eradicated from the U.S. Army by strict sanitary precautions and vaccination, offered free vaccinations to its citizens. Dr. Armstrong, health commissioner of La Crosse, Wisconsin, called the lack of unvaccinated children "appalling," noting the people held no theories; they were not anti-vaccinationists, but "just lazy and careless." But should an epidemic manifest itself, "personalities will not be regarded," and he would immediately institute compulsory vaccination.[31]

The *Washington Post* (October 16, 1919) went further in praising compulsory vaccination that all but eliminated smallpox from the armed forces: "It would seem obvious that if these results can be obtained by American medicine in war time through military organization, similar results for the civilian population could at least be approximated by a strong peacetime Federal health organization."

Compulsory Vaccination Argued Before the United States Supreme Court and Subsequent Legal Cases

In his review of "State Laws on Compulsory Immunization in the United States"[32] Charles L. Jackson presented the legal base for vaccination:

> The power inherent in the State to enact and enforce laws and to protect and promote the health, safety, morals, order, peace, comfort, and general welfare of the people is known as police power. It means that the State has the power to advance the public welfare by restraining the use of liberty and property. Health laws, which usually specify what a person may or may not do, fall into this category. In general, they prohibit acts that might endanger the health of others in the community. Compulsory immunization is a health law with a different twist. It differs because it requires a person to submit himself to a specific personal procedure that he may not desire.

Following numerous challenges to compulsory vaccination, "it became an established principle of law that State legislatures may, under certain conditions, require vaccination." Principle, however, was not law, and in 1905, the case of *Jacobson v. Massachusetts*, 197 U.S. 11, clarified the question. The complaint stemmed from a decree on February 27, 1902, when the board of health of Cambridge, MA, "being of the opinion that it was necessary for the public health and safety, required the vaccination and revaccination of all the inhabitants thereof." On July 17, 1902, the defendant "refused and neglected to comply with such requirement." He was tried, found guilty and fined $5. The case, involving the validity, under the Constitution of the United States, of certain provisions in the statutes of Massachusetts relating to vaccination, was argued before the United States Supreme Court December 6, 1904.

The defendant argued that section 137, chapter 75, of the Revised Laws of Massachusetts was in derogation of the rights secured by the Preamble of the Constitution of the United

States and under the 14th Amendment (specifically, that the State shall not deprive any person of life, liberty or property without due process of law) and the Massachusetts law was opposed to the spirit of the Constitution.

The decision, John Marshall Harlan II writing for the court, February 20, 1905, upheld the constitutionality of the statute and affirmed the defendant's conviction and fine for refusing to be vaccinated. Two justices, David Brewer and Rufus Peckham, dissented.[33] The decision read, in part: "The liberty secured by the constitution of the United States does not impart an absolute right in each person to be, at all times and in all circumstances, wholly freed from restraint. Real liberty for all could not exist which recognizes the right to use his person or his property, regardless of the injury that may be done to others."[34]

In 1921 and 1922, a more deadly strain of smallpox ravaged the Midwest. As jurists tended to rule more favorably toward compulsory vaccination during epidemics, proponents were fortunate that a second challenge was brought before the Supreme Court. In 1922, under the heading, "A Foolish Case," the *Laredo Weekly Times,* October 22, advised, "A case from San Antonio which is now before the United States supreme court will settle a question which has been agitated by many insurgents all over the country." The article predicted, "The case will be decided in favor of the municipality, for there is nothing in our constitution which forbids a city from enacting its own police laws."

The case concerned the ordinance of San Antonio, Texas, requiring all pupils attending public school to be vaccinated. Parents of the plaintiff Rosalyn (Rosalind) Zucht contended that the city council had acted beyond its authority in delegating such power to the board of health and that such action was an infringement of personal rights and liberties. The argument set forth that while society has the right to take such measures against individuals as are necessary for the protection of the whole, vaccination did not come under that classification, "since it is held to be impossible to prove that vaccination results in benefits to the community."[35]

The case of *Zucht v. King,* 260 U.S. 174 (1922) was argued October 20, 1922, and quickly decided November 13, 1922. The Supreme Court did not accept the arguments as convincing or applicable to the point at issue and associate justice Louis D. Brandeis, who wrote the opinion, declared the 14th Amendment gave state and municipal authorities all necessary rights to make and enforce health laws. "The decision simply reaffirms the right of the public to protection from communicable diseases by whatever means science has demonstrated to be effective," and in view of a prior decision (*Jacobson v Massachusetts,* 1905), "a contrary contention presents no substantial constitutional question."[36]

A pithy summary appeared in newspapers around the country:

Health Ordinances Declared Valid
[By Associated Press]

Washington.— Municipal ordinances, authorizing boards of health to enforce vaccination against small pox and take other precautions to prevent epidemics are valid, the supreme court held.[37]

Interestingly, the *Star Journal* (Sandusky, OH), November 16, 1922, observed, "Oddly enough, some people who have been very active in the fight for prohibition of the liquor traffic, and who would not concede that prohibition infringes on personal liberty, were most anxious to see compulsory vaccination made illegal, and doubtless many who argue for personal liberty in drinking would, at the same time, maintain that a general health measure, such as vaccination, is a matter for the state rather than the individual to control."

As clear as these two cases appeared to be, there were always those who found a way around the law. In 1924, when smallpox threatened Columbus, Ohio, the board of health ordered compulsory vaccination for all citizens. The matter was referred to city attorney Charles A. Leach, who declared that the United States Supreme Court vested the state with the authority to enforce compulsory vaccination but did not find for either the local boards of education or health with such authority. He further stated that while boards of education did not have the authority to enforce vaccination in schools, it was empowered to exclude from schools all unvaccinated students. In light of Leach's decision, the proposal for compulsory vaccination was abandoned.[38]

Other cases of law were equally complex. In 1924, when the Pennsylvania State Health Department notified the Lehigh Coal and Navigation Company that all its employees must be vaccinated due to a case of smallpox, authorities were put in a quandary, as the majority of the 6,000–8,000 miners were of foreign birth and had always fought against vaccination and other medical measures. In 1926, a case in Wisconsin concerned the question of whether an employer became liable for benefits under the Workman's Compensation Act for the death of an employee following compliance with the employer's order for compulsory vaccination. Commissioner L.A. Tarrell of the Wisconsin Industrial Commission heard the case of Josephine Mentzel of Shiocton against Menasha Printing & Carton Company. The widow claimed her husband, Albert, died January 13, 1926, after being vaccinated on January 2. The company countered by claiming Mentzel died of heart trouble.

Two years later, in 1928, another Wisconsin case dealt with a family seeking compensation from the city of Appleton, claiming vaccination was forced upon them. When a visitor to the family contracted smallpox, F.P. Dohearty, city physician, informed them they would have to submit to vaccination or quarantine. They opted for the latter, but several days later changed their minds and freely submitted to vaccination. They subsequently claimed to have been forced to submit. After a hearing by the city council, the case was brought to the board of health, where the nurse and Dr. Dohearty were questioned. The board went on record as approving the action of the doctor and denied claim if a lawsuit was started against the city.[39]

Old-Fashioned Smallpox

In 1921, a more virulent strain of smallpox struck Kansas City; during September, October and November; no fewer than 100 deaths were reported from the disease. Only one fatal case occurred to a person with a successful vaccination scar and that procedure had been administered 32 years previously. The *Kansas City Star,* November 15, reported that in schools where the majority of children were of foreign parentage, the response to the vaccination order was almost 100 percent, "as alien-born persons were accustomed to vaccination."[40]

Fear of the "old fashioned Smallpox" (also known as Asiatic or European smallpox) quickly spread to other midwestern and western states. With the death rate in Kansas City reaching 36 percent (103 dying out of 290 infected), preparations in Ohio were made to institute compulsory vaccination. Prior to this, Ohio had suffered only from mild visitations (known as the "American form"), resulting in a near total neglect of protection. They had reason to fear, as railroads and automobiles linked the two industrial centers and cross-contamination was considered highly likely. If such were to happen, smallpox would "spread like wildfire, and thousands of deaths would result before it could be controlled."[41] Acknowledging such on a national level, postmaster general Work offered free vaccination for the 333,000 members of the postal service.[42]

In Oklahoma, the State Department of Health warned, "The indifference of the populace to the danger [of virulent smallpox] remained unpenetrated until the visitation of the calamity which now grips Oklahoma.... That the situation abounds in pathos is apparent when we remember that no less than 38 lives have already been the price of the awakening." Unfortunately, appropriations for the control of smallpox epidemics had not kept pace with the growth in population, with funds having remained stationary since statehood in 1907.[43]

When addressing the issue of illnesses being derived from vaccination, Superintendent Richeson of Decatur, Illinois, made the observation that while the operation "does make an occasional person very sick ... this is the kind of person that would die of smallpox" if not protected.[44] During the eradication programs of the mid–20th century, the World Health Organization would recommend that no contraindications to vaccination should be considered sufficient. Their rationale was twofold: the risk of smallpox was greater than the risk of complications and, as vaccinations were carried out by nonmedical persons, those persons could not be expected to correctly diagnose complicated diseases and withhold vaccination.[45]

Chiropractors persisted in their anti-vaccination efforts. In 1921, an advertisement from Missouri promised, "Chiropractic Adjustments will remove the cause of the unhealthy conditions which make you a fit subject for Smallpox, and thereby prevent the disease.[46] A chiropractic ad from 1922 did that one better by promising, "If you are in good health, you won't get it anyway."[47] Unfortunately, a 1923 report from Southern California stated that after several chiropractors "undertook to control the disease by their system of therapeutics," they were responsible for 15 cases and "Chiropractor Griswold died of smallpox."[48] Iowa chiropractors warned, "We must defeat the efforts of a group who would make sick an entire community of well people in the fear that a small portion of it may get sick."[49]

In 1926, the board of managers of the State Charities Aid Association, New York, took a stand against the

As a group, chiropractors were a vocal opponent of vaccination, believing their "adjustments" were safer and more effective in preventing smallpox. From the *Chillicothe Constitution* [MO], November 30, 1921.

Esmond bill to license chiropractors to practice medicine on the grounds "the practitioners of chiropractic attack the modern health program by denying the germ origin of disease wholesale"; they denied "vaccination for smallpox, oppose the treatment of diphtheria by antitoxin, condemn surgery and reject the treatment of diabetes by insulin."[50] Compulsory vaccination also continued to be "a bone of contention" to Christian Scientists, who brought a case opposing the law to the Iowa State Supreme Court in 1921.[51]

"Black," or hemorrhagic smallpox, broke out in Michigan, killing a man who had proclaimed he would "rather have smallpox" than be vaccinated. His death on February 13, 1922, was quickly followed by 28 fresh cases, resulting in 8 deaths. By April 1, the disease was reported in half the counties of the state. Dr. R.M. Olin, commissioner of health, drolly commented, "Personal liberty grants anyone the right to contract smallpox—and die with it—if he does not believe in vaccination, but it does not give him the moral right to leave helpless children unprotected."[52]

In March 1921, the United States Public Health Service declared that the anti-vaccination campaign to be one cause of the widespread prevalence of smallpox. More than 3,000 cases were reported in the first week of February, with California, Minnesota, Wisconsin and Illinois having the highest numbers.

Smallpox Cases by State for the Week Ending February 5, 1921

Alabama	110	Montana	49
Arkansas	31	Nebraska	145
California	262	New Jersey	1
Florida	49	New York	8
Illinois	302	North Carolina	100
Indiana	186	South Dakota	50
Iowa	169	Texas	105
Kansas	117	Vermont	44
Louisiana	76	Virginia	3
Maine	5	Washington	104
Maryland	5	West Virginia	22
Massachusetts	2	Wisconsin	298
Minnesota	482	District of Columbia	1
Missouri	195	Kentucky	69[53]

New York authorities feared the importation of smallpox from Canada and Connecticut and reported 12 cases in the western portion of the state traced to Ohio. Twenty-nine cases were also reported at the St. Regis Reservation. Indian chiefs and clergymen aided health officers with "energetic measures" to prevent further spread.[54] In Connecticut, disagreement over the classification of the disease led to wildly conflicting reports and townspeople followed the governor's personal representative, Dr. Locke, from case to case, seeking verification of their suspicion that the disease was not smallpox. One physician called the outbreaks "wart pox" (an obscure term not widely recognized, meaning the mildest form of smallpox); another, the suspended health officer, declared it to be "light smallpox" and a third diagnosed the affliction as "walking smallpox," meaning those afflicted were not confined to bed. In any case, the Danbury hat factory laid off 50 workers because of their refusal to be vaccinated. While the city commissioner moaned that adverse publicity cost Bridgeport $1,000,000, anti-vaccinationists turned council meetings into a crusade against the merits of vaccination.[55]

In fairness to physicians, it was difficult to differentiate smallpox from other diseases.

The Bridgeport Department of Health published a short card, "How to Tell if You Have Symptoms of Smallpox." Briefly, it stated that the "prodromal," or first period, lasted from 2½–4 days, during which time the patient suffered from severe headaches, vomiting, constipation, and severe pains in the back of the head and in the lumbar region of the back. A high fever then developed, lasting from the second until the fifth day, with symptoms resembling the grip (influenza). The patient then appeared to recover for several days before the appearance of a little red rash. Thereafter, the rash became "babular," progressing another 4–5 days before becoming pustular, sometimes with a rise in temperature. It was stated a doctor should be called at the first appearance of these symptoms.[56]

Although well meaning, this information was probably less than helpful. Using unknown words (prodromal, babular) and odd variations (pustular) was confusing, and likely nothing definite could be used to diagnosis smallpox until distinctive lesions appeared. Calling a physician "at the first appearance of symptoms" was safe advice, but did little to counter anti-vaccinationists' claims that treating spurious smallpox was a medical scheme to make money.

A more effective way to educate people was through the developing field of mass media. The film *One Scar or Many* was produced by the Utah State Board of Health, in cooperation with the medical profession and theatres. Nearly 1,500 persons attended the premiere in Salt Lake City, learning about the preparation of vaccine and the necessity of vaccination. After a "considerable showing," it was to be included in theatre programs throughout the state.[57] The same year, New York State commissioner of health, Dr. Matthies Nicoll, Jr., spoke on a broadcast from the General Electric radio station WGY in Schenectady. He stated that a modification of the state's vaccination act in 1915, mainly restricting compulsory vaccination of schoolchildren to "first and second class cities," had caused neglect of vaccination in rural areas. This meant vaccination of the general public rested in the hands of the people themselves, "and in the last analysis upon them rests the responsibility of keeping smallpox out of the state."[58]

This echoed a 1921 report of the United States Public Health Service, indicating that "Smallpox by Public Vote" held sway: when people supported and voted for strong compulsory laws, smallpox was negligible, but when local authorities were given discretionary power, or when laws lacked the compulsory feature, rates tended to rise. Eastern states had demonstrated a low smallpox curve for the past six years, while seven southern and six central states showed high curves, although the central states' curve was twice that of the southern. The curve for the three Pacific Coast states revealed a "most extraordinary increase in the disease" from 1915 to 1920.[59]

It is also important to note that the public airwaves also served as a medium through which anti-vaccinationists got across their message. A case in 1930 charged radio station owner/operator Norman Baker of "making scurrilous attacks" upon physicians and prominent citizens in Muscatine, Iowa, as well as upon the American Medical Association and state officials, over station KENT, by attacking their pro-vaccination stance and "assailing the so-called 'medical trust.'" The case was eventually brought to the federal radio commission on Baker's request to renew his license. Baker protested his innocence, in part by claiming "the sole owner of a radio station could do as he pleased if the public liked it."[60]

36

International Public Health

> International public health, then, came into being at a time of great contrasts and
> upheavals in which unprecedented material prosperity went hand-in-hand with
> grossly insanitary conditions in the spreading but overpopulated towns.[1]

The spirit of cooperation between nations in the 19th century came to fruition in 1851,
when two significant events took place: the first International Sanitary Conference, Paris,
(detailed in chapter 14) and the International Exhibition, London, where over 6,000,000
visitors viewed the scientific wonders of the age. In addressing members of the former, the
French foreign minister remarked that at such gatherings "all the industries of the universe
seemed to have forgotten their former rivalries to join hands."

During the six-month period the conference was in session, delegates discussed maritime quarantine and the newest threat to public health: cholera, which had reached Western
Europe a mere 20 years before. Little permanent success was achieved, but with the importance of international cooperation recognized, a second conference was held in Paris in 1859,
and a third at Constantinople in 1866. The fourth conference, held after the opening of the
Suez Canal, ran the month of July 1874, and as in all previous instances, cholera was the
primary concern. Delegates approved an international treaty establishing maritime quarantine for ships traveling from east to west through the canal.

The first International Sanitary Conference in which the United States participated
was convened in Washington, DC, in 1881, where the United States proposed that every
ship entering its ports be required to have a certified bill of health. The motion failed. The
idea of a "permanent International Sanitary Agency of Notification" was also proposed, as
delegates recognized the need for an international and reliable system of epidemiological
reporting. Cholera, yellow fever and the plague represented the primary concerns and these
topics dominated future conferences in Rome (1885), Venice (1892), Dresden (1893), Paris
(1894) and Venice (1897).

Sanitary conferences in the 1800s had concentrated on two basic issues: the removal
of hindrances to trade and transport by quarantine and the creation of a barrier by which
the spread of cholera across Europe could be prevented. Many of the arguments put forth
were contentious and outmoded; with germ theory still in its infancy, few proposals of a
scientific nature were agreed upon.[2]

By the end of the 19th century, four international health councils were established in
Alexandria, Egypt; Constantinople, Turkey; Tangiers, Morocco and Tehran, Persia. The
International Sanitary Bureau, later renamed the Pan American Sanitary Bureau (PASB)
and eventually the Pan American Health Organization (PAHO) came into being at Washington in 1902. A year later, the 11th Sanitary Conference was held in Paris, where it was

agreed that a permanent health bureau should be created. In 1909, the decision was made to create an international public hygiene office that became the Office International d'Hygiene Publique (OIHP) in 1909. This organization disseminated information on communicable diseases and their control, meeting every two years except for a five-year period during World War I. OIHP performed the preparatory work for the International Sanitary Conference 1911–1912, and was involved in the convention of 1926, where, for the first time, provisions against smallpox and typhus were included.

The president of the Permanent Committee of the OIHP, Professor Rocco Santoliquido, stated that that the chief guarantee of international security from disease lay in the standard of public health of each national unit. He added that erecting barriers of disease (quarantine) were outmoded and "endemic foci of communicable disease should be circumscribed and obliterated." Toward that end, "the masses must accept the necessity for measures taken" through education. As described by the World Health Organization (WHO), "Thus were formulated for the first time in an intergovermental meeting, on 3 June 1919, the precepts which have since become a corner-stone of international health work."

After World War I, President Woodrow Wilson championed the League of Nations. One task he envisioned for it was to "endeavour to take steps in matters of international concern for the preservation and control of disease."[3] Despite Wilson's support, the United States refused to join. Consequently, the Health Organisation arm of the League of Nations was established in Geneva, Switzerland. The OIHP continued its independent work from Paris, while two regional health organizations (PASB and another in Alexandria) also continued their operations. National and international travel remained a problem in regard to the transmission of disease, and cooperation between states and nations was needed. In 1910, a 17-year-old immigrant boy suspected of having smallpox caused 2,700 passengers aboard the North German Lloyd steamship *Main* to undergo compulsory vaccination. The ship, out of Bremen, discharged the youth at the government quarantine island of Reedy and after the diagnosis was confirmed, 800 immigrants, who had already departed on the Baltimore & Ohio Railroad, had to be intercepted and returned, while the 45 cabin passengers were traced to their homes.[4] Cross-country contamination of smallpox in the United States became so acute in 1924 that the surgeon general requested the American Automobile Association (AAA) to alert its 500,000 members to get vaccinated. If motorists did not comply, he suggested federal intervention in interstate travel could result.[5]

The United States continued its support of the PASB and in 1926, Dr. Hugh S. Cumming, U.S. surgeon general, Public Health Service (as well as director of the PASB), wrote, "One of the most important events in recent years in the field of international health regulations was the signing at Havana, Cuba, on Nov. 14, 1924, of the Pan-American sanitary code, which provides for the collection and dissemination of information concerning the incidence of communicable diseases and prescribes and standardizes the measures necessary to prevent their transmission from one country to another." He added, "The importance of this international sanitary treaty as a health measure and as an aid to commerce in the avoidance of costly delays to ships in quarantine can hardly be over-estimated."[6]

A Sad Commentary on the United States

In the 1920s, the entire world was looking at the United States, not for guidance but in horror at the prevalence of smallpox. In 1921, there were 108,135 cases reported, with

764 deaths; in 1922, there were a total of 27,822 reports of smallpox; in 1923, the number was 26,731, hardly a substantial decrease. In 1924, the country headed the list of civilized nations in the number of cases reported. That year, there were 825 known deaths from 35 of the 48 states in the union from which reports were received, marking an increase in all cases of 75 percent over 1923, with a 628 percent increase in deaths. Between 1911 and 1926, there were over 700,000 reported cases of smallpox, as reported by Dr. Chapin, president of the American Health Association. In 1925, there were 39,636 cases (one-fifth of all smallpox in the world), "more than any country furnishing statistics, except British India. Even Soviet Russia, with a larger population, had only half as many cases." The 8,000 deaths in Mexico suggest it was proportionately higher in that country, but actual statistics were lacking. This led to the observation, "It is a sad commentary upon the United States that its smallpox prevalence must be compared only with countries whose standards of intellectual and scientific developments are regarded as distinctly inferior."[7]

In a comparison among states, it was reported New York required all schoolchildren in first- and second-class cities (ranked on population) to be vaccinated. In consequence, New York ranked lowest among 20 of the most populous states between 1915 and 1920 at 0.026 per thousand, compared to 2,000 for Kansas. In Michigan, 3,500 smallpox cases were reported between January and August 1924, with 146 deaths. In 1924, Wisconsin reported 1,300 cases with 121 deaths; Minnesota registered 500 deaths. The total number of smallpox deaths for 1925 was 702, with nearly 42,000 cases reported. Dr. Frederick Eberson, assistant professor of medicine, University of California, observed, "The people of California were given the privilege of enjoying 'all the smallpox they want' when the teeth of the compulsory vaccination law were pulled in [1911 and] 1923." Since the change in laws, California saw an increase of more than 800 percent in smallpox cases. Figures revealed an average of 511 cases during 1912–1916, and an increase in average to 2,682 a year from 1917 to 1921, and to 4,263 a year from 1922–1926.[8]

The year 1925 brought bad news to Washington, DC, as 19 out of 54 suffering from smallpox in the city died between January and April. In consequence, Dr. Hugh S. Cummin of the Public Health Service ordered 62,000 government employees to be vaccinated, starting with those from the Veterans' Bureau. Despite the fact mortality had reached 31 percent, immediately after his order, picketers appeared with signs declaring "many hundreds had been murdered by vaccination."

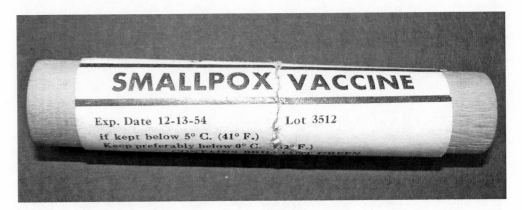

This is an actual smallpox vaccination container as issued to practitioners in the 20th century (from the authors' collection).

"VOTE YES"   *"VOTE YES"*

The Truth About Amendment No. 6

The California State Board of Health in an official bulletin makes the statement that 80 per cent of the parents of California school children are opposed to the practice of vaccination and will not consent thereto. It is because the present law does not amply protect those who object to vaccination and does not control the University that an amendment to the constitution is offered for adoption. In many instances there have been unwarranted exclusions of children, hundreds being deprived of school privileges for which their parents pay taxes, and Amendment No. 6 is designed to assure the fulfillment of the intent of our State Legislature when it enacted the present law of preferential exemption.

Amendment No. 6 does not prohibit vaccination or inoculation; it simply prohibits COMPULSORY vaccination and inoculation

MEDICAL AUTHORITIES DISAGREE on the PROTECTIVE VALUE of VACCINATION

Stating that medical authorities disagreed on the protective value of vaccination, the Public School Protective League ran the editorial "The Truth About Amendment No. 6." The purpose of the amendment was not to prohibit vaccination, but to prohibit the compulsory vaccination of schoolchildren. The debate over compulsory vaccination and "conscience clauses" was prevalent in California for decades and led to increased cases of smallpox (from the *Oakland Tribune,* October 31, 1920).

Protestors had reason for concern. In Madrid, where several cases brought out 300,000 persons willing to undergo the operation, manufacturing establishments were unable to keep up with demand; that supplied was infected with pus germs, causing swellings and "even lymphangitis" (inflammation of lymph vessels). Fortunately for a foreign ambassador who contracted the disease, he was spared the pesthouse, being rushed to the newly built but as yet unopened King's Hospital for Infectious Diseases by the director general of public health, Dr. Murillo, where he recovered in splendid surroundings.

In Paris, matters took on a different perspective as a smallpox epidemic threatened to wreak havoc on spring fashions: if ladies were vaccinated on the arm, they could not wear their sleeveless evening gowns and if vaccinated on the leg, their participation in the Charleston was "enough to make all South Carolina burst into sobs." The problem was, in some respects solved, by wearing decorative scarlet ribbons as proof of vaccination, while gauze dressings were embroidered in colors to match frocks.

With the disease spreading along sections of the northern and eastern industrial belt of the United States, it was humorously noted "it takes six years to get an idea through Congress, but it is a sad truth that it sometimes takes generations to get an idea through public consciousness." At a time when it would have been beneficial for Calvin Coolidge to step up and set a positive example, White House physician J.F. Coupal refused to say whether the president had undergone the procedure. On a more positive note, Dr. Mervyn Gordon announced from London that Drs. W.E. Gye and J.E. Bernard had succeeded in photographing smallpox germs, which, it was hoped, would permit a close study of the disease.[9]

In 1926, a reported 33,752 smallpox cases, with 380 deaths, occurred in the United

States, leading to two droll comments: "We have more smallpox because we have more cheerful idiots opposing vaccination which prevents smallpox," and, "It is enlightening to read that smallpox is more frequent where opposition to vaccination is strongest, Southern California and Northern England." In an effort to "redeem our country from this unenviable record," health agencies across the country designated November and December 1926 as a "period of public enlightment regarding the nature of smallpox and its prevention." Little was achieved, as surgeon general Cumming reported to Congress in 1929 that the United States "had the unenviable distinction of reporting more cases of smallpox during the year than any other country in the world from which reports were received except India." The total number for 1928 was estimated between 33,000 and 34,000, "testimony to the neglect of the people to utilize vaccination, the known means of preventing the disease."[10]

While large yellow and black posters appeared in St. Paul, Minnesota, proclaiming "black smallpox" (Minnesota had no compulsory vaccination laws), North Carolina's approach was to eliminate quarantine and rely entirely on vaccination of those who came in contact with the disease. Dr. Sears, the state health officer observed, "If you want to catch smallpox you are welcome to; the State affords vaccination against the disease and it is the assumption that those who do not care for vaccination wouldn't particularly mind the disease."

In Jackson, Mississippi, reports for the first seven months of 1926 revealed 134 cases among whites and 371 among blacks, compared to 425 and 544 in 1925. The 1925 statistics were better in North Carolina, where all the "colored schools, practically all the white schools and most of the large Indian schools" were vaccinated. Unfortunately, protection for Native Americans lagged. In Decatur, Nebraska, in 1926 a mild epidemic on the reservation turned severe, spreading the disease into the surrounding area. In 1927, a severe epidemic broke out at the Seminole oil field in Oklahoma. In this case, medical personnel were funded by the Indian Territory Illuminating Oil Company and the Empire Company, large operators in the Seminole field. A bill appropriating $5,000 to combat the epidemic was also introduced in the state senate. Smallpox also appeared on the Allegany Indian Reservation, New York, in 1927. A massive vaccination program reached 372 residents, or 67 percent of the population, "making it one of the best vaccinated areas in the state."[11]

The dangers of a smallpox epidemic were also apparent during massive flooding within seven states along the Mississippi Valley. More than 100,000 of the 173,566 refugees in 60 concentration camps were immunized with typhoid and smallpox vaccine, while the Red Cross hastened to vaccinate all persons in the flood zone, since the recession of the waters was expected to accentuate danger from disease. Vaccination was also extended to those who elected to remain in their homes within flooded towns.[12]

Day-to-Day Life with Smallpox

In a lecture to the Kiwanis on April 22, 1930, Dr. Andy Hall, director of the Illinois department of health, observed, "Illinois has more people in high schools and centers of learning than any other state, save one; Chicago is the medical center of the nation if not of the world and yet, for all this development we have more to fear from smallpox than any nation in the world."[13] Statistics bore him out.

Surgeon general H.S. Cumming reported to Congress in January 1930, that 38,000 cases of smallpox were reported in the United States during the past fiscal year; in 1929, there were 38,062 cases reported (numbers including only 44 states and the District of Columbia), showing a marked increase over 1927, when 35,000 were reported.[14]

According to the Iowa State Department, smallpox grew steadily in the state:

Smallpox in Iowa, 1925–1930

Year	No. of Cases	Deaths
1925	645	442
1926	1131	2
1927	1279	2
1928	1894	4
1929	1913	5
1930	3044	3

This represented an increase of 430 percent over the figures between 1929 and 1925. The cases from 1930 caused 880 persons to lose a combined 43 years in quarantine.[15] While the fatalities reflect low numbers after 1925, indicating that variola minor was the prevalent strain of smallpox, they caused Dr. C.E. Dakin of the State Department of Health to observe, "It appears that like the poor, we shall have smallpox always with us."[16]

The only good news came in 1933, when the Metropolitan Life Insurance Company reported that prevalence in the United States and Canada was decreasing. According to their figures, which included 44 states, the District of Columbia and 8 Canadian provinces, there were a combined total of 46,654 cases in 1930; 29,493 in 1931; and 13,121 in 1932, representing a 37 percent decrease. Significantly, among all those included, South Dakota alone reported almost 1,800 cases and Vermont, the fourth smallest state in respect to population, had reported over 900 cases during the previous four years, or 70 cases for every 100,000 inhabitants. The report noted Vermont had no compulsory vaccination law. While the disease was of the mild type, with an average case-fatality of 3 per 1,000 cases, the exception was Vancouver, BC. During the early months of 1932, there were 56 cases of smallpox, 29 of which were definitely identified as the confluent, virulent type. Before the outbreak was brought under control, 29 persons died.[17]

Vermont was not the only state without vaccination laws: due to the ever-present force of anti-vaccinationists, by the 1930s, four states had laws prohibiting compulsory vaccination, 28 had no vaccination laws, six provided for a local option and only 10 had compulsory laws.[18] Complicating the picture, by 1931 the American Medical Association warned that nearly 14 percent of all vaccinations would lose their protective power after only one year and 33 percent after two years. After 5 years, half of those vaccinated would again be susceptible and after ten years, the rate rose to nine-tenths. Additionally, the association advised that "Negroes" lost the protective effects more rapidly than white people.[19] To aid in anti-smallpox programs, the Christmas Seals Organization sponsored a vaccination drive in 1935.[20]

Variola major was eliminated as an endemic disease in the United States in 1927; variola minor remained endemic until the latter part of the 1940s.[21] This brings up an important distinction between endemic, epidemic and outbreaks of smallpox, with statistics telling one story and the daily lives of individuals quite another. While endemic (ever-present) and epidemic (an accountable beginning and end) smallpox were eliminated, "outbreaks" (small and localized cases) continued to strike terror among those exposed to the disease.

Residents of Fitchburg, Massachusetts, in 1932, likely had no awareness of the distinction between the words endemic, epidemic and outbreak. All they knew was that 15 cases of smallpox had been reported (all but one were adults) and that supplies of vaccine were so low motorcycle police were dispatched to Boston for more. Men, women, children and babies in arms stood in long lines waiting their turn to be vaccinated. Their fear was real and as the number of cases climbed to 60, their world revolved around survival.[22] After mass compulsory vaccination finally eliminated the threat, daily life returned to normal. In assessing this and other minor events in the post-endemic phase, it is always important to remember that when relying solely on numbers to establish the long, sustained and short-term appearance of disease, they cannot, by themselves, tell the story. Only by witnessing (in the case of smallpox, through retrospective study), the panic and effect on individuals, can the real tragedy be comprehended and the numbers put in perspective.

The Foci of Smallpox

Although without cooperation or assistance from the United States, the Health Organisation of the League of Nations received financial support from the Rockefeller Foundation to augment funding by the league. In the years between the world wars, international unity was particularly important due to a pandemic of influenza in 1918–1919, that killed 15–18 million people, and an epidemic of typhus in 1919–1920 that swept through Eastern Europe. On August 22, 1928, the Smallpox Vaccination Commission of the league opened discussion on reports from England and the Netherlands that in some cases "sleeping sickness" (encephalitis; an inflammation of the brain most commonly caused by viruses and as an aftereffect of systemic viral diseases, such as influenza, measles and chicken pox)[23] occurred after vaccination. Concern was so great in the Netherlands that compulsory vaccination in schools was suspended for a year. By August 27, the commission voted that despite the development of occasional sleeping sickness, there was no reason to discontinue vaccination.[24]

This did not alleviate concern that smallpox or vaccination or both played a role in the development of sleeping sickness. During a high and rapidly escalating outbreak in St. Louis and the Midwest in 1933, medical science of the time attributed the infection to "one of those living disease organisms too small to be caught in filters, or seen under microscopes." Noting that it had been 221 years since the recognition of epidemic encephalitis and 15 years since an almost worldwide search began for its cause, precursors including smallpox and vaccination were still considered viable threats.[25]

Later research indicated that the incidence of post-vaccinial encephalitis likely stemmed from differing strains of seed vaccinia virus. Strains used in laboratories around the world for the production of vaccine were arbitrary and varied considerably in their biological properties. Production and maintenance also influenced the strength, efficiency and safety of the end product. However, it was not until 1967 that international recommendations specifying which strains should be used were established.[26]

International success of vaccination was proven when Austria, Belgium, Bulgaria, Danzig, Denmark, Switzerland, Ireland, Latvia, Lithuania, Malta, Scotland and "Jugo-Slavia" reported no cases of smallpox during 1931 and the first half of 1932. Emphasis shifted to smallpox control in three specific areas:

1. Soviet Russia, where smallpox was unusually severe and appeared to be on the increase, even though there had been a considerable reduction following World War I;

2. The endemic mild form of smallpox prevalent in England. During the first 32 weeks of 1933, there were 1,712 cases (more than half in London), compared with 4,784 cases during 1931;

3. Spain and Portugal, where Spain suffered from variola minor, and Portugal, the more severe type of variola major. The disease appeared to be on the increase in both countries.

British India was typically cited as an example of what happened when vaccination was not enforced: 88,380 cases were reported in 1931, with nearly 19,000 deaths. In North America, Mexico remained the country with the highest incidence, reporting 9,971 deaths in 1931.[27] The League of Nations data, garnered from 26 countries, revealed in 1936 that, covering the decade from 1920 to 1930, the United States showed the second-highest number of cases, with Canada facing similar conditions.[28] A 1936 survey of 9,000 families in 130 localities in 18 states of the Union revealed that only 58 percent of people of all ages had been vaccinated or had suffered from smallpox; the younger the person, the higher the percentage. Rural areas fared worse, with only a 40 percent vaccination rate compared to 80 percent of adults in cities. Revaccination was seldom practiced.[29]

Advancements in Technique and Preservation of Lymph

Selection of a vaccinifer (the animal to be inoculated for production of lymph) had traditionally been the cow, but during World War I, the Lister Institute of Preventive Medicine in Elstree, England, began employing sheep for the procedure. Around the same time, water buffaloes were used in India, Indochina and Indonesia. Strains of seed (the material used for inoculation of animals to produce vaccine pulp) varied significantly in titre (strength), biological properties and in methods of preservation. Without any international consensus as to standardizing vaccinia strains or to dictate procedures, techniques of individual laboratories varied from country to country.

In an effort toward standardizing vaccine, the Smallpox and Vaccination Commission of the Health Organisation, League of Nations, began collecting information in 1926 from vaccine producers regarding production, testing, standardization, storage and delivery of vaccine. France, Germany, the Netherlands, Switzerland and the United Kingdom participated. New standards having been completed in 1927, the UK incorporated them into the Therapeutic Substances Regulations the same year. The regulations included qualifications of staff, animals to be used and their housing, precautions to be observed during the production process, specifications for final containers to hold the vaccine, labeling and testing for the absence of anaerobic organisms and streptococci. Significantly, international standards were not established until after 1967.[30]

During the 19th century, testing of potency of lymph was done solely by observation of the success rate of human "takes." A. Calmette and C. Guérin developed a method of potency testing by rabbit inoculation in 1901, later improved by Guérin, who introduced the inoculation of serial dilutions of virus, enabling the vaccine lymph to be titrated with some accuracy.

In 1902, F.R. Blaxall dried calf lymph in porcelain dishes over sulfuric acid, allowing it to be prepared in bulk. A. Carini described a similar method in 1906, with the refinement of storage of dried material in vacuo.[31]

Liquid glycerolated vaccine continued to be the favored method of distribution but it proved entirely unsatisfactory for use in tropical countries. In 1909, two scientists, R. Wurtz and L. Camus, working at the Vaccine Institute in Paris, developed a new procedure of drying lymph in thin layers over sulfuric acid, adding 10 percent gum arabic to facilitate reconstitution that demonstrated a greater ability to retain potency. During World War I, their freeze-dried vaccine were sent to French colonies in Africa, and the Paris Vaccine Institute continued to annually supply 10,000,000 doses between 1920 and 1940. After the First World War, Wurtz and Camas worked on the technique of drying lymph with the aid of refrigerants; L. Otten followed, working along the same lines. His methods were credited with the elimination of smallpox from the Netherlands East Indies (Indonesia) in 1937.[32]

During the smallpox scare in England in 1929 the Pasteur Institute was taxed almost to its limit to produce vaccine. The use of refrigeration, allowing sera to be made and stored in vast quantities was a solution for just such an emergency.[33] Reconstitution of dried lymph proved difficult, however, and techniques varied between individuals, producing mixed results. The danger also existed that when grinding dried lymph into powder before reconstitution, airborne scatter could prove dangerous.[34]

During the 1920s, lanolin and Vaseline were added to liquid lymph because they were considered suitable inert vehicles, but by the 1930s, egg white was added as a buffering agent. Another use of eggs originated in 1929, when it was discovered that egg-cultured vaccinia survived with undiminished titre after six weeks' storage at 25C. Freeze-drying was first described by L.F. Shackell in 1909, and from 1935 onward the technique was used for the preservation of many liable biological agents, including viruses, bacteria and blood plasma. In 1937, M. Kaiser's studies on freeze-dried vaccinia were published, and dried vaccine prepared in this manner was used extensively by the German army during World War II.[35]

With guarded optimism that the day was approaching when mankind could be immunized against all contagious diseases, the Pasteur and Curie Institutions and the Academy of Medicine, Paris, concentrated their efforts on discovering vaccines. Citing the success of smallpox vaccine in France, where the disease had entirely disappeared as endemic, occurring only rarely in scattered cases, Professor Lereboulet of the French Academy observed, "Our vaccination work has been so successful and the public has accepted it so heartily that today it is safe to say France has no fears of smallpox."[36]

The four chief points in vaccination during the 1930s were the use of potent vaccine, clean technique, restriction to a very small area and rapid drying of the vesicle. The "multiple pressure method" was considered by many to be the best method of encompassing these requirements. As described by the state board of health, Indiana, the technique consisted of shallow pricking of the skin with a sterile needle, then adding a drop of vaccine covering an area not greater than ⅛" in diameter. The needle was not thrust into the skin but was held parallel to the arm, with the side of the needle point pressed firmly and rapidly into the skin approximately 30 times without ever being lifted. By this method, vaccine was carried into the deeper layers of the skin without injury or bleeding. All evidence of vaccination faded away within several hours. After the pressures were made, excess vaccine was wiped off with a sterile gauze to complete the vaccination. The idea of omitting any dressing was also suggested. Authorities recommended that vaccine be kept on ice or in a refrigerator to maintain potency. The optimal time for primary vaccination was as soon after birth as practicable, with revaccination every five to ten years.[37]

The British Medical Research Council announced the discovery of a new smallpox serum on July 10, 1931. Based on the work of Professor William Tulloch and Dr. James Craigie, the serum was described as a "flocculation reaction" obtainable in cases of smallpox, which enabled a definite diagnosis when symptoms were otherwise doubtful. Results also indicated that the serum might give immediate protection to persons in contact with small-pox, acting more quickly than the current vaccination method.[38]

G. H. Eagles and D. McClean studied the use of virus propagated in embryonated eggs in 1929, in the hope it could be preserved for extended periods.[39] By 1933, United States surgeon general Hugh S. Cumming reported that this British method would not only be cheaper and simpler, but would also silence the anti-vaccination groups who objected to using the "pus" of a cow.[40] The same year, Dr. Thomas M. Rivers and S.M. Ward experimented with the freeze-dried method for preserving vaccinia, adding egg albumin or gum arabic before drying. This was successfully used to immunize humans by the intracutaneous route.[41] Two years later, the American Public Health Association reported on a new vaccine developed at the Rockefeller Institute, New York. As explained by Dr. Rivers, it was "made by giving smallpox to a laboratory test tube instead of a calf." The important difference was freedom from contamination, with the new serum so pure it could be "injected hypodermically underneath the skin," resulting in no soreness and no scar. Four thousand persons were tested with this vaccine and found to be immune.[42]

Although by 1935, most Americans believed smallpox had been eradicated from the country, outbreaks and prevention continued to appear in the newspapers. Before the June 1937 Boy Scout Jamboree in Washington, DC, Dr. James E. West, Grand Panjandrum of the association, proclaimed compulsory vaccination for all attendees. Anti-vaccinationists objected to the order. The same year, druggists promoting the procedure advertised the following: "Smallpox Vaccine is made by Parke, Davis & Co. under the most careful supervision possible. There is no risk and very little discomfort with modern vaccination."[43]

During the Great Depression, after thousands of American farmers lost their land, many moved west to pick fruit and cotton. Outbreaks of smallpox were blamed on these migrant workers, particularly in California's Imperial Valley, deepening unrest throughout the state. While indigents were offered free vaccinations, authorities in neighboring states warned locals to receive vaccination in case the disease spread.[44]

World War II and Its Aftermath

In the period between the World Wars, one editorialist noted, "We have not reached the day of diseaseless wars just yet, but the time has come when parents can see their sons march away without knowing that the terrors of typhoid and smallpox are more to be dreaded than the bullets from the guns of the enemy."[45] In fact, smallpox played a minor role during the Second World War in Europe, but that did not mean the consequences of variola major and minor were not felt throughout the world.

World War II brought an end to international public health works, limiting the Health Organisation to publishing the *Weekly Epidemiological Record* and supplying information on health matters. In the United States, tensions and suspicions ran high when dealing with foreign powers. In 1942, there were 1,510 Americans aboard the Swedish liner *Gripsholm* being brought home under an exchange agreement with Japan who were informed that physicians would not recognize vaccination certificates issued by Japanese physicians: all would be required to undergo new vaccinations or be subject to quarantine upon reaching American soil.[46]

International cooperation remained at a standstill until 1941–1942, when President Franklin D. Roosevelt and Prime Minister Winston Churchill put forth proposals resulting in the creation of the United Nations Relief and Rehabilitation Administration (UNRRA) in 1943. Its mission "was to provide support for countries once the war had ended. In November 1943, forty-four allied and associated nations signed an agreement establishing this "'United Nations' agency, which in effect became the first truly international relief agency in world history." UNRRA was disbanded in 1946, having contributed invaluable work for what would become the World Health Organization (WHO).[47]

In contrast to worldwide epidemics of smallpox after World War I, outbreaks after World War II were isolated. Variola minor was imported into Italy from North Africa in 1944, producing over 6,000 cases before it was eliminated, while variola major occurred in Turkey during the war (over 12,000 cases), moving from there into Greece. Colonial powers including France, Portugal, Belgium and the Netherlands suffered importations of smallpox from their overseas holdings, exacerbated by aerial travel that eliminated the time lapse of long sea voyages. Germany suffered almost no smallpox outbreaks during World War II but in its aftermath importations occurred in 18 of the 36 years between 1922 and 1958. Spain and Portugal contained both variola major and minor between 1944 and 1948, but numbers were low. Thereafter, only cases of variola minor were reported and smallpox was eliminated as an endemic disease by the early 1950s. From 1920 onward, most countries in Central America were free of endemic smallpox, although small outbreaks continued to erupt.[48]

Although England sustained a relatively quiet period between 1939 and 1945, at least 15 outbreaks occurred in 1946–1947, due, in part, to soldiers returning in 1946 from overseas posts and the influx of postwar students from Africa and Asia. Additionally, alone among advanced industrial nations, the United Kingdom did not require overseas travelers entering the country to produce a valid international vaccination certificate. (This did not change until 1963.) With low vaccination rates in infancy due to strong anti-vaccination forces and the failure to regularly vaccinate hospital workers, the infection was easily passed from one person to another and initiated outbreaks. Most cases were of variola minor but health authorities in the UK (as well as the U.S.) did not take them seriously, resulting in 35 outbreaks in 14 out of 24 years between 1935 and 1958. The largest occurred in 1947, when 48 cases were reported.[49]

Statistics reported by the United States surgeon general's office (1943) stated that during World War I, with 4 million men under arms, 853 cases of smallpox were reported. Between 1940 and 1943, smallpox cases occurred at a rate "too small to record graphically." The acceptance of young men entering the armed services receiving "shots" as a matter of course to protect against smallpox and typhoid fever greatly increased public awareness and acceptance. Unfortunately, that did not stop the anti-vaccinationist fervor of the Committee for Medical Freedom, which continued to protest against compulsory vaccination on the grounds that during World War I, 2,000 soldiers at Fort Devens died of vaccination and that it was "covered up" by reports that the deaths were caused by influenza. Dr. Roy F. Feemster, director of the Division of Communicable Diseases, and Dr. Frederick F. Russell, professor of preventive medicine at Harvard, denied the charges.[50] Postwar incidence of smallpox was slightly more discouraging.

Rapid demobilization of troops through Honolulu to San Francisco presented the danger of soldiers carrying smallpox and in March 1946, California state health authorities announced an outbreak from the Orient, calling on the public to undergo vaccination promptly.[51] By March 31, doctors reported 7 cases of "black," or Oriental, smallpox, carried by soldiers from Japan. In fear that the disease would spread, military officials quarantined two transports with heavy personnel loads, both of which reported a smallpox case aboard.[52] In Oakland, 10,000 people rushed to be vaccinated after smallpox was discovered aboard the navy transport *LaSalle* off Treasure Island. Additionally, three merchant seamen aboard the *Marine Devil* were discovered to have smallpox, while another transport from Jinsen, Korea, had two cases and was quarantined.[53] In light of this scare, vaccination clinics as far away as Herkimer, New York, were opened to counter the malignant smallpox brought in from servicemen returning from Korea.[54]

The same year, a soldier returning to the United States from Japan introduced smallpox into Seattle. By March, the death toll from this importation stood at 5, and was called "the worst in the nation since 1913." Vaccine from Philadelphia was brought in to help fight the threat.[55] Alerts went out to cities as far away as San Diego, Los Angeles, Portland and Vancouver, urging citizens to get vaccinated. Volunteers from the army, navy, U.S. Public Health Service, the state department of health and the Red Cross manned volunteer stations in Seattle.[56] The outbreak ultimately resulted in 51 cases and 16 deaths.

In February 1947, a 47-year-old merchant who had lived in Mexico City for 6 years boarded a bus for New York City. Along the way, he developed headaches, pain in the back of his neck and a rash. The journey lasted 6 days and he resided in a Manhattan hotel four more days before entering a hospital. He died March 10, of hemorrhagic smallpox, after having infected 12 others. In the resultant panic, Mayor William O'Dwyer telephoned Secretary Forrestal, who sent one quarter of a million units of vaccine from naval stores, and police commissioner Arthur W. Wallander arranged to have 82 police precincts functioning as vaccination clinics. By April 20, more than 3,300,000 persons had taken advantage of the protection and ultimately over 6 million were vaccinated, including the revaccination of schoolchildren and 10,000 state employees in Albany.

Twelve persons eventually contracted the disease and two died. Public health authorities traced the route of the bus, and everyone who might have come in contact with passengers was urged to receive vaccination. By September 1947, new regulations were established, requiring vaccination certificates of all persons entering or departing Mexico.[57]

A further outbreak of smallpox occurred in Cameron County, Texas, when a man named Salvador Leal came down with the disease in February 1949. A vaccination campaign was immediately put in operation, although Christian Scientists opposed the order on the grounds it violated religious freedom. Authorities supposed that Mexican nationals who were frequent visitors at the Leal home were the carriers. Eight cases and 1 death were reported. A Cuban tourist returning from Mexico in March 1949 was blamed for a smallpox scare in that nation and in April, 7 Cuban baseball players trying out for the Abilene Blue Sox (Class C West Texas–New Mexico League) were hospitalized following smallpox vaccinations. So great was the fear that laws were enacted in Wisconsin forbidding funerals for victims of smallpox and mourners were required to submit to vaccination before attending services.[58]

Variola major was eliminated as an endemic disease in the United States by 1927, but in states without vaccination laws, variola minor persisted into the latter half of the 1940s.[59]

Epidemics of variola major were seen in Colombia in 1943 and 1947, in Bolivia in the 1940s and in Ecuador up to 1962. The last outbreak was in Peru during 1941–1943, where nearly 10,000 deaths were reported. Over the next 20 years, variola minor became the predominant form of smallpox, with several thousand cases reported every year; Brazil continued to be a major exporter of variola minor until smallpox was eradicated in the whole Western Hemisphere in 1971.[60]

Thailand had a major epidemic of smallpox in 1945–1946, with more than 62,000 cases; Malaysia suffered outbreaks in the early 1940s, and it was not eliminated until 1949. The disease spread into the Philippines in 1948, but was again eliminated in 1949. Korea reported 20,000 cases in 1946, with a major epidemic in 1951. Smallpox was reintroduced into Indochina in 1947, reaching epidemic proportions in 1949.

After a major epidemic in 1908, smallpox went into decline in Japan and in 1918, vaccination was made mandatory for all 1-year-olds and revaccination upon entry to school. Between 1927 and 1944, only 5,412 cases were reported. With the end of World War II and repatriation of soldiers, smallpox broke out again, with 1,614 cases in 1945 and 17,800 in 1946. Control measures were further strengthened and smallpox ceased to be endemic in Japan in 1951.[61]

Following the war, major epidemics of smallpox were seen in the Netherlands East Indies, with high incidences in 1950 and 1951. By 1941, primary vaccination was compulsory in India, but revaccination was compulsory only in Madras. By 1944, over 60 million vaccinations were given annually. After 1947, when the partition of British India into Pakistan (East and West) and India occurred, vaccinations were undertaken but most were ineffective due to low potency of vaccine.

An epidemic in Iraq in 1940–1941 reached over 3,000 cases and spread westward into Syria, Lebanon, Turkey, Palestine and Jordan and eastward into Iran. In 1943, a major outbreak occurred in Turkey. Endemic smallpox was eliminated in that country in 1951, but cases continued to be reported in Iran and Iraq until the late 1950s.

Fighting during the Second World War led to severe outbreaks in all 5 countries of Northern Africa. The only outbreak of smallpox in Europe happened in Italy in 1944–1945, due to importation of variola major from North Africa. Smallpox continued to be a factor in Northern Africa until 1948, when improved health services brought about a significant decrease in cases.

Extensive vaccination campaigns in Western, Central and Eastern Africa from 1941 to 1946 brought smallpox under control, with fewer than 250 cases a year reported. The exception was South Africa, where the migration of the black population between 1940 and 1941 due to wartime activities resulted in the spread of variola minor. In 1943, an outbreak of variola major, probably imported from India, occurred in Natal, spreading into Transvaal. Whites as well as blacks were stricken, with a case-fatality rate as high as 30 percent. Vaccination was made compulsory and the epidemic ended in 1947. Scattered epidemics of variola minor continued through the 1940s, with numbers declining in the 1950s.[62]

With the immediate postwar era coming to an end, significant advances had been achieved in the control of smallpox. The Chinese were making a determined effort at vaccination, and India and Africa remained the two major hot spots, with Middle Eastern countries and Mexico, Central America and South America remaining sources of infection. It was finally time for international health organizations to step up and take action. But like everything else connected with smallpox, there were to be no shortcuts between desire and accomplishment.

37

A New Biological Philosophy

> Were it possible to vaccinate successfully all persons of all countries at one and the same time then smallpox would become a memory only. Were all children vaccinated during the first year of life, smallpox would not get much of a foothold at all unless introduced from the outside.[1]

Formally established on April 7, 1947, when its constitution was entered into force, the World Health Organization (WHO), medical arm of the United Nations, made a serious attempt to combat smallpox in 1950 through its regional affiliate, the Pan American Sanitary Bureau (PASB). Dr. Soper, director of the PASB, first became interested in such a program in 1947, when a minor outbreak of smallpox precipitated mass panic in New York City (see chapter 36). Seeking help from the United States (the bureau's largest contributor), Soper was directed to the U.S. National Institutes of Health. They referred him to William Gebhardt at the Michigan State Health Department Laboratory. (Established in 1873, the Michigan laboratory was the 5th oldest state health agency in the nation. Under a grant from the legislature in 1921, biologic products (including vaccine for smallpox) produced in the laboratory were provided free to state health officers and physicians. In 1933, the lab isolated one of the three polio viruses, naming it the "Lansing" strain, and in 1949, it was designated as one of four regional Salmonella Identification Centers in the United States, linked with the international agency in Copenhagen, established a year earlier by WHO.)[2] Scientists at the Michigan lab developed new techniques for freeze-drying vaccine that were piloted in Peru in 1950, under the direction of Dr. Abraham Horwitz. Positive results led to discussion and ultimate agreement on a regional program to eradicate smallpox from the Americas. In 1952, delegates voted $75,000 for the program and another $144,000 in 1954. By 1958, smallpox was on the verge of being interrupted in all countries of the Americas except Brazil, Colombia and Ecuador.

Contiguous with vaccination programs for typhus, typhoid and cholera, WHO sponsored a smallpox campaign in Korea in 1950, with programs against smallpox in Inchon and Seoul. Native physicians performed the service under the supervision of the WHO United Command, which supplied equipment.[3]

If proof were needed that Europe was not exempt from contagion, an outbreak of "eastern smallpox" appeared in Glasgow in early April 1950. The scourge was brought to the Scottish lowlands by an Indian seaman from Bombay, and it killed 26-year-old Dr. Janet Fleming and infected 20 others, who were sent to isolation wards in Robroyston Hospital. Dr. Stuart Laidlaw, Glasgow health officer, warned travelers not to leave without vaccination certificates. The United States Public Health Service responded by ordering ships that had touched Great Britain to vaccinate all passengers. The order affected 2,000 passengers aboard three ships bound for America: the *Queen Elizabeth* (carrying actresses Peggy Cummins and Virginia Mayo), *Caronia* and *Media*. In January 1951, during the holiday season in Brighton, another outbreak of 32 confirmed cases and 8 deaths caused the vaccination of over 80,000 people.[4]

Further discussion at WHO on smallpox control occurred in 1953, 1954 and 1955. To put the term "control" in historical perspective, it is important to underscore that the concept of "eradication," or the total elimination of a living organism, was not universally accepted as practicable or even possible during the first half of the century.

According to the World Health Organization, the term "eradication" was first used in 1884, in connection with a United States program developed to control bovine contagious pleuropneumonia, a highly fatal disease introduced into New York from Europe in 1843. The disease spread to the Midwest and eventually foreign countries embargoed the meat. Congress established the Bureau of Animal Industry in 1884, with the specific aim of eliminating pleuropneumonia. After an intensive 5-year campaign, it was eliminated in the United States.

Success against this bovine disease led Dr. Charles Chapin to speculate in 1889 that if preventive measures were undertaken, they could actually lead to eradication. Use of the word eventually became more common, but with significant differences: to some, "eradication" was used in reference to the extinction of a disease pathogen, while others used it in conjunction with a reduction to levels where it ceased to be a public health problem.[5] The *Concise Oxford Dictionary* defines it as to "remove or destroy completely," taken from the Middle English, "tear up by the roots."[6] In 1965, Dr. René Dubos further stated the case in his text, *Man Adapting*:

> At first sight, the decision to eradicate certain microbial diseases appears to constitute but one more step forward in the development of the control policies initiated by the great sanitarians of the nineteenth century, which have been greatly expanded since the beginning of the microbiological era. In reality, however, eradication involves a new biological philosophy. It implies that it is possible and desirable to get rid of certain disease problems of infection by eliminating completely the etiological agents, once and for all.[7]

At the 11th World Health Assembly, 1958, held in Minneapolis, Professor Viktor Zhdanov, Deputy Minister of Health for the USSR, postulated that the eradication of smallpox was theoretically possible within ten years. His report proposed that vaccination and revaccination be made compulsory throughout the endemic world beginning in 1959. His plan, based on the Leicester system, consisted of "surveillance-containment activities," or prompt identification, notification, isolation, quarantine and disinfectant measures.

Pointing to the success of the USSR's anti-smallpox program, Zhdanov offered 25 million doses of freeze-dried vaccine to WHO, as well as assistance to Burma, Cambodia, Ghana, Guinea, India, Indonesia, Iraq and Pakistan. Cuba offered 2 million doses of glycerolated vaccine. The delegates endorsed the proposal and called for the director-general to study and report on the implementation.

His report, presented in January 1959, suggested a global program of mass vaccinations operated by a smallpox eradication service, "integrated with the general public health services" of the infected countries, but "directed, or at least co-ordinated, centrally." Suggesting freeze-dried vaccine for tropical areas, the data indicated that 977 million people lived in endemic areas. Based on a formula using $0.10 per person, the estimated cost was $97.7 million dollars. The program did not include the People's Republic of China, which was not a WHO member. No mention was made of an end date.[8]

The timing of the smallpox proposal proved unfortunate, as it coincided with the implementation of WHO's global malaria eradication program. In fact, by 1959, WHO had already attempted two previous eradication programs: for hookworm in 1909, and yellow fever soon after. Animal carriers (reservoirs) or insects transmitted these diseases to humans and although the malaria, hookworm and yellow fever programs eventually achieved some success, it became apparent there was no way to eliminate animal carriers or insects, making the end goal of eradication impossible.

The only other eradication program sponsored by international organizations was for yaws. After the discovery that a single injection of long-lasting penicillin proved a cure, successful yaws control occurred in Haiti in 1948–1949. In the mid–1950s, the PASB and UNICEF supplied support for a mass treatment program for syphilis and yaws, which again proved successful, but the disease was eliminated in only a few of the smaller countries.[9]

Smallpox eradication followed other eradication programs for two reasons: because variola minor had become the primary form of the disease and was not considered a major health concern and because it was so widespread. In 1959, it was probable that smallpox was endemic in 59 countries and territories in Africa, South America and Asia, encompassing 1,734,921,000 persons, or 59 percent of the world's population. The proposal at the 12th World Health Assembly, 1959, envisioned national campaigns achieving 80 percent vaccination and revaccination rates in affected populations, with local governments assuming responsibility for administration, execution and much of cost. To the detriment of the smallpox program, between 1959 and 1966, little was achieved, as WHO's primary emphasis lay in the malaria eradication program. The failure to achieve eradication of hookworm, yellow fever and malaria greatly damaged WHO's credibility and major financial backers such as UNICEF refused to become involved in smallpox, fearing another disappointment.

Continuing its work throughout the Western Hemisphere, the Pan American Health Organization worked with a budget of $13,178,869 in 1962 to assist governments in carrying out 303 health projects. Already reporting success against smallpox, statistics for 1960 indicated that in 7 North American nations, 4,792 cases were reported. While this was an increase of 28 cases over 1959, it represented a significant decrease from 10 years previous when 9,301 cases were reported. From January to August 1961, there were 978 incidents of smallpox, 631 occurring in Rio de Janeiro and 317 in Ecuador.[10]

Regional programs not substantially supported by WHO proved successful in Bolivia and Paraguay, where smallpox was eliminated in 1960; Ecuador followed in 1963. During the years 1959–1963, Africa was torn by internal strife and health authorities were powerless to conduct any meaningful control. Algeria was the only country in Northern Africa where the disease was epidemic but as the civil wars quieted, it successfully eliminated smallpox as endemic in 1961. In former French colonies where freeze-dried vaccine had been introduced, the Central African Republic (1955), the Congo (1954) and Gabon (1956) were free from the disease, but open borders invited importation. Other countries, including Burma, Colombia, India, Pakistan and Peru also conducted strenuous vaccination campaigns, with positive results.[11]

In western Asia, smallpox was eliminated in Iraq (1959), Democratic Yemen (1960), Saudi Arabia (1961) and Iran (1963) but, similar to Africa, importation of smallpox continued, primarily from countries bordering the Persian Gulf. Working in conjunction with Britain, the Soviet Union and WHO, in 1962 India launched a national smallpox eradication program costing $15,000,000. Thirteen vaccine-producing institutes were created, while the Soviet Union offered 250 million doses of freeze-dried vaccine to aid the cause of vaccinating all 3,000,000 persons living in New Delhi. Of equal importance, female social workers made special efforts to overcome a major handicap by convincing peasant women to accept vaccination. Two years later, Britain gave 4 million does of freeze-dried vaccine after an appeal from WHO.[12]

By 1962, there were thought to be 44 countries with endemic smallpox, of which 14 were conducting eradication programs, 22 had programs that had not yet started and 8 had done nothing. In January 1964, the WHO Expert Committee of Smallpox raised the vaccination/revaccination requirements for eradication to 100 percent and outlined a 10-point attack:

WHO Eradication Program

Attack phase
Vaccination target (100%)
Primary vaccination (newborns)
Revaccination in schools, industry and cities
Production and supply of vaccine
Training of vaccinators
Health education
Vaccination records
Evaluation
Eradication[13]

As noted above, China was not a WHO member and thus was not included in the global eradication program, despite suffering epidemics in 1930–1934, 1936–1939 and 1946–1948. In 1950, during another two-year epidemic (1950–1951), health authorities from the People's Republic of China launched a program stressing vaccination/revaccination. As part of the initiative, China produced calf vaccine of the "Temple of Heaven" strain at 5 locations: Beijing, Shanghai, Dalian, Kunming and Lanzhou. Success in eliminating the disease was achieved in all large cities and major towns within 5 years. Outbreaks believed to be precipitated by the old standard of inoculation occurred in 1958, and a second phase began the same year, with technical aid provided by the USSR. This campaign ran until 1958. After several cases due to importation were reported in 1959, another mass program, this time concentrating on the border areas, was started. By 1961 the goal of eliminating smallpox throughout China had been achieved.[14]

The United States Takes a Stand

Dr. Karel Raska, an epidemiologist from Czechoslovakia, was elected as director of the division of Communicable Diseases for WHO. His election was significant in that he believed smallpox eradication was possible and the establishment of the Smallpox Eradication Unit in 1965 was a giant step forward.

In the United States, internal programs proved a valuable backdrop. In late 1962, legislators warned that the immunization levels in the country were "dangerously low," making the country susceptible to importation. Within a month the American Medical Association sent smallpox information to more than 6,000 individuals and organizations. The precautions proved successful when, in 1965, a smallpox case was identified in Washington, DC, Health authorities correctly diagnosed and vaccinated all who came in contact with the victim.[15]

Dr. Raska was to have important aid with the United States' development of the jet injector, which made it possible for 500 or more vaccinations to be performed without replenishing the vaccine, enabling as many as 1,000 persons to be vaccinated per hour. The jet injector gun for intradermal injections was field-tested by the Centers for Disease Control (CDC) in Tonga (a constitutional monarchy under British protection), where the medical staff gave away toy metal crickets (clickers) as a reward for being vaccinated. The simple tactic worked, as 44,390 persons were vaccinated.[16] Of even greater import was the commitment of the United States to expand its popular field trials of a measles vaccination program in Western and Central Asia (begun in 1961), to include smallpox eradication.

April 7, 1965 (the anniversary of WHO's constitution), was celebrated as World Health Day. "Smallpox — Constant Alert" was chosen as the theme that year in recognition of an importation of smallpox into Europe in 1962 and 1963. Dr. Benjamin Blood and Dr. James Watt of the U.S. Public Health Service proposed to President Lyndon Johnson that he involve the nation in the global eradication of smallpox. Johnson pledged financial support for the Pan American Health Organization's efforts and on November 23, 1965, his staff issued a press release, promising to help protect 105 million people in 18 African countries; under the program, over 90 million people were to be given smallpox vaccination and 29 million were to receive inoculations against measles.[17]

Encouraged by the United States' participation, member countries of WHO meeting in Geneva issued a report May 13, 1966, unanimously approving a 10-year program designed to eliminate smallpox (1967–1977). It was estimated 1.8 billion vaccinations would be required to eradicate smallpox zones in Asia, Africa and the Americas. Noting that 12 countries had succeeded in eliminating endemic smallpox since 1959, observations of the 18th World Health Assembly included:

1. In many endemic countries, other health concerns overrode smallpox control.
2. Administrative and supervisory support was required.
3. Large amounts of freeze-dried vaccine, transport, refrigeration and equipment were needed.
4. Revaccination (continuing vaccination) was necessary.

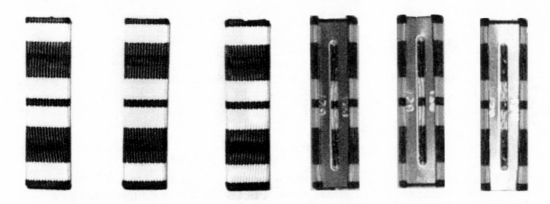

Left: These Smallpox Eradication Ribbons were awarded to any member of the United States Public Health Service who served for at least 90 days between January 1, 1966, and October 26, 1977, in the Smallpox Campaign (from the authors' collection). Right: Smallpox ribbons, rear view.

5. Pilot projects were needed to determine strategy.
6. Independent assessment of vaccination success rates.
7. Contiguous endemic countries must start campaigns simultaneously.

The cost of vaccination was still calculated at $0.10/single dose and it was believed funding of $25–36 million would be required, of which $2.4 million for the first year of the campaign was approved for 1967, representing a substantial increase in WHO's smallpox budget. A problem immediately arose when the United States objected, issuing the opinion that WHO provide only technical assistance and advice. The U.S. believed financial support should come from the United Nations and voluntary contributions. When UNICEF declined to become involved for fear of another WHO eradication program failure, money became a serious issue. Notwithstanding, the 18th Assembly issued its firmest stance by declaring "the world-wide eradication of smallpox to be one of the major objectives of the Organization."[18]

The following year, when it became obvious voluntary contributions would not be enough, the director-general decided on a two-part plan: a regular budget allocation and a special fund of $2.4 million, designated solely for smallpox eradication. By 1968, the aim was to have programs in 41 countries, including Afghanistan, Burma, India, Indonesia, Nepal, Pakistan, Brazil, Colombia, Peru and substantially all of Africa south of the Sudan. Learning from past mistakes, principles for eradication and a reporting system were presented up front instead of retrospectively and ongoing research was encouraged.

With the understanding that 220 million persons were to be vaccinated in 1967, the plan took for granted that South American countries and Pakistan would produce vaccine for their own needs, while the USSR would supply Afghanistan, Burma and India. Under its Western and Central African program, the United States was expected to provide 30–40 million doses per year.

Costs estimates escalated rapidly. The sum of $180 million was now considered necessary for complete success. WHO contributed 4.7 percent of its budget. International support between 1967 and 1979 amounted to $98 million: of this, only 5 countries — the United States ($16.6 million), USSR ($7.1 million), Federal Republic of Germany ($3.5 million), United Kingdom ($3.4 million) and France ($2.9 million)— contributed 5 percent or more of the budget. In addition, the USSR supplied 25 million doses of vaccine each year, continued throughout the global program. Minimal financial assistance came from international organizations, including UNICEF, the League of Red Cross and Red Crescent Societies and the World Food Programme.

By May 1966, with formal approval of the program and a budget approved by WHO's Health Assembly, work began in earnest, with an unofficial timetable of 10 years. With current data then indicating a total of 31 countries with endemic smallpox, encompassing a population of 1,078,775,000, "the Intensified Smallpox Eradication Programme was thus conceived in an atmosphere of sanguine rhetoric overshadowed by real doubts about its ultimate success."[19]

International Travel in the Age of the Jet Airplane

Underscoring a new threat in the spread of contagion, a headline from 1959 warned, "Disease Gets Around Fast in Jet Age." Referencing the current edition of the *American*

Medical Association, Dr. Wesley W. Spink, of the University of Minnesota Medical School, noted, "In this era of missiles and jet travel a medical problem in Madras, India, today, may be that of New York City's tomorrow."

He related a case of a German physician traveling from India to Ceylon, where he thought he contracted influenza. The doctor continued by plane to Switzerland and then by train to Heidelberg, Germany. There, he was correctly diagnosed with smallpox, having infected 13 persons in Europe along the way. Clearly, in the age of steamers, his disease would have been evident long before he arrived in Europe, but with the rapidity of travel, infected persons covered thousands of miles, unknowingly spreading disease before they could be quarantined. Adding to the danger, smallpox was rare enough that physicians often misdiagnosed it. Using the American training program established during World War II to train doctors in unfamiliar tropical diseases as an example, Dr. Spink suggested a regular postgraduate course for physicians, worked out through the U.S. Public Health Service or WHO.[20]

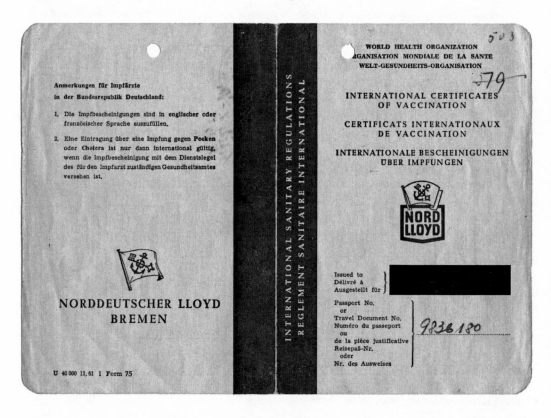

Above and opposite: This is the front and back of an original World Health Organization International Certificate of Vaccination, issued to Olga Markschat, issued in 1963. It bears the approval stamp from Gesehen der Amtsarzt (from the authors' collection).

The inside text reads, "International Certificate of Vaccination or Revaccination Against Smallpox," and includes the invdividual's name, date of birth, signature and date of revaccination. The bottom text reads, "The validity of this certificate shall extend for a period of three years, beginning eight days after the date of a successful primary vaccination, or, in the event of a revaccination, on the date of that revaccination. The approved stamp mentioned above must be in a form prescribed by the health administration of the territory in which the vaccination is performed. Any amendment of this certificate, or erasure, or failure to complete any part of it, may render it invalid" (from the authors' collection).

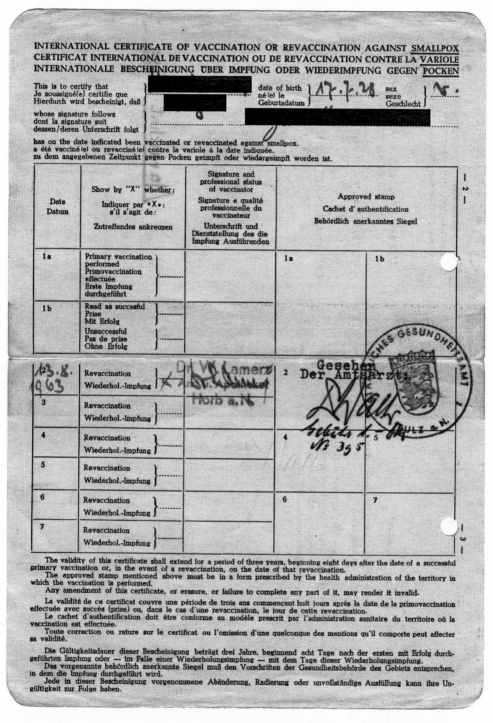

INTERNATIONAL CERTIFICATE OF VACCINATION OR REVACCINATION AGAINST SMALLPOX
CERTIFICAT INTERNATIONAL DE VACCINATION OU DE REVACCINATION CONTRE LA VARIOLE
INTERNATIONALE BESCHEINIGUNG ÜBER IMPFUNG ODER WIEDERIMPFUNG GEGEN POCKEN

This is to certify that
Je soussigné(e) certifie que
Hierdurch wird bescheinigt, daß

date of birth
né (e) le
Geburtsdatum

sex
sexe
Geschlecht

whose signature follows
dont la signature suit
dessen/deren Unterschrift folgt

has on the date indicated been vaccinated or revaccinated against smallpox.
a été vacciné (e) ou revacciné (e) contre la variole à la date indiquée.
zu dem angegebenen Zeitpunkt gegen Pocken geimpft oder wiedergeimpft worden ist.

Date Datum	Show by "X" whether: Indiquer par «X»: s'il s'agit de: Zutreffendes ankreuzen	Signature and professional status of vaccinator Signature e qualité professionnelle du vaccinateur Unterschrift und Dienststellung des die Impfung Ausführenden	Approved stamp Cachet d' authentification Behördlich anerkanntes Siegel
1a	Primary vaccination performed Primovaccination effectuée Erste Impfung durchgeführt	1a	1b
1b	Read as succesful Prise Mit Erfolg / Unsuccessful Pas de prise Ohne Erfolg		
23.8. 1963	Revaccination Wiederhol.-Impfung X	2	
3	Revaccination Wiederhol.-Impfung		
4	Revaccination Wiederhol.-Impfung	4	5
5	Revaccination Wiederhol.-Impfung		
6	Revaccination Wiederhol.-Impfung	6	7
7	Revaccination Wiederhol.-Impfung		

The validity of this certificate shall extend for a period of three years, beginning eight days after the date of a successful primary vaccination or, in the event of a revaccination, on the date of that revaccination.
The approved stamp mentioned above must be in a form prescribed by the health administration of the territory in which the vaccination is performed.
Any amendment of this certificate, or erasure, or failure to complete any part of it, may render it invalid.

La validité de ce certificat couvre une période de trois ans commençant huit jours après la date de la primovaccination effectuée avec succès (prise) ou, dans le cas d'une revaccination, le jour de cette revaccination.
Le cachet d'authentification doit être conforme au modèle prescrit par l'administration sanitaire du territoire où la vaccination est effectuée.
Toute correction ou rature sur le certificat ou l'omission d'une quelconque des mentions qu'il comporte peut affecter sa validité.

Die Gültigkeitsdauer dieser Bescheinigung beträgt drei Jahre, beginnend acht Tage nach der ersten mit Erfolg durchgeführten Impfung oder — im Falle einer Wiederholungsimpfung — mit dem Tage dieser Wiederholungsimpfung.
Das vorgenannte behördlich anerkannte Siegel muß den Vorschriften der Gesundheitsbehörde des Gebiets entsprechen, in dem die Impfung durchgeführt wird.
Jede in dieser Bescheinigung vorgenommene Abänderung, Radierung oder unvollständige Ausfüllung kann ihre Ungültigkeit zur Folge haben.

In order to protect Americans, the United States utilized a disease reporting system jointly undertaken by many countries through WHO. Daily radio messages detailing instances of disease were sent over powerful WHO transmitters in Geneva, enabling countries to take immediate action. Quarantine inspectors stationed at major airports vaccinated foreigners entering the country from infected areas who did not have the proper clearance. The program proved so successful, between 1953 and 1959 the nation remained free of smallpox.[21] This precaution applied to Americans, as well, as they were warned that once they left the country, proof of vaccination within the prior three years was required to reenter. As it was long past the age of inspecting scars, travelers were required to present a certificate on an approved WHO card, called an "International Certificate of Vaccination."[22]

Other nations were not as fortunate. According to statistics provided by WHO, during the year ending June 30, 1959, smallpox was imported into 11 countries through international travel that included 11 ships and 2 aircraft. The colony of Aden reported 132 cases imported from Yemen; Ceylon reported 27 cases and 2 deaths on Leydon Island, imported by boat from India; Germany reported 18 cases at Heidelberg, transmitted from the physician described above; Ghana had 3 cases and 1 death; Iran reported 3 cases by persons crossing into the country at unauthorized checkpoints; Malaya, Pakistan, Nigeria, the Philippines and United Arab Republic reported imported cases, as did England, with 1 case in Liverpool, source unidentified. In total for 1958, 247,000 smallpox cases were reported, 88 percent in India and Pakistan. In comparison, the annual average between 1952 and 1957 was fewer than 150,000 reported cases.[23]

As though they were jewel thieves instead of unsuspecting victims, infected passengers became the object of international manhunts. In 1960, for instance, WHO alerted Ceylon, India, Iran, Turkey and Italy of possible contagion by an airline passenger en route from Ceylon to London. When finally "apprehended" after a visit to Wormwood Scrubs Prison in London, the smallpox suspect was hospitalized. His route to England had taken him through five countries, incidentally contaminating Malayan cabinet ministers and representatives of 22 countries in the Malayan capital on his way from Colombo. A companion, who continued from London to Oslo, became the object of another search as newspapers and radio broadcasts urged him to contact health authorities.[24]

Reports from the 1960s continued to reflect fear from importation. In 1962, two Pakistani immigrants introduced the disease into London, while an outbreak of smallpox in West Germany was traced to a German family returning from Liberia. The same year, all persons who boarded the North German liner *Bremen* when it docked in New York had to submit to vaccination due to outbreaks in Germany, Britain and Switzerland.[25] Near panic occurred in August 1962, when a boy named James Orr, infected with a highly malignant form of smallpox, passed through Idlewild Airport. The son of a missionary, en route from Brazil to Canada, he spent hours at Grand Central Station before boarding a train to Canada. As the family held yellow cards as "protection in depth" (a warning in the event of illness that the holder had been in a smallpox area) and also possessed valid certificates, it was conjectured the boy had been improperly vaccinated. International calls to anyone who may have come in contact with him were immediately issued. WHO also warned that vaccination and certificates were only valid for three years. It was ultimately charged that a physician in Brazil issued certificates without actually inoculating the Orrs and that he failed to use the proper WHO certificates. In defense, Brazilian authorities charged the air carriers and airport officials for accepting substandard certificates, noting "blame is to be largely shared by them."[26]

As late as 1967, a smallpox scare in the United States occurred after an India Air Line flight from Bombay to New York via Frankfurt, Germany, was found to have carried a passenger infected with smallpox. Health officials in Maryland, Texas, Wisconsin, Virginia and

Puerto Rico tracked down contaminated passengers who entered their jurisdictions and kept them under observation for 16 days.[27]

Isolated Instances of Smallpox in the Eradication Era — United States

The last officially acknowledged case of smallpox in the United States occurred in 1949, but as the following reports indicated, local authorities believed their municipalities were visited by the disease as late as 1953. Whether they were actually chicken pox, as Federal authorities speculated, was not clarified. One fact remained clear, however: as late as the 1930s, the incidence and mortality from variola was high, with almost 49,000 cases reported in 1930. The virtual elimination of the disease was, by and large, the result of school vaccination requirements and immigration regulations.[28]

By the 1950s, most doctors in the United States had never seen a case of active smallpox, but with the threat of importation ever possible, vaccination remained critical. This, however, exacerbated the inherent dangers of the procedure. In a report from 1951, a mother from Kansas City complained that after mass vaccinations in Reedsburg, her baby became ill, as it had suffered from eczema at the time and should not have undergone the procedure. The public health physician, Dr. Neupert, pointed out that due to the large number of recipients, physicians did not have time to examine all persons before the operation. He added that "the threat of smallpox was greater than the threat of possible reactions to the vaccination against it." The story played in the newspapers, but significantly, the point made was that instead of ignoring her complaint, the health officer made the effort to explain it. The newspaper added, "In one swift stroke, he forestalled any sub-voice criticism that might develop and at the same time answered a complaint in forthright fashion. When you let the people have the facts, you inoculate against rumors, too."[29]

In allaying fears of pain and scarring, people were also educated to the fact that modern vaccination was performed by taking a small drop of vaccine and placing it on the arm, where it was then gently tapped into the skin or inserted by a subcutaneous prick, leaving no visible mark and eliciting only a slight fever. Those with scars the "size of nickels" received vaccination the "old fashioned" way.

The ease of vaccination had nothing to do with allaying the objections of anti-vaccinationists. In 1953, a law outlawing compulsory vaccination in Arkansas came before legislators, vigorously supported by the Health Freedom League.[30] If one of their arguments had to do with the fact that smallpox was eradicated from the United States, they needed look no further than Beaver Crossing, Nebraska, where 2 cases were reported among schoolchildren, setting off a wave of vaccinations for more than one-half the town's population of 425. The same year, from Wisconsin, an 18-year-old college freshman and student-athlete bitterly complained that, as her father had refused to have her vaccinated as a youth, she later contracted the disease, which left her face rough and scarred.[31]

On the lighter side, before the Miss Universe Pageant to be held in Long Beach, California, on July 23, 1954, "Miss Cuba" refused the required smallpox vaccination on the grounds she "might get sick and not be able to compete." Rather than be disqualified, she was required to be examined daily by the Long Beach Health Department.[32]

The development of other vaccines quickly proved successful, particularly for infants and children.

Generally Approved Immunization Schedule, 1965

Age	Preparation
2 months	DTP (diphtheria, tetanus, pertussis) plus Type 1 oral polio vaccine
3 months	DTP plus Type 3 polio vaccine
4 months	DTP plus Type 2 polio vaccine
9 months	Measles vaccine
12 months	Smallpox vaccine
15 months	Boosters of DTP and the 3 types of polio vaccine
4 years	DTP booster
5–6 years	Smallpox revaccination
8 years	Adult type tetanus-diphtheria booster[33]

Isolated Instances of Smallpox in the Eradication Era — International

In March 1953, an epidemic of smallpox broke out in Northern England; a month later, it claimed its fifth victim. Centered in the textile manufacturing districts of Yorkshire and Lancashire, isolated reports originated in at least six towns. Investigation into the cause was completed in 1954; from the conclusions drawn, it was "apparent that the risk of smallpox is greater than it has been for generations." In commenting on the findings, the *Manchester Guardian* noted that the entire attitude of the United Kingdom required reconsideration. Proving the point, in 1958, 700 store clerks were vaccinated after it was revealed a woman who had made an extensive shopping tour in Liverpool on May 10 subsequently died of the disease.

Typically, smallpox exposure originated with immigrants. In 1962, a confirmed case was attributed to a Pakistani who arrived January 4, bringing cries for stricter controls over those entering the country from that nation and India. This was important, for under the National Health Act, valid certificates were not required for entry. With the number of infections rising to 16, WHO characterized England as having a legitimate epidemic. Thousands rushed to be vaccinated although the Ministry of Health stated there was no need for mass vaccinations. The United States sent half-a-million vaccine inoculations to Britain, the Pentagon reporting the cost was paid by the British government. During the same period, WHO reported mild outbreaks in West Germany and Switzerland, although stating there was little immediate danger of smallpox spreading to other countries.

These outbreaks did not prevent anti-vaccinationists from protesting. The same year, in response to death statistics from England, a protest against the procedure was published in Texas, warning that there was "no scientific evidence" in favor of vaccination, but "an abundance of proof" that sanitation, isolation and refrigeration were the answer.[34] Depressingly, there seemed no end of smallpox reports, but by the 1950s, international awareness and cooperation was more prevalent.

Major epidemics of cholera and smallpox persisted in East Pakistan during 1958. That spring, Dr. T. Aidan Cockburn arrived in Dacca to set up a department for the treatment of infectious diseases under the International Cooperative Assistance Program. In a letter, he observed that he was faced with an "enormous epidemic of smallpox and cholera, with 2,000 people dying every week." By December, Cockburn, along with two American medical teams, one Afgan team and one Russian group, "rode out the epidemic," and Dacca "settled back into its normal somnolence."

In 1959, the Indonesian government promised to vaccinate 5 million people in Northern Java to stop a smallpox epidemic. Interestingly, in Thailand, S.M. Keeny, a director of UNICEF researching leprosy, discovered that villagers were willing to undergo examinations only if they received free smallpox vaccination. Keeny reported UNICEF supplied the necessary medicines for the "package deal," and that the new campaign reached 2 million a year. Keeny's team was assisted by a local doctor who used magic while performing 2,400 vaccinations a year. Relying primarily on herbs, he used his magic in more difficult cases, getting about 70 percent cures.

Better results were obtained in the Republic of Vietnam, where Dr. Le Cuu Truong, Vietnamese delegate to WHO, Pacific Region Conference, reported that between 1935 and 1959, that nation had 60,000 cases and 10,000 deaths, but with the compulsory vaccination campaign, none had been reported since. Reports from Singapore were more grim: during 1951–1952, a total of 500,000 persons contracted smallpox, with a mortality of 150,000 in surrounding Asian countries, while in North Korea, authorities accused Allied planes of dropping vermin, containers of spiders and bed bugs over Communist territories in special artillery shells. While it was difficult to determine the extent of disease, a report dated 1951, by Brigadier-General Crawford E. Sams, chief of the Army Far Eastern Public Health and Welfare Section, stated "hundreds of thousands" of Communist troops and civilians died of typhus, smallpox and typhoid fever. He also found cases of hemorrhagic smallpox and estimated that disease among North Koreans and Chinese took the lives of 3,000,000.[35] Asia remained a major area of contagion. A smallpox epidemic in January claimed 50 lives in Saigon, while in December 1957, agency reports indicated 600 had died of smallpox in the East Pakistan university town of Rajsahi, forcing schools and colleges to close.[36]

An officer for the Indian government's smallpox eradication program reported that since the operation began in late 1962 more than 50 percent of India's population had been vaccinated. The program was carried out with vaccine donated by the Soviet Union and funds and technical assistance from the United States and WHO.

Smallpox epidemics generally went in 3-year cycles; 1964 was an especially bad year and worse was expected in 1967, but numbers were atypically low in Madras. Dr. A. Ramachandra Rao, public health officer, traced the break in the cycle back to 1960. Finding a large number of infants suffering from smallpox at the Infectious Disease Hospital, he went against conventional wisdom and vaccinated all those from 3 days to 6 months, successfully proving that even at such a young age, vaccination worked.[37]

On a larger scale, Dr. Rao praised the work of Dr. C. Henry Kempe for bringing significant advances for the eradication of smallpox into India. In 1952, Dr. Kempe (born in Breslau, Germany, April 6, 1922), of the University of California, went to India, where he studied blood samples of recently vaccinated individuals, discovering they contained high concentrations of antibodies working against the virus used in vaccination. Dr. Kempe then devised a new serum that it was hoped would prevent complications which sometimes followed vaccination. The serum, called "vaccinia hyperimmune gamma-globulin," was tested in Madras in 1953 and again in March–April 1960. Results proved that when administered prophylactically to individuals coming in close contact with the infection, the incidence of disease was reduced to about a quarter of that in the controls. Due to the limited supply of the serum, its use was likely to be restricted to high-risk individuals.

After conducting research in 1960, Dr. Kempe, by then head of the Department of Pediatrics at the University of Colorado, and Dr. A.W. Downie, professor of bacteriology, University of Liverpool, assigned students to a 3-month tour at the hospital. Along with

Ms. L. St. Vincent, a virologist from the University of Colorado, the team supplied modern equipment the hospital could not afford, paid for by grants from WHO, the National Institutes of Health, U.S.A., and the University of Colorado. Health officers from around the world later trained there in the detection of smallpox. Dr. Kempe was nominated for the Nobel Prize for his work on a safer smallpox vaccination.[38]

In 1965, officials reported epidemics in Buldana and Bhandara districts of Madhya Pradesh, a state 500 miles south of New Delhi, and in the community of Ghaziabad, a few miles east of the capital. In New Delhi, 54 cases were reported in January, of which 21 proved fatal. A WHO spokesman suggested the high number of cases and unusual number of deaths were due to drought and food shortages, which forced inland populations into major cities, spreading disease and lowering people's stamina. Overcrowding was also rampant at Allahabad, 400 miles east of New Delhi, as several million people gathered in January for the religious bathing festival known as Khumb Mela.

In 1956, there were 38 cases of smallpox reported in Beirut, compelling the Lebanon authorities to ask WHO for smallpox vaccine. In 1960, five years after the last reported case in the Soviet Union, a Soviet artist brought the disease home from India and started a small outbreak in Moscow. More than 120 Americans were among those vaccinated, while tourists were refused rooms until they showed a valid certificate. Formal notification was reported to WHO, with the assurance, "all necessary steps" were being taken to prevent the spread of disease.[39]

While the number of smallpox cases in Mexico had greatly declined by 1954, U.S. Public Health inspectors were stationed at border crossings to check vaccination certificates. In 1953, vaccinations, totaling 354,000, were made on the border from Brownsville to the California line; at the Santa Fe street bridge, 70,000 vaccinations were given to those crossing from Mexico to El Paso. By the end of 1954, it was estimated 500,000 more vaccinations would have been performed. In addition, migrant workers (braceros) were vaccinated every year whether they had a current certificate or not. Each person was issued a slip showing proof of vaccination; after being checked to see the procedure had "taken," slips were then exchanged for an International Smallpox Certificate at the U.S. Public Health Service offices.

The vaccine used was sent from medical supply houses, packed in dry ice and kept under refrigeration until needed; it gave better than a 95 percent take. In 1957, the task of vaccinating fell to the U.S. Public Health Service, Division of Foreign Quarantine. Of the 6 quarantinable diseases (smallpox, yellow fever, typhus, cholera, plague and relapsing fever), only the first two were checked at the Mexican border. U.S. citizens were not examined or vaccinated unless they had been in a disease area or had come in contact with an infected person.[40]

Sandwiched between world outbreaks came the 1959 headline, "Bolivian Smallpox Hit by Mass Vaccinations." In a joint project carried out by the Serivicio Cooperative De Salud Publico and the U.S. Public Health Service, nearly 2,500,000 persons, or three-fourths of the population, were vaccinated in less than two years, virtually eliminating the disease. At the start of the campaign in 1957, Bolivia had the highest rate of smallpox in the world. While the presence of the disease threatened all the Americas, success appeared almost impossible, as there were few roads to reach the aboriginal population.

The assembled 11 teams traveled by river through torrid jungles, covering as much as 100 miles a day, and they broadcast through loudspeakers the purpose of the trip as they approached villages. Using the Province of Cochabama as a focus where an epidemic in 1957 resulted in 87 cases, secondary teams followed the primary teams, making sure the vaccinations had been done properly. Upon completion, Drs. Harald Frederiksen, Torres Munos and Jauregui Molina, directors of the work, hoped their success would prove a model for similar campaigns. Proving much work remained, WHO reported an annual average of 178,000 cases between 1951 and 1955.[41]

Asian countries continued to provide about four-fifths of all smallpox cases, with Africa following as the second major exporter of smallpox. An engineer returning from a business trip to Nigeria introduced smallpox into Duesseldorf, Germany, in 1962, causing WHO to declare the city a "locally infected area." Airports receiving passengers from Duesseldorf were required to check vaccination certificates before allowing visitors into their countries. In 1963, the Polish press reported 93 cases of smallpox and several deaths during the first week of August.[42]

The situation in Africa was complicated by intense poverty, military actions and lack of education. Numerous accounts point to "witch doctors" using "mumbo jumbo" to (ineffectually) treat smallpox patients, but one from Lagos, Nigeria, presented a slightly different "take." When Dr. Albert Helsher, an American missionary, saw a local practitioner (babaloyo) pricking the skin and applying his own "vaccine" concoction, he offered him a packet of needles and the correct vaccine, suggesting he could do better with "magic needles." The man complied, and it "wasn't long before other witch doctors were doing the same — and we were able to avert a serious epidemic."[43]

On the opposite end, in 1962, despite African superstitions, medical authorities announced plans to vaccinate the entire population of Leopoldville after 53 smallpox cases were reported, 90 percent of causalities being children under 12.[44] Smallpox continued to appear within its traditional boundaries during the remainder of the decade, with numbers fluctuating between positive and negative. In 1967, for example, WHO reported 60,941 cases for the first 7 months of the year, up from 43,509 in 1966. Asia reported the most victims, followed by Africa and South America.[45]

In 1969, Richard Nixon's White House announced the 100-millionth vaccination against smallpox in Niger under a program of the United States Agency for International Development (AID). President Nixon added that the success was due to people from 20 nations of Central and West Africa coming together with AID and WHO.[46]

The Decade of the 1970s —
Conflicting Reports

[If smallpox] comes now in an isolated outbreak, we can get rid of it. This is the
first disease ever to be eradicated and there won't be another in our lifetime.[1]

As late as 1970 (proving that as long as smallpox existed in the world, no country, however efficient its health service, was ever safe), doctors vaccinated 100,000 persons after two deaths and more than 200 patients were quarantined in Germany's Ruhr Valley. As in most other outbreaks, this was introduced by a vacationer, Bernd Klein, returning from Pakistan. While Klein's family were receiving death threats, Czechoslovakia, East Germany, Britain, Portugal and Spain imposed precautionary measures, while East German border guards set up checkpoints on the highway linking West Germany with West Berlin.[2]

Half the 20,000,000 citizens of the Congo-Kinshasa were vaccinated for smallpox from 1967 to 1969; but proving the difficulty of the situation, more than 300 cases were reported in March 1970. In all, statistics revealed that between 15,000 and 25,000 Africans died of the disease every year.[3]

Assisting in the global effort against smallpox was the Centers for Disease Control (CDC), Atlanta, established July 1, 1946, under the Public Health Service. Originally created to control malaria, by 1971 the agency coordinated a national attack on a wide range of diseases that spread from person to person and from animals and nature to humans. The CDC soon developed into a major world center for research, operating field stations across the United States and Puerto Rico.

When the CDC was notified of an outbreak of smallpox in Accra, Ghana, a busy international seaport, director Dr. David J. Spencer contacted the appropriate staff from his 3,800 person staff and arranged for systematic vaccination in village-by-village visits by medical teams. Such teamwork inspired Dr. William H. Foege, in speaking of WHO's goal of eradicating smallpox by 1976, to boldly proclaim, "We're going to get rid of it before then." He elaborated by stating that from the time of massive vaccinations in 20 West African nations there had been no reported cases (since May 1969) where once there had been 1,000 cases yearly.[4]

Responding to a request from WHO in 1970, Canada pledged $145,000 annually for the next four years. The funds were to purchase up to 17,000 vials yearly of a special vaccine suitable for the jet injector method of vaccination. The vaccine was to be produced by the Connaught Medical Research Laboratories of the University of Toronto, one of the world's foremost sources of this high-quality vaccine and one of two WHO international Reference Centres for smallpox vaccine. Canada also contributed nearly $2,230,000 Canadian into the regular WHO budget.[5]

The year 1970 also witnessed the first substantiated episode on record where smallpox germs were carried by air currents, causing a long-range epidemic. According to epidemic specialists of WHO, this was the first clear indication that smallpox could be transmitted by other than face-to-face contact (see also below). An investigation at the Meschede Hospital, West Germany, revealed that a patient had been admitted in January with what was believed to be typhoid fever. He was kept isolated, but by January 16, his symptoms were diagnosed as smallpox. Seventeen patients eventually came down with smallpox 7–17 days after the first victim was admitted. It was determined the disease was carried through corridors and up stairwells to other floors, and even up the outer façade of the building. Twenty people were eventually infected, with four deaths.[6]

The danger of outbreaks was brought home to the world in the winter of 1972, when Yugoslavia reported a discovery of smallpox to WHO headquarters in Geneva. Considering Yugoslavia sent approximately 700,000 workers to Germany, Italy, Switzerland, France and Sweden, the danger became instantly apparent. In March, when the presence of smallpox became widely known, tourists from the Continent immediately cancelled their Easter travel plans, potentially crippling the economy. Additionally, the potential for disaster loomed for Germany, which had just spent $600 million preparing for the Olympic Games to be held in August.

The outbreak began in the southern province of Kosovo, and was eventually traced to an Albanian Moslem who had returned home from Mecca and Medina, stopping in Baghdad along the way to buy second-hand clothes. Within a month, 75 cases of smallpox were reported, 8 had died and 800 were quarantined. An American team flew into the country, carrying with them 24 automatic vaccination jet injector guns at a cost of $825 each. Within days, it was estimated, 18 million Yugoslavs underwent the procedure and on April 14, WHO announced the last case of smallpox, indicating the outbreak was over.[7]

On January 1, 1971, WHO announced a revised list of quarantinable diseases: smallpox, plague, cholera and yellow fever, while in March, the U.S. Public Health Service modified its regulations, stating, "Although the United States can require evidence of smallpox vaccination from all persons entering the United States, this will only be enforced for those who within the past 14 days have been in countries reporting smallpox. Persons inquiring about immunization requirements should be informed that it is desirable and recommended that they be vaccinated prior to departure." It was further stated that the change was a modification only, "not an elimination of the requirement for proof of immunization against smallpox." Vaccinations were required to be registered on the official certificate and signed by the holder, showing the name of the manufacturer and batch number of the vaccine and validated by the authorized stamp of local health authorities.[8]

On May 14, 1971, the world celebrated the 175th anniversary of the first vaccination against smallpox. At that time, it was estimated that by the end of 1971 only 6 countries in the world would continue to report smallpox. During the first 4 months of 1971, fewer than 14,000 cases were reported to WHO, by 13 countries, over half of which were from Ethiopia, with the rest spread over Africa, Asia, South America and a few in Europe. It was estimated that for the entire year, 25,000 cases would be reported, a substantial decrease from 1967, the first year of the worldwide Smallpox Eradication Program.[9]

The estimate would prove optimistic. As of June 6, 1972, there were 30,763 cases of smallpox reported to WHO, compared to 22,968 the previous year. Rather than seeing it as a setback, Dr. Foege of the CDC considered the increase a result of an improved surveillance system. He cited West Africa as having significantly improved its reporting system and because of it, smallpox was considered eliminated in that part of the world. With the disease no longer a threat in Yugoslavia, areas of concern continued to be Bangladesh, where 3,290 cases had been reported since the reintroduction of smallpox from India in January.[10]

Eradication would not come quickly or easily. In September 1972, the Centers for Disease Control (CDC) indicated a 38 percent increase in smallpox cases around the world. During the first 7½ months of 1972, a total of 47,872 cases were reported to WHO, compared with 34,697 from the same period in 1971.[11] Even so, increasing optimism was spreading through the world health community. The same month the above statistics were given, experts at CDC announced their belief that it was "only a matter of years" before smallpox was eradicated from the world. Already eliminated from the Western Hemisphere, Dr. Donald A. Henderson (formerly of the CDC), in charge of the smallpox eradication program for WHO, predicted it would only require 18 months before the disease was eliminated altogether.

To reach that goal, work needed to be done. During the first 9 months of 1972, there were 35,599 cases of smallpox reported in India, Pakistan, Bangladesh and Nepal. By March 1973, a 2-month epidemic killed thousands in Bangladesh, including 2,500 in Dacca, alone. The *Dacca Morning News* reported 60–70 persons were dying daily, with widespread disease across the fledgling nation, and as many as 5,000 infected. Dr. N. Ward of WHO characterized the disease as being fatal to one-third of those who contracted it and authorities sent 40,000 health workers into service to give vaccinations throughout the country.

Speaking for WHO, Dr. Halfdan Mahler, a 50-year-old Dane who had become head of the organization in July 1973, warned that if the epidemic in India was not controlled within two years, it would pose a serious threat to the rest of Southeast Asia and possibly the world community. The Bihar State in eastern India was pinpointed as being the most infected area and despite massive efforts, by June 1974, between 10,000 and 30,000 fatalities had been reported, making it the worst epidemic in more than half a century. Health authorities reported that some Bihar rivers were polluted with the bodies of smallpox victims, as some Hindus did not follow the custom of cremation out of fear the smallpox goddess, who entered the body along with smallpox, would also be destroyed. Furthermore, village medicine men advised patients to wear magic stones around their necks to ward off disease, promising, "no evil spirits will enter your body."[12]

While WHO authorities were reluctant to comment on reasons behind the epidemic for fear of antagonizing Indian agencies whose cooperation they required, Indian government authorities blamed "serious inadequacies in the Bihar administration's anti-smallpox programs" for some of the problems. Editors of the British publication *Lancet* went further, blaming WHO for "losing ground" by not being sufficiently aggressive in its war on disease.

By June 1974, foreign health experts working in India sharply criticized WHO, declaring that, "By publicly minimizing the scope of the epidemic, the WHO is simply encouraging the Indian government to sit back on its haunches." Dr. Donald A. Henderson of WHO took issue with the comments, denying the current crisis could not be classified as "the worst in recent history" because, "compared to other years, the numbers are not comparable."

Efforts at control were centered around the Tatanagar Railway Station, 150 miles west of Calcutta, where more than 15,000 people passed through a day, carrying smallpox into other areas. Vaccination there was made compulsory and the plan worked well for 3 weeks, until a local official objected to having his family checked for vaccination. By the end of July, massive vaccination drives had made headway in breaking the smallpox cycle.[13]

Tragedy on a smaller scale struck London, where a 23-year-old female technician contracted smallpox while working on a WHO project. A married couple visiting her in the hospital contracted the disease, the woman later dying. This prompted WHO to declare London a "smallpox zone," requiring travelers leaving England to have a valid vaccination certificate. British Airlines reported a massive demand for inoculations. Heathrow Airport was forced to send out an urgent demand for serum as supplies dwindled, while Gatwick authorities indicated only one airline had serum left. Even Westminster Hospital, London, experienced critical shortages because of great demand.[14]

To Vaccinate or Not to Vaccinate

Although smallpox had been eradicated in North America for years, in August 1973, the disease was officially declared "dead" in the Western Hemisphere. Dr. Joseph Millar, director of the Bureau of State Services, CDC, along with doctors from Canada, Venezuela, Portugal and Brazil, comprised a 5-man commission that investigated medical records and performed two weeks of spot examinations. Their research determined that with the success of WHO's eradication program in Brazil, the time had come for a formal announcement.[15]

The news was stunning proof of the success of global cooperation, but it also evoked new discussions on a recent quandary: to continue vaccinating all children as a matter of public health policy or to eliminate the requirement in the face of decreasing need. Two major factors were involved in the decision: the expense of vaccination, which had the potential to cripple budgets of smaller countries, states or communities and the actual danger to susceptible individuals from the vaccine. In the United States, from 1951 to 1970, there were 37 deaths from smallpox, but 100 fatalities were blamed on vaccination; complications were most likely in individuals with blood disorders, eczema and cancer.

In the United States, the CDC had already recommended the elimination of routine vaccinations, with all but four states quickly complying. In October 1971, this and other reports to the surgeon general resulted in the elimination of universally required vaccination. (The order did not pertain to military personnel, who were required to have a smallpox vaccination every 3 years.)[16] By October 1972, fewer than 40 percent of children received vaccination. The abandonment of vaccination for entry into the United States saved Washington $150 million a year in vaccine alone.[17]

Great Britain also discontinued routine vaccinations, although health care professionals, members of the armed forces and travelers visiting countries where the disease was present were required to be vaccinated.[18] In Canada, Health and Social Development minister Laurent L. Desjardins issued a statement in February 1976, advising that "the need for vaccination is virtually nonexistent because smallpox has been virtually eradicated from the world," adding, "It is now considered in Canada that there is more danger to persons vaccinated, especially to children, from the vaccine — which can cause complications — than there is from smallpox itself." The only requirement for vaccination applied to persons who had been in an infected area.[19]

Following WHO's strategy of surveillance and containment in areas where smallpox still existed, efforts were directed at Ethiopia. Teams, including volunteers from the Peace Corps, crossed mountains and valleys, reaching between 800 and 1,500 persons per day. Aiding the cause in another way, the United States contributed $200,000 to WHO to support two helicopters used to reach isolated areas. With an intensive program aimed at "zero smallpox" to run for 3 months, Dr. Mahler asked for additional contributions of $2.2 million to support the anti-smallpox campaign for 1975. With that, he hoped the disease would be wiped out, a result going down in history "as a true public health miracle."[20]

"Smallpox: Point of No Return"

That was the rallying cry of World Health Day, April 7, 1975. With smallpox in Ethiopia expected to reach "nil" by March, and reported cases in Bangladesh and India expected to end within months, the world awaited the end of a scourge that had plagued humans "from time immemorial." Unfortunately, unanticipated outbreaks in Bangladesh in February 1975 threatened to push back the date, although Dr. Henderson predicted, "If we really make a major effort here, then the goal of world eradication will be delayed only a few months."

By April, however, Dr. Stanley O. Forster, WHO director for the country, reported that over 1,500 people had perished since January 1, with fatalities running at 30 percent of those infected. A massive campaign, involving 40,000 workers, achieved "spectacular success," and by May it was hoped that "indigenous" cases would be eradicated in a matter of weeks. By July, headlines read, "India wipes out feared smallpox," which Dr. Henderson called "a fantastic achievement," perhaps "the greatest accomplishment" to date in WHO's global eradication program. Within the week, Indian and WHO officials announced India free from smallpox "for the first time in recorded history."[21]

Dr. Mahler then explained that in two years, an international team of experts would revisit India, with hopes of certifying the country free from smallpox. Should that prove to be the case, it was said, "Two years from now he hopes smallpox will officially be eradicated from the world's landscape." Continuing the good news, at the dawn of 1976 Bangladesh was reported free of smallpox and by April, WHO announced that 15 countries of West Africa (Benin, Gambia, Ghana, Guinea, Guinea-Bissau, Ivory Coast, Liberia, Mali, Mauritania, Niger, Nigeria, Senegal, Sierra Leone, Togo and Upper Volta) were free from smallpox. The only known cases left in the world were in 34 remote villages in Ethiopia; as of May 12, 1975, WHO reported only 45 active cases in these areas.[22]

While medical laboratories around the world began destroying stocks of smallpox virus used to make vaccine to prevent an accidental revival of the disease, a report of smallpox in Somalia was reported by WHO in February 1977. One case of variola minor was reported in Mogadishu, while others were found in a wide area northeast of the capital, covering the Bay, Hiran and lower Shebelle regions, as well as Kenya. By May, Dr. Isao Arita, director of WHO's smallpox eradication program, termed the outbreak "serious" as the number of infected persons reached 280.

Nearly a year after it was believed the last smallpox case had been eliminated, WHO asked for $3.9 million in emergency funds and vaccines to fight the resurgence, calling the epidemic a "considerable danger for adjacent countries." With 3,000 health workers searching villages and vaccinating inhabitants, the outbreak was ended in November 1977.[23]

On Tuesday, December 13, 1977, during a ceremony in Dacca, Bangladesh, the World Health Organization announced that variola major had been completely eradicated except for half a dozen laboratory samples preserved under strict security. The last known case of variola major occurred in 1975. The victim was a 3-year-old girl, Rahima Banu, of Kuralia, on the island of Bhola in the Ganges delta. She recovered from the disease and "for the last two years has made her family quite wealthy by posing for pictures." The last known death was a 10-year-old Somali child who contracted variola minor October 10, 1977. Subsequent reports indicated the last case was Ali Maow Maalin, a 24-year-old cook from Merka, Somalia, on October 26, 1977.[24] The last casualty, however, had yet to be claimed.

The Last Tragedies

In March 1973, a 23-year-old unvaccinated laboratory technician named Ann Algeo was working at the Mycological Research Laboratory at the London School of Hygiene and Tropical Medicine. She was present when a researcher harvested variola grown in eggs, and she unknowingly became infected. After developing symptoms that were not immediately diagnosed as smallpox, she was hospitalized in an open ward, infecting two people visiting a patient in an adjacent bed and a nurse. The nurse survived, but the others became the first smallpox fatalities in Great Britain in over a decade.

A more serious incident occurred in 1978. Janet Parker was a 40-year-old employee of the University of Birmingham Medical School, UK. She had an office and a darkroom one floor above a laboratory where research on live smallpox virus was conducted. Although she had been vaccinated in 1966, on August 11, 1978, she developed a rash, concurrent with headache and muscle pains. On August 24, she was admitted to East Birmingham (later Heartlands) Hospital and diagnosed by Professor Alasdair Geddes and Dr. Thomas Henry Flewett as having variola major. The diagnosis was confirmed the following day by electron microscopy on fluid from her rash and she was transferred to Catherine-de-Barnes, an isolation hospital.

Between the time of exposure and her isolation, Parker came in contact with numerous persons, over 300 of whom were tracked down, vaccinated and quarantined. Only her mother, Hilda Witcomb, contracted smallpox and she recovered. Her father, Frederick Witcomb, became a concurrent victim, dying from cardiac arrest when visiting his daughter in the hospital.

Janet Parker died of smallpox on September 11, 1978, making her the last official victim of the speckled disease that had plagued mankind for so long. Thirteen nations immediately began requiring vaccination certificates from Britons traveling abroad, but after WHO advised against the necessity, four nations dropped the requirement.

The official report, conducted by Professor R.A. Shooter, detailed incidents around the case. In 1977, WHO had informed Dr. Henry Bedson, head of the microbiology department at Birmingham, that his application to become a Smallpox Collaborating Centre had been refused on the grounds there had been several safety violations and on the fact WHO desired to limit the number of laboratories that worked with the virus. On two occasions, the Dangerous Pathogens Advisory Group had inspected Bedson's laboratory and determined facilities fell far short of those required by law and poorly trained technicians were allowed to handle the smallpox virus. Ultimately, however, research was allowed to continue.

Shooter's report also indicated that Bedson misrepresented his smallpox work to WHO authorities, claiming it had declined since 1973, when, in fact, it had risen dramatically as he hurried to finish his studies before the lab was closed. The report also indicated that as 12 years had elapsed between her vaccination and the accident, Parker was not adequately protected from smallpox.

Conclusions of the investigation determined that Parker had probably been infected with a strain of smallpox called "Abid," named after a 3-year-old Pakistani boy who had been an earlier victim, when it was handled on July 24–25, 1978. It was speculated the virus traveled on air currents up a ventilator and service duct or that she may have had face-to-face contact with one of the laboratory workers.

Compounding the tragedy, Professor Henry Bedson committed suicide on September 6 by slitting his throat at his home. He died at the Queen Elizabeth II Hospital in Birmingham, leaving a note saying, "I am sorry to have misplaced the trust which so many of my friends and colleagues have placed in me and my work." The contamination tragedies were debated in Parliament and led to changes in how dangerous pathogens were handled in the United Kingdom. The university was prosecuted by the Health and Safety Executive for breach of health and safety legislation, but it was exonerated in court.[25]

39

Stamping Out Smallpox

> In terms of magnitude of importance, in terms of saving lives, I would rate the eradication of smallpox to the discovery of penicillin and polio vaccine.— Dr. Donald Hopkins, assistant operations director, Centers for Disease Control.[1]

The January 13, 1978, edition of *Weekly Epidemiological Record of the World Health Organization,* Geneva, declared, "As of 10 January, 1978, the organization has recorded zero smallpox incidence worldwide for the last 11 weeks, since a patient was reported from Somalia with onset of rash on 26 October, 1977."

To celebrate the victory, on March 31, 1978, the United Nations issued four commemorative stamps to mark the Global Eradication of Smallpox. A 13-cent and a 31-cent stamp were issued for use at the United Nations New York headquarters. Designed by H. Auchli of Switzerland, the stamps pictured a smallpox virus seen through a microscope. The virus was black against a pink and blue background. An 80-centime and a 1.10 franc-stamp were issued for use at the U.N.'s European offices in Geneva. Designed by E. Weishoff of Israel, they were four-colored, showing two globes. One globe was smallpox-infected, the other smallpox-free. (For collectors' information, sheets of 50 stamps were vertical.)

Cacheted first-day covers were created for the World Federation of United Nations Associations (WFUNA) by Irish painter Liam Roberts. His acrylic work showed four semi-abstract human figures stamping out smallpox with viruses at their feet. The African nations of Togo and Lesotho also issued commemoratives: Togo issued four stamps with two designs, one of Edward Jenner and the other showing children being vaccinated. Lesotho's stamps depicted Dr. Jenner vaccinating a child and a native child against a WHO emblem.[2]

On October 26, 1978, the United Nations and the national Centers for Disease Control both planned special observations to celebrate the passage of one year without a documented case of smallpox. One interesting adjunct was the publication by the CDC of an offer already in place by WHO: a $1,000 reward for the discovery of a documented case of smallpox anywhere in the world during the next year. In 1979, if no cases were reported, WHO planned to declare field (as opposed to laboratory) smallpox eradicated from the Earth.

During the eradication years beginning in 1967, the CDC sent more than 300 doctors and technicians overseas who administered over 1 billion vaccinations at a cost to the world of $250 million and to the United States alone of $27 million. With the virtual elimination of the disease, the CDC smallpox quarantine service was reduced from 200 to 20 and Dr. J. Michael Land, head of the bureau, announced that the name would eventually be changed and the remaining personnel shifted to other international programs.

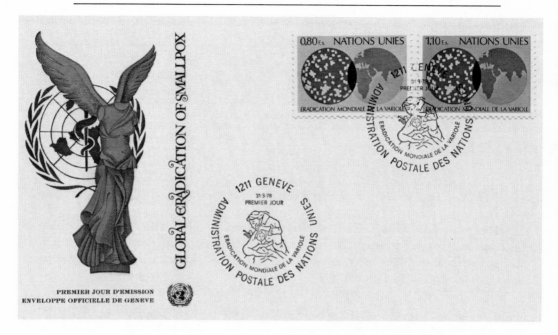

First Day Cover, Geneva, 1978 (from the authors' collection).

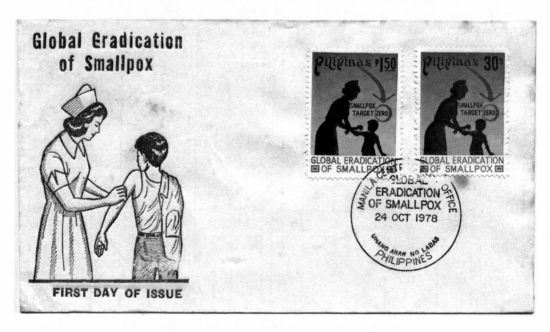

First Day Cover, Philippines, 1978 (from the authors' collection).

For their work in fighting smallpox, Dr. William Foege, then director of the CDC, and Dr. Donald Henderson, then on the staff of Johns Hopkins, were presented the J.C. Wilson Award for Achievement in International Affairs, accompanied by $10,000 prizes.[3] Henderson was also awarded the Albert Schweitzer International Prize for Medicine in 1985.[4]

The Last Great Risk

With the elimination of field smallpox, the greatest risk of reemergence was posed by laboratory accidents. In 1975, at least 75 labs possessed infective variola. Recognizing potential danger, WHO officials began prompting lab authorities to destroy their stock or ship them to central locations, recommending that only centers in Atlanta, London, Moscow, Japan and the Netherlands keep the virus. Researchers complied and by 1977, only 18 labs reported retention of smallpox.[5]

Fear of laboratory accidents and the greater threat of germ warfare against an entirely unvaccinated global population prompted world health authorities to suggest the idea of utterly destroying all remaining smallpox virus. This was not an easy decision to make, nor did the scientific community unanimously support it. Dr. Bernard Dixon, writing in *New Scientist* magazine, argued that in future years researchers might need the variola microbe in the fight against other diseases:

> Sooner of later we may have special need of it to help us in fighting disease and for other practical purposes. And the complex structure of even such a minuscule life form as this ... could never be rebuilt in the laboratory. The end product of millions of years of organic evolution is totally unique.
>
> Within a few decades, with the disappearance of both smallpox vaccination and the disease itself, all traces of immunity in the world population will have disappeared. The prospect in such a situation of the accidental (or indeed conscious) release of smallpox virus into a totally vulnerable community is horrifying.
>
> There is, of course, no disagreement about the need to retain stocks of vaccina (the virus used in preparing smallpox vaccine) in the foreseeable future.
>
> What we can be certain about is that, as time passes, the dangers inherent in such decisions will increase remorselessly.[6]

Two years later, despite WHO's desire to limit the number of laboratories retaining repositories of smallpox virus to four, 15 labs were believed to hold the virus. Three were in the United States: at the CDC in Atlanta, the U.S. Army Research Institute of Infectious Diseases (which specialized in developing techniques for handling biological warfare) and the American Type Culture Collection, a nonprofit scientific group. The Walter Reed Army Institute of Research voluntarily gave up its stockpile in early 1978.

Under the WHO plan, only the CDC would keep its specimens, taken from the last known major outbreaks in India and Bangladesh in 1976. The virus was kept in freezers at 94°F below zero. The freezers were constantly bathed with ultraviolet light strong enough to kill any microbes that escaped. Workers entering the lab must have been vaccinated against smallpox and every garment worn was sterilized before reuse. Workers were also required to shower thoroughly and blow their noses when leaving the lab. This step was necessary to ensure that germs that may have thawed, escaped and withstood the ultraviolent light did not leave the room in the workers' nasal cavities.[7]

The Pentagon resisted the idea to remove stock from the Army Research Institute, citing concerns that a two-year period was insufficient to prove smallpox had been eliminated. The Department of Defense further stated that vaccination was still a requirement for the military and that "the decision to eliminate smallpox vaccination for civilians may be premature at this time."

In addition to military concerns, Karl Western, chief of communicable diseases for WHO's Pan American office, noted that "the pride of laboratory directors" might be a bigger factor in limiting the number of laboratories holding smallpox virus. Likening them to "string savers" or stamp collectors, he said they were reluctant to break up a complete set. WHO received better compliance with laboratories in Brazil and Peru, which voluntarily destroyed their smallpox viruses or transferred them to other countries, leaving only two South American labs in the Western Hemisphere outside the United States known to store smallpox.[8]

Fear of a different type arose in March 1979, when 12 ampules of infectious smallpox were discovered by accident at the California State Department of Health Services while workers were cataloging the lab's stock, leaving open the question as to whether other laboratories unknowingly held stock. The 12 ampules were autoclaved (destroyed by steam heat) but the CDC called on centers worldwide to check their records to be certain no viruses remained.[9] This problem would arise again in October 2001, when "a nearly forgotten stockpile" consisting of 120 liters of smallpox vaccine was discovered at a remote mountainside lab in the Poconos, stored at minus 20°C. Owned by the French company Aventis, the supply, thought to be effective even after 30 years of cold storage, was to be donated to the federal government. Transferred from the Swiftwater, PA, laboratory to an undisclosed location, it was believed to be worth about $150 million and contain enough to vaccinate 85 million people.[10]

The debate over what to do with the last remaining active smallpox virus continues to the present day (2012). Despite WHO's pronouncement on May 18, 1980, that smallpox had been completely eradicated, isolated reports continued to make headlines. In 1980, an Italian engineer from Milan was said to have contracted it.[11] A 1983 photo of a girl under the heading "Smallpox Strikes Again" appeared in Patna, capital of Bihar State, India[12] and WHO reported 21 cases of suspected cases in 1984.[13] All were determined to be chicken pox or other diseases.

Monkeypox and AIDS

After the discovery of "whitepox" (monkeypox) found in apparently healthy monkeys, Dr. Charles Rondle, senior lecturer in medical microbiology at the London School of Hygiene and Tropical Medicine, warned that "if there are dormant or latent smallpox viruses, then an animal reservoir of smallpox does exist. If the smallpox viruses can be reactivated, the whole eradication program is in jeopardy."

In 1979, Professor Keith Dumbell of St. Mary's Hospital, London, remarked that as a variation of smallpox had been found in monkeys, cattle and mice, a mutation might make the animal virus dangerous to humans.[14] In light of the monkeypox discovery, the CDC agreed that "we should keep sample viruses for the foreseeable future. Now that smallpox is gone, we're finding other pox viruses that we didn't see before. It is essential to be able to differentiate between these." The center emphasized that after 1980, smallpox virus would be authorized only at the CDC, at St. Mary's Hospital, London, the National Institute of Health, Tokyo, and Moscow's Laboratory of Smallpox Prophylaxis.[15]

Between February 1996 and October 1997, there were 551 cases of monkeypox reported in the Congo, with the resulting death of 10 children. The disease caused fever, breathing problems, horrific blistering and scarring on the face and hands, but was not considered as contagious as smallpox. WHO spokesman David Heymann reported that it was not believed the disease would spread over a wider area. He added that there was no present need to reintroduce smallpox vaccination that had proven effective against monkeypox, but was phased out when smallpox was declared eradicated in 1980. A further argument against vaccination was that it could be deadly to persons suffering from AIDS, which was widespread in much of Africa.[16]

In 1987, Daniel Zagury of the University of Paris injected himself with an experimental Acquired Immune Deficiency Syndrome (AIDS) vaccine, created from a smallpox vaccine genetically engineered to include fragments of the AIDS virus. The vaccine "produced immunity to two very different strains of the virus," reported Dr. Robert Gallo of the National Cancer Institute.[17] The following year, the *Manitoba Gazette Reporter* (February 3, 1988) questioned whether the global smallpox eradication program had "activated a latent AIDS virus," also spread through the reuse of vaccination needles. A consultant to WHO told the *London Times,* "I believe the smallpox vaccine theory is the explanation to the explosion of AIDS." David McConkey, author of the article, noted this may be a "silver lining" in words similar to those used to describe smallpox victims two hundred years ago: "Many people would like to blame AIDS on someone else — foreigners or those who live different lifestyles. Some even believe that AIDS is a punishment from God. But if research shows that the smallpox vaccine was the spark which ignited the AIDS fire, then the 'blame' suddenly would shift from 'them' (especially homosexuals) to 'us.'"

Interestingly, in 1989, a strain of virus used in Europe as a smallpox vaccine was suggested as a preventive of rabies.[18]

The Circuitous Route Back to Germ Warfare

We go from silver lining to depressing familiarity. In the debate on whether to destroy the last remaining smallpox viruses, the question of smallpox use in germ warfare surfaced repeatedly. In a 1987 editorial, one author wrote, "There's another scary reason why some scientists want to keep the virus on ice. They say it is better for the superpowers to keep their stocks of smallpox virus aboveboard and in sight rather than risk the possibility of some country's keeping secret stocks for use in biological warfare."[19]

Although smallpox is not considered an ideal biological weapon, the threat of its being released on an unvaccinated world raised unmitigated fears. In a 1998 article for the *New England Journal of Medicine,* Drs. Donald Henderson and Joel Breman (National Institutes of Health) wrote that the short supply of vaccine against smallpox would make any outbreak "catastrophic," as facilities for making vaccine had been dismantled or converted to other uses. They recommended that WHO "call on all countries to destroy immediately all stocks" as a message that the use of the virus "would be the most reprehensible of crimes." They added, "The threat posed by the possible use of smallpox as a terrorist weapon is genuine." They estimated about 1 in 4 people who contracted smallpox would die of it."[20]

President Nixon dismantled the large U.S. biological weapons program in 1969, permitting, by treaty, only defensive research. Dr. Henderson noted that the destruction of the Soviet Union's stockpile of smallpox had never been verified. Graham Pearson, former head of the Porton Down Center, which housed Britain's dismantled bioweapons program, expressed his own concern, remarking, "Russia worries me. It is a big problem."[21]

September 11, 2001, changed the landscape and direction of American fears, summoning new fears of biological warfare. The Centers for Disease Control and Prevention quickly put together a plan, outlining step-by-step directions for state health workers in case of a biological attack on American soil. With 15.4 million doses of smallpox vaccine on hand, Homeland Security director Tom Ridge stated that the federal government proposed to buy an additional 300 million.[22] By November, President George W. Bush's administration announced it had signed a contract with a British pharmaceutical company to manufacture 155 million doses of smallpox vaccine, to be delivered by the end of 2002. This action by the United States "led to a lot of confusion about what's appropriate and what should be done in Canada," causing that country to draft a contingency plan to immunize front-line workers.[23]

Writing from the heart, an editorialist for the *Post-Standard* (NY), October 25, 2001, made this observation of the possible threat: "That such a scenario is even within the bounds of the imagination is a sad commentary on humanity. If the day ever arises when forces of hatred and violence use this virus as a weapon, it will signal a terrifying step backward in human evolution."

The same month, WHO reported it was preparing for possible new outbreaks of small-pox as a result of terrorism. Dr. David Heymann, executive director for communicable dis-eases at WHO, remarked that the unpredictability of smallpox could have a "boomerang effect," infecting many of the same people in whose name the terrorists said they were fight-ing, a scenario that raised this question: "Would Osama bin Laden's al-Qaida network unleash a disease that could end up killing millions of Muslims?"

In January 2002, President Bush proposed a $3.7 million increase for the National Institutes of Health, $1.5 million of which was to go toward bioterrorism research.[24]

While research conducted by Jeffrey Frelinger at the University of North Carolina, Chapel Hill, revealed that the immune cells of people vaccinated against smallpox decades ago still reacted strongly to a related virus, suggesting "resistance is waning, but not rapidly,"[25] fear levels remained high. Elisa Harris, a biological weapons expert on the National Security Council under President Bill Clinton, remarked, "It's highly possible Iraq retains stocks of the smallpox virus (from that outbreak) into the '80s and '90s and beyond." The CIA believed that four other nations other than the U.S. possessed samples of smallpox — Iraq, North Korea, Russia and France.[26]

On December 13, 2002, President Bush announced that up to 500,000 health care responders would be vaccinated nationwide as early as late January 2003. Two problems immediately arose: cost and health problems. The Onondaga County Health Department estimated it would cost more than $475,000 — or $792 per person — to comply with the first phase of Bush's plan, with money coming out of reductions in county public health programs. In Pennsylvania, the state's largest health care union, District 1199P of the Service Employee's International Union, advised its members to refuse the vaccine until better safe-guards were in place.

A study by Dr. Perry Smith and Hwa-Gan Chang of the New York Health Department and Dr. Kent Sepkowitz of the Memorial Sloan-Kettering Cancer Center, New York, pub-lished in the *Journal of the American Medical Association,* confirmed the risks involved, stating that more than half New York's hospitalized patients would be at increased risk of compli-cations with smallpox-vaccinated health care workers. By March 2003, two medical per-sonnel had died from heart attacks after receiving vaccination and 17 more suffered cardiac problems. Plans to compensate people disabled or killed by smallpox vaccine reached Capitol Hill, where Democrats and Republicans argued over appropriate financial awards. A deal was eventually reached, offering a lump sum of $262,100 to families of those who were killed by the vaccine.[27]

A U.S. Military study, 2003, reported that out of 230,734 military personnel vaccinated between December 2002 and mid–March 2003, eighteen cases of myopericarditis (inflammation of the pericardium and cardiac muscular wall)[28] were found, more than triple the expected rate of nonvaccinated people, translating into at least 78 cases per million. Updated figures showed 37 cases out of 450,293 military personnel vaccinated through May 28, 2003 — a similar rate. The study cited other side effects, including soreness at the injection site, fever and muscle aches, widespread skin rash and, rarely, encephalitis, or inflammation of the brain. Fewer than 40,000 civilians received the vaccine and by the summer of 2003, the program had all but ceased.[29]

Exercise Global Mercury, 2003, a multi-country exercise simulation (Canada, France, Germany, Italy, Japan, Mexico, Britain and the U.S.) of biological warfare, proved the difficulty of coordination. Conducted over a 56-hour period between September 8 and 10, the test revolved around terrorists infecting themselves with smallpox then traveling to different parts of the globe to spread the disease. Computer servers crashed, language barriers proved insurmountable and it was discovered no one had a master list of emergency contact numbers. While the outcome was less than expected, a WHO spokesman called the test "a useful exercise."

Coordinated with WHO and the Global Health Security Initiative, member nations of the G-8 group of major industrialized nations called for stockpiling of smallpox vaccines. In 2005, preceded by major sales to the U.S. and Canada, the Cangene Corporation agreed to supply the United Kingdom with vaccinia immune globulin (VIG) estimated to be worth $17 million. (Cangene's VIG was the only product approved by the U.S. Food and Drug Administration; Cangene's agent outside the U.S. and Israel was Acambis, a British pharmaceutical company.) A year later, the U.S. Army Medical Research Institute of Infectious Diseases at Fort Detrick signed a cooperative Research and Development Agreement with Chimerix, Inc., a biotechnological company developing orally available, targeted medicines to treat smallpox and other viral infections.

In 2006, U.S. cabinet secretaries participated in a drill that simulated a smallpox attack by terrorists. Dana Perion, White House spokesperson, noted, "While there's a concern, we do not have any concern that a smallpox attack is imminent."[30]

The Biodiversity Debate

Kenneth Herrmann, deputy director of the CDC's viral diseases division, remarked in 1991 that "the inertia of politics" was responsible for delaying the destruction of the smallpox virus, adding, "There's no scientific justification at this point to retain the viable smallpox virus." In a poll taken by WHO two years earlier, only 5 of 58 leading virologists supported keeping the virus. "No strong case can be made" for maintaining the stockpiles, WHO continued, as the virus itself served no useful purpose, as vaccines were made from the related virus vaccinia.[31]

A different case was argued in 1978, when an editorialist for the *New York Times* wrote:

> The issue of what to do with the virus is one that science has never had to face before, even though many species of living things have become extinct and mankind, inadvertently, may have killed off more than a few. There simply has never before been a case in which the extermination of a living species has been both possible and seriously considered as a deliberate policy. The issue is both practical and philosophical. It is also a matter of public health and of ecology....

There is also, among some persons, a deep reluctance to destroy the last sample of the virus simply because it represents a living species and is irreplaceable. No one would suggest total eradication of the Bengal tiger or even the king cobra, for instance, so why put a different standard on the smallpox virus?[32]

In 1993, armed with newly developed maps of the molecular structure of the virus, WHO called for simultaneous destruction of the remaining stocks by New Year's Eve. The continuing rift among scientists prompted WHO to delay its order — but not for long. Headlines in 1994 read, "Smallpox's final day scheduled," "Smallpox on death row" and "Smallpox will be burned like a witch at the stake."

Yet again, the date was postponed. WHO set June 30, 1999, as the new date of destruction, and again it retreated. By 2002, the 32-member executive board of the United Nations Health Agency endorsed a recommendation by WHO director-general Gro Harlem Brundtland to delay setting a final date, requiring a report on the progress of research, to be submitted in 2011.[33]

Research progressed quickly. In 2002, army scientists from Fort Detrick succeeded in fatally injecting monkeys with smallpox at the federal Centers for Disease Control and Prevention in Atlanta. Experts reported this was the first time animals had developed smallpox that resembled the disease found in humans. Previously, scientists had been able to inject only animals with similar diseases, such as monkeypox and mousepox. A team at Virginia's George Mason University reported in 2003 that in a laboratory setting, blood cells from people vaccinated against smallpox were four times less likely to become infected with AIDS. Basing their study on a published report in 1999 that showed a relative of smallpox, myxoma poxvirus, used the same cellular doorway — the CCR5 receptor — to infect a cell the same way AIDS did, Ken Alibek, a bioterrorism and smallpox expert at George Mason, reported, "Our outcomes are very encouraging."

In 2003, Jeffrey Schlom of the National Cancer Institute genetically engineered vaccinia into a milder form and added a gene that made an antigen, or marker, called CEA. Adding three immune-boosting molecules to a booster (Tricom), he found that the altered smallpox plus boosters increased survival of half the patients in the first small trial at Georgetown University. A year later, Dr. Sharon Frey, St. Louis University, was named principal investigator to test the next generation of smallpox vaccine, where two new investigational vaccines, manufactured by Acambis, Inc., were to be compared with existing smallpox vaccine, known as Dryvax.

Based in part on these studies, WHO sent "shock waves" through the scientific community in 2004 by announcing its recommendation that researchers be permitted to conduct genetic-engineering experiments with the smallpox virus with the idea that this was the best way to combat a disease considered a leading bioterrorism threat. The idea was supported by Dr. Ken Alibek (a former top scientist in the Soviet biological weapons program who defected in 1992), who responded, "It's absolutely the right decision." He added that the "bad guys" already knew how to genetically engineer smallpox to render current vaccines useless, "so why prohibit legitimate researchers to do research for protection."[34]

The End Without an End

After two days of heated debate, the 193-nation World Health Assembly issued a statement May 24, 2011, postponing the destruction of variola for three more years. A spokesman stated that the decision-making assembly of WHO "strongly reaffirmed the decision of previous assemblies that the remaining stock of smallpox (variola) virus should be destroyed when crucial research based on the virus has been completed."

The topic will come up for review in 2014, but whatever decision they reach is not legally binding. The actual political and ethical issues ultimately rest in the hands of authorities from the United States and Russia.[35]

It is perhaps fitting that the continuation or eradication of a unique living organism that has plagued mankind for centuries should hinge on the complex fabric of human nature: curiosity, fear and morality. What we decide will mark us well.

A Glossary of Medicine
in the 19th Century

Acne A small pimple or hard tubercle on the face; a small pustule or pimple, which arises usually about the time the body is in full vigor.

Alastrim (Variola minor) A mild form of smallpox. In the early 20th century great debates raged over whether this disease was actually smallpox or a separate disease probably related to chicken pox. Improper diagnoses led to delays in proper treatment and generalized vaccination. Also known as Kaffir pox, Cuban itch, milkpox, pseudosmallpox, pseudovariola, West Indian smallpox and whitepox.

Amaas A term used in Africa during the end of the 19th century and into the 20th century, referring to a mild form of smallpox, later identified as variola minor.

American form of smallpox In the 1920s this term referred to the mild (typically non-lethal) form of smallpox then present in most states.

"Anatomist's snuff-box" A site on the dorsum (back or posterior) of the hand at the base of the metacarpal of the thumb, the site used for inoculation in Africa, Afghanistan and Persia in the 19th century.

Antisepsis From the late 19th century: destroying microbes and septic matter.

Arm-to-arm transfer The passage of lymph from an infected person to a healthy one for the purpose of conveying immunity by inducing a mild form of smallpox (variation) or cowpox (vaccination). The virus was inserted under the skin, usually on an ivory point or needle.

Asafetida (*Ferula Asafoetida*); an ill-smelling plant gum used in cases of hysteria, dyspepsia, flatulent colics and as an anti-spasmodic.

Asiatic or European smallpox In the 1920s these two terms were used to indicate a virulent or deadly form of smallpox as opposed to the mild form then found in most states.

Black measles A severe form of measles characterized by dark, hemorrhagic eruptions accompanied by headache, chills and fever and a characteristic rash on arms, legs and trunk; occasionally mistaken for smallpox.

Black smallpox Confluent smallpox; the most virulent form of the disease.

Black snake root (*Cimicifuga*) The root of the *Actaea racemosa* plant grown in the United States; used by the Indians as a treatment for rheumatism and later by local physicians for the same illness as well as dropsy and hysteria. It was considered a mild diuretic and moderately toxic. When taken as a tea, it was considered a preventive of smallpox. Also known as "black cohosh."

"Buying pocks"   An 18th century English expression used when children were sent to buy smallpox crusts for use in variolation, or who were "bedded" with other children suffering from the malady in the hope that by bringing them in contact with those stricken they would contract a mild form of the disease.

Caustic   An agent that destroys living tissue.

Chicken pox   *see*   **Varicella.**

Collodion   A sticky substance that hardens in the air, used to cover wounds.

Confluent smallpox   A condition of smallpox where the pustules run into one another; the prognosis is typically grave

Cosmo-telluric influence   A term used in the late 1870s and 1880s signifying "laws of Nature" (from *Daily Gleaner*, March 17, 1879).

Croton   The name of the ricinus or castor-oil berry, from its likeness to a tick; *Oleum tiglii*; a fixed oil expressed from the seed of the croton plant, *Croton tiglium*. Croton oil was used as a powerful cathartic. The oil has a yellowish hue, a faint small and an acrimonious taste. It is toxic to the skin, heart, muscle and gastrointestinal tract.

"Cuban itch"   Slang used by lay people when describing a mild, eruptive disease denied by them as being smallpox but actually representing the true disease. This term came into use after the Spanish-American War. Other slang terms originating around the same time were "Spanish itch," "Georgia bumps" (used primarily in the South) and "Bold chicken pox." When in denial over the diagnosis, a vague expression, "the disease," was commonly employed (*see also* Alastrim).

Diphtheria   A bacterial infection identified by the formation of a membrane over the tonsils and soft palate. The word came into general use around 1859. Before that, the disease was commonly diagnosed as sore throat, croup or scarlatina.

Dysentery   Frequent stools, chiefly mucus, sometimes mixed with blood, combined with loss of appetite and nausea. It was known to occur chiefly in summer and autumn and was "often occasioned by much moisture succeeding quickly intense heat, or great drought, whereby the perspiration was suddenly checked, affecting the intestines. It was believed to be caused by unwholesome and putrid food and by noxious exhalations and vapors. A peculiar disposition of the atmosphere seems often to predispose, or give rise, to dysentery, in which case it prevails epidemically."

Eczema   An itchy, red skin rash that weeps or oozes serum.

Encephalitis   An inflammation of the brain most commonly caused by viruses and as an after-effect of systemic viral diseases such as influenza, measles and chicken pox. In the 1920s it was thought the disease could be brought on by smallpox vaccination.

Endemic   Referring to a disease that occurs continuously, or is ever-present in sections of the population, as opposed to an epidemic that has a fixed beginning and end.

Engrafting   *see*   **Variolation.**

Epidemic   The introduction of smallpox into a populated area not previously, or not recently, afflicted with an outbreak. With few individuals unprotected by immunity (either natural or acquired), people of all ages were susceptible.

Epidemic years   The recurrence of smallpox after a period of years, typically when the adult population had already developed immunity from previous outbreaks. Thus, a disproportionate number of children who had not been previously exposed or vaccinated were the primary victims.

Equination   Vaccination by horsepox, or "grease."

Erysipelas   A skin infection commonly mistaken for smallpox. It caused a red rash on the face or legs, accompanied by fever, chills, swelling and tenderness. When matter was mistakenly taken from patients with this condition and used for vaccination, the outcome could prove fatal.

Erythema   Reddening of the skin due to irritation, injury or inflammation.

"Fall fever"   A term used in the United States to designate typhoid fever because it typically came with the fall of the leaves.

Fluor albus   A white secretion from the vagina, similar to that of gonorrhea.

Flux   The common term for "dysentery," meaning loose stools. Often used in conjunction with "bloody," indicating diarrhea tinged with blood (*see also* Dysentery).

Fomites   A term mostly applied to substances imbued with contagion.

Gaselier   Lighting; similar to a chandelier, but utilizing gas for fuel.

Glycerol   (Glycerine) A trihydric alcohol present in chemical combinations of all fats. It was used to stabilize smallpox vaccine virus and at the same time served as an antibacterial preservative, while allowing for the maintenance of the vaccine in liquid form, ensuring long term survival of the active virus. Dr. Copeman's use of glycerol came into popular use in the 1890s.

"God's sickness"   A term used by the Russian peasantry who believed that if a child died of smallpox it would immediately become an angel.

Golden root   (*hydrastis canadenis*) A woodland plant primarily found in the Ohio Valley. Also known as goldenseal, orange root, yellow root and yellow puccoon, it was used as an astringent, anti-inflammatory and mild laxative in the treatment of various diseases, including smallpox. It was introduced into Great Britain in 1760 and by 1850 had become a major export to Europe where it was known as Warnera.

Grease   *see*   **Horsepox.**

Horsepox   A rare disease of horses similar to cowpox. Commonly called "Grease," it involved an inflammation of the fetlocks. Virus obtained from grease was occasionally used in place of cowpox with success, particularly in France.

Immunity, acquired   Protection from smallpox by either variolation or vaccination.

Immunity, natural   Protection from smallpox by an individual having undergone and survived an attack of the disease acquired by exposure through air or incidental contact with an infected person.

Impetigo   A skin disease characterized by red, hard, dry prurient spots on the face, neck, and sometimes over the whole body, occasionally mistaken for smallpox.

Inoculation   The transfer of dead or weakened disease matter into the body of another with the aim of producing immunity from that disease. The material injected is referred to as the vaccine. In the early 18th century in Great Britain, the term "inoculating the smallpox" or "inoculation" referred to the transfer of smallpox matter from one human into the skin of another (*see also* Vaccine inoculation).

Insertion   An 18th century term for variolation

Insufflation   The Chinese method of variolation, achieved by inhaling dried smallpox scabs to induce a mild form of the disease.

Jenner Mode   Vaccination with kine or cowpox matter (lymph).

Kaffir pox   *see*   Alastrim.

Kine pox   Cowpox.

Lazaretto   Another word for quarantine.

Lichen   A disease with extensive eruptions of papulae affecting adults connected with internal disorder, usually terminating in scurf; recurrent, not contagious.

Lockjaw   Tetanus.

Lymph   Pustule matter (smallpox).

Lymphangitis   Inflammation of lymph vessels.

Marasmus   Emaciation, or a generalized wasting of the body caused by malnutrition.

Miasma   Pollution, corruption or defilement generally; contagion. The application of any poisonous matter to the body, applied to those very subtle particles arising from putrid substances that communicate disease. Miasma was produced by moist vegetable and animal matter in the stage of decomposition. The virus of plague, smallpox, measles, chincough (pertussis; whooping cough), cynanche maligna, scarlet fever, and typhus were believed to be transmitted through the poisoned atmosphere.

Multiple pressure method   A technique recommended in the 1930s for vaccination, using the side of a needle to make up to 30 small pricks in an area ⅛" large before adding a drop of vaccine.

Nettles/ Nettle rash   An eruption on the skin producing little elevations, often appearing instantaneously, especially if the skin is scratched. They continue for an hour or two and then typically disappear; so called for its similarity to the rash caused by the sting of the common nettle plant.

Nidus   Focus of infection.

Nosology   The doctrine of the names of diseases; the arrangement of diseases into classes, orders, genera, species, etc.

Nuisance   Used in the mid–19th century to indicate a troublesome or dangerous situation or person (smallpox sufferers were considered "nuisances") as opposed to the more common usage of "annoying."

Opthalmia   Severe irritation of the eye.

Orange root   (*Hydrastis canadenis*) A herb also known as goldenseal, orange root, yellow root and yellow puccoon. It was used topically and internally to modify symptoms of smallpox. It was a woodland plant found in the Ohio Valley during the 19th century, and Native Americans used it for a variety of medical conditions. The herb was introduced into Great Britain in 1760 where it was known as Warnera. By 1850 it had become an important export from the United States to Europe.

Orthopoxvirus   The genus under which variola, vaccinia, cowpox, monkeypox, Ectromelia, camelpox, taterapox, raccoonpox and Uasin Gishu disease are included.

Overlaid   Expression primarily used when compiling statistics, indicating two or more disease processes were involved in causing a fatality; for example, if a patient suffered from pneumonia and smallpox, with both contributing to the death, they were considered to be overlaid.

Pesthouse   The name given to a quarantine area, usually for smallpox victims.

Phenol   A crystalline derived from the distillation of coal tar, dangerous because of its rapid corrosive action on tissues. Phenol was used to prepare the skin before injections in the early part of the 20th century and was later developed for use to accelerate the lowering of bacterial counts in active vaccinia vaccine.

Phlogogenic Producing inflammation; antophlogistic, meaning to reduce inflammation.

Phthisis A wasting away; pulmonary tuberculosis/consumption.

Pitts/Pitting Smallpox scars; also spelled "pits."

Plague A term in general use during the 1800s to indicate any disease of epidemic proportions.

"Points" The common term for doses of vaccine; derived from the fact vaccine was administered from the point of a lancet or sharp object.

"Points" (2) Used at the turn of the 20th century in England to indicate an area where vaccination was performed: "there should be vaccination in several points" as proof of success.

"Portuguese disease" Slang for syphilis.

Pratique A French nautical word meaning "freedom from quarantine."

Prurigo A chronic skin disease marked by papules.

Purified virus Concentrated lymph possessing a crystal clear appearance as opposed to clarified (contaminated) lymph.

Pustule A small pimple on the skin usually the size of a peppercorn.

"Queen's mark" An expression used on the Caribbean Inlands in the early 20th century in reference to the vaccination scar.

Roentgen rays Better known as X-rays, discovered by Wilhelm Konrad Roentgen (1845–1923), a German physicist. He won the Nobel Prize in physics in 1901.

Scarifier An instrument used to vaccinate containing one or more ivory points.

Scarlatina Scarlet fever; an acute contagious disease characterized by pharyngitis and a pimply red rash, followed by fever and chills, abdominal pain and malaise. Typically a disease of children, the tonsils become swollen and the tongue turns from what is characterized as a "white strawberry" color to that of a "red strawberry."

Scotch fiddle The itch. A vulgar expression of the 17th–19th centuries typically associated with diseases of the genitalia.

Scrofula (aka "the king's evil") Characterized by hard, indolent tumors, particularly found in the neck, behind the ears and under the chin, which degenerate into ulcers from which a curdled white matter is discharged. Nineteenth century clinicians considered it a hereditary disease of children that was seldom fatal but very debilitating. Modern science has identified it as a form of extrapulmonary tuberculosis.

Scurf Small exfoliations of the cuticle, which takes place after some eruptions on the skin, a new cuticle being formed underneath during the exfoliation.

Seed The material used for inoculating the vaccinifer. This was the second stage in obtaining vaccine lymph (20th century).

Sloughing Separation of dead from living tissue as in an ulceration.

Titre/titer A standard of strength.

Transplantation An 18th century English term for variolation, derived from the horticultural process of inserting a bud into a plant.

Typhoid fever A severe infectious disease marked by fever and septicemia caused by salmonella, transmitted through contaminated human waste and oral secretions. Patients experience a rash followed by abdominal pain, marked fever, GI ulcers and shock with frequent damage to the liver and spleen. In rare cases a recovered person may become a carrier.

Unprotected person   A person who has not been vaccinated.

Vaccination, primary   This refers to the first time a person was vaccinated.

Vaccine inoculation   A term used early in the 1800s to distinguish the Jenner Method of injecting matter taken from infected cows from the earlier method of transferring matter from human to human.

Vaccine lymph   The clarified suspension obtained from the vaccine pulp. This was the fourth stage in obtaining vaccine lymph. Clarification removed the denser debris from the procedure but remained a milky color due to the presence of cells and bacteria.

Vaccine pulp   The material reaped from scarified skin of the vaccinifer. This was the third stage in obtaining vaccine lymph.

Vaccine/vaccination   The term originally referred only to smallpox. It came into wide use in the 19th century after Dr. Edward Jenner developed the cowpox vaccine as a means of preventing smallpox by introducing disease matter derived from cows into humans. While providing immunity from smallpox, it did not make the recipient a carrier of the disease.

Vaccinia   (Variola vaccinia) Another term for cowpox in the 19th century; at the turn of the 20th century it was defined as "smallpox robbed of its virulence or attenuated by its passage through the resistant tissues of the cow through successive generations of animals."

Vaccinifer   The animal from which vaccine was produced. The inoculation of an animal was the first stage in the process of obtaining lymph in the 19th and early 20th centuries (*see also* Seed; Vaccine lymph; Vaccine pulp).

Varicella   Chicken pox; sometimes called variola spuria because it resembled smallpox. In the U.S. the disease was also known as waterpox, glasspox, sheep-pox and crystal-pox because of a resemblance of the blisters to the substances mentioned. The varicella-zoster virus is not related to smallpox.

Variolation   A method of protection from smallpox by introducing matter from an infected human smallpox blister into the body of a healthy person, either by inhalation or through a small open wound. The procedure created a mild form of the disease; upon recovery, the individual would then be immune from a full-blown attack. Practiced by various cultures around the world for centuries, variolation posed a grave risk to those who had not undergone the operation, as those who had become unwitting carriers were capable of infecting others and starting epidemics. "Variolation" and "inoculation" were used interchangeably. Other terms used in the 18th century were "engrafting," "small-pox inoculation," "insertion," and "transplantation," derived from agricultural vocabulary.

Variolinum   An oral vaccine developed by homoeopathists as a substitute for bovine vaccine virus. The question regarding acceptance of this method raged in courts throughout the early 20th century.

Varioloid, Variola   A term originating in England in 1818, used in reference to a phenomenon believed to occur when smallpox operated on human systems in which some change had previously been produced by vaccination. For some time it was believed to be a mutant or new form of smallpox. Also, "smallpox after vaccination," or a mild form of the disease contracted by vaccinated persons.

Vesicular   The development of small blisters.

Walking smallpox   A term used to describe smallpox victims not ill enough to be confined to bed.

Warnera *see* **Golden root.**

Wart pox   A quasi-medical term used in the 1920s to refer to the "most mild" form of smallpox.

Weep/to weep   The oozing of the vaccine lymph after the scab was removed.

White plague   An early 20th century term for tuberculosis.

Yaws   (Framboesia) A skin disease caused by a spirochaete, *Treponema pertenus,* thought to originate in Africa, closely resembling smallpox in appearance but of a non-fatal nature, although often producing chronic, deforming and incapacitating lesions. In the early 1900s medical authorities believed yaws was transmitted to the United States by contact with Malay nations. In the 20th century, long-acting penicillin provided a cure.

Zymotic   Related to or produced by fermentation. Used in the 19th century to refer to epidemic, endemic and contagious diseases, coming into general use around 1848.

Chapter Notes

Preface

1. The *Key West Citizen,* September 30, 1932.

Chapter 1

1. Lettsom, John Coakley, "Observations on the Cow Pox," *European Magazine,* London, February 1, 1802.
2. Hooper, Robert, *Lexicon Medicum, or Medical Dictionary* (New York: Harper & Brothers, 1842, pages not numbered) (hereinafter cited as *Lexicon*).
3. Fenner, F., Henderson, D.A., Arita, I., Jezek, Z., Ladnyi, I.D., "Smallpox and Its Eradication" (Geneva: World Health Organization, 1988), chapter 2, pp. 215, 229 (hereinafter cited as "WHO").
4. *New York Evening Post,* reprinted in the *Daily Milwaukee News,* February 16, 1865.
5. WHO, chapter 2, pp. 72–75.
6. "What Is Smallpox?," Health-cares.net, http://skin-care.healthcares.net/smallpox.php.
7. *Atlanta Constitution,* reprinted in the *Kane Republican* (PA), May 4, 1894.
8. WHO, chapter 2, p. 119.
9. *Times and Gazette* (WI), August 2, 1884.
10. WHO, chapter 2, p. 210.
11. WHO, chapter 2, p. 210; Best, M., Neuhauser, D., Slavin, L., "Heroes and Martyrs of Quality and Safety," *Qual Saf Health Care* (2004), 82–83.
12. "Ayurveda," http://en.wikipedia.org/wiki/Ayurveda.
13. WHO, Chapter 5, p. 211.
14. WHO, Chapter 7, pp. 211, 214.
15. *Marble Rock Journal,* January 16, 1902.
16. WHO, Chapter 7, pp. 225–226.
17. Ibid., 226–227.
18. Ibid., 225.
19. WHO, Chapter 5, pp. 233–235.
20. Ibid., 214–215.
21. Ibid., 214–229.
22. William Black (M.D.), *Observations, Medical and Political, on the Small Pox,* 8 vol., 2nd ed. (London: 1781) (from *European Magazine,* London, March 1, 1805).
23. *Marble Rock Journal,* January 16, 1902.
24. *Logansport Daily Journal* (IN), March 7, 1882; see also *Weekly Standard* (NC), March 11, 1863, for a similar history.
25. *Bucks County Gazette* (PA), September 29, 1892.
26. *Iowa Liberal,* November 27, 1878.
27. WHO, Chapter 5, p. 219.
28. Lack, Evonne, "The Story of Smallpox from Variolation to Vaccine," 2010, www.babycenter.com; "Edward Jenner," *World of Microbiology and Immunology,* bookrags.com/biography/edward-jenner-wmi.
29. Letter from J. De Carro, dated Vienna, August 25, published in the *Philosophical Magazine* (London), January 1, 1804.
30. Health-cares.net.
31. Haggard, Howard W., *From Medicine Man to Doctor* (Minneola, NY: Dover, 2004), 220–232.
32. *Eau Claire News* (WI), December 2, 1882.
33. *New York Daily Times,* March 15, 1853.
34. WHO, Chapter 5, p. 228.
35. *Evening Independent* (OH), October 23, 1920.
36. *Wilmington & Delaware Advertiser,* August 31, 1826.

Chapter 2

1. *European Magazine* (London), March 1, 1805.
2. WHO, Chapter 5, p. 219.
3. *The Newes, Published For Satisfaction and Information of the People with Privilege* (London), February 4, 1663.
4. *Protestant Mercury* (London), July 29, 1681.
5. *The Spectator* (London), March 10, 1712.
6. *Monthly Mirror* (London), September 1, 1803.
7. Cohn, David V., "Lady Mary Montagu," http://pryamid.spd.louisville.edu/~eri/fos/lady_mary_montagu.html.
8. *European Magazine* (London), March 1, 1805.
9. Ibid.
10. *Banner of Liberty* (NY), May 16, 1860.
11. WHO, Chapter 6, p. 254.
12. *London Journal,* May 29, 1725.
13. Melville, Lewis, *Lady Mary Wortley Montagu: Her Life and Letters, 1689–1762* (Boston: Indy, 54–55).
14. WHO, Chapter 6, p. 255.
15. *Lloyd's Evening Post* (London), August 20–22, 1781.
16. *Penny London Post,* June 3–6, 1748.
17. *Ipswich Journal,* April 16, May 14, 21, 1757.
18. Ibid., October 1, 1757.
19. Ibid., September 15, 1759.
20. Ibid., December 19, 1761.
21. Van Zwanenberg, David, "The Suttons and the Business of Inoculation," *Medical History* 22 (1978), 71–8219, 78–82, citing Sutton, Robert, *The Inoculator or Suttonian System of Inoculation, Fully Set Forth in a Plain and Familiar Manner.*
22. Van Zwanenberg, "The Suttons," citing Creighton, C., Strutt Papers, *A History of Epidemics in Britain, 1666–1893,* 2 vol., Cambridge: Cambridge University Press, 1894), 609.
23. Ibid.
24. *Lexicon.*
25. Van Zwanenberg, "The Suttons," citing Houlton, R., *Indisputable Facts Relative to the Suttonian Art of Inoculation, with Observations on Its Discovery, Progress, Encouragement, Opposition, etc.* (Dublin: W.G. Jones, 1768).

26. Van Zwanenberg, "The Suttons," citing Houlton, R., "A Sermon on Inoculation," 1766.

27. *Ispwich Journal,* June 21, 1766.

28. Van Zwanenberg, "The Suttons," citing Houlton, *Indisputable Facts.*

29. Ibid., citing Abraham, J.J., *Lettsom, His Life, Times, Friends and Descendents,* (London: Heinemann, 1933).

30. Ibid., citing Houlton, *Indisputable Facts.*

31. *Dublin Journal,* February 18–21, 1769.

32. Ibid., March 7–9, 1769.

33. Ibid., December 9–12, 1769.

34. Ibid., December 14–16, 1769.

35. *European Magazine and London Review,* May 1, 1782.

36. *Dublin Journal,* October 21–24, 1769.

37. Ibid., February 3–6, 1770.

38. *Morning Herald and Daily Advertiser* (London), May 17, 1782.

39. Van Zwanenberg, David, "The Suttons and the Business of Inoculation," Medical History, Vol. 22, 1978, pp. 77–82.

40. *European Magazine,* March 1, 1805.

41. *St. James's Chronicle, or the British Evening-Post,* November 17–20, 1787. The letter from Milan was dated October 24.

42. *Lloyd's Evening Post* (London), August 20–22, 1781.

43. Jenkins, J.S., M.D., FRCP, "The English Inoculator: Jan Ingen-Housz," *Journal of the Royal Society of Medicine* 92 (October, 1999), www.nchi.nlm.gov/pmc/articles/pmcl29398/pdf/jrsomed0004–0046.pdf.

44. "Smallpox Timeline," www.historyofvaccines.org/content/timelines/smallpox.

45. Zwanenberg; Bishop, W.J., "Thomas Dimsdale, M.D., F.R.S. (1712–1800), and the Inoculation of Catherine the Great of Russia," *American Medical Journal* 4, New Series (1932), 321–338.

46. . Jenkins, J.S., M.D., FRCP, "The English Inoculator: Jan Ingen-Housz," *Journal of the Royal Society of Medicine* 92 (October, 1999), www.nchi.nlm.gov/pmc/articles/pmcl29398/pdf/jrsomed0004–0046.pdf.

47. *London Evening-Post,* July 21–23, 1767.

48. *Gentleman's Magazine* (London), February 1, 1783.

49. *London Evening-Post,* January 30–February 1, 1759.

50. Ibid., December 24–27, 1763.

51. Ibid., February 27–March 1, 1753.

52. WHO, Chapter 6, p. 256.

Chapter 3

1. *Monthly Miscellany,* March 1774.

2. *Thatcher's Medical Biography,* vol. 1, p. 43.

3. *European Magazine,* March 1, 1805.

4. WHO, Chapter 5, p. 236.

5. Ibid., 236–237.

6. *Kane Republican* (PA), May 4, 1894, reprinted from the *Atlanta Constitution;* Morton, Henry H., "Smallpox," *Journal of the American Medical Association* 22 (1894).

7. *Portsmouth Herald* (NH), June 24, 1903.

8. Fenn, Elizabeth A., *Pox Americana, The Great Smallpox Epidemic of 1775–82,* (New York: Hill and Wang, 2001), 23–24.

9. WHO, Chapter 5, pp. 238–239.

10. Wilson, Samuel M., "On the Matter of Smallpox," *Magazine of Natural History* 103, no. 9, (September 1994), 64–66.

11. Tandy, Elizabeth C., "Local Quarantine and Inoculation for Smallpox in the American Colonies, 1620–1775," Committee on Dispensary Development, United Hospital Fund, New York City, www.ajph.alphapublications.org/cgil/reprint/13/3/203.pdf, citing Davis, W.T. ed., "Bradford's History of the Plymouth Plantation, 1620–1647," Original Narratives of American History Series, vol. 6, pp. 312–312, http://www.swarthmore.edu/SocSci/bdorseyl/41docs/14-bra.html.

12. Tandy, citing Winthrop, John, "Winthrop's Journal, or a History of New England," ed. J.K. Hosmer, Original Narratives of American History Series, Vol. v, [1]. p. 119.

13. d'Errico, Peter, "Jeffrey Amherst and Smallpox Blankets," http://www.nativeweb.org/pages/legal/amherst/lord_jeff.html: reference: *The Conspiracy of Pontiac and the Indian War after the Conquest of Canada,* vol. 2 (Boston: Little Brown, 1886), 39.

14. d'Errico, citing Long, J. C., "Lord Jeffrey Amherst: A Soldier of the King" (New York: Macmillan, 1933), 186.

15. d'Errico.

16. Berreto, Luis, and Rutty, Christopher J., "Speckled Monster: Canada, Smallpox and Its Eradication," *Canadian Journal of Public Health* 93, no. 4 (2002), 12–25.

17. Pesanmbbee, Michelene E., "When the Earth Shakes: The Cherokee Prophecies of 1811–12," *American Indian Quarterly* 17, no. 3, p. 308.

18. WHO, Chapter 5, p. 238; Berreto and Rutty, "Speckled Monster."

19. Fenn, Elizabeth, "The Great Smallpox Epidemic of 1775–82," *History Today* 53, no. 8 (August 2003), 10–14.

20. "MacKenzie's Travels and Voyages," reprinted in *European Magazine,* September 1, 1802.

21. Ibid.

22. Starna, William A., "The Biological Encounter: Disease and the Idiological Domain," *American Indian Quarterly* 16, no. 4 (1992), 513.

23. Fenn, *History Today.*

24. Dobyns, Henry F., and Euler, Robert C., "Pai Cultural Change," *American Indian Quarterly* 23, no. 3/4 (1999), 151.

25. Starna, "Biological Encounter."

26. Tandy, citing Records of the Town of East Hampton, Long Island, vol. 1, p. 201.

27. Ibid., citing Salem Town Records, Essex Institute Historical Collection, 1913.

28. Ibid., citing Massachusetts Provincial Statutes, 1701–1702, chapter 9.

29. Ibid., citing Massachusetts Provincial Statutes, 1731–1732, chapter 13.

30. Ibid, citing Massachusetts Provincial Statutes, 1764–1765, chapter 12.

31. Ibid., citing South Carolina Provincial Statutes, 1738, chapter 653.

32. Ibid., citing New York Provincial Statutes, 1755, chapter 990.

33. Ibid., citing Huntington, New York Town Records, Vol. 2, p. 512.

34. Tandy, "Local Quarantine."

Chapter 4

1. Farmer, Laurence, M.D., "When Cotton Mather Fought Smallpox," *American Heritage Magazine,* August 1957; excerpt from Cotton Mather's diary, August 24, 1721, http://www.americanheritage.com/articlces/magazine/ah/1957_5_40.shtml.

2. Celebrate Boston: Heroes and Martyrs, "First Inoculation in America," www.celebrateboston.com/first/inoculation.htm.

3. "Cotton Mather," www.nndb.com/people/377/000048233/.

4. "Celebrate Boston: Zabdiel Boylston," *European Magazine*, March 1, 1805.
5. Ibid.
6. Timonius, Dr. Emanuel, and Pylarinus, Jacobus, *Some Account of What Is Said of Inoculating or Transplanting the Small Pox* (Boston: 1721), 2–3.
7. Wilson, "On the Matter of Smallpox."
8. *European Magazine* (London), December 1, 1794.
9. Celebrate Boston, "First Inoculation"; *European Magazine,* March 1, 1805.
10. Timonius.
11. Farmer.
12. *European Magazine* (London), December 1, 1794.
13. Beall, O.T. and Shryock, R.H., *Cotton Mather: First Significant Figure in American Medicine* (Baltimore: Johns Hopkins Press, 1954).

Chapter 5

1. Letter of John Adams to James Warren, Philadelphia, July 24, 1776.
2. Markel, Howard, "Life, Liberty and the Pursuit of Vaccines," February 28, 2011, http://www.nytimes.com/2011/03/01/health/01smallpox.html.
3. Project Staff, "Library Treasures: Benjamin Franklin, Smallpox Pamphleteer," March 19, 2010 http://www.historyof vaccines.org/content/blog/library-treasures-benjamin-franklin-smallpox-pamphleteer.
4. Markel.
5. WHO, Chapter 6, p. 244.
6. Berman, Michele R., M.D., "George Washington, Smallpox, and the American Revolution," www.celebrity-diagnosis.com/2011/george-washington-smallpox-and-the-american-revolution; Fenn, *Pox Americana.*
7. "Smallpox inoculation and quarantine in Colonial America," http://inpropiapersona.com.
8. "Inoculation: Thomas Jefferson," www.monticello.org/site/research-and-collections/inoculation.
9. Berreto.
10. Thompson, Mary V., "George Washington's Mount Vernon: More to dread ... than from the Sword of the Enemy," Mount Vernon Annual Report, 2002, amended 5/16/2001, www.mountvernon.org.
11. Fenn, *History Today.*
12. Thompson.
13. Fenn, *PoxAmericana,* 49–51.
14. Fenn, *History Today.*
15. "Small Pox," *Black Loyalist,* www.blackloyalist.info.new-informationpage; Purdie's *Virginia Gazette,* June 15, 1776.
16. *Black Loyalist*; *Virginia Gazette,* May 31, 1776.
17. *Black Loyalist*; *Virginia Gazette,* July 17, 1776.
18. Thompson.
19. Russell, T. Triplett, and Gott, John K., *Faquier County in the Revolution* (Westminster, MD: Heritage Books, 1977), 177–178.
20. Fenn, *History Today.*
21. Wilentz, Sean, *Andrew Jackson"* (New York: Time Books, Henry Holt, 2005), 16–17.
22. WHO, Chapter 6, p. 246.

Chapter 6

1. Haggard, 229; see also *St. Joseph Herald* (MO), February 5, 1870.
2. Venes, Donald, ed., *Taber's Cyclopedic Medical Dictionary,* 20th ed. (Philadelphia: F.A. Davis, 2001), 115 (hereinafter cited as *Taber's*).

3. "Edward Jenner," http://jennermuseum.com.
4. Ibid.
5. *Lexicon.*
6. WHO, Chapter 6, p. 265.
7. *Lexicon.*
8. WHO, Chapter 2, p. 108.
9. Hammarsten, J.F., Tattersall, W., and J.E. Hammarsten, "Who Discovered Smallpox Vaccination — Edward Jenner or Benjamin Jesty?," discussion notes between Dr. Hammarsten (Atlanta) and Dr. Bean (Galveston); Text from the *American Clinical and CLimatological Association Journal,* 90 (1970), 44–55, http://www.ncbi.nlm.gov/pmc/articles/PMC2279376/?page=11.
10. Ibid.
11. Jenner Museum.
12. WHO, Chapter 7, p. 295.
13. Pearson, George, "A Statement of the Progress in the Vaccine Inoculation and Experiments to Determine Some Important Facts Belonging to the Vaccine Disease," *Philosophical Magazine*, August 1, 1799 (London).
14. WHO, Chapter 6, pp. 246, 252.
15. Jenner, Edward, *An Inquiry into the Causes and Effects of the Variolae Vaccinae* (1798).
16. Jenner Museum.
17. WHO, Chapter 7, pp. 296, 299.
18. Jenner Museum.

Chapter 7

1. Brandon, Isaac, "Address to Dr. Jenner on the Anniversary of his Birth," at the First Annual Festival of the Governors and Friends of the Royal Jennerian Society, May 17, 1803.
2. *London Star,* June 14, 1800.
3. *London Observer,* October 26, 1800.
4. *London Echo,* January 2, 1880.
5. *Philosophical Magazine* (London), January 1, 1801: Professor De Carro to Dr. Pearson, Vienna, October 22, 1800; report of C. Nowell, M.D., Boulogne-fur-Mer, December 3, 1800.
6. *Edinburgh Advertiser,* May 26–May 29, 1801.
7. *Monthly Magazine* (London), August 1, 1802.
8. Berreto, citing McIntyre, John W.R., and Houston, Stuart, "Smallpox and Its Control in Canada," *CMAJ,* August 1, 1902.
9. *Monthly Magazine,* January 20, 1802.
10. *London Times,* September 24, 1801.
11. *Monthly Magazine,* Supplementary Number, January 20, 1802.
12. *The Star,* London, March 15, 1800.
13. *Edinburgh Advertiser,* February 10–13, 1801.
14. "The Three Original Publications on Vaccination by Edward Jenner," *Harvard Classics* 38, no. 4, http://lachlan.bluehaze.com.au/lit/jeff06.html.
15. *Monthly Magazine,* April 1, 1802.
16. *London Courier and Evening Gazette,* January 7, 1802.
17. *Philosophical Magazine,* February 1, 1802.
18. *Repertory of Arts, Manufactures, and Agriculture* (London), November 1, 1802.
19. *Adams Centinel* (PA), January 2, 1805.
20. Ibid., May 4, 1803.
21. "Smallpox Timeline," www.historyofvaccines.org/content/timelines/smallpox; Wilson, 64–66; Cook, S.E., "Smallpox," *Journal of the History of Medicine* (1941).
22. Wilson.
23. *Edinburgh Weekly Journal,* September 15, 1802.

24. *Philosophical Magazine,* January 1, 1804.
25. *Gentleman's Magazine and Historical Chronicle* 74, January 1, 1804.
26. *Edinburgh Weekly Journal,* July 9, 1806.
27. Ibid., May 23, 1804.
28. Jenner Museum.

Chapter 8

1. Leavell, Byrd S., "Thomas Jefferson and Smallpox Vaccination," Department of Medicine, University of Virginia School of Medicine, Charlottesville, VA, citing Dunglison, Robert, "The Autobiographical ANA of Robert Dunglison, M.D.," *Trans. American Philosophical Society* 53, no. 8 (1963), New Series, ed. Samuel X. Radbill, M.D.
2. Leavell.
3. "Benjamin Waterhouse," http://en.wikipedia.org/wiki/Benjamin_Waterhouse.
4. Powell, Alvin, "The Beginning of the End of Smallpox," *Harvard University Gazette,* http://news.harvard.edu/gazette/1999/05.20/waterhouse.html.
5. Ibid.
6. *Providence Impartial Observer* (RI), July 18, 1801, reprinted in the *Waterloo Daily Courier* (IA), May 9, 1902.
7. Leavell, citing Blanton, W.B., *Medicine in Virginia in the Eighteenth Century* (Richmond: Garrett and Massie, 1931), 192–194.
8. *Adams Centinel,* January 2, 1805.
9. Leavell, citing Malone, D., *Jefferson the President: First Term* (Boston: Little-Brown, 1970), 173–174.
10. Leavell.
11. *Adams Centinel,* January 2, 1805.
12. *European Magazine,* February 1, 1802.
13. "Little Turtle," http://en.wikipedia.org/wiki/Little_Turtle.
14. *European Magazine,* April 1, 1802.
15. Ibid., September 1, 1802, letter of John Coakley Lettsom (italics and capitalization in original).

Chapter 9

1. *Adams Centinel* (PA), January 2, 1805.
2. Martin, Henry A., "Jefferson as a Vaccinator," *North Carolina Medical Journal* (January 1881).
3. "Vaccination," *Encyclopaedia Britannica: A Dictionary of Arts, Sciences, and General Literature,* vol. 10, ed. Thomas Spencer Baynes (J.M. Stoddart, 1889), 727.
4. *Monthly Magazine* (London), March 1, 1804.
5. *Encyclopaedia Britannica,* 727.
6. *Daily Star* (NY), http://old.thedailystar.com/news/community/obits/2003/11/ob1104.html.
7. "Vaccination," *Texas State Journal of Medicine* 11 (1916), 243.
8. *New York Daily Times,* March 20, 1857.
9. "Inoculation," www. Monticello.org.
10. *Adams Centinel, May 4, 1803* (italics and capital letters in original).
11. *London Courier and Evening Gazette,* February 28, 1801.
12. Fenn, *Pox Americana,* 41.
13. *Adams Centinel,* January 2, 1805.
14. Ibid., April 27, 1808.
15. "Inoculation," www. Monticello.org.
16. Letter from Thomas Jefferson, http://lachlan.bluehaze.com.au/lit/jeff06.htm.
17. WHO, Chapter 9, pp. 366–367.

Chapter 10

1. *World* (NY), November 5, 1893, the epitaph on Edward Jenner's tomb.
2. *Bell's Weekly Messenger* (London), January 1, 1800.
3. *London Observer,* March 9, 1802.
4. *Adams Centinel* (PA), September 1, 1802 quoting the British House of Commons of June 3, 1802.
5. *London Times,* October 22, 1802.
6. WHO, Chapter 7, p. 293.
7. *British Press, or Morning Literary Advertiser* (London), May 18, 1803; *Gentleman's Magazine* (London), March 1805; *British Press* (London), May 17, 1805.
8. *Edinburgh Weekly Journal,* August 17, 1803.
9. *Edinburgh Weekly Advertiser,* January 1, 1814.
10. *Edinburgh Advertiser,* July 1, 1814; *Daily Wisconsin Patriot,* June 1, 1858.
11. *Edinburgh Advertiser,* April 10, 1818.
12. *Lexicon.*
13. *Torch Light and Public Advertiser* (MD), February 12, 1822.
14. Ibid., February 19, 1822.
15. *Berreto.*
16. *London Courier,* September 13, 1822.
17. *Republic Compiler,* December 19, 1821.
18. "Jenner," www.bookrags.com.
19. Jenner Museum.
20. WHO, Chapter 6, p. 265.
21. *London Times,* February 18, 1823.
22. *Edinburgh Advertiser,* May 9, 1823.
23. WHO, Chapter 7, p. 302.
24. Rolleston (M.D.), J.D., "The Smallpox Pandemic of 1870–1874," November 24, 1933, citing F. Parsons, "Isolation Hospitals," 1914. www.ncbi.nlm.gov/PMC/articles/PMC22.
25. *London New Times,* October 29, 1821.

Chapter 11

1. *Galveston Daily News* (TX), March 15, 1868.
2. *London Courier and Evening Gazette,* October 28, 1801.
3. *London True Sun,* April 29, 1835.
4. "Smallpox," www.historyofvaccines.org/content/timelines/smallpox.
5. *Berkshire County Eagle* (MA), March 22, 1860.
6. *Evans and Ruffy's Farmers' Journal and Agricultural Advertiser* (London), May 17, 1830.
7. *Hagerstown Mail* (MD), September 11, 1829.
8. *London Courier,* September 3, 1830, citing *Welsh's Reminiscences.*
9. *London New Times,* January 12, 1828.
10. *London Courier,* January 10, 1840.
11. *Hagerstown Mail,* December 11, 1840.
12. *Weekly Gazette and Free Press* (WI), January 1, 1864.
13. *Ohio Repository,* September 11, 1829.
14. *London Atlas,* January 5, 1839.
15. *London Evening Star,* February 24, 1843.
16. *Amateur and Working Gardener's Gazette* (London), February 1, 1845.
17. *Churchman's Newspaper* (London), January 24, 1845.
18. "Edward Jenner," www.historylearningsite.co.uk/edward_jenner.htm.
19. *London Atlas,* June 17, 1848.
20. *London Patriot,* January 11, 1849.
21. *London British Banner,* July 3, 1850.
22. *Whitewater Register* (WI), February 27, 1858.
23. Rolleston.

24. *Tallis's London Weekly Paper,* July 23, 1853.
25. *Lloyd's Weekly Newspaper* (London), August 28, 1853.
26. "Vaccination Act," http://en.wikipedia.org/wiki/Vaccination/Vaccination_acts.
27. Rolleston.
28. *London Nonconformist,* January 24, 1855.
29. *Evening Star,* May 23; *London Nonconformist,* April 2, 1856.
30. *Evening Star,* May 23, 1856.
31. *London Nonconformist,* April 2, 1856.
32. Ibid., February 11, 1857.
33. *Patriot,* March 12, 1858.
34. *New York Daily Times,* June 3, 1854.
35. *London Illustrated Times,* September 18, 1858.
36. *London Press,* August 15, 1863.
37. *London Nonconformist,* September 7, 1859.
38. *Evening Star,* September 17, 1859.
39. *Civilian and Gazette* (TX), August 4, 1857.
40. *Berkshire County Eagle* (MA), March 22; *World* (NY), July 19, 1860.
41. *London Penny Newsman and Weekly Advertiser,* July 1, 1860.
42. *Evening Herald,* September 22, 1864.
43. *Patriot,* December 28, 1865.
44. *New York Times,* June 9, 1861.
45. *London Nonconformist,* July 17, 1861.

Chapter 12

1. *Ohio Repository,* February 14, 1822, reprinting news from a North Carolina newspaper.
2. "Constitution of New York Vaccine Institute, 1802," from *Early American Reprints,* Second Series, Fiche 2789.
3. Singla, Rohit K., "Missed Opportunities: The Vaccination Act of 1813," May 1, 1998, www.leda.law.harvard.edu/leda/data/229/rsingla.pdf.
4. "The Introduction of Inoculation into Maryland Historically Considered," Address of J.R. Quinan, M.D., Baltimore, 1883.
5. *Encyclopaedia Britannica,* 727.
6. Singla, citing "The Cow-Pox Act," Smillie, Wilson, *Public Health: Development of Public Health in the United States, 1607–1914* (1955), 31.
7. Ibid., citing James Smith letters, Early American Imprints, Second Series, Fiche 45729.
8. Ibid., citing CPI Conversion Factors, 1996, p. 41, http://www.orst.edu/Dept/poil_sci/sahr/cpi96.htm.
9. Kotar, S.L., and Gessler, J.E., *The Steamboat Era: A History of Fulton's Folly on American Rivers* (Jefferson, NC: McFarland, 2009), 198.
10. Singla, citing Smith, Two Letters, 3, p. 41; *Encyclopaedia Britannica,* 727.
11. Ibid., citing Smith, Two Letters; Of Senate of Pennsylvania, 1809–1810, p. 42.
12. Ibid, citing James Smith, Prospectus of a Permanent National Vaccine Institution 2 (1818), microfilmed on Early American Imprints, Second Series, Fiche 45728, 19, p. 42.
13. Ibid.
14. Ibid, citing Smith Prospectus, 20–21; "An Act for the Free Distribution of Genuine Vaccine Matter, 1814," Virginia Acts, chapter 14.
15. Singla, citing Smith Prospectus, 24.
16. Kotar and Gessler, 244.
17. Singla, citing Smith Report.
18. Ibid, citing Duffy, John, *History of Public Health in New York City* (1968), 248.
19. Ibid., citing "Act for Establishing the *New York* Vac-
cine Institution, 1816 and 1817," *Early American Imprints,* Second Series, Fiche, 38419.
20. Ibid., citing James Smith Memorial 6 (1816), *Early American Imprints,* Second Series, Fiche 38948.
21. Ibid., citing Smith, 1816 Memorial.
22. Singla, 64.
23. Ibid., citing Annals of Congress, 1457 (1816).
24. Ibid, citing Annals of Congress, 1455 (1816); 10 House J.767 (1816), p. 65.
25. Ibid., citing Annals of Congress, 469, 470 (1817), p. 67.
26. Ibid., citing Letter from Frances Le Barron, Surgeon, U.S. Army to Dr. James Smith, November 5, 1816; letter from James Smith to Senator Horsey, January 26, 1821.
27. Ibid., citing H. Doc. No. 19–90, 1826; Letter from Samuel Southard to House Representatives, March 8, 1826; *American State Papers,* Class 6, Naval Affairs, Vol. 2, doc. 301, 1860.
28. Ibid., citing Letter from James Smith to Senator Horsey, 6–7, p. 68.
29. Ibid., citing Annals of Congress, 299 (1818); Archives, Senate Documents, Box iSA-C1, House Bills, p. 58.
30. Ibid., citing Smith Report.
31. Ibid., citing Smith Prospectus, p. 52 (italics added).
32. Ibid., citing Smith Report, 4, p. 62.
33. Ibid.
34. Ibid., citing Smith Prospectus 5–6, P. 69.
35. Ibid.
36. *Ohio Repository,* July 16, 1819 (italics in original).
37. Singla, Smith Report, 2, 7, 11, Abridgement of the Debates of Congress 8 (1820), p. 63.
38. Ibid., citing Letter from James Smith to Senator Lloyd, April 25, 1822, appended to H. Rep. No. 17–48, 1822, pp. 62–63.
39. Singla, 71.
40. Ibid.
41. Ibid., citing the five issues of the *Vaccine Inquirer,* February 1822–June 1824, issued by James Smith, allegedly published by a Society of Physicians in Baltimore, but clearly under Smith's direction. In them, Smith published, unedited, numerous documents associated with the Tarboro Tragedy, hoping to set the record straight.
42. *Torch Light and Public Advertiser* (MD), February 19, 1822.
43. Ibid.
44. Ibid.
45. Singla, citing "The North Carolina Accident," 3 Vaccine Inquirer 111 (1822); open letter from Dr. Ward, February 7, 1822.
46. Ibid., citing 3 Vaccine Inquirer, 143.
47. Ibid., citing Smallpox in the Town of Tarborough, 1 Vaccine Inquirer 111 (1822); letter of Dr. Ward, February 7, 1822.
48. Ibid., citing open letter from Dr. Ward, February 7, 1822.
49. *Torch Light and Public Advertiser,* February 19, 1822; letter of James Smith, Baltimore, January 24, 1822.
50. Singla, citing 39 Annals of Congress, 1638 (1822).
51. *Torch Light and Public Advertiser,* February 12, 1822 (italics in original).
52. Ibid., citing Annals of Congress, 1382 (1822), p. 78.
53. Ibid., citing Letter from James Smith to Senator Lloyd, April 25, 1822.
54. *Torch Light and Public Advertiser,* February 10, 1822.
55. Singla, citing Annals of Congress, 1634 (1822), pp. 80–81.

56. *Ohio Repository,* February 21, 1822, reprinted from the *Genius of Liberty.*
57. Ibid.

Chapter 13

1. *Adams Centinel* (PA), January 11, 1826.
2. *Ohio Repository,* August 22, 1822.
3. Singla, citing James Smith Memorial to Congress (1824), from the *Vaccine Inquirer,* 1824.
4. Ibid., citing Smith, Catechism, 20.
5. Ibid., citing Affidavit of James Smith, 5–7, Smith, Catechism.
6. Ibid., citing H. Rep. No. 18–78, 2 (1824); H. Rep. No. 19–95 (1827).
7. *Torch Light and Public Advertiser,* August 5, 1832, reprinted from the *Olive Branch.*
8. *Star and Adams County Republican Banner* (PA), December 13, 1831, reprinted from the *New York Journal of Commerce.*
9. *Hagerstown Mail* (MD), April 9, 1830 (italics added).
10. *Hagerstown Mail and Washington County Republican Advertiser* (MD), February 18, 1831.
11. *Bangor Daily Whig and Courier,* June 2, 1838.
12. *Republican Compiler* (PA), July 6, 1830.
13. *Hagerstown Mail and Washington County Republican Advertiser,* December 24, 1830.
14. Seaton, Edward Cator, "A Handbook of Vaccination" (London: MacMillan, 1868), http://books.google.com; Rumsey, Henry Wyldbore, "Essays on the State of Medicine," *London Medical Gazette* 23 (Ayer, 423–424; reprnt., New York: Arno, 1977).
15. *Adams Sentinel,* January 21, 1839.
16. Seaton, "Sixth Report of Medical Officer of Privy Council," *A Handbook of Vaccination,* 10.
17. Rumsey (italics in original).
18. Seaton.
19. *New York Daily Times,* February 7, 1853.
20. *Lorain Republican* (OH), May 29, 1844.
21. *Montreal Gazette,* May 3; *Colonial Gazette* (London), June 1, 1844.
22. *Daily Sentinel and Gazette* (WI), August 29, 1846.
23. *Taber's,* 735.
24. *Huron Reflector* (OH), January 29, 1850.
25. *Tri-Weekly Galveston News,* March 27, 1856.
26. *Civilian and Gazette* (TX), May 5, 1857.
27. *Sheboygan Journal* (WI), March 19, April 2, 1857.
28. *Fort Wayne Sentinel* (IN), July 11, 1857.

Chapter 14

1. *Alton Observer* (IL), March 15, 1838.
2. *Republican Compiler* (PA), April 17, 1832.
3. Pearson, J. Diane, "Lewis Cass and the Politics of Disease," *Wicazo Sa Review* 18, no. 2, (Autumn 2003), 9–35.
4. Ibid., citing "Vaccination of the Indians," April 17, 18, 1832, *Gales and Seaton's Register of the Debates of Congress, 1831–1832;* Senate 795–797, Washington, D.C., Historical Documents Institute, 1830.
5. Ibid., citing April 24, 1832, Sen. 834.
6. Ibid., citing Lewis Cass circular, "Indian Vaccination Act Instructions," May 10, 1832.
7. Ibid., citing Lewis Cass, Letter to Major John Dougherty, May 9, 1832 in *Letters Sent by the Office of Indian Affairs, 1824–1881* (Washington, DC: National Archives and Records Administration).

8. Bergen, Evans, *Dictionary of Quotations* (New York: Delacourt, 1968), 345.
9. Pearson, Diane J., citing Kappler, "Treaties Drawn with Indian Nations," *Indian Affairs: Laws and Treaties* 2:139–289.
10. Kotar, *Steamboat Era.*
11. Pearson, Diane J., citing H.R. Schoolcraft, "Schoolcraft's Expedition to Indians of the Northwest," June 6, 1832, from the New American State Papers, Indian Affairs, 4, pp. 269–322; J. Allen, "A Map and Report of Lt. Allen's and H.B. [*sic*] Schoolcraft's Visit to the Northwest Indians in 1832," May 9, 1832.
12. *Huron Reflector,* August 2, 1836.
13. Reprinted in the *Republican Compiler,* March 20, 1838.
14. *Alton Telegraph,* March 14; *Alton Observer,* March 15, 1838, from the *St. Louis Commercial Bulletin.*
15. Pearson, Diane J., citing Allis, S., *The Dunbar-Allis Letters on the Pawnee,* ed. W. Wedell New York: Garland, 1985), 701.
16. *Bangor Daily Whig and Courier,* July 31, 1838, reprinted from the *St. Louis Republican.*
17. Pearson, J. Diane, "Lewis Cass and the Politics of Disease," Wicazo Sa Review, Vol. 18, No. 2, Autumn 2003, pp. 9–35.
18. *Wisconsin State Journal,* July 16, 1853.
19. *Newport Daily News* (RI), June 16; *Prairie Du Chien Patriot* (WI), March 19, 1847; *Wisconsin Tribune,* July 19, 1850; *Weekly Wisconsin,* May 7, July 2 (reprinted from the *St. Louis Republican*); *Sheboygan Lake Journal,* August 20, 1851.
20. *Independent American* (WI), March 17; *Wisconsin State Journal,* May 3, 1854.
21. *Janesville Gazette* (WI), June 16, 1855; *Daily Hawk-Eye and Telegraph* (IA), November 16, 1856; *Sheboygan Journal,* February 5, 1857; *Linn County Register* (IA), June 5, 1858; *Janesville Morning Gazette,* September 9, 1859.
22. *Compiler* (PA), March 7, 1859.

Chapter 15

1. *Janesville Morning Gazette* (WI), July 15, 1857.
2. *Western Times* (WI), July 15, 1857.
3. *Lexicon.*
4. *Adams Sentinel* (PA), August 3, 1846.
5. *New York Daily Times,* July 14, 1854.
6. *New York Times,* June 30, 1859.
7. Ibid.
8. WHO, "The First Ten Years of the World Health Organization," Geneva, 1958, p. 4.
9. *Evolution of International Public Health,* "The International Sanitary Conferences," http://whglibdoc.who.int/Publications/a38153_(Ch1).pdf.
10. "International Public Health Organizations Before WHO," http://ocp.hul.harvard.edu/Contagin.
11. *New York Daily Times,* March 15, 1853.
12. Ibid., April 7, 1857.
13. *Civilian and Gazette* (TX), April 28, 1857.
14. *New York Daily Times,* May 13, 1857.
15. Ibid., May 15, 1857, reprinted from *Philadelphia Evening Journal,* May 14, 1857.
16. *New York Daily Times,* May 16; *Syracuse Daily Courier,* May 18, 1857.
17. *Taber's,* 1303.
18. *New York Daily Times,* February 1, 1853.
19. Ibid., January 9, 1854.
20. Ibid., February 2, 1857.
21. *New York Times,* June 3, 1858.

Chapter 16

1. *New York Times,* September 3, 1858.
2. *New York Daily Times,* May 8, 1857.
3. Ibid., May 16, 1857.
4. Spann, Edward K., *The New Metropolis* (New York: Columbia University Press, 1981), 162.
5. All accounts of the arson, unless specifically indicated, were from the *New York Times,* September 3, 4, 1858.
6. Ibid., September 4, 1858.
7. *Christian Cabinet* (London), December 8, 1858.
8. *Racine Daily Journal* (WI), January 12, 1860.
9. *Boston Daily Globe,* August 19, 1887.
10. *World* (NY) August 14, 1860.
11. *Weekly Chronicle and Register* (London), October 16, 1858.
12. *New York World,* July 20, 1860.
13. *New York Times,* May 17, 25, June 3, 13, 24, 25, 30, July 16, 1859.
14. Ibid., May 25, 1859.
15. Ibid., January 9, 1860.
16. Ibid., March 12, 1860.
17. Ibid., January 28, 1861.
18. *Berkshire County Eagle* (MA), February 23, 1860.
19. *Weekly Gazette and Free Press* (WI), February 10; *Daily Argus and Democrat* (WI), July 9, 16; *Janesville Daily Gazette* (WI), July 9, 1860.
20. *New York World,* September 26; *Daily Argus and Democrat,* November 1, 1860.
21. *Weekly Gazette and Free Press,* August 31, 1860.
22. *Mauston Star* (WI), August 8, 1860.
23. *Daily Argus and Democrat,* September 10, 1860.

Chapter 17

1. *Racine Journal* (WI), May 21, 1896.
2. *London Evening Herald,* February 4, 1863.
3. *London Miner,* May 2, 1863.
4. *London Evening Herald,* May 20, 1863.
5. *London Nonconformist,* April 29; *:London Evening Herald,* April 29, 1863.
6. *New York Times,* March 29, 1861; *Madison County Courier* (IL), November 23, 1865.
7. *London Nonconformist,* February 18, 1863.
8. *London Evening Herald,* September 28, 1864.
9. *Alton Weekly Courier* (IL), December 17, 1857, reprinted from the *Washington Union;* see also the *Indiana Messenger* (PA), November 15, 1871, where a Pennsylvania physician claimed that if administered before pustules appeared, they failed to develop. The idea of curing whooping cough also received public attention in July 1857 when an Atlanta doctor claimed to have incidentally cured that disease after administering vaccination for smallpox (see chapter 13).
10. *Horicon Argus* (WI), March 5, 1858.
11. *Penny Newsman* (London), May 3, 1863 reprinted from the *Scotsman.*
12. *Democratic Expounder and Calhoun County Patriot* (MI), September 29, 1842 reprinted from the *New York Union.*
13. *Dubuque Daily Herald* (IA), November 30, 1871.
14. *Dawson's Fort Wayne Daily Times* (IN), March 25, 1864.
15. *Adams Sentinel* (PA), May 18, 1840.
16. *Waterloo Courier* (IA), March 3, 1870.
17. Reprinted in the *La Crosse Daily Republican* (WI), February 19, 1860.
18. *Lloyd's Weekly Newspaper* (London), May 10, 1863.

Chapter 18

1. *New York World,* December 12, 1860.
2. Ibid.; *Daily People's Press and News* (WI), December 18; *Banner of Liberty* (NY), December 5, 1860.
3. *Grant County Herald* (WI), January 12, 1861.
4. *Janesville Gazette* (WI), March 20, 1866.
5. *Janesville Daily Gazette* (WI), September 2, 1861, reprinted from the *Chicago Journal.*
6. Denney, Robert E., *Civil War Medicine: Care and Comfort of the Wounded* (New York: Sterling, 1994), 10, 60.
7. *Janesville Daily Gazette,* December 10, 1861.
8. *Newport Daily News* (RI), June 13, 1862.
9. *Peninsular News and Advertiser* (DE), November 8, 1861.
10. *Oconto Pioneer* (WI), October 31, 1861.
11. Denney, 62–63.
12. *Janesville Daily Gazette,* January 11, 1865.
13. *Iowa State Register,* May 25, 1864.
14. *New York Times,* June 9, 1861.
15. Ibid., June 17, 1861.
16. Ibid., July 23, 1861.
17. Ibid., August 15, 1861.
18. *Janesville Daily Gazette,* August 6, 1861 reprinted from a special dispatch to the *Chicago Tribune.*
19. *New York Times,* August 8, 1861.
20. Ibid., August 26, 1861.
21. *Marysville Tribune* (OH), November 13, 1861.
22. *Janesville Daily Gazette,* December 10, 1861.
23. *New York Times,* August 26, 1861.
24. *M'Kean Miner* (PA), October 29, 1861.
25. Leech, Margaret, *Reveille in Washington, 1860–1865* (New York: Carroll & Graf, 1941), 215.
26. *Weekly Gazette and Free Press,* February 14, 1862.
27. *Janesville Daily Gazette,* March 27, 1862.
28. *Weekly Gazette and Free Press,* April 18, 1862.
29. *Janesville Daily Gazette,* April 26, 1862.
30. *Athens Messenger* (OH), May 1, 1862.
31. *Janesville Daily Gazette,* August 4, 1862.
32. *London Press,* August 15, 1863.
33. *Adams Sentinel* (PA), June 3, 1862.
34. *New York Times,* July 3, 1862.
35. Ibid., January 3, 1864, letter of George T. Strong dated December 28, 1863.
36. *Adams Sentinel,* September 1, 1863.
37. *Dubuque Democratic Herald* (IA), September 26, 1863.
38. *New York Times,* August 6, 1862.
39. Ibid., January 24, 1862.
40. Ibid., February 1, 1862.
41. *Janesville Daily Gazette,* February 7, 1862 reprinted from the *New York World.*
42. *Peninsular News and Advertiser* (DE), May 2, 1862.
43. *New York Times,* March 8, 1862.
44. Ibid., April 14, 1862.
45. Ibid., February 28, 1862.
46. Ibid., June 5, 1862.
47. Ibid., February 20, 1863.
48. Denney, 66.
49. Ibid., 143.
50. Reprinted in the *Richland County Observer* (WI), January 2, 1863.
51. *Weekly Standard* (NC), January 14, 1863.
52. Ibid., May 13, 1863.
53. *Morning Oregonian,* January 15, 1863.
54. *Janesville Daily Gazette,* February 4, 1863.
55. Leech, 247, 249, 251.
56. *Weekly Standard,* March 4, 1863.
57. Denney, 254.

58. *Lexicon.*
59. *Burlington Weekly Hawk-Eye* (IA), February 14, 1863.
60. *Wisconsin State Journal,* June 10, 1863.
61. *Ripon Weekly Times* (WI), March 27, 1863.
62. *Semi-Weekly Wisconsin,* November 21, 1863.
63. Denney, 236, 238.
64. Ibid., 246.
65. Ibid., 252; *Semi-Weekly Wisconsin,* December 16, 1863.

Chapter 19

1. *Daily Milwaukee News,* February 16, 1865 reprinted from the *New York Evening Post.*
2. Thomas, Benjamin P., *Abraham Lincoln: A Biography* (New York: Alfred A. Knopf, 1952), 403.
3. Leech, 283.
4. *Allen County Democrat* (OH), December 23, 1863.
5. Reprinted in the *Janesville Daily Gazette,* January 19, 1864.
6. Reprinted in the *Galveston Twi-Weekly News,* February 24, 1864.
7. *Janesville Weekly Gazette,* August 5, 1864.
8. Denney, 320.
9. Ibid., 62–63.
10. *Hornellsville Tribune* (NY), May 23, 1867.
11. *New York Times,* January 23, 1865.
12. *Janesville Daily Gazette,* April 18, 1866.
13. *Mason City Globe-Gazette* (IA), September 28, 1943.
14. *Janesville Daily Gazette,* July 15, 1864.
15. *London Evening Herald,* September 27, 1862.
16. *Janesville Daily Gazette,* March 2, 1864.
17. *Democratic Expounder* (MI), December 15, 1864.
18. *Adams Sentinel,* March 21, 1865.
19. *Semi-Weekly Wisconsin,* January 6, 1864.
20. *Cedar Valley Times* (IA), May 26, 1864.
21. *Union* (DE), March 16, 1865.
22. *Democratic Expounder,* June 12, 1864.
23. *New York Times,* June 12, 1864.
24. Ibid., April 18, 1864.
25. Ibid., April 22, 1865.
26. *The Englishman/The Atlas* (London), April 29, 1865.
27. *New York Times,* April 22, 1865.
28. Ibid., January 31, 1865.
29. Ibid., February 3, 1865.
30. Ibid., April 28, 1865.
31. Ibid., April 29, 1865.
32. *Herald and Torch Light* (MD), January 11, 1865.
33. *New York Times,* January 16, 1864.
34. *Semi-Weekly Wisconsin,* January 13, 1866.
35. *New York Times,* January 29, 1872.
36. *Elyria Republican* (OH), August 7; *Daily Journal* (IN), September 18, 1879.
37. *Daily Index* (VA), July 18; *Janesville Daily Courier,* July 20, 1865.
38. *Daily Index,* August 10; *Cedar Falls Gazette,* October 20; *Janesville Gazette,* December 7, 1865.
39. *New York Times,* February 12, 1866.
40. *Burlington Daily Hawk-Eye* (IA), March 23, 1866.
41. *Adams Sentinel,* May 1, 1866.

Chapter 20

1. *London Echo,* April 14, 1870.
2. *London Commonwealth,* July 7, 1866.
3. *London Weekly Chronicle,* December 1, 1866.
4. *New York Times,* March 13, 1867 reprinted from the Legislative Chambers in Paris.

5. WHO, Chapter 7, 296.
6. *Freeport Weekly Journal* (IL), January 24, 1866.
7. *London Nonconformist,* January 31, 1866.
8. *Lloyd's Weekly Newspaper* (London), January 6, 1867.
9. Ibid., January 20, 1867.
10. Rolleston.
11. *London Atlas,* April 27, 1867.
12. *London Nonconformist,* September 29, 1869.
13. *Edinburgh Evening Courant,* December 27, 1869.

Chapter 21

1. *London Echo,* April 1, 1870.
2. Smallman-Raynor, Matthew, and Cliff, Andrew D., "The Geographical Transmission of Smallpox in the Franco-Prussian War: Prisoner of War Camps and Their Impact upon Epidemic Diffusion Processes in the Civil Settlement System of Prussia, 1870–71," http://www.questia.com/reader/printPaginator/176.
3. Rolleston.
4. *New York Herald,* May 31, 1870.
5. *London Echo,* June 14; *Wisconsin State Journal,* June 4, 1870.
6. *Janesville Gazette,* June 29, 1870.
7. *New York Herald,* September 9, 1870.
8. *London Nonconformist,* November 30, 1870.
9. Rolleston, citing Prinzing, F., *Epidemics Resulting from Wars* (London: 1916).
10. *Janesville Gazette,* October 1, 1870.
11. Smallman-Raynor.
12. Reprinted in the *Wisconsin State Journal,* October 21, 1870.
13. Reprinted in the *London Nonconformist,* January 11, 1871.
14. Rolleston.
15. *Decatur Local Review* (IL), July 10, 1873.
16. Edwardes, E.J., *Vaccination and Smallpox in England and Other Countries* (1892), 31–45.
17. Rolleston.
18. *Australian and New Zealand Gazette* (London), May 8, 1869.
19. *Burlington Daily Hawk-Eye* (IA), November 16, 1871.
20. Munk, W., and Marson, J.I., "Smallpox Cases at Highgate Hospital," *Medical Times and Gazette* (London: 1871), vol. 1, p. 70.
21. 36th Annual Rep. Registrar-General's Report (London), 1875, p. 46.
22. Seaton.
23. Rolleston.
24. *Medical Times and Gazette* 1 (1871), 634.
25. Powell, Allan, *The Metropolitan Asylums Board and Its Work, 1867–1930* (1930), 31.
26. *London Echo,* April 14, 1870.
27. *Week's News* (London), February 11, 1871.
28. Metropolitan Asylums Board Minutes, 1872–1873 (London), vi., 262–267.
29. *British Medical Journal,* no. 2 (1879), 895.
30. *Brief: The Week's News* (London), January 31, 1879; Rolleston.
31. *London Echo,* May 25, 1870.
32. Ibid., December 7, 1870.
33. *Wandsworth and Battersea District Times* (London), December 24, 1870.
34. *London Nonconformist,* February 1, 1871.
35. *London Week's News,* February 4, 1871.
36. *London Central Press,* February 6, 1871.
37. *Titusville Morning Herald* (PA), February 6, 1871, reprinted from the *London Times;* see also *London Week's*

News, April 22, 1871, for confirmation on the protection of health care workers by revaccination. The chairman of the Liverpool Health Committee also stated he did not know of a single case of smallpox reccurring after revaccination.

38. *Newport Daily News* (RI), July 20, 1871.
39. *Lloyd's Weekly Newspaper,* April 16, 1871.
40. *Wandsworth and Battersea District Times,* April 22, 1871.
41. *Herald and Torch Light* (MD), March 9, 1870. As an indication of how skeptical the newspaper regarded this "perfect cure," the paragraph was run under an article describing the "Kintolochus Rex," a 25-foot-long prehistoric skeleton, and over a recipe for obtaining the fine brown color so desirable in buckwheat cakes.
42. *Adams Sentinel,* January 30, 1866.
43. *New York Times,* March 4, 1871.
44. *London Weekly News,* October 7, 1871.
45. *London Sun and Central Press,* November 21, 1871.
46. *Lloyd's Weekly Newspaper,* April 30, 1871.
47. *Week's News,* February 18, May 20, July 1, 15, 29, September 30, October 7, December 30; *Lloyd's Weekly Newspaper,* July 23, November 5, 26, December 3, 31, 1871.
48. *Week's News,* March 4, 1871.
49. Rolleston.
50. *Sun and Central Press,* September 5; *Boston Daily Globe,* July 9, 1872.
51. *Week's News,* March 11, 1871.
52. Rolleston.
53. Seaton, E.C., "A Handbook of Vaccination," 1868.
54. Rolleston.

Chapter 22

1. *Waterloo Courier,* March 12, 1868; Dr. Middleditch, writing about himself.
2. *Morning Oregonian,* November 12 & 14, 1870.
3. *Sparta Eagle* (WI), May 1, 1867.
4. *New York Herald,* May 14; *New York Times,* August 1, 1869.
5. *New York Herald,* December 29, 1870.
6. *Alton Weekly Telegraph* (IL), November 24, 1871, reprinted from *New York World.*

Chapter 23

1. *New York Herald,* January 22, 1870.
2. *Morning Oregonian,* December 19, 1868.
3. *Mendocino Herald* (CA), November 20, 1868.
4. *Morning Oregonian,* December 16, 19, 1868.
5. Letter dated January 12, 1869, printed in the *New York Sun.*
6. *Mendocino Herald,* January 15, 1869.
7. *Lafayette Advertiser* (LA), February 6, 1869.
8. *Mountain Democrat* (CA), December 26, 1868.
9. *Fort Wayne Daily Gazette* (IN), January 9, 1869.
10. *Tioga County Agitator* (PA), May 10, 1871.
11. "Goldenseal in Profile," http://b-and-t-world-seeds.com.htm.
12. *Waukesha Freeman* (WI), December 26, 1872.
13. *Galveston Daily News,* January 6, 1869.
14. *Freeport Journal* (IL), February 17, 1869, reprinted from the *New York Sun.*
15. *Mountain Democrat,* March 20, 1869.
16. *New York Herald,* January 22, 1870.
17. Reprinted in the *Waukesha Plaindealer* (WI), February 13, 1872.
18. *Indiana Progress* (PA), February 15, 1872.

19. *New York Times,* July 16, 25, 1871.
20. *Berkshire County Eagle* (MA), June 3, 1859.
21. *Cedar Falls Gazette* (IA), December 22, 1871.
22. *Gettysburg Compiler* (PA), April 19, 1872.
23. *Iowa Liberal,* September 19, 1877; *Huntingdon Journal* (PA), February 22, 1878; *Reno Evening Gazette,* November 1880.
24. *Indiana Weekly Messenger,* May 2, 1888, reprinted from the *Philadelphia Times.*
25. *London Echo,* July 4, 1896.
26. *North China Herald* (Shanghai), October 6, 1893.

Chapter 24

1. *Sparta Eagle* (WI), May 12, 1871.
2. *Defiance Democrat* (OH), January 18, 1873, reprinted from the *Cleveland Plain Dealer.*
3. *Janesville Gazette,* August 24, 1878; *Richwood Gazette* (OH), January 19, 1882.
4. *Davenport Daily Gazette* (IA), July 26, 1879.
5. *Janesville Gazette,* November 24, 1877.
6. *Indiana Progress* (PA), November 16, 1871.
7. *Waukesha Freeman* (WI), May 16, 1872.
8. *Hornellsville Weekly Tribune* (NY), December 12, 1873.
9. *Logansport Weekly Journal* (IN), March 19, 1870.
10. *Edwardsville Intelligencer* (IL), May 23, 1872.
11. *Janesville Gazette,* December 22, 1876.
12. *Oakland Daily Evening Tribune,* August 17, October 31, 1876.
13. Ibid., September 21, 1876.
14. *Galveston Daily News,* September 22, 1876, reprinted from the *Morning Call.*
15. Ibid., April 24, 1877.
16. *Iowa Liberal,* November 27, 1878.
17. *Marysville Tribune* (OH), January 22, 1879, reprinted from the *San Francisco Chronicle.*
18. *Jackson Sentinel* (IA), January 20, 1876.
19. *Nevada State Journal,* August 26, 1876.
20. *Weekly New Mexican,* January 26, 1878.
21. *Helena Independent* (MT), January 26, 1878.
22. *Galveston Daily News,* May 22, July 9, September 4, 14, 1879.
23. *New York Sun,* October 14; *New York Evening Gazette,* October 14, 1879.
24. *Iowa Liberal,* December 10, 1879.

Chapter 25

1. *Biddeford Daily Journal* (ME), December 5, 1885.
2. *Daily Milwaukee News,* January 27, 1869; *Morning Oregonian,* June 8, 1875.
3. *Oakland Daily Evening Tribune* (CA), October 12, 1876.
4. *Manitoba Daily Free Press,* November 30, 1876.
5. Ibid., November 25, 1876.
6. Ibid., Match 5, 1877.
7. *Fitchburg Daily Sentinel* (MA), November 28; *Manitoba Daily Free Press,* November 25, December 8, 1876, March 5, 1877.
8. *Manitoba Daily Free Press,* December 27, 1876.
9. Ibid., March 5, 1878.
10. *Democrat* (NY), May 22; *New York Times,* May 30, 1883; *Manitoba Daily Free Press,* June 14, 1883, March 20, 1884; *Sioux County Herald* (IA), June 28, 1883.
11. *Newark Daily Advocate* (OH), November 22; *New York Times,* November 26, 1884.
12. *Manitoba Daily Free Press,* June 17; *Salt Lake City*

Tribune (UT), August 21; *Syracuse Daily Standard* (NY), August 15, 1885.

13. *New York Times,* August 22, 1885.

14. *Sunday Herald* (NY), September 13, 1885.

15. Berreto.

16. *Dover Weekly Argus* (OH), July 1, 1881, reprinted from the *Chicago Tribune* and carried by numerous newspapers for several years.

17. *Oxford Mirror* (IA), October 2, 1885.

18. Reprinted in the *Morning Review* (IL), October 21, 1885.

19. *Daily Northwestern* (WI), September 30, 1885.

20. *Daily Leader* (WI), October 6; *Morning Review,* October 7, 1885.

21. *Titusville Morning Herald,* September 18, 1885.

22. *New York World,* October 9, 1885.

23. *Indian Journal* (Muskogee, Indian Territory, OK), October 22, 1885.

24. *Fresno Republican* (CA), December 12, 1885.

25. *Manitoba Daily Free Press,* March 15, 1886.

26. *Colonies and India* (London), May 26, 1877.

27. *Week's News* (London), June 15, 1878.

28. Ibid., January 13, 1877.

29. *London Guardian,* May 23, 1877.

30. *London Daily Express,* July 4, 1877.

31. *London Guardian,* April 10, 1878.

32. *Mountain Democrat* (CA), May 24, 1879, reprinted from *The Traveller.*

33. Reprinted in the *Indiana Progress* (PA), November 8, 1877.

34. *London Centaur,* December 13, 1879.

35. *London Brief News and Opinion,* March 26, 1881.

36. Ibid., May 21, 1881.

37. Ibid., September 10, 1880.

38. *Galveston Daily News,* June 23, 1883, reprinted from the *London Times.*

39. *Brief News and Opinion,* May 14, June 8, 25; *Guardian,* October 4, 18, 25, November 1, 15, 1882.

40. *Chelsea Herald* (London), May 31, 1884.

41. *Athens Messenger* (OH), March 4, 1875.

42. *Alton Weekly Telegraph* (IL), May 16, 1873.

43. *Le Mars Daily Sentinel* (IA), May 30, 1884; *Edmonton and Tottenham Weekly* (London), June 5, 1885.

44. *Lloyd's Weekly Newspaper,* March 16, 1884.

45. *Guardian,* June 25, 1884.

46. *New York Times,* December 7; *Chelsea Herald,* July 12; *London Nonconformist and Independent,* September 11, 1884.

47. *Guardian,* January 7, May 20, June 10, 24, 1885.

48. *Huntingdon Journal,* September 12, 1884; *Edmonton and Tottenham Weekly,* February 6, 1885.

49. *London Evening Sentinel,* April 25, 1885, reprinted from the *New York Times.*

50. *New York Times,* March 7, 1886, reprinted from the *London Daily News.*

51. *London Daily Mail,* October 17, 1901.

52. Reprinted in the *Waukesha County Democrat* (WI), October 16, 1875.

Chapter 26

1. *Daily Gleaner* (Jamaica), "Small-Pox: A few Words of Advice to the People of Jamaica," February 24, 1879.

2. *Galveston Daily News,* November 23, 1869; *New York Herald,* July 29, 1870.

3. *New York Times,* July 21; *Galveston Daily News,* September 20, 1878; *Morning Oregonian,* September 6, 1880.

4. *Daily Gleaner,* February 24, 1879.

5. *Boston Daily Globe,* July 21, 1883.

6. *Daily Gleaner,* March 29, 1881.

7. *Logansport Daily Journal* (IN), November 14, 1882.

8. *Daily Gleaner,* February 24, 1879.

9. Ibid., March 17, 1889 (capitalization and italics in original).

10. Ibid., May 10, 1881.

11. WHO, Chapter 7, p. 292.

12. *Daily Gleaner,* September 8, 1881.

13. WHO, Chapter 7, p. 292.

14. *Janesville Gazette,* October 31; *Morning Oregonian,* November 18, 1871; *Daily Republican* (IL), June 18, 1872.

15. *Bangor Daily Whig and Courier* (ME), December 30, 1878.

16. Reprinted in the *Decatur Daily Review,* February 28, 1879.

17. *Racine Daily Herald,* March 13, 1879, reprinted from the *Chicago Inter Ocean;* see also *Bucks County Gazette* (PA), March 20, 1879.

18. *Daily Gleaner,* May 10, 1881.

19. *The Colonies and India,* July 14, 1877.

20. WHO, Chapter 5, p. 241.

21. *Australian and New Zealand Gazette,* September 14, 1878; August 13, 20, October 8, 15, 22, 29, November 5, 26, December 3, 1881, January 21, April 29, July 15, 1882; *The Colonies and India,* September 19, 1884.

22. *Australian and New Zealand Gazette,* January 18, 1875.

23. *The Colonies and India,* August 21, 1880.

24. Reprinted in the *ManChester Guardian;* see *Galveston Daily News,* April 8, 1875.

25. *Daily Free Press* (Winnipeg), March 23, 1875.

26. *Waukesha County Democrat,* May 8, 1875, reprinted from the *Shanghai Gazette.*

27. *Indian Journal* (Indian Territory, OK), November 13, 1879.

28. *North-China Herald* (Shanghai), May 18, 1880, March 29, 1881, May 19, 1882.

29. WHO, Chapter 5, p. 227.

30. *Galveston Daily News,* September 20, 1878.

31. *The Colonies and India,* April 4, 11, 1884.

32. Reprinted in the *Belleville Telescope* (KS), October 9, 1884.

33. *Marion Daily Star* (OH), August 20, 1881.

34. *The Colonies and India,* May 8, 1884.

35. WHO, Chapter 5, pp. 233–235.

36. *The Colonies and India,* February 8, 1879.

37. *Evening Light* (TX), September 28, 1882.

38. *New York Times,* December 31, 1882.

39. *Lowell Weekly Sun* (MA), January 6, 1883; *Decatur Morning Review,* August 26, 1884.

40. WHO, Chapter 6, p. 258.

41. *Alton Weekly Telegraph,* December 20, 1872.

42. *Freeborn County Standard* (MN), March 25, 1880.

43. *Defiance Democrat* (OH), May 11, 1872.

44. *Evening Gazette* (NY), August 2, 1879.

45. *Chester Daily Times* (PA), November 28, 1879, reprinted from the *London Ledger.*

46. *Newport Mercury* (RI), May 20, 1882.

47. *Atlanta Constitution,* August 11, 1882.

48. *San Antonio Light,* August 23, 1883.

49. *Alton Review,* December 5, 1884.

50. *Eau Claire News* (WI), January 2, 1886.

51. *Galveston Daily News,* January 26, 1886.

52. *Atchison Daily Globe* (KS), October 10, 1887.

53. *London Echo,* October 11, 1890.

54. *Indian Journal,* June 5, 1879.

55. *Sioux County Herald,* April 4, 1878.

56. *Galveston Daily News,* August 8, 1878.
57. *Hornellsville Tribune,* February 14, 1879.
58. *Indiana Weekly Messenger,* September 30, 1885.

34. *Edwardsville Intelligencer* (IL), January 16, 1889.
35. *Jackson Sentinel* (IA), September 25, 1884.
36. *Fort Wayne Daily Sentinel,* April 9, 1883.

Chapter 27

1. *Galveston Daily News,* December 3, 1881.
2. *Reno Evening Gazette,* November 9, 1880.
3. *Galveston Daily News,* January 8, 1882; *Fitchburg Sentinel,* May 8, 1883.
4. *Evening Gazette* (IA), May 24, 1883.
5. *Weekly Gazette* (CO), April 2, 1881.
6. *Galveston Daily News,* November 10; *Hopewell Herald* (NJ), November 16; *Helena Independent,* November 18, 1881; *Daily Gazette* (CO), April 21, 1882; *Decatur Weekly Republican,* March 17, 1887.
7. *Janesville Daily Gazette,* January 31, 1881.
8. *Decatur Daily Review,* July 4, 1881.
9. *Atlanta Constitution,* December 8, 1881.
10. *Fitchburg Daily Sentinel* (MA), January 3, 1882.
11. *Ohio Democrat,* January 5, 1882.
12. *Waterloo Courier* (IA), March 1, 1882; *Fort Wayne Daily Gazette,* July 28; *New York Times,* October 13, 1883.
13. *Fort Wayne Sunday Gazette,* March 23, 1884.
14. *Indiana Weekly Messenger* (PA), August 24, 1881; *New York Times,* November 18, 1882.
15. *Galveston Daily News,* January 8, 1882; *Evening Gazette* (NY), February 10, March 8; *Fitchburg Daily Sentinel,* February 17; *Pottsville Review* (IA), February 26; *Chester Daily Times* (PA), February 17, 1881.
16. *Pottsville Review,* January 21; *New York Times,* January 21, 1882.
17. *Burlington Daily Hawk-Eye* (IA), July 9, 1882.
18. *Decatur Morning Review,* September 9, 1884; *Lowell Weekly Sun* (MA), April 8, 1882; *Fitchburg Daily Sentinel,* July 30, 1887; *Decatur Daily Dispatch,* December 31, 1889.
19. *Morning Review* (IL), September 13, 1882; *New York Times,* June 27, 1883.
20. *Fort Wayne Daily Gazette,* January 18; *Helena Independent,* January 20; *Richwood Gazette* (OH), March 2, 1882.
21. *Atchison Globe* (KS), January 30, 1882.
22. *Daily Journal* (IN), April 25; *Fitchburg Sentinel,* March 18, 1882; *Evening Herald* (NY), August 19, 1887; *Stevens Point Daily Journal* (WI), March 3, 1888.
23. *San Antonio Daily Light,* January 25, 1886.
24. *New York World,* November 18, 1885; *Salt Lake City Tribune,* March 9, 1888.
25. *Ohio Democrat,* February 9, 1882; *Dunkirk Observer-Journal* (NY), February 16, 1889; *New York Times,* January 19, 1882.
26. *Burlington Daily Hawk-Eye,* March 8; *Newport Daily News,* January 16, 1882; *New York Times,* April 20, 1889.
27. Wilson.
28. Ibid.
29. *European Magazine,* March 1, 1805, reprinted from Dr. Black, "Observations, Medical and Political, on the Small Pox," with information drawn from Rhazes; Avicenna ("the prince of Arabian philosophers," born in Assena A.D. 978); Gregory Abulpharagius (an Armenian physician, born A.D. 1226) and Zabdiel Boylston (Boston philosopher, born at Brookline, near Boston, 1684).
30. Wilson.
31. *New York Times,* March 9, 1884.
32. *Syracuse Daily Standard,* August 26, 1885.
33. Medical Record, reprinted in the *Stevens Point Daily Journal,* November 21, 1885.

Chapter 28

1. *Racine Daily Journal,* June 14, 1894: extract from the address of President Hibbard at the opening of the American Medical Association held at San Francisco, June 1894.
2. *Logansport Daily Pharos,* June 16, 1892; Bradford *Era* (PA), July 4, 1892; *Logansport Daily Reporter,* June 2, 1893.
3. *Decatur Daily Republican,* July 9, 1892; *Galveston Daily News,* September 3, 1892.
4. *Weekly Gazette and Stockman* (NV), May 4; *Fort Wayne Gazette,* May 17; *New York World,* October 28, 1893.
5. *Waterloo Daily Courier,* May 10; *Warren Ledger,* November 10, 1893.
6. *Lima Times-Democrat* (OH), December 8, 1893.
7. *Manitoba Morning Free Press,* April 25, 1894.
8. *Logansport Daily Journal,* May 13; *Iola Register* (KS), November 2; *Republic County Freeman* (KS), November 1, 1894.
9. *Cedar Rapids Evening Gazette,* September 20; *Iola Register,* March 15, 1895; *Evening Herald* (NY), April 16, 1896.
10. *Cherokee Advocate* (OK), December 8, 1882.
11. *Fitchburg Sentinel,* November 16; *Boston Daily Globe,* November 19, 1891.
12. *San Antonio Daily Light,* November 28, 1893; *Republic County Freeman,* May 17, 1894.
13. *News* (MD), January 8, 1895.
14. *Atlanta Constitution,* October 17, 1897.
15. *Trenton Evening Times* (NJ), October 4, 1898.
16. *Daily Index* (VA), August 21, 1865.
17. *Daily Milwaukee News,* September 1, 1865.
18. *St. Joseph Herald,* October 23; *Daily Milwaukee News,* November 9, 1869; *Wisconsin State Journal,* February 8; *Titusville Morning Herald,* February 21, 1870.
19. *Santa Fe Daily New Mexican,* February 25; *New York Herald,* March 11; *New York Times,* March 11, 14, April 17, 1870; "On This Day in History," http://nativenewsonline.org/history/hist0123.html.
20. *Daily Gazette and Bulletin* (PA), April 20; *Wisconsin State Journal,* June 8, July 12; *Ohio Democrat,* August 26; *Indiana Democrat,* July 28; *Fort Wayne Daily Gazette,* October 14; *Morning Oregonian,* November 15; *Cambridge City Tribune,* December 1, 1870.
21. *Freedom County Standard* (NM), May 18; *Dubuque Daily Herald,* August 10; *Edwardsville Intelligencer,* November 23; *Hagerstown Mail,* November 24, 1871; *Stevens Point Journal,* September 4, 1880; *Hutchinson News,* December 29, 1881; *Burlington Daily Hawk-Eye,* June 24; *Galveston Daily News,* June 27; *Our Brother in Red,* December 1, 1882.
22. *Alton Telegraph,* May 31; *Iowa Postal Card,* June 5; *Logansport Daily Journal* (IN), August 14; *Indian Journal,* April 24, 1884; *Huntingdon Journal,* October 2, 1885; *Manitoba Daily Free Press,* April 26; *Star and Republican Banner* (PA), May 1; *Bradford Era,* October 11, 19; *The Ledger,* October 26, 1888; *Newark Daily Advocate,* August 28, 1890.
23. *Manitoba Daily Free Press,* August 3, 1892.
24. *Daily Gazette* (WI), May 17, 1894.
25. *Weekly Gazette and Stockman* (NV), January 2, 1896.
26. *Weekly Northwestern* (WI), January 8, February 23, 24; *Weekly Wisconsin,* October 30, 1897.
27. *Daily Review* (IL), May 13; *Oakland Tribune,* January 22, 1897.

28. *Lima Daily Times,* November 7, 1892.

29. *Salt Lake City Tribune,* January 27, 1900.

30. *Evening Democrat* (PA), May 16, 1898.

31. *Post-Standard* (NY), April 24, 1899.

32. Reprinted in the *Racine Daily Journal,* June 14, 1894.

33. *Fort Wayne Journal-Gazette,* November 8, 1899.

34. *LeMars Semi-Weekly Sentinel* (IA), March 30, 1893.

Chapter 29

1. *Daily Kennebec Journal* (ME), August 31, 1898.

2. *London Echo,* August 22, 1893; *Lexicon.*

3. *London Echo,* August 9, 1893.

4. *Guardian,* May 31, 1893.

5. Ibid., May 29, 1893.

6. Ibid., April 26, 1893.

7. *London Echo,* April 10; *Guardian,* April 22, 1896.

8. *Church Weekly,* April 17; *London Echo,* April 20, 1896.

9. *Guardian,* April 29, 1896.

10. Ibid., August 19, 26, 1896.

11. *Blackheath Gazette,* September 25, 1896.

12. *Middlesex Courier,* January 25, 1896 (italics in original).

Chapter 30

1. *London Echo,* August 26, 1890.

2. *London Iron,* October 21, 1887.

3. *Bradford Era,* October 14; *Manitoba Free Press,* October 14, 1891, February 10, 1892.

4. *Manitoba Free Press,* July 12, 18, August 1, 11, October 21, 1892; April 26, 1893; November 9, 1897; *Bradford Era,* July 14; *Muskogee Phoenix* (OK), July 21; *Salt Lake Tribune,* August 28, 1892; *Alexis Visitor* (IL), February 16, 1898.

5. *New York Times,* August 2; *Daily Gleaner,* March 23, July 8, 29, August 5, October 25, November 5, 22, December 1, 1886; January 7, July 18, 1887; July 26, 1894; March 25, 1895; August 6, September 19, 1896 (here called the *Tri-Weekly Gleaner*); April 20, October 19, 1898; *The Colonies and India,* December 3, 1886; July 25, 1888; *The World,* April 22, 1887.

6. *Galveston Daily News,* May 26; *Fitchburg Daily Sentinel,* July 29; *Bangor Daily Whig and Courier,* August 10; *Daily Gleaner,* October 26, 1887; *Fort Wayne News,* May 6; *The New Era* (IA), July 1, 1896; *Landmark* (NC), May 18; *Adams County Union* (IA), July 1; *Daily Iowa Capital,* December 8, 1897; *Galveston Daily News,* May 29, 1898.

7. *Pottsville Review* (IA), January 16; *Galveston Daily News,* July 9, 1886; *San Antonio Daily Light,* January 13, 1887; *Cedar Rapids Evening Gazette,* September 24, 1891; *McKean Democrat* (PA), September 9, 1892; *Fort Wayne Gazette,* February 3, 1893.

8. *New York Times,* July 14, August 2, 1886; *Manitoba Daily Free Press,* June 15, 1889; *Logansport Daily Reporter,* August 27; *Indiana Democrat,* December 18; *Centralia Enterprise and Tribune* (WI), December 20, 1890; *Herald and Torch Light,* April 9, 1891.

9. WHO, Chapter 8, p. 358.

10. *Evening Journal* (WI), June 20, 1890.

11. WHO, Chapter 8, p. 358.

12. Stanley, Henry M., *In Darkest Africa, or the Quest, Rescue and Retreat of Emin, Governor of Equatoria,* 2 vol. (New York: Charles Scribner' Sons, 1890), vol. 1, p. 73; vol. 2, pp. 20, 24, 28–29, 31, 34–35.

13. *Church Weekly,* September 9, 1898; *Jackson Sentinel,* June 26, 1890; Westminster Budget (London), September 3, 1897.

14. *Hawaiian Gazette,* April 17, August 4, October 23, 1896; March 15, 1898.

15. "The Report on Sanitary Measures In India, 1890–1891," Army Sanitary Commission, Vol. 24, p. 181; Vol. 18, p. 203.

16. Ibid., Vol. 19–24.

17. *London Echo,* August 5, 1891.

18. Ibid., August 5, 1891; August 18, 21, 1893; July 30, 1896; *The Colonies and India,* September 14, 1895; November 28, 1896; *London Daily Mail,* July 15, 1896.

19. *LeGrand Record* (IA), December 4, 1885; *Van Wert Republican* (OH), August 2, 1888; *North-China Herald,* January 20, March 30, April 7, October 6, 1893; December 28, 1894; *Massilon Independent* (OH), October 13, 1898.

20. *Marion Daily Star* (OH), March 4, 1886; *North-China Herald,* January 27, 1893; *Hawaiian Gazette,* November 20, 1896.

21. WHO, Chapter 8, p. 343.

22. *Atlanta Constitution,* December 16, 1901.

23. *St. Joseph Herald,* September 11, 1886; *London Echo,* August 26, October 11; *Evening Herald* (NY), October 3, 1890; *Hutchinson Daily News,* February 5, 1891; *Fitchburg Daily Sentinel,* June 12, 1897.

24. *Hutchinson News,* December 15, 1891.

25. *Daily Mail* (London), May 23, 1896.

26. *Standard* (VT), May 2, 1894.

27. WHO, Chapter 8, pp. 316, 328.

Chapter 31

1. *Salt Lake City Tribune* (UT), January 27, 1900.

2. Ibid., January 11, 1900.

3. *Lowell Sun* (MA), January 20, 1900.

4. *Muskogee Phoenix* (OK-Indian Territory), January 18, 1900.

5. *Webster City Tribune* (IA), March 9, 1900.

6. *New York Times,* February 5; *Cedar Rapids Evening Gazette,* December 26, 1900.

7. *Syracuse Herald,* May 14, 1909.

8. WHO, Chapter 9, pp. 386–387.

9. *Cedar Rapids Evening Gazette,* June 2, 1900.

10. *Webster City Tribune* (IA), June 15, 1900.

11. *Taber's,* 2364.

12. *Emmet County Republican* (IA), March 28; *Daily Gazette and Bulletin* (PA), April 1; *Newark Advocate* (OH), November 5, 1901; *Washington Post,* May 17, October 29; *Titusville Morning Herald* (PA), February 1, 1905; *Pointer* (IL), February 7, 1908.

13. *Portsmouth Herald* (NH), January 15, 1909.

14. *Dubuque Telegraph-Herald* (IA), December 20, 1901.

15. *Anaconda Standard* (MT), September 4, 1908.

16. *Fort Wayne Journal-Gazette,* October 27, 1909.

17. *New York Times,* January 4, 1901.

18. *Daily Gazette* (WI), January 7; *Post-Standard* (NY), January 15; *Daily News* (MI), January 7, 1901.

19. *Hawaiian Gazette,* April 19, 1901.

20. *Elyria Daily Reporter* (OH), January 10, 1901.

21. *Waukesha Freeman* (WI), January 31, 1901, reprinted from the *Syracuse Palladium.*

22. *New York Times,* December 24, 1900.

23. *Fort Wayne Journal-Gazette,* October 31, 1900.

24. *Cedar Rapids Evening Gazette,* August 28, 1901.

25. *Grand Rapids Tribune,* August 31, 1901.

26. *Marshfield Times* (WI), August 30, 1901.

27. *Salt Lake City Tribune,* September 6, 1901.

28. *Cedar Rapids Evening Gazette,* October 24, November 6, 7, 1901.

29. *Waterloo Daily Courier,* October 18; *Des Moines Daily News,* October 28, 1901.

30. *Cedar Rapids Evening Gazette,* November 6; *Buffalo Center Tribune* (IA), November 15, 1901.

31. *Waterloo Times-Tribune,* December 6, 1901.

32. *Cedar Rapids Evening Gazette,* November 22, 1901.

33. *Marion Register* (IA), September 27; *Cedar Rapids Evening Gazette,* October 2; *Janesville Daily Gazette* (WI), October 9; *Sault News-Record* (MI), October 3; *Ironwood News Record* (MI), October 12; *Marshfield Times* (WI), November 15; *Racine Daily Journal,* October 10; *Narka News* (KS), October 18; *Manitoba Morning Free Press,* November 15, 1901.

34. *Marble Rock Journal* (IA), December 19, 1901.

35. *Indianapolis Star,* October 6, 1923.

36. *Atlanta Constitution,* May 15, 1901.

37. *Washington Post,* February 7, 1906.

38. *Robesonian* (NC), March 1, 1920.

39. *Moberly Weekly Monitor* (MO), August 2, 1923.

40. *Anniston Star* (AL), August 29, 1927; *Lowell Sun,* August 21, 1924, July 18, 1925; *Appleton Post-Crescent* (WI), June 8, 1927; *Evening Independent* (OH), August 31, 1926; *Steubenville Herald-Star* (OH), February 7, 1933.

41. *Anaconda Standard,* December 17, 1900.

42. MacNalty, Sir Arthur Salusbury, K.C.B., "The Prevention of Smallpox: From Edward Jenner to Monckton Copeman," pp. 1–13, presented as the Inaugural Monckton Copeman Lecture, delivered at Apothecaries' Hall, London, March 30, 1967; citation from the Milroy Lectures, "Vaccination — Its Natural History and Pathology," 1898, Chapter IV, January 1968, www.ncbi.nlm.nih.gov/PMC/articles/PMC.

43. WHO, Chapter 7, p. 283.

44. MacNalty.

45. *Weekly Call* (IL), March 3, 1900.

46. WHO, Chapter 8, p. 320.

47. *Manitoba Morning Free Press,* April 26, 1902.

48. *Lima Times Democrat* (OH), March 13, 1905.

49. *Upper Des Moines Republican* (IA), March 19, 1913.

50. *Kingsport Times* (TN), January 23, 1928.

51. *Clovis News-Journal* (NM), December 22, 1950.

Chapter 32

1. *Oelwein Daily Register* (IA), March 27, 1914.

2. *Indiana Weekly Messenger* (PA), October 11, 1905.

3. *News* (MD), January 8, 1905.

4. Youngman, C.W., "Report of the PA Board of Health," March 1, 1901, reprinted from the *Daily Gazette and Bulletin* (PA), April 1, 1901.

5. *Wellsboro Agitator* (PA), January 10, 1906.

6. *Lock Haven Express* (PA), January 4, 1906.

7. *New Castle News* (PA), December 19, 1905.

8. *San Antonio Sunday Light,* January 21, 1906.

9. *Lowell Sun,* May 23, August 9, 1900.

10. *Boston Daily Globe,* September 4, 1900.

11. Anaconda *Standard,* November 25, 1900.

12. Washington *Post,* May 17, 1905.

13. *Weekly Telegram* (WI), July 15, 1904.

14. *Oakland Tribune* (CA), January 5, 1905.

15. *The Courier* (PA), July 24, 1906.

16. Altoona *Mirror,* December 5, 1906.

17. Indiana *Evening Gazette* ((PA), February 1, 1907.

18. Altoona *Mirror,* February 18; Titusville *Morning Herald,* March 23, April 20; Indiana *Evening Gazette,* June 12, 1907.

19. Coshocton *Age,* May 1, 1903.

20. *Cedar Rapids Republican,* February 8, 11, 1902.

21. Carroll *Herald* (IA), February 12, 1902.

22. Denton *Journal* (MD), April 27, 1901.

23. *Daily Kennebec Journal* (ME), November 30, 1901.

24. *Boston Daily Globe,* October 15, 1904.

25. *Lowell Sun,* January 22, 1903.

26. *Semi-Weekly Iowa State Reporter,* February 21; May 6; *Waterloo Daily Courier,* November 7, 1902; *The Daily Times-Tribune* (IA), January 18; *Semi-Weekly Waterloo Courier,* February 23, 1906.

27. *Emporia Gazette* (KS), January 29, reprinted from *Saturday Review; Racine Daily Journal,* June 18; *Waterloo Daily Courier,* July 31, 1909; *Waterloo Evening Courier,* March 15, 1911.

28. *Atlanta Constitution,* April 2; *Brownsville Daily Herald* (TX), April 3; *Hawarden Independent* (IA), June 11, 1903; *Star and Sentinel* (PA), January 25, 1905.

29. *Terril Tribune* (IA), January 30, 1903.

30. *Boston Daily Globe,* January 29, 31, February 10; *New York Times,* February 9, March 10, 1902; Lloyd, James Hendries, ed., *Philadelphia Medical Journal* 9, January–June 1902 (Philadelphia: Philadelphia Medical, 1902).

31. *Trenton Times* (NJ), January 3, 1902.

Chapter 33

1. *Fort Wayne Sentinel,* December 20, 1900.

2. *Post-Standard* (NY), July 10; *New York Times,* October 17, 1902; *Daily Palladium* (MI), January 17, 1903; *Daily Gazette and Bulletin* (PA), June 1, 1904; *Stevens Point Journal* (WI), March 3, 1906; *Morning Herald,* November 8, 1907; *Marshfield Times,* December 20, 1911; *Burlington Hawk-Eye* (IA), March 9, 1915.

3. *Washington Post,* May 17, 1905.

4. *Mills County Tribune* (IA), April 19, 1910, April 28, 1911.

5. *Robesonian,* March 20, 1911.

6. *Landmark* (NC), July 14, 1908; *Weekly Democrat* (MS), August 12, 1909; *Pomery Herald* (IA), June 16, 1910.

7. *Waterloo Weekly Courier,* June 15, 1909.

8. *Middleton Daily Times-Press* (NY), June 28, 1910.

9. *Landmark,* February 11, 1910.

10. *Newport Daily News,* December 24, 1910.

11. *Olean Evening Times* (NY), December 14, 15, 19, 22, 28, 1911; January 16, 25, March 1, 1912; *Middleton Daily Times-Press,* February 11; *Orange County Times-Press* (NY), February 12, 1915; *Olean Evening Herald,* May 22, 1917; *Middleton Daily Times-Press,* February 1, 1918.

12. *La Crosse Tribune* (WI), October 22; *Janesville Daily Gazette,* October 22; *Logansport Pharos-Reporter* (IN), October 22, 1914.

13. Ibid., November 27; *San Antonio Light,* December 9, 1915.

14. *Oakland Tribune,* November 19, 1911; *La Crosse Tribune,* January 7, 1913.

15. *Oakland Tribune,* December 17, 1916.

16. *Chester Times,* December 6, 1911.

17. *Middleton Daily Times-Press,* December 20, 1912.

18. *Titusville Herald,* November 29, 1915.

19. *Alton Evening Telegraph* (IL), April 9, 17, 1918.

20. *Portsmouth Herald* (NH), March 14; *Washington Post,* March 22; *Lima Times-Democrat,* April 12, 1913.

21. *Anaconda Standard,* April 11; *Manitoba Morning Free Press,* April 11, 1913.

22. *Lake Park News* (IA), February 21, 1918.

23. Stevens (M.D.), George M. "Vaccination for Small-

pox: The Three-Point Chisel Method" (Los Angeles: Department of Epidemiology of the Los Angeles City Health Department, 1933), 243–246.

24. "John Nivison Force, Hygiene," Berkley, 1938, http://texts.cdlib.org/view?docId=hb0g50035s&chunk.id=div0005&brand=calisphere&do.

25. *Oakland Tribune,* December 17, 1916.

26. *Coshocton Tribune,* May 7, 1918.

27. *Xenia Daily Gazette* (OH), June 9, 1917.

Chapter 34

1. *Hackney Express and Shoreditch Observer* (London), October 5, 1901.

2. Ibid., January 6, February 2, 1900.

3. *London Daily Mail,* January 20, 1900.

4. *London Echo,* June 21, 1901.

5. *London Daily Mail,* January 13, 1902.

6. *Chicago Daily Herald/Cook County Herald,* February 1, 1902; *Daily Mail,* April 15, 16; *Shoreditch Observer,* January 22, 1910.

7. *London Mercury,* August 30, 1902.

8. *Church Weekly* (London), September 27; *Daily Gleaner* (Jamaica), September 30, 1901.

9. *Church Weekly,* December 13, 1901.

10. *Daily Mail,* December 13, 1901.

11. *Austin Daily Herald* (MN), February 20, 1902; *Iola Daily Register,* June 4, 1913.

12. *Daily Mail,* October 19, 1901.

13. *New York Times,* January 12, 1902.

14. *Daily Mail,* April 8, 1903.

15. WHO, Chapter 8, p. 324.

16. *Daily Mail,* February 3, 1902.

17. *British Medical Journal,* "Vaccination and Exemption in 1908," October 16, 1909.

18. *Daily Mail,* November 6, 1922.

19. *British Medical Journal,* "Vaccination and Exemption in 1908" (October 16, 1909).

20. *Emporia Gazette* (KS), January 29, 1909.

21. *Shoreditch Observer,* January 18, 1908.

22. *Washington Post,* February 25, 1909.

23. *Daily Mail,* April 23, 1908.

24. *Daily Gleaner,* September 7, 1920.

25. *Daily Mail,* October 31, November 1–3, 6–10, 14, 22, December 6, 11, 1922.

26. *Daily Gleaner,* April 10, 1924.

27. "Alastrim," http://medical-dictionary.thefreedictionary.com/alastrim.

28. *Daily Gleaner,* July 18, 27, 1923.

29. *North-China Herald* (Shanghai), August 25; *Daily Gleaner,* September 28, 1923; *Charleston Gazette* (WV), January 12, 1930.

30. *Daily Gleaner,* October 11, 1923.

31. WHO, Chapter 8, p. 324.

32. *Charleston Gazette,* January 13, 1926; *Lethbridge Herald* (Alberta, Canada), January 18; *Daily Gleaner,* August 6, 1927.

33. *Sioux City Journal* (IA), April 17; *North Adams Transcript* (MA), April 17, April 22, 1929.

34. *Manitoba Morning Free Press,* January 21, 1902.

35. *Daily Gazette* (WI), May 24, 1901.

36. *Manitoba Morning Free Press,* October 10, November 15, December 24, 1901; May 7, 1902.

37. Ibid., January 14, 1905; *Lethbridge Herald,* June 24, 1911.

38. *Manitoba Morning Free Press,* December 20, 1912, June 19, 1914.

39. Berreto, 4.

40. *Alaska Citizen,* May 15; *Fairbanks Daily Times,* July 12; *Fairbanks Sunday Times,* July 16, 1911.

41. *La Crosse Tribune and Leader-Press,* November 22, 1919; *Manitoba Free Press,* January 8, 1920, January 21, 1921, January 30, 1924; *North-China Herald,* February 14, 1920; *Lethbridge Daily Herald,* January 25, March 19, 1921; *London Daily Mail,* February 12, 1921; *Steubenville Herald-Star,* May 28, 1924; *Traverse City Record-Eagle,* March 3, 1924.

42. *Manitoba Free Press,* October 27, 1927, March 26, 1930; *Lethbridge Herald,* December 27, 1929.

43. WHO, Chapter 7, pp. 278–280.

44. *Fitchburg Sentinel,* August 18, 1923.

45. WHO, Chapter 8, p. 339.

46. *North-China Herald,* November 26, 1902.

47. Ibid., March 11; May 13, November 4, 1904.

48. Ibid., April 15, May 27, December 16, 1904; March 3, November 10, 1905; January 24, 1908; May 29, July 3, 1909; *Daily Kennebec Journal,* September 8, 1922.

49. *North-China Herald,* September 2, 1911; *London and China Telegraph,* February 12, 1917.

50. *North-China Herald,* December 10, 1921, February 11, December 16, 1922; January 13, October 20, 1923; *Daily Kennebec Journal,* December 27, 1921; *Cook County Herald,* March 14, 1924; *Hammond Times* (IN), June 21, 1939.

51. WHO, Chapter 8, pp. 348–349.

52. Ibid., 344.

53. *Daily Gleaner,* April 10, September 20, October 6, 11, 1902.

54. Ibid., October 11, 1902, reprinted from *London Echo.*

55. Reprinted in the *Daily Gleaner,* May 5, 1903; *Daily Mail,* October 25, 1901.

56. *Daily Gleaner,* March 21, June 30, August 26, 1903.

57. Ibid., October 10, 1903; June 11, September 30, 1904; August 18, 1905; September 7, 1906; February 3, 1911.

58. Ibid., September 29, 1911.

59. Ibid., September 27, October 2, 1920; February 16, September 21, 1921; August 4, September 29, 1922; September 15, 19, October 10, 23, 1923.

60. Ibid., February 10, 12, 22, March 6, 11, April 22, August 20, 1930; May 23, 1939.

61. Ibid., January 12, July 21, 1906; *New York Times,* September 9, 1906.

62. *Daily Gleaner,* March 2, 1915, November 13, 1916; December 3, 1917.

63. Ibid., August 23, 1923.

64. *New York Times,* November 10, 1901; *Oakland Tribune,* June 7, 1902; *Washington Post,* September 17, 1907.

65. *Daily Gleaner,* May 25; Bakersfield *Californian,* July 3, 1916.

66. *Daily Gleaner,* February 25, 1911.

67. Nevada State *Journal,* November 22, 1914.

68. *Daily Gleaner,* October 31, 1919.

69. Ibid., February 16; *Port Arthur News* (TX), April 18, 1929.

70. *Altoona Mirror,* April 29; *Daily Gleaner,* May 27, 1930.

71. *Daily Gleaner,* May 27, 1930.

72. *Lima News,* November 6, 1921.

73. WHO, Chapter 8, pp. 333–335.

74. *San Antonio Light,* January 25, 1916.

75. "From the Front, Vera Cruz, July 3, 1914," *Journal of the American Medical Association* 63 (HighWire Press, 1914); *Bismark Daily Tribune,* September 4, 1914; *Atlanta Constitution,* January 18, 1915; *North Adams Transcript* (MA), September 15, 1917.

76. WHO, Chapter 8, p. 333.

77. *San Antonio Express,* January 23, 1924.

78. *Corsicana Daily Sun* (TX), July 11, 1926; *Billings Gazette* (MT), April 3, 1930.

79. WHO, Chapter 8, p. 333.
80. Ibid, pp. 351, 361.
81. *Daily Mail,* November 1, 1922.
82. WHO, Chapter 8, pp. 358–359.
83. *San Antonio Light,* September 11, 1937.
84. WHO, Chapter 8, p. 361.
85. *Daily Mail,* September 8, 1903.
86. WHO, Chapter 8, p. 361.
87. *Fort Wayne News,* March 30; *Bucks County Gazette,* April 10, 1908; *Pomeroy Herald* (IA), June 16, 1910; *New Castle News* (PA), April 14, 1911.
88. WHO, Chapter 8, p. 346.
89. *Daily Kennebec Journal,* September 8, 1922.
90. *Hawaiian Gazette,* April 19, 1901, March 20, 1903.
91. WHO, Chapter 8, p. 362.
92. *Washington Post,* September 7, 1910.
93. *Daily Mail,* August 29, 1907.
94. *Daily Gleaner,* May 13; *Muskogee Times-Democrat* (OK), May 2, 1913.
95. *Middletown Daily Times-Press* (NY), June 25, 1925.

Chapter 35

1. *Checotah Times* (OK), January 27, 1922.
2. *Boston Sunday Globe,* July 13, 1902.
3. *Emporia Gazette* (KS), January 22, 1904.
4. *Racine Daily Journal,* October 6, 1905.
5. *Galveston Daily News,* March 28, April 8; *Brownsville Herald* (TX), October 23; *Haskell News* (OK), December 3, 1914.
6. *Hutchinson News,* July 11; *Oelwein Daily Register* (IA), July 19, 1914.
7. *Daily News Record* (VA), May 31, 1917.
8. *Waukesha Freeman,* September 24, 1914.
9. *Titusville Herald,* December 22, 1914.
10. *Wellsboro Agitator,* November 7; *Altoona Mirror,* November 1, 1917.
11. *Appleton Post-Crescent,* March 20, 1920.
12. WHO, Chapter 7, pp. 283, 292.
13. *Atlantic News-Telegraph* (IA), January 27, 1928.
14. WHO, Chapter 8, p. 326.
15. *Racine Journal-News,* December 24, 1915.
16. *Landmark,* September 15, 1914.
17. *Brownsville Herald,* June 5, 1914.
18. *Fitchburg Daily Sentinel,* June 10, 1918.
19. WHO, Chapter 8, pp. 321–322, 327.
20. *Capital Times* (WI), March 3, 1921.
21. WHO, Chapter 8, p. 326.
22. Ibid., pp. 359, 361.
23. *Fort Wayne Journal-Gazette,* August 25, 1916.
24. *Hutchinson News,* July 25, 1927.
25. WHO, Chapter 8, p. 326.
26. *Chester Times,* December 29, 1932.
27. *North-China Herald,* December 24, 1926; *San Antonio Light,* February 26, 1929; *Joplin Globe,* March 23, 1932.
28. WHO, Chapter 8, pp. 317, 320–232.
29. *Capital Times,* March 5, 1921.
30. *Daily Northwestern* (WI), July 14, 1924.
31. *Lake Park News* (IA), February 21; *Galveston Daily News,* December 12; *Evening Gazette* (OH), December 30, 1918; *Daily Republican-News* (OH), January 20; *New Castle News,* July 29, 1919; *Corsicana Daily Sun,* January 24; *La Crosse Tribune,* September 22, 1919.
32. Jackson, Charles L., "State Laws on Compulsory Immunization in the United States," *Public Health Reports* 84, no. 9 (September 1969).
33. *Jacobson v. Massachusetts,* 197 U.S., Justia.com,

http://supreme.justia.com/us/197/11/index.html; "*Jacobson v. Massachusetts*— Significance, Compulsory Vaccination Lawful, Court Defers to Legislature, Exemption for Unfit Adult? Impact," http://law.jrank.org/pages/12780/Jacobson-v-Massachusetts.html.
34. *Helena Independent,* February 19, 1927.
35. *Daily Courier* (PA), November 16, 1922.
36. "*Zucht v. King,*" 260 U.S. 174, http://justia.com/us/260/174/.
37. *Janesville Daily Gazette,* November 13, 1922.
38. *Portsmouth Daily Times,* September 24, 25, 1924.
39. *Lebanon Daily News* (PA), August 19, 1924; *Appleton Post-Crescent,* May 12, 1926, December 4, 1928.
40. *Lenox Times-Table* (IA), February 23, 1922, reprinted from the *Journal of Iowa State Medical Society.*
41. *Coshocton Tribune,* January 23; *Mansfield News* (OH), January 25, 1922.
42. *Portsmouth Herald,* January 20, 1923.
43. *Checotah Times,* January 27, 1922.
44. *Decatur Daily Review,* August 29, 1923.
45. WHO, Chapter 7, p. 307.
46. *Chillicothe Constitution* (MO), November 30, 1921.
47. *Mansfield News,* January 29, 1922.
48. *Santa Fe New Mexican,* June 29, 1923.
49. *LeMars Globe-Post* (IA), November 24, 1924.
50. *Salamanca Republican-Press* (NY), February 26, 1926.
51. *Vindicator and Republican* (IA), May 25, 1921.
52. *Ironwood Daily Globe and News Record* (MI), April 5, 1922.
53. *Bismark Times,* March 17, 1921.
54. *Syracuse Herald,* October 1, 1922.
55. *Bridgeport Telegram,* March 15, 16, May 12, 1922.
56. Ibid., January 12, 1922.
57. *Salt Lake City Tribune,* February 13, 1923.
58. *Evening Tribune-Times* (NY), December 17, 1923.
59. *Iola Daily Register,* October 10, 1921.
60. *Stevens Point Daily Journal,* October 21; *Muscatine Journal* (IA), October 23, 1930.

Chapter 36

1. "Evolution of International Public Health," Part I, p. 3, http://whglibdoc.who.int/Publications/a38153_(Ch1).pdf.
2. Ibid.; "Contagion: International Sanitary Conferences," Harvard University Open Library Collections Program, http://ocp.hul.harvard.edu/contagions/sanitaryconferences.hyml.
3. Covenant of the League of Nations, Article XXIII (f), cited in "International Public Health Organizations Before WHO," Chapter 1, p. 5, http://ocp.hul.harvard.edu/(Contagion).
4. *Mansfield News,* May 5, 1910.
5. *San Antonio Sunday Light,* August 24, 1924.
6. *Altoona Mirror,* April 13, 1926.
7. *Lowell Sun,* November 12, 1926; *Altoona Mirror,* April 13, 1926; *Lockhart Post-Register* (TX), November 18, 1926; *Appleton Post-Crescent,* February 9, 1925; *Kingsport Times* (TN), November 21, 1926; *Tipton Daily Tribune* (IN), March 20, 1925.
8. *Kingston Daily Freeman* (NY), May 5, 1925; *Wakefield Advocate* (MI), August 23, 1924; *Daily Northwestern,* December 26, 1925; *Titusville Herald,* January 28, 1927; *Oakland Tribune,* July 15, 1929.
9. *Daily Gleaner,* May 8, 1925; *La Crosse Tribune and Leader-Press,* May 14, 1926; *Lubbock Morning Avalanche* (TX), May 2, 1925; *Helena Independent,* May 20, 1927;

Lawrence Daily Journal-World (KS), April 30, 1925; *Star Journal* (OH), July 18, 1925.

10. *McIntosh* (OK), November 25, 1926; *Laredo Daily Times,* May 10, 1927; *Manitowoc Herald-News* (WI), December 14, 1927; *Helena Independent,* January 5, 1929.

11. *Fitchburg Sentinel,* August 15, 1925; *Syracuse Herald,* April 3, 1927; *Laurel Daily Leader* (KS), September 14, 1926; *Robesonian,* May 25, 1925; *Waterloo Evening Courier,* October 23, 1926; *Ada Evening News* (OK), February 11; *Salamanca Republican-Press,* October 3, 1927.

12. *Salamanca Republican-Press,* May 7, 1927.

13. *Decatur Daily Review,* April 23, 1930.

14. Ibid., August 12; *Corsicana Daily Sun,* January 28; *Moravia Union* (IA), January 16, 1930.

15. *LeMars Globe-Post* (IA), November 13, 1930.

16. *Mason City Globe-Gazette* (IA), October 10, 1931.

17. *Santa Fe New Mexican,* June 30, 1933.

18. WHO, Chapter 8, p. 331.

19. *Palo Alto Tribune,* August 12, 1931.

20. *Spencer Daily Report* (IA), October 25, 1935.

21. WHO, Chapter 8, p. 332.

22. *Lowell Sun,* January 14; *Fitchburg Sentinel,* February 25, 1932.

23. *Taber's,* 696.

24. *Daily Gleaner,* August 30, September 5, 1928.

25. *Salamanca Republican-Press,* August 26, 1933.

26. WHO, Chapter 7, pp. 281–282.

27. *Freeport Journal-Standard,* March 22, 1933.

28. *Winnipeg Free Press,* July 17, 1936.

29. *Evening Independent* (OH), September 15, 1936.

30. WHO, Chapter 7, pp. 279, 281, 289.

31. Collier, L.H., "The Preservation of Vaccinia Virus," Vaccine Lymph Unit, Lister Institute of Preventive Medicine, Elstree, Hertfordshire, England, p. 77, http://ncbi.nlm.nih.gov/PMC/articles/PMC18/pdf/bactrev00017-0081.pdf.

32. WHO, Chapter 7, p. 286; Collier, 78.

33. *Renwick Times* (IA), June 27, 1929.

34. Collier, pp. 77, 79.

35. Ibid., pp. 81–82.

36. *Renwick Times,* June 27, 1929.

37. *Tipton Daily Tribune* (IN), May 2, 1930.

38. *Daily Gleaner,* July 22, 1931.

39. Collier, 80–81.

40. *Syracuse Herald,* November 19, 1933.

41. Collier, 82.

42. *Daily Mail* (MD), October 9; *Ada Evening News,* October 9, 1935.

43. *Winnipeg Free Press,* February 13, 1935; *Evening Huronite* (SD), May 10; *Monessen Daily Independent* (PA), June 8, 1937.

44. *Yuma Daily Sun,* January 7, 1938.

45. *Joplin News Herald,* September 2, 1924.

46. *Salt Lake City Tribune,* July 30, 1942.

47. *International Public Health Organizations Before WHO.*

48. WHO, Chapter 8, p. 326.

49. Ibid., 323–326.

50. *Mason City Globe-Gazette,* September 28; *Muscatine Journal,* April 24; *Berkshire Evening Eagle* (MA), April 2, 1943.

51. *Galveston Daily News,* March 23, 1946.

52. *Nevada State Journal,* March 31, 1946.

53. *Oakland Tribune,* April 2, 1946.

54. *Syracuse Herald-Journal,* May 4, 1946.

55. *Hutchinson News-Herald,* March 29, 1946.

56. *Nevada State Journal,* March 31, 1946.

57. *Laredo Times,* January 12, 1948; *Lowell Sun,* April 14; *Berkshire Evening Eagle,* April 15; *Dunkirk Evening Observer,* April 16; *Kingston Daily Freeman,* April 18; *Syracuse Herald American,* April 20; *Kokomo Tribune* (IN), April 24; *Ogden Standard-Examiner,* (UT), April 30; *Galveston Daily News,* September 12, 1947.

58. *Valley Morning Star* (TX), February 27; *San Antonio Light,* March 18; *Titusville Herald,* March 26; *Corsicana Daily Sun,* April 14, 1949; *Wisconsin State Journal,* December 15, 1948.

59. WHO, Chapter 8, p. 332.

60. Ibid., 334–335.

61. Ibid., 344.

62. Ibid., 361.

Chapter 37

1. *Daily Courier* (PA), March 8, 1926.

2. *Traverse City Record Eagle* (MI), March 24, 1960.

3. *Clatskanie Chief* (OR), November 3, 1950.

4. *Mason City Globe-Gazette,* April 3; *Pacific Stars and Stripes* (Japan), April 13, 1950; *Greeley Daily Tribune* (CO), January 17, 1951.

5. WHO, Chapter 7, p. 371.

6. Pearsall, Judy, ed., *The Concise Oxford Dictionary,* 10th ed. (New York: Oxford University Press, 1999), 483.

7. WHO, Chapter 9, p. 388.

8. Ibid., 371.

9. Ibid., 386–387.

10. *Ames Daily Tribune* (IA), December 8, 1961.

11. WHO, Chapter 9, pp. 405–406.

12. *Lethbridge Herald,* June 28; *Independent* (CA), February 5, 1964.

13. WHO, Chapter 9, pp. 388, 394–402.

14. Ibid., Chapter 8, p. 340.

15. *News Journal* (OH), June 22, 1965.

16. *Titusville Herald,* January 27, 1965.

17. *Arizona Republic,* November 26, 1965.

18. *Daily Gleaner,* May 14, 1966; WHO, Chapter 9, pp. 405–409.

19. WHO, Chapter 9, pp. 410–419.

20. *El Paso Herald-Post,* April 24; *Post-Register* (ID), April 27, 1959.

21. *McKean County Democrat* (PA), November 19, 1959.

22. *Redlands Daily Facts* (CA), May 23, 1961; *Arcadia Tribune* (CA), February 26, 1962.

23. *Portsmouth Herald,* December 16, 1959.

24. *Joplin Globe,* October 8; Abilene *Reporter,* October 9, 1960.

25. *Arcadia Tribune,* February 26; European edition of *Stars and Stripes* (Germany), January 13, 1962.

26. *Aiken Standard and Review* (SC), August 20; *Bennington Banner* (VT), August 25; *Winnipeg Free Press,* August 30, 1962.

27. *Corpus Christi Times,* April 3, 1967.

28. *Anderson Herald* (IN), January 27, 1962.

29. *Wisconsin State Journal,* September 2, 1951.

30. *Northwest Arkansas Times,* February 5, 1953.

31. *Beatrice Daily Sun* (NE), April 14; *Wisconsin Rapids Daily Tribune,* June 22, 1953.

32. *Ironwood Daily Globe,* July 16, 1954.

33. *Lowell Sunday Sun,* August 15, 1965.

34. *Newport Daily News,* April 18, 1953; *Lethbridge Herald,* January 20, 1954; *Ogden Standard-Examiner,* May 28, 1958; *Anderson Herald* (TN), January 27; *Light* (TX), June 8, 1962.

35. *Syracuse Herald-Journal,* May 31; *Berkshire Eagle,* December 12, 1958; *Logansport Pharos-Tribune,* December 24, 1959; *Simpson's Daily Leader-Times* (PA), February 23, 1961; *Pacific Stars and Stripes* (Japan), September 24, 1965;

Abilene Reporter-News, November 11, 1952; *Daily News* (PA), March 10, 1952.

36. *Chester Times,* February 6, 1954; *Pacific Stars and Stripes* (Japan), January 13, 1958.

37. *San Antonio Express,* February 4, 1966.

38. *Humboldt Standard* (Canada), December 17, 1953; *Fitchburg Sentinel,* January 24, 1968; Kempe, C.H., "The Use of Vaccinia Hyperimmune Gamma-Globulin in the Prophylaxis of Smallpox," Bulletin of WHO, 1961, Geneva, pp. 41–48.

39. *Arizona Republic,* January 23, 1960.

40. *El Paso Herald-Post,* November 1, 1954, May 24, 1957.

41. *Steubenville Herald-Star,* October 28, 1959.

42. *Wisconsin State Journal,* August 8, 1963.

43. *Lethbridge Herald,* May 28, 1960; see also *Nevada State Journal,* September 18; *Corpus Christi Times,* November 9, 1960; *Oneonta Star* (NY), July 13, 1961; *Hutchinson News,* February 6, 1962.

44. *Kingsport Times-News* (TN), February 11, 1962.

45. *Troy Record* (NY), November 2, 1967.

46. *Abilene Reporter-News,* December 1, 1969.

Chapter 38

1. *Hutchinson News,* March 14, 1971; comment of Dr. William H. Foege.

2. European *Stars and Stripes,* January 7, 1962; *Tucson Daily Citizen,* February 3, 1970.

3. *Winnipeg Free Press,* July 23, 1970.

4. *Hutchinson News,* March 14, 1971.

5. *Daily Gleaner,* October 23, 1970.

6. *Arizona Republic,* November 3, 1970.

7. Walker, Connecticut, "How to Treat an Epidemic," *Charleston Sunday Gazette-Mail* (WV), June 18, 1972.

8. *Provo Daily Herald,* May 12, 1971.

9. *Commerce Journal* (TX), June 10, 1971.

10. *Albuquerque Journal,* July 18, 1972.

11. *Times Recorder* (OH), September 10, 1972.

12. *Lethbridge Herald,* September 18, 1973; *Indiana Evening Gazette,* April 29; *Ogden Standard-Examiner,* June 5; Pacific *Stars and Stripes* (Japan), June 7; *Hutchinson News,* June 8; *Frederick Post* (MD), June 15; *Fairbanks Daily News-Miner* (AK), June 14, 1974.

13. *Times Standard* (CA), June 10; *Winnipeg Free Press,* June 13; *Independent* (CA), July 23, 1974.

14. *Arizona Republic,* November 3, 1972; *Gastonia Gazette* (NC), March 1; *Lubbock Avalanche-Journal,* April 7; *The Bee* (VA), April 11; *Kingsport Times-News* (TN), April 8, 1973.

15. *Lima News,* August 29, 1973.

16. *Stars and Stripes* (Germany), April 13, 1973.

17. *Hutchinson News,* February 16, 1975.

18. *Daily Review* (CA), September 17; *Daily Mail* (MD), October 11, 1972.

19. *Stonewall Argus* (Manitoba), February 4, 1976.

20. *Las Vegas Optic,* April 22; Pacific *Stars and Stripes* (Japan), July 13; *Salt Lake City Tribune,* November 14, 1974.

21. *Buffalo Grove Herald* (IL), February 19; *Winnipeg Free Press,* February 25; *Oakland Tribune,* April 7; Pacific *Stars and Stripes,* April 9; *Brandon Sun* (Manitoba), May 2, 1975.

22. *Charleston Daily Mail,* August 15, 1975; *Simpson's Leader-Times,* January 2; Pacific *Stars and Stripes,* April 17; *Bakersfield Californian,* May 19, 1976.

23. *Bakersfield Californian,* September 28, 1976; *Lubbock Avalanche-Journal,* April 22; *Independent* (CA),

May 16; *Daily News-Record* (VA), May 18; *Des Moines Register,* December 14, 1977.

24. *Des Moines Register,* December 14, 1977; *Ironwood Daily Globe,* May 4, 1978.

25. *Altoona Mirror,* September 11, 1978; Koplow, David A., *Smallpox: The Fight to Eradicate a Global Scourge* (Berkeley: University of California Press, 2003), 25–26, http://en.wikiperia.org/wiki/Janet_Parker.

Chapter 39

1. *Daily News* (PA), October 25, 1978.

2. *Winnipeg Free Press,* March 21, 1978.

3. *Daily News* (PA), October 25, 1978.

4. *Chronicle-Telegram* (OH), March 13, 1985.

5. Koplow.

6. Pacific *Stars and Stripes,* March 13, 1976.

7. European *Stars and Stripes,* August 17, 1978.

8. *Winnipeg Free Press,* August 22, 1978.

9. European *Stars and Stripes,* April 23, 1979.

10. *Daily News* (TX), March 31, 2002.

11. *Lethbridge Herald,* April 23, 1980.

12. *Burlington Hawk-Eye,* June 19, 1983.

13. European *Stars and Stripes,* May 29, 1985.

14. *Burlington Hawk-Eye,* June 15, 1979.

15. *Galveston Daily News,* December 20, 1978.

16. *Texas City Sun,* December 3, 1997.

17. *Indiana Progress,* June 3, 1987.

18. *Aiken Standard,* July 3, 1989.

19. *Gazette* (IA), November 7, 1987.

20. *Daily Herald* (IL), August 21, 1998.

21. *Santa Fe New Mexican,* December 13, 1998.

22. *Daily Globe,* October 19, 2001.

23. *Daily Herald* (IL). November 29, 2001; *Lethbridge Herald,* December 30, 2002.

24. *Star-Herald* (NE), October 27; *Altoona Mirror,* November 14, 2001; *Rederick Post,* January 26, 2002.

25. *Salina Journal,* August 29, 2002.

26. *Hays Daily News* (KS), October 8; *Del Rio News-Herald* (TX), November 5; *Post-Standard* (NY), November 18, 2002.

27. *Post-Standard,* December 29, 2002; *Intelligencer* (PA), February 11; *Telegraph* (IL), March 26; *Gazette* (IA), March 28; *Indiana Gazette,* April 1; *Salina Journal,* April 12, 2003.

28. *Taber's,* 1420.

29. *Salina Journal,* June 25; *Indiana Gazette,* October 3, 2003.

30. *Medicine Hat* (Alberta), December 31, 2003; *Winnipeg Free Press,* September 20, 2005; *Frederick News-Post,* April 19; *Aiken Standard,* March 19, 2006.

31. *Syracuse Herald-Journal,* May 28, 1991.

32. *Cedar Rapids Gazette,* December 25, 1978, reprinted from the *New York Times* Service.

33. *Hutchinson News,* August 30; *Santa Fe New Mexican,* November 27, 1993; *Gazette* (IA), October 30; *Hutchinson News,* November 8; *Texas City Sun,* November 2, 1994; *Syracuse Herald-Journal,* January 25, 1995; *Altoona Mirror,* January 18, 2002.

34. *Sunday Capital* (MD), January 27, 2002; *Salina Journal,* April 1; *Daily Herald* (IL), September 15, 2003; *Telegraph Sunday* (IL), March 14 (article by Dr. Sharon Frey); *Post-Standard* (NY), November 12, 2004.

35. "The U.N. Puts off Destroying Last Smallpox Viruses," *Manila Bulletin,* May 25, 2011.

Bibliography

Abraham, J.J. *Lettsom, His Life, Times, Friends and Descendents.* London: Heinemann, 1933.

"Alastrim": http://medical-dictionary.thefreedictionary.com/alastrim.

"Ayurveda." http://en.wikipedia.org/wiki/Ayurveda.

Baynes, Thomas Spencer, ed. "Vaccination." *Encyclopædia Britannica: A Dictionary of Arts, Sciences, and General Literature,* Vol. 10. London, J.M. Stoddart, 1889.

Beall, O.T., and R.H. Shryock. *Cotton Mather: First Significant Figure in American Medicine.* Baltimore, Johns Hopkins Press, 1954.

"Benjamin Waterhouse." http://en.wikipedia.org/wiki/Benjamin_Waterhouse.

Berman, Michele R. "George Washington, Smallpox, and the American Revolution." www.celebritydiagnosis.com/2011/george-washington-smallpox-and-the-american-revolution.

Berreto, Luis, and Christopher J. Rutty. "Speckled Monster: Canada, Smallpox and Its Eradication." *Canadian Journal of Public Health* 93, no. 4 (2002).

Best (M.D.), Neuhauser, and L. Slavin. "Heroes and Martyrs of Quality and Safety." *Qual Saf Health Care,* 2004.

Black (M.D.), William. *Observations, Medical and Political, on the Small Pox.* 2nd ed. London: 1781 (from *European Magazine,* March 1, 1805).

Blanton, W.B. *Medicine in Virginia in the Eighteenth Century.* Richmond: Garrett and Massie, 1931.

"Bradford's History of the Plymouth Plantation, 1620–1647." *Original Narratives of American History* 6. www.swarthmore.edu/SocSci/bdorsey1/41docs/14-bra.html.

Celebrate Boston: Heroes and Martyrs. "First Inoculation." www.celebrateboston.com/first/inoculation.htm.

Cohn, David D. "Lady Mary Montagu." http://pyramid.spd.louisville.edu/~fos/lady_mary_montagu.html.

Collier, L.H. "The Preservation of Vaccinia Virus:" http://ncbi.nlm.nih.gov/PMC/articles/PMC18/pdf/bactrev00017-0081.pdf.

"Contagion: International Sanitary Conferences." Harvard University Open Library Collections Program. http://ocp.hul.harvard.edu/contagions/sanitaryconferences.html.

"Covenant of the League of Nations." Article XXIII (f). http:ocp.hul.harvard.edu/(Contagion).

Creighton, C. Strutt Papers. *A History of Epidemics in Britain, 1666–1893.* 2 vols. Cambridge: Cambridge University Press, 1894. www.openlibrary.org/books/OL18919376M.

Denney, Robert E. *Civil War Medicine: Care and Comfort of the Wounded.* New York: Sterling, 1994.

d'Errico, Peter, "Jeffrey Amherst and Smallpox Blankets." http://www.nativeweb.org/pages/legal/amherst/lord_jeff.html.

Dobyns, Henry F., and Robert C. Euler. "Pai Cultural Change." *American Indian Quarterly* 23, no. 3/4 (1999).

"Edward Jenner." *World of Microbiology and Immunology.* www.bookrags.com/biography/edward-jenner-wmi.

"Edward Jenner." www.historylearningsite.co.uk/edward_jenner.htm.

"Evolution of International Public Health." The International Conferences. http://whglibdoc.who.int.Publications/a38153_(Ch1).pdf.

Farmer, Laurence. "When Cotton Mather Fought Smallpox." *American Heritage,* August 1957. http://www.americanheritage.com/articles/magazine/ah/1957_5_40.shtml.

Fenn, Elizabeth. "The Great Smallpox Epidemic of 1775–82." *History Today* 53, no. 8 (August 2003).

_____. *Pox Americana: The Great Smallpox Epidemic of 1775–82.* New York: Hill and Wang, 2001.

Fenner, F., D.A. Henderson, I. Arita, Z. Jezek, and I.D. Ladnyi. "Smallpox and Its Eradication." Geneva: World Health Organization, 1988.

"From the Front: Vera Cruz, July 3, 1914." *Journal of the American Medical Association* 63. HighWire, 1914.

"Goldenseal in Profile." http://b-and-t-world-seeds.com.htm.

Haggard, Howard W. *From Medicine Man to Doctor.* Mineola, New York: Dover, 2004.

Hammarsten, J.F., W. Tattersall, and J.E. Hammarsten. "Who Discovered Smallpox Vaccination — Edward Jenner or Benjamin Jesty?" *Amer-*

ican Clinical Climatological Association Journal 5, no. 90 (1970.) http://www.ncbi.nlm.gov/pmc/articles/PMC2279376/?page=11.

Hooper, Robert. *Lexicon Medicum, or Medical Dictionary.* New York: Harper & Brothers, 1842.

Houlton, R. *Indisputable Facts Relative to the Suttonian Art of Inoculation, with Observations on Its Discovery, Progress, Encouragement, Opposition, etc.* Dublin: W.G. Jones, 1768.

"International Public Health Organizations Before WHO." http://ocp.hul.harvard.edu/Cantagion.

Jackson, Charles L. "State Laws on Compulsory Immunization in the United States." *Public Health Reports* 84, no. 9 (September 1969).

"*Jacobson v Massachusetts.*" http://supreme.justia.com/us/197/11/index.html.

"*Jacobson v Massachusetts*: Significance, Compulsory Vaccination Lawful, Court Defers to Legislature, Exemption for Unfit Adult? Impact." http://law.jrank.org/pages/12780/Jacobson-v-Massachusetts.html.

Jenkins, J.S. "The English Inoculator: Jan Ingen-Housz." *Journal of the Royal Society of Medicine* 92 (October 1999).

"Jenner." www.bookrags.com.

"John Nivison Force, Hygiene." Berkley, 1938. http://texts.cdlib.org/view?docID=hb0g50035&chunk.id=div0005&brand=calisphere&do.

Kempe, C.H. "The Use of Vaccinia Hyperimmune Gamma-Globulin in the Prophylaxis of Smallpox." Bulletin of WHO. Geneva: 1961.

Koplow, David A. *Smallpox: The Fight to Eradicate a Global Scourge.* Berkeley: University of California Press, 2003.

Kotar, S.L., and J.E. Gessler. *The Steamboat Era: A History of Fulton's Folly on American Rivers.* Jefferson, NC: McFarland, 2009.

Lack, Evonne, "The Story of Smallpox from Variolation to Vaccine." 2010. www.babycenter.com.

Leavell, Bryd S. "Thomas Jefferson and Smallpox Vaccine." *American Philosophical Society* 53, no. 8 (1963). New Series.

Leech, Margaret. *Reveille in Washington, 1860–1865.* New York: Carroll & Graf, 1941.

"Letter from Thomas Jefferson." http://lachlan.bluehaze.com.au/lit/jeff06.htm.

Lettsom, John Cockley. "Observations on the Cow Pox." *European Magazine* (London), February 1, 1802.

"Little Turtle." http://en.wikipedia.org/wiki/Little_Turtle.

Lloyd, James Hendries, ed. "Dr. Emmanuel Pfeiffer." *Philadelphia Medical Journal* 9 (January–June 1902). Philadelphia: Philadelphia Medical, 1902.

Long, J.C. *Lord Jeffrey Amherst: A Soldier of the King.* New York: Macmillan, 1933.

MacNalty, Sir Arthur Salusbury, "The Prevention of Smallpox: From Edward Jenner to Monckton

Copeman." Milroy Lectures, January 1968. www.ncbi.nlm.nih.gov/PMC/articles/PMC.

Markel, Howard. "Life, Liberty and the Pursuit of Vaccines." February 28, 2011. http://www.nytimes.com/2011/03/01/health/01smallpox.html.

Martin, Henry A. "Jefferson as a Vaccinator." *North Carolina Medical Journal* (January 1881).

McIntyre, John W.R., and Stuart Houston. "Smallpox and Its Control in Canada." *CMAJ* (August 1, 1902).

Melville, Lewis. *Lady Mary Wortley Montagu: Her Life and Letters, 1689–1762.* Boston: Indy Publish.com.

Morton, Henry H. "Smallpox." *Journal of the American Medical Association* 22 (1894).

Munk, W., and J.I. Marson. "Smallpox Cases at Highgate Hospital." *Medical Times and London Gazette.* London: 1871.

"On This Day in History." http://nativenewsonline.org/history/hist0123.htm.

Pearsall, Judy, ed. *The Concise Oxford Dictionary.* 10th ed. New York: Oxford University Press, 1999.

Pearson, Allis S. *The Dunbar-Allis Letters on the Pawnee.* Edited by W. Wedell. New York: Garland, 1985.

Pearson, George. "A Statement of the Progress in the Vaccine Inoculation; and Experiments to Determine Some Important Facts Belonging to the Vaccine Disease." *Philosophical Magazine,* August 1, 1799. London.

Pearson, J. Diane. "Lewis Cass and the Politics of Disease." *Wicazo Sa Review* 18, no. 2 (Autumn 2003).

Pesanmbbee, Michelene E. "When the Earth Shakes: The Cherokee Prophecies of 1811–1812." *American Indian Quarterly* 17, no. 3.

Powell, Alvin. "The Beginning of the End of Smallpox." *Harvard University Gazette.* http://news.harvard.edu/gazette/1999/05.20/waterhouse.html.

Project Staff. "Benjamin Franklin, Smallpox Pamphleteer." March 19, 2010. Library Treasures. http://www.historyofvaccines.org/content/blog/library-treasures-benjamin-franklin-smallpox-pamphleteer.

"Report on Sanitary Measures in India, 1890–1891." Vols. 18, 24. Army Sanitary Commission, 1892.

Rolleston, J.D. "The Smallpox Pandemic of 1870–1874." November 24, 1933. www.ncbi.nlm.gov/PMC/articles/PMC22.

Rumsey, Henry Wyldbore. "Essays on the State of Medicine." *London Medical Gazette* 23. Ayer; reprnt., Arno, New York, 1977.

Russell, T. Triplett, and John K. Gott. *Faquier County in the Revolution.* Westminster, MD: Heritage Books, 1977.

Seaton, Edward Cator. "A Handbook on Vaccination." London: MacMillan, 1868.

Singla, Rohit K. "Missed Opportunities: The Vaccination Act of 1813." May 1, 1998. www.leda. law.harvard.edu.leda/date/229/rsingla.pdf.

Smallman-Raynor, Matthew, and Andrew D. Cliff. "The Geographical Transmission of Smallpox in the Franco-Prussian War: Prisoner of War Camps and Their Impact upon Epidemic Diffusion Processes in the Civil Settlement System of Prussia, 1870–71." http://www.questia.com/ reader/printPaginator/176.

"Small Pox." *Black Loyalist.* www.blackloyalist.info. new-informationpage.

"Smallpox Inoculation and Quarantine in Colonial America." http://inpropiapersona.com.

"Smallpox Timeline." http://historyofvaccines.org/ content/timelines/smallpox.

Spann, Edward K. *The New Metropolis.* New York: Columbia University Press, 1981.

Stanley, Henry M. *In Darkest Africa, or the Quest, Rescue and Retreat of Emin, Governor of Equatoria.* 2 vol. New York: Charles Scribner' Sons, 1890.

Starna, William A. "The Biological Encounter: Disease and the Ideological Domain." *American Indian Quarterly* 16, no. 4 (1992).

Stevens, George M. "Vaccination for Smallpox: The Three Chisel Method." Los Angeles: Department of Epidemiology of the Los Angeles City Health Department, 1933.

Tandy, Elizabeth C. "Local Quarantine and Inoculation for Smallpox in the American Colonies, 1620–1775." New York: Committee on Dispensary Development, United Hospital Fund, NYC. www.ajph.alphapublications.org/cgil/reprint/13/3/ 203.pdf.

Thatcher, James. *A Medical Biography of Eminent American Physicians and Surgeons.* Indianapolis: Hollenbeck, 1898.

Thomas, Benjamin P. *Abraham Lincoln: A Biography.* New York: Alfred A. Knopf, 1952.

Thompson, Mary V. "George Washington's Mount Vernon: 'More to dread ... than from the Sword of the Enemy.'" Mount Vernon Annual Report, 2002. www.mountvernon.org.

"The Three Original Publications on Vaccination by Edward Jenner." *Harvard Classics* 38, no. 4. http://lachlan.bluehaze.com.au/lit/jeff06.html.

Timonius (Dr.), Emanuel, and Jacobus Pylarinus. *Some Account of What Is Said of Inoculating or Transplanting the Small Pox.* Boston: Dr. Zabdiel Boylston, 1721.

"Vaccination Act." http://en.wikipedia.org/wiki/ Vaccination/Vaccination_acts.

"Vaccination." *Texas State Journal of Medicine* 2 (1916).

Van Zwanenberg, David. "The Suttons and the Business of Inoculation." *Medical History* 22 (1978).

Venes, Donald, ed. *Taber's Cyclopedic Medical Dictionary.* 20th ed. Philadelphia: F.A. Davis, 2001.

Walker, Connecticut, "How to Treat an Epidemic." *Gazette Mail* (WV), June 18, 1972.

"What is Smallpox?" Health-cares.net. http://skin-care.health-cares.net/smallpox.php.

Wilentz, Sean. *Andrew Jackson.* New York: Times Books, Henry Holt, 2005.

Wilson, Samuel M. "On the Matter of Smallpox." *Natural History* 103, no. 9 (September 1994).

"Winthrop's Journal, or a History of New England." Edited by J.K. Hosmer. In *Original Narratives of American History Series* 7.

World Health Organization. "The First Ten Years of the World Health Organization." Geneva: 1958.

Zall, Paul, "Franklin on Franklin." http://www. historyofvaccines.org/content/timelines/smallpox.

"Zucht v. King." http://justia.com/260/174/.

Zwanenberg (Bishop), W.J. "Thomas Dimsdale, M.D., F.R.S. (1712–1800), and the Inoculation of Catherine the Great of Russia." *American Medical Journal* 4 (1932). New Series.

Newspapers and Magazines

Abilene Reporter (KS)
Abilene Reporter-News (KS)
Ada Evening News (OK)
Adams Centinel (Sentinel) (PA)
Adams County Union (IA)
Aiken Standard and Review (SC)
Alaska Citizen
Albuquerque Journal (NM)
Alexis Visitor (IL)
Allen County Democrat (OH)
Alton Observer (IL)
Alton Telegraph (IL)
Alton Weekly Courier (IL)
Alton Weekly Telegraph (IL)
Altoona Mirror (PA)
Amateur and Working Gardener's Gazette (London)
American Heritage Magazine
American Indian Quarterly
American Medical Journal
Ames Daily Tribune (IA)
Anaconda Standard (MT)
Anderson Herald (TN)
Anniston Star (AL)
Appleton Post-Crescent (WI)
Arcadia Tribune (CA)
Arizona Republic
Atchison Daily Globe (KS)
Athens Messenger (OH)
Atlanta Constitution
Atlantic News-Telegraph (IA)
Atlas (London)
Austin Daily Herald (MN)
Australian and New Zealand Gazette (London)
Bakersfield Californian
Bangor Daily Whig & Courier (ME)

Banner of Liberty (NY)
Beatrice Daily Sun (NE)
Bee (VA)
Belleville Telescope (KS)
Bell's Weekly Messenger (London)
Bennington Banner (VT)
Berkshire County Eagle (MA)
Biddeford Daily Journal (ME)
Billings Gazette (MT)
Black Loyalist (VA)
Blackheath Gazette (London)
Boston Daily Globe
Bradford Era (PA)
Brandon Sun (Manitoba)
Bridgeport Telegram (CT)
Brief News & Opinion (London)
Brief: Week's News (London)
British Banner (London)
British Medical Journal
British Press: or, Morning Literary Advertiser
Brownsville Daily Herald (TX)
Bucks County Gazette (PA)
Buffalo Center Tribune (IA)
Burlington Daily Hawk-Eye (IA)
Burlington Weekly Hawk-Eye (IA)
Cambridge City Tribune (IN)
Capital Times (WI)
Carroll Herald (IA)
Cedar Falls Gazette (IA)
Cedar Rapids Evening Gazette (IA)
Cedar Valley Times (IA)
Centralia Enterprise and Tribune (WI)
Central Press (London)
Centaur (London)
Charleston Daily Mail (SC)
Charleston Gazette (SC)
Checotah Times (OK)
Chelsea Herald (London)
Cherokee Advocate (OK)
Chester Daily Times (PA)
Chillicothe Constitution (MO)
Christian Cabinet (London)
Chronicle-Telegram (OH)
Church Weekly (London)
Churchman's Newspaper (London)
Civilian and Gazette (TX)
Clatskanie Chief (OR)
Cleveland Plaindealer (OH)
Clovis News-Journal (NM)
Colonies and India (London)
Commerce Journal (TX)
Commonwealth (London)
Compiler (PA)
Cook County Herald (IL)
Corpus Christi Times (TX)
Corsicana Daily Sun (TX)
Coshocton Age (OH)
Coshocton News (OH)

Courier (London)
Courier (PA)
Courier and Evening Gazette (London)
Daily Argus and Democrat (WI)
Daily Courier (PA)
Daily Free Press (Winnipeg)
Daily Gazette (WI)
Daily Gazette and Bulletin (PA)
Daily Gleaner (Jamaica)
Daily Hawk-Eye & Telegraph (IA)
Daily Herald/Cook County Herald (IL)
Daily Index (VA)
Daily Iowa Capital
Daily Journal (IN)
Daily Journal (Logansport, IN)
Daily Kennebec Journal (ME)
Daily Leader (WI)
Daily Mail (London)
Daily Mail (MD)
Daily Milwaukee News (WI)
Daily News (MI)
Daily News Record (VT)
Daily Northwestern (WI)
Daily Palladium (MI)
Daily People's Press and News (WI)
Daily Republican (IL)
Daily Republican-News (OH)
Daily Review (IL)
Daily Sentinel and Gazette (WI)
Daily Star (NY)
Daily Times–Tribune (IA)
Davenport Daily Gazette (IA)
Dawson's Fort Wayne Daily Times (IN)
Decatur Daily Dispatch (IL)
Decatur Daily Republican (IL)
Decatur Daily Review (IL)
Decatur Local Review (IL)
Decatur Morning Review (IL)
Decatur Weekly Republican (IL)
Defiance Democrat (OH)
Del Rio News-Herald (TX)
Democrat (NY)
Democratic Expounder and Calhoun County Patriot
   (MI)
Denton Journal (MD)
Des Moines Daily News (IA)
Des Moines Register (IA)
Dover Weekly Argus (OH)
Dublin Journal
Dubuque Daily Herald (IA)
Dubuque Democratic Herald (IA)
Dubuque Telegraph-Herald (IA)
Dunkirk Evening Observer (NY)
Dunkirk Observer-Journal (NY)
Eau Claire News (WI)
Echo (London)
Edinburgh Advertiser
Edinburgh Evening Courant

Edinburgh Weekly Advertiser
Edinburgh Weekly Journal
Edmonton and Tottenham Weekly Guardian
Edwardsville Intelligencer (IL)
El Paso Herald-Post (TX)
Elyria Daily Reporter (OH)
Elyria Republican (OH)
Emmet County Republican (IA)
Emporia Gazette (KS)
Englishman (London)
European Gazette (London)
Evans and Ruffy's Farmers' Journal and Agricultural Advertiser (London)
Evening Gazette (IA)
Evening Gazette (NY)
Evening Herald (London)
Evening Huronite (SD)
Evening Independent (OH)
Evening Journal (WI)
Evening Light (TX)
Evening Post (London)
Evening Sentinel (London)
Evening Star (London)
Evening Tribune-Times (NY)
Fairbanks Daily News-Niner (AK)
Fairbanks Sunday Times (AK)
Fitchburg Daily Sentinel (MA)
Fort Wayne Daily Gazette (IN)
Fort Wayne Journal-Gazette (IN)
Fort Wayne News (IN)
Fort Wayne Sentinel (IN)
Fort Wayne Sunday Gazette (IN)
Frederick Post (MD)
Freeborn County Standard (MN)
Freeport Journal-Standard (IL)
Freeport Weekly Journal (IL)
Fresno Republican (CA)
Galveston Daily News (TX)
Galveston Daily Times (TX)
Gastonia Gazette (NC)
Gazette (IA)
Gentleman's Magazine (London)
Gettysburg Compiler (PA)
Grand Rapids Tribune (MI)
Grant County Herald (WI)
Greeley Daily Tribune (CO)
Guardian (Manchester)
Hackney Express and Shoreditch Observer (London)
Hagerstown Mail (MD)
Hagerstown Mail and Washington County Republican Advertiser (MD)
Hammond Times (IN)
Haskell News (OK)
Hawaiian Gazette
Hawarden Independent (IA)
Hays Daily News (KS)
Helena Independent (MT)
Herald (Buffalo Grove, IL)

Herald & Torch Light (MD)
History Today
Horicon Argus (WI)
Hornellsville Tribune (NY)
Hornellsville Weekly Tribune (NY)
Humboldt Standard (Canada)
Huntingdon Journal (PA)
Huron Reflector (OH)
Hutchison News (KS)
Hutchison News-Herald (KS)
Illustrated Times (London)
Impartial Observer (Providence, RI)
Independent (CA)
Independent American (WI)
Indian Journal (Muskogee, Indian Territory, OK)
Indiana Democrat
Indiana Evening Gazette
Indiana Messenger
Indiana Progress
Indiana Weekly Messenger
Indianapolis Star (IN)
Inter Ocean (Chicago, IL)
Iowa Liberal
Iowa Postal Card
Iowa State Register
Iola Register (KS)
Ipswich Journal (MA)
Iron (London)
Ironwood Daily Globe (MI)
Ironwood Daily Globe and News Record (MI)
Ironwood News Record (MI)
Jacksonville Sentinel (IA)
Janesville Daily Gazette (WI)
Janesville Gazette (WI)
Janesville Morning Gazette (WI)
Joplin Globe (MO)
Joplin News Herald (MO)
Journal of Iowa Medical Society
Journal of the History of Medicine
Kingsport Times (TN)
Kingsport Times-News (TN)
Kingston Daily Freeman (NY)
Kokomo Tribune (IN)
La Crosse Daily Republican (WI)
La Crosse Tribune (WI)
La Crosse Tribune and Leader-Press (WI)
Lafayette Advertiser (LA)
Lake Park News (IA)
Landmark (NC)
Laredo Daily Times (TX)
Las Vegas Optic (NV)
Laurel Daily Leader (KS)
Lawrence Daily Journal-World (KS)
Lebanon Daily News (PA)
LeGrand Record (IA)
Le Mars Daily Sentinel (IA)
Le Mars Globe-Post (IA)
Le Mars Semi-Weekly Sentinel (IA)

Lenox Times-Table (IA)
Lethbridge Herald (Alberta)
Light (TX)
Lima Times-Democrat (OH)
Linn County Register (IA)
Lloyd's Evening Post (London)
Lloyd's Weekly Newspaper (London)
Lock Haven Express (PA)
Lockhart Post-Register (TX)
Logansport Daily Journal (IN)
Logansport Daily Pharos (IN)
Logansport Daily Reporter (IN)
Logansport Pharos-Reporter (IN)
Logansport Weekly Journal (IN)
London and China Telegraph
London Daily News
London Journal
London Medical Gazette
London Review
Lorain Republican (OH)
Lowell Weekly Sun (MA)
Lubbock Avalanche-Journal (TX)
Lubbock Morning Avalanche (TX)
Madison County Courier (IL)
Magazine of Natural History
Manitoba Daily Free Press
Manitoba Morning Free Press
Manitowoc Herald-News (WI)
Mansfield News (OH)
Marble Rock Journal (IA)
Marion Daily Star (OH)
Marion Register (IA)
Marshfield Times (WI)
Marysville Tribune (OH)
Mason City Globe-Democrat (IA)
Mason City Globe-Gazette (IA)
Massilon Independent (OH)
Mauston Star (WI)
McIntosh (OK)
McKean Democrat (PA)
Medical Times and Gazette (London)
Medicine Hat (Alberta)
Mendocino Herald (CA)
Mercury (London)
Middlesex Courier (England)
Middleton Daily Times-Press (NY)
Mills County Tribune (IA)
Miner (London)
M'Kean Miner (PA)
Moberly Weekly Monitor (MO)
Monessen Daily Independent (PA)
Monthly Magazine (London)
Monthly Mirror (London)
Monthly Miscellany (London)
Montreal Gazette
Moravia Union (IA)
Morning Herald and Daily Advertiser (London)
Morning Oregonian (OR)

Morning Review (IL)
Mountain Democrat (CA)
Muscatine Journal (IA)
Muskogee Phoenix (OK)
Narka News (KS)
Nevada State Journal
Newark Daily Advocate (OH)
New Era (IA)
New Castle News (PA)
Newport Daily News (RI)
Newport Mercury (RI)
New Times (London)
New York Daily Times
New York Evening Post
New York Journal of Commerce
New York Sun
News (London)
News (MD)
News Journal (OH)
Nonconformist (London)
Nonconformist & Independent (London)
North Adams Transcript (MA)
North Carolina Medical Journal
North-China Herald (Shanghai)
Northwest Arkansas Times
Oakland Daily Evening Tribune (CA)
Observer (London)
Oconto Pioneer (WI)
Oelwein Daily Register (IA)
Ogden Standard-Examiner (UT)
Ohio Democrat
Ohio Repository
Olean Evening Times (NY)
Olive Branch Torch Light and Public Advertiser (PA)
Oneonta Star (NY)
Our Brother in Red (OK)
Oxford Mirror (IA)
Palo Alto Tribune (CA)
Patriot (London)
Penny London Post
Penny Newsman, And Weekly Advertiser (London)
Philadelphia Medical Journal
Philosophical Magazine (London)
Pointer (IL)
Pomery Herald (IA)
Port Arthur News (TX)
Portsmouth Herald (NH)
Post-Register (ID)
Post-Standard (NY)
Pottsville Review (IA)
Prairie Du Chien (WI)
Protestant Mercury (London)
Provo Daily Herald (UT)
Racine Daily Herald (WI)
Racine Daily Journal (WI)
Redlands Daily Facts (CA)
RenoEvening Gazette (NV)
Renwick Times (IA)

Repertory of Arts, Manufactures, and Agriculture (London)
Republican Compiler (PA)
Republic County Freeman (KS)
Richland County Observer (WI)
Richwood Gazette (OH)
Ripon Weekly Times (WI)
Robesonian (NC)
St. James's Chronicle; or the British Evening-post (London)
St. Joseph Herald (MO)
St. Louis Commercial Bulletin (MO)
St. Louis Republican (MO)
Salamanca Republican-Press (NY)
Salina Journal (KS)
Salt Lake Daily Tribune (UT)
San Antonio Express (TX)
San Antonio Light (TX)
San Antonio Sunday Light (TX)
San Francisco Chronicle
Santa Fe Daily New Mexican (NM)
Sault News–Record (MI)
Semi-Weekly Iowa State Reporter
Semi-Weekly Wisconsin
Shanghai Gazette
Sheboygan Journal (WI)
Sheboygan Lake Journal (WI)
Shoreditch Observer (London)
Simpson's Daily Ledger-Times (PA)
Sioux County Herald (IA)
Sparta Eagle (WI)
Spectator (London)
Spencer Daily Report (IA)
Standard (VT)
Star (London)
Star and Republican Banner (PA)
Star and Sentinel (PA)
Star Journal (OH)
Stars and Stripes (European edition: Germany)
Stars and Stripes (Pacific edition: Japan)
Steubenville Herald-Star (OH)
Stevens Point Daily Journal (WI)
Stonewall Argus (Manitoba)
Sun & Central Press (London)
Sunday Herald (NY)
Syracuse Daily Courier (NY)
Syracuse Daily Standard (NY)
Syracuse Herald (NY)
Syracuse Herald American (NY)
Syracuse Palladium (NY)
Tallis's London Weekly Paper
Telegraph (IL)
Terril Tribune (IA)
Texas City Sun (TX)
Times (London)
Times (NY)

Times and Gazette (WI)
Times Recorder (OH)
Times Standard (CA)
Tioga County Agitator (PA)
Tipton Daily Tribune (IN)
Titusville Morning Herald (PA)
Torch Light & Public Advertiser (MD)
Traverse City Record Eagle (MI)
Trenton Evening Times (NJ)
Tribune (Chicago)
Tri-Weekly Galveston News (TX)
Troy Record (NY)
True Sun (London)
Trans-American Philosophical Society
Tucson Daily Citizen (AZ)
Union (DE)
Upper Des Moines Republican (IA)
Valley Morning Star (TX)
Van Wert Republican (OH)
Vindicator and Republican (IA)
Wakefield Advocate (MI)
Wandsworth & Battersea District Times (London)
Washington Post
Waterloo Daily Courier (IA)
Waterloo Evening Courier (IA)
Waterloo Times-Tribune (IA)
Waukesha County Democrat (WI)
Waukesha Freeman (WI)
Waukesha Plaindealer (WI)
Webster City Tribune (IA)
Weekly Call (IL)
Weekly Chronicle (London)
Weekly Chronicle and Register (London)
Weekly Democrat (MS)
Weekly Gazette (CO)
Weekly Gazette and Free Press (WI)
Weekly Gazette and Stockman (NV)
Weekly New Mexican
Weekly Northwestern (WI)
Weekly Standard (NC)
Weekly Telegram (WI)
Weekly Wisconsin
Week's News (London)
Wellsboro Agitator (PA)
Western Times (WI)
Westminster Budget (London)
Whitewater Register (WI)
Wilmington & Delaware Advertiser
Winnipeg Free Press (Canada)
Wisconsin Rapids Daily Tribune
Wisconsin State Journal
Wisconsin Tribune
World (NY)
Xenia Daily Gazette (OH)
Yuma Daily Sun (AZ)

Index